AF339267

APPLIED BIOMEDICAL ENGINEERING

Edited by **Gaetano D. Gargiulo**
and **Alistair McEwan**

Applied Biomedical Engineering
Edited by Gaetano D. Gargiulo and Alistair McEwan

CBS, Edition **2016**

Published by InTech
Janeza Trdine 9, 51000 Rijeka, Croatia

Publishing Process Manager Romina Krebel

Technical Editor Teodora Smiljanic

Cover Designer InTech Design Team

Image Copyright Leigh Prather, 2010. Used under license from Shutterstock.com

Additional hard copies can be obtained from orders@intechopen.com

Applied Biomedical Engineering, Edited by Gaetano D. Gargiulo and Alistair McEwan
p. cm.
ISBN 978-953-307-256-2

Contents

Preface

The field of biomedical engineering has expanded markedly in the past few years; finally it is possible to recognize biomedical engineering as a field on its own. Too often this important discipline of engineering was acknowledged as a minor engineering curriculum within the fields of material engineering (bio-materials) or electronic engineering (bio-instrumentations).

However, given the fast advances in biological science, which have created new opportunities for development of diagnosis and therapy tools for human diseases, independent schools of biomedical engineering started to form to develop new tools for medical practitioners and carers.

The discipline focuses not only on the development of new biomaterials, but also on analytical methodologies and their application to advance biomedical knowledge with the aim of improving the effectiveness and delivery of clinical medicine.

The aim of this book is to present recent developments and trends in biomedical engineering, spanning across several disciplines and sub-specializations of biomedical engineering such as biomedical technology, biomedical instrumentations, biomedical signal processing, bio-imaging and biomedical ethics and legislation.

In the first section of this book, Biomedical Technology, advances of new and old technologies are applied to the biomedical science spanning from LED application to human tissues, to osteoporosis prevention via ultrasound stimulation up to investigation in affordable home care for patients. In the second section of this book, Biomedical Instrumentations, concepts of medical engineering are reviewed together with advances in bio instrumentation such as the measurement of pressure, the optimization of wireless power links and new sensor development for electrophysiology monitoring. Highlights of bio-imaging processing and general biomedical signal processing are presented in the third and fourth section of the book, Biomedical Signal Processing and Bio-imaging, spanning from the Brain Computer Interface to the development of neural network for biomedical signal processing and the application of bio-impedance for novel tomography techniques.

As Editors and also Authors in this field, we are honoured to be editing a book with such interesting and exciting content, written by a selected group of talented researchers.

Gaetano D. Gargiulo
Alistair McEwan

"Federico II" The University of Naples, Naples, Italy
The University of Sydney, NSW, Australia

Part 1

Biomedical Technology

1

Application of High Brightness LEDs in the Human Tissue and Its Therapeutic Response

Mauro C. Moreira, Ricardo Prado and Alexandre Campos
Federal University of Santa Maria/UFSM
Brazil

1. Introduction

The peculiarities of the light emitting diode, such as low power consumption, extremely long life, low cost and absolutely secure irradiation power is a attracting many researchers and users. With the advancement and the emergence of new applications of LEDs on health manufacturers of these solid-state devices, they have improved in all parameters of interest to its applicability as the evolution of performance in the maintenance of lumen (photometric unit), several categories of power, availability and reliability of the color spectrum and wavelength.

The high intensity LEDs plays an important role in therapeutic application, aggregating the technology of solid-state devices and a variety of electronic converters that supplying these long-lifetime devices for controlling the output current, output power, duty cycle and other parameters that directly interfere in luminous efficiency in the wavelength and the response of treatments applied to human health.

In skin, the red light has restorative action, healing and analgesic, while blue has bactericidal action. The intensity of the beams of light emitted by LEDs on the skin is lower, since its cells maintain a good interaction with the light (Elder, D. et al., 2001). In addition to speeding up the cell multiplication, the light beam favorably act in the recovery of the skin affected by acne. A major advantage of LEDs is the emission of light in a broad spectrum, from ultraviolet to the near infrared.

Bearing in mind the important issues referred above, this work describes a wide study of the state of the art on this topic in concert with proposals of driver topologies and preliminary results based on ongoing experiments. The study has been motivated by the important benefits already mentioned and need of improvement of the driver topologies in this prominent field of study.

2. LED application in human tissue

The applications of LEDs in health are emerging as a wide interest filed in the scientific community due to its advantages, low cost and long lifetime of these devices.

2.1 Penetration of light generated by LEDs in human tissue

The process of refraction and reflection is intense in organic substrates. This process is responsible for the dispersion of light as shown in Figure 1. A detailed evaluation of this process is very peculiar, because the composition of substrates varies from person to person.

Despite the high spread, the degree of penetration is considerable, with approximately 50% of all incident radiation reaching the substrates immediately below of the skin (Yoo, B. H. Et al., 2002). By submitting the skin to the LED light in red (visible light) or near infrared (Arsenide of Gallium) radiation, a small portion is absorbed by the dermis and epidermis. This is due to the presence of these layers photoreceptors. As an example of photoreceptors present in these layers, we can mention the amino acids, the melanin, and other types of acids. Normally each type of photoreceptor is sensitive to a particular wavelength.

Thus, the light can be absorbed, depending on the color and the wavelength, so selective or not, depending on the need to which it applies. For example, the red light, near the infrared, easily penetrates the fabric because they are not blocked by blood and water as other wavelengths do.

Wavelengths of less than 630nm such as yellow, blue and green are considerably blocked by the hemoglobin in the blood, so they do not penetrate deeply (Marques C. et al., 2004). You can check this, for example, as a bright light through your fingers (the wavelength in red can cross).

Wavelength greater than 900nm are blocked by liquid from the skin and connective tissues. Many possible wavelengths in this range emit a large amount of energy away from the infrared that cannot be seen by the human eye, these type of radiation also starts to produces a certain amount of heat when interacting with the human skin (HTM, 2007).

2.2 Action of color and depth of penetration in human tissue

The blue is in the range of 430 to 485nm. The green is in the range of 510 to 565nm. The yellow is between 570 to 590nm. The red is in the range of 620nm to 700nm to the point that does not become more visible, in the range of 740nm.

Some companies that manufacture LEDs say that the yellow light helps remove wrinkles.

There is also some interesting research, which emphasize that the application of blue light helps in the elimination of bacteria that cause some forms of acne.

The phototherapy with the narrow band blue light seems to be a safe treatment and one additional effective therapy for treatment of mild and moderate acnes. Some researchers suggest that the green LED light can help against cancer, but this color cannot penetrate more than the skin.

3. Adequate wavelengths

There is some evidence that a wavelength provide better biological response than another. Some research indicates that 620, 680, 760, and 820nm could be the most appropriate wavelength (Heelspurs, 2007) for health treatments. The LEDs commercially available emit light in some certain wavelengths, for example, at 630, 660, 850, and 880nm. These values are not exact, as may change during real operation and system unpredictable parameters (such as temperature and abnormal variation in the input current). There is a certain range of LEDs available with more biologically active action wavelengths. The wavelength of 630nm generated by certain LED can affect the peak of 620nm and the wavelength of 660nm generated by the LED is approaching the peak of 680nm, 850nm, and at the peak of 820nm. By operating the LEDs with currents in the range of mA, it is possible to improve the input waveform. It will be necessary to conduct a study before diagnosing which is the ideal wavelength for realizing the application and order which is intended. The best array of LEDs will be whatever the mixture a wavelength generated by LEDs and a non-pulsed,

although some wavelengths and with generation of pulses may reach deeper tissues (Heelspurs, 2007).
For the healing of cuts, wounds and ulcers to red light has a better performance in terms of its wavelength. The range of 800 to 850nm shows excellent healing characteristics acting to subcutaneous tissue.

3.1 Depth of penetration in human tissue depending on the wavelength
The penetration of light in human tissue is linked to the wavelength, that is, the greater the length greater will be their interaction in human tissues, since these wavelenghts respect the range of visible light (Heelspurs, 2007). Therefore, the application of a particular wavelength directly connected with the color to be used will depend on the application you want to achieve in the desired tissue segment, as shown in Figure 1.
The wavelength is controlled by tuning of the duty cycle of the converter. The value of the desired wavelength is measured by a spectrometer.

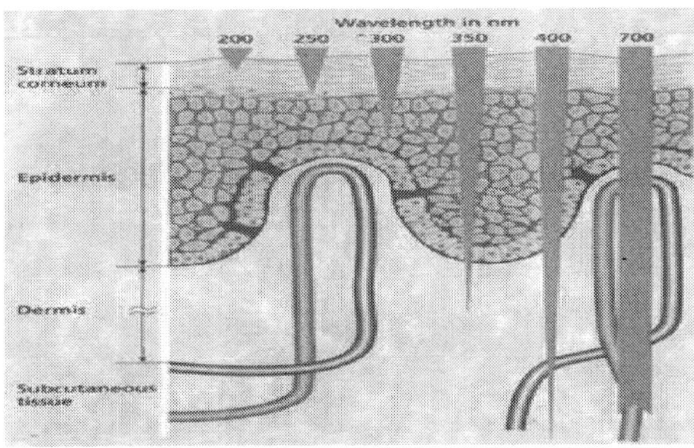

Fig. 1. Action of color and depth of penetration in human tissue.

4. Changing the wavelength peak

Control brightness study (N. Narendran, et al., 2006) demonstrates that the light output of each LED junction temperature can be controlled by the output current reduction (RCC - Reduction of Direct Current) or reducing duty cycle (PWM). The Figure 2 illustrates the change of the peak of wavelength depending on the level of current and duty cycle for the four types of LEDs.
The LEDs of white light show peaks for the blue and may have portions converting to yellow. However, the change of the peak of wavelength to the peak of yellow can be reduced.
Therefore, only the peak of wavelength of the blue was considered. For the Red LED AlInGaP (Figure 2a), the peak of wavelength decreased, or changed to blue, with the reduction of current or duty cycle. These changes were very similar. For InGaN LEDs based on the green (Figure 2b), in blue (Figure 2c) and white (Figure 2d), the peak of wavelength increased with the reduction of the current or the reduction of duty cycle. The change of wavelength was reduced with the reduction of the current or the reduction of duty cycle in a

LED that emits red light, in the remaining tested cases the opposite was verified (N. Narendran, et al., 2006).

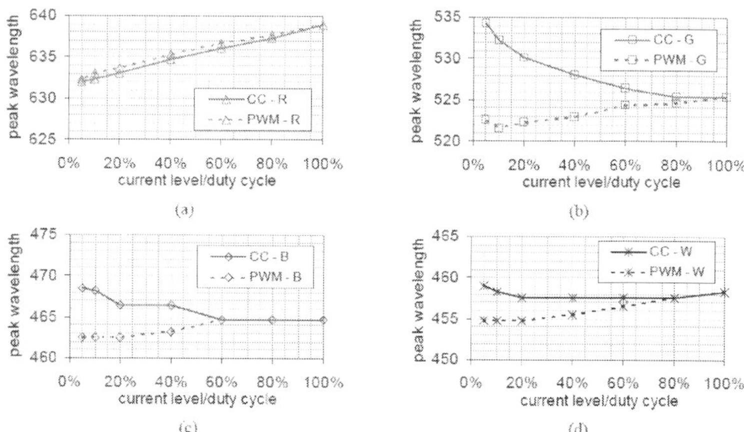

Fig. 2. Peak wavelength shift as a function of current level or duty cycle for (a) red, (b) green, (c) blue and (d) white LEDs.

5. Converters DC/DC applied in high-brightness LEDS

The application of switched converters in high-brightness LEDs is interesting, because these converters have higher efficiency than the linear converters. Thus, the main possibilities of implementing the isolated and non-isolated DC-DC converters. This analysis will facilitate the understanding of the effects of these converters and its influence on the high-brightness LEDs (Sá Jr., E. M., 2007). Resonating converters assist in the reduction of peak power; have low losses in switching and low electromagnetic interference. Therefore, these topologies are also of interest to applications with LEDs. The LEDs can also be fed by current chopper. Compared to a pure DC signal and this increases the peak value of the LED current. Moreover, the LED pulsing current contains high-frequency components. Some harmonics can cause problems of electromagnetic interference if the LEDs are separated from the converter. It is therefore of interest to quantify the generation of harmonics.

5.1 Converters not isolated commonly used for supply LEDs
The buck converter, shown in Figure 3, is widely used as power source for high-brightness LEDs.
The attribute of the source of current output makes such devices interesting electronic converters, mainly because its output current can be continuous.
Thus, the output capacitor C_{out} may have a small capacitance and it is unnecessary to use an electrolytic capacitor, which has the characteristic of a lifetime considerably smaller (Sá Jr., E. M., 2007).
The inductance output L_1, can be projected for the acquisition of a small ripple in the current wave, maintaining a stable optical characteristics and suitable temperature of the LED junction.

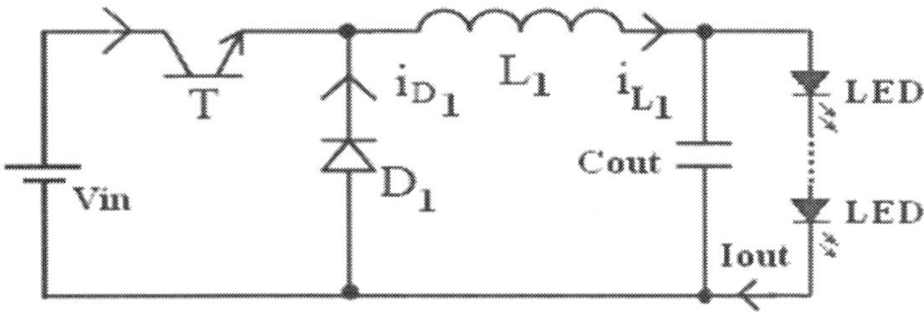

Fig. 3. Buck converter.

If the output capacitor is removed from the basic DC/DC converters, the current in the LEDs is no longer purely DC, but contains a pulsating component. For Boost or Buck-Boost converters the load of the LED is powered by an almost squared wave with a sufficiently high reactance. The CUK electronic converter is composed by a boost converter entry in series with a Buck converter in the output and a merger of two converters in series using only one controlled key. The composition of these two converters in series allows the input and output to operate in continuous mode. The gain of such static converter is the same as the Buck-Boost converter. The buck converter used in the output stage, allows to obtain a low ripple current in the LED, even for a small amount of C_{out} (Sá Jr., E. M., 2007). The Zeta converter consisting of a Buck-Boost input converter in series with a Buck converter in the output. Similarly to the CUK converter, the buck converter allows the output to obtain a low current wave of the LED. The SEPIC converter is composed of a boost input converter in series with a Buck-Boost output converter. The discontinuity of current output in this configuration does not make it attractive to be used in conjunction with high-brightness LEDs (Sá Jr., E. M., 2007).

5.2 Converters not isolated commonly used for supply LEDs

Currently, there is a considerable range of converters that can be used to supply LEDs, such as that with galvanic isolation. This sort of application employ the Flyback, Push Pull, Forward and resonant converters (Moreira, M.C., et al. 2008). The Figure 4 shows a system for supplying power to LEDs using galvanic isolation.

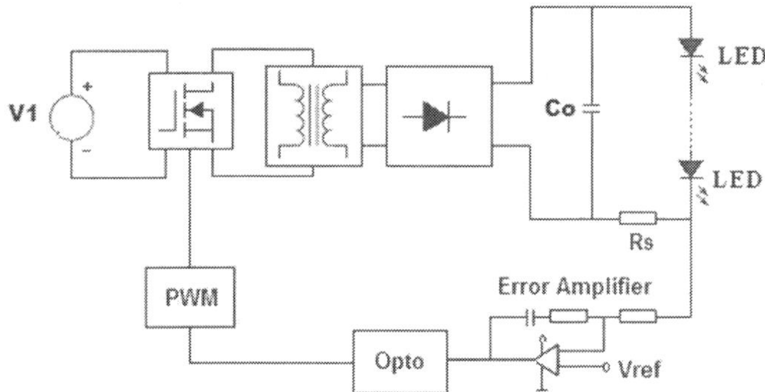

Fig. 4. Representation of a supply system for LEDs with galvanic isolation.

6. Topology proposals

After reviewing several possible topologies for LEDs power supply and control, four topologies are proposed for this study, considering their easy implementation and control of current making them attractive its use. Four converters have been developed. Flyback, Buck, Buck-boost and Sepic converters.

The Flyback converter was more robust and has the advantage of being isolated, but had some noise in the form of wave. The Buck converter controls the current and offers good response, but has the disadvantage of not being isolated.

The Buck-boost converter showed good response and a bit of noise. The Sepic converter showed a good response for current and stability.

In short, the Flyback converter was the most beneficial to the supply arrangements of LEDs. Will be presented the results of Buck and Flyback converters who had a good response (Moreira, M.C., et al. 2008).

6.1 Flyback converter

The Flyback converters of levels below 100W of power are widely used for the several applications and also for lighting with LED, normally, operating in discontinuous mode. This mode of operation is appropriate to control of current. The proposed topology is observed in Figure 5 and was developed to supply the array of LEDs, which produce red light (Moreira, M.C., et al. 2008).

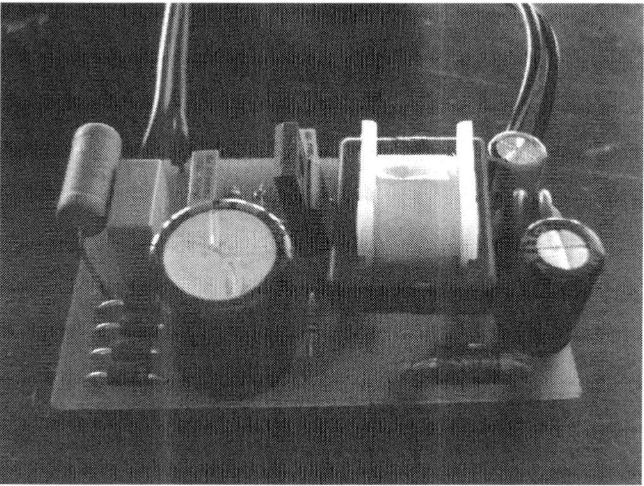

Fig. 5. LEDs powered by a Flyback converter.

The red color has a greater wavelength (in the range of 647 to 780nm) and penetrates more deeply into the tissue. Thus, it is indicated for healing and recovering deep tissues (Moreira, M.C., et al. 2008).

The Flyback converter employed in the experiments owns a universal voltage input and its maximum output voltage is 5V.

The maximum output current is 2A. His frequency of switching is 100kHz.

The proposed arrangement of red LED contains 30 high-intensity LEDs of 5mm, with wavelength in the range of 725 to 730nm. The current in each LED is around 20mA.

The source was designed to support up to 100 LEDs.

The Figure 6 shows a picture of the implementation of red LEDs in a patient who suffered a suture of 6 points.

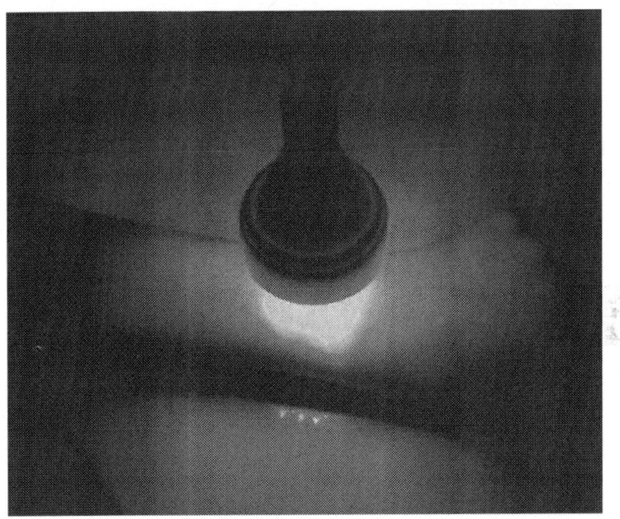

Fig. 6. Implementation of red LEDs in a patient who suffered a suture of 6 points.

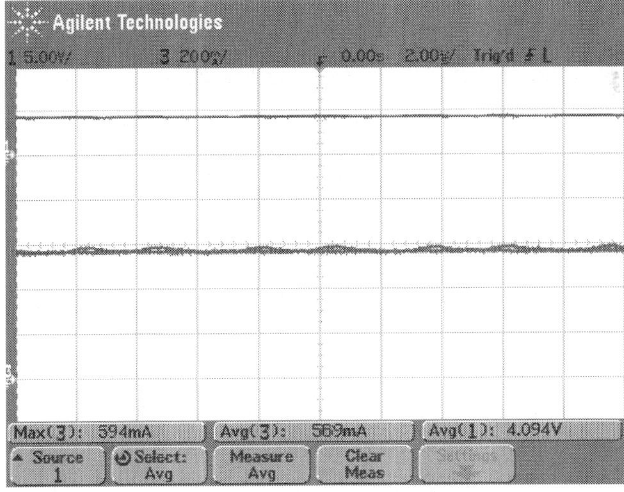

Fig. 7. Waveforms of voltage and current of the Flyback Converter - LEDs that emit the color red.

The estimate is that in 5 sessions (5 continuous days), 20 minutes each, the healing is complete, reducing the time for healing by 50% (Moreira, M.C., et al. 2008).

These tests are being conducted in patients with proper authorization and with the participation of two doctors, a surgeon and a dermatologist, in the West Regional Hospital in Chapecó, SC - Brazil.

Figure 7 shows the waveform of voltage and current of the Flyback Converter on the arrangement red. The voltage produced on the LED was 4.1V and current on the LEDs around 570mA.

The values obtained were close to the simulation and design (Moreira, M.C., et al. 2008).

6.2 Buck converter

The second converter developed has the Buck configuration as shown in Figure 8, with the following characteristics: Input Voltage DC-13V (after one stage rectified by with a Flyback converter) and the output voltage reaches 6V and maximum output current reaches 1A. The frequency of switching is 52kHz. The source has total isolation, even on short-circuit conditions in its terminals (Moreira, M.C., et al. 2008).

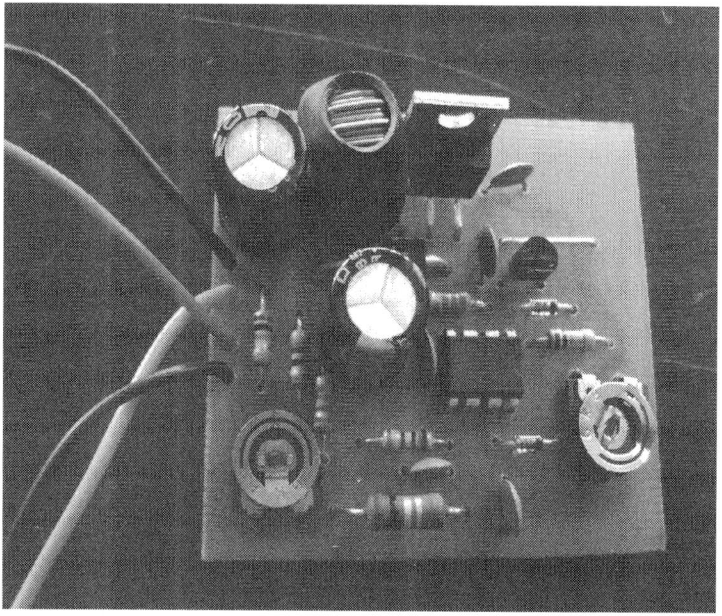

Fig. 8. Buck converter.

This topology has the same versatility of Flyback converter and supply the array of LEDs.

Figure 9 shows the waveform of voltage and current of the Buck Converter on the arrangement red.

The voltage produced on the LED was 3.8V and current on the LEDs around 580mA. The values obtained were close to the simulation and design.

Figure 10 shows the prototype in the laboratory.

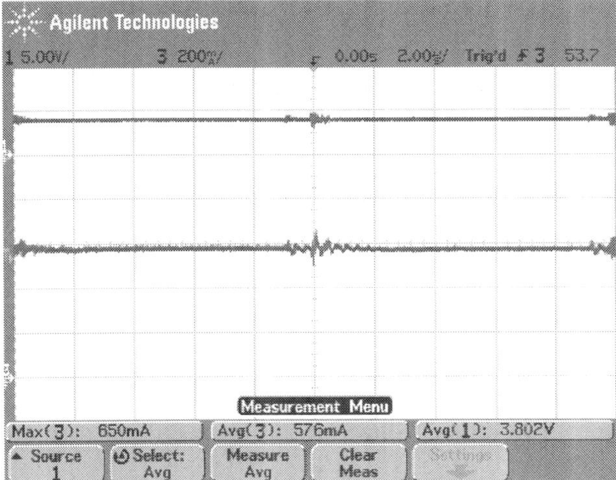

Fig. 9. The waveforms of voltage and current in the Buck converter - LEDs that emit red light.

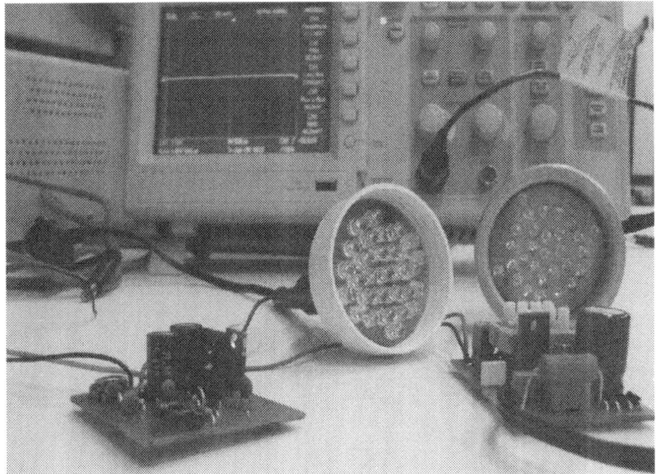

Fig. 10. Assembly of prototypes in the laboratory.

6.3 Dosage implementing the arrangement of LEDs

The concentration of light from the LED bulb can concentrate the same to a certain point that may have a high proportion in millicandelas, but passing through the skin undergoes a dispersion of its light concentration. The rate control devices is important because the total light energy emitted by the LED or energy in Watts per square centimeter, in units of mW/cm^2 is essential.

If the designer to use his knowledge to choose less expensive to manufacture power supply, then the power converter should be about 2 or 3 times more than the total of its light energy. The maximum light output of the output device is the source of half the power (W = Volt x Amps) of the transformer. The mW/cm² is the total light energy in mW divided by the length and breadth of the array of LEDs in cm.

7. Criteria, control and response to treatment of the patients who were treated by red light emitted by high-brightness LEDs

Patients who are subject to treatment will be properly classified with criteria established by the doctors who assist in the implementation of therapy. Among them, age, sex, physical condition and mental health. The therapy was performed with LEDs in the Western Regional Hospital in the city of Chapecó-SC, Brazil. An orthopedic surgeon and researcher will be responsible for the applications. The sessions were 40 minutes. Applications may be daily or not. Will depend on the type of cut or injury. Several may be twenty to forty sessions. Figures below are presented pictures of patients who are undergoing treatment. Figures 11 and 12, are of a patient who had leprosy and ostemeolite. Still has low immunity. After twenty sessions of 40 minutes the ulcer has reduced by 70% its size and depth, as shown in Figure 12 (Moreira, M. C., 2009). In this procedure was used the Buck converter who supply the LEDs that emit red light. The response of this converter was very good, because it presents a fine control of electrical current which is directly linked to the control of the wavelength.

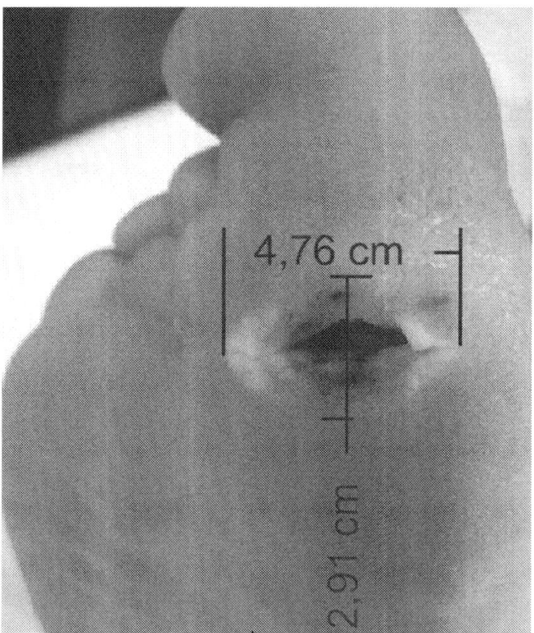

Fig. 11. Patient with ulcer in the sole of the foot before of therapy.

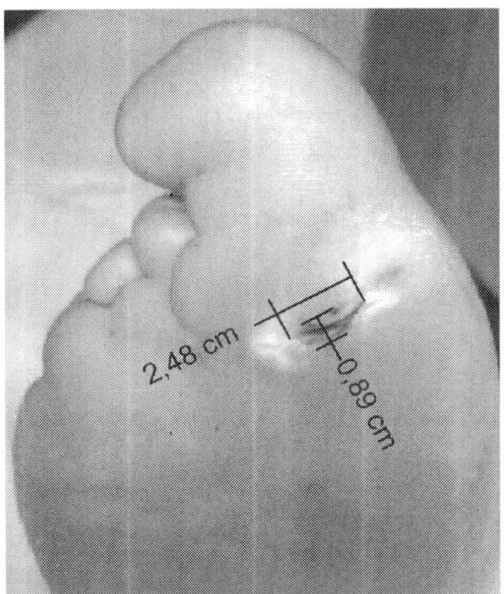

Fig. 12. Patient with ulcer in the sole of the foot after twenty sessions of LEDtherapy.

Photos 13, 14 and 15 show a patient who had an ulcer for more than two years.
The treatment lasted 50 days with applications of 40 minutes per day.
The patient had tried numerous types of treatment and was not successful.
During treatment with LEDs she did not use any kind of medication just LEDtherapy.
In this procedure was used the Flyback converter who supply the LEDs that emit red light
(Moreira, M. C., 2009).

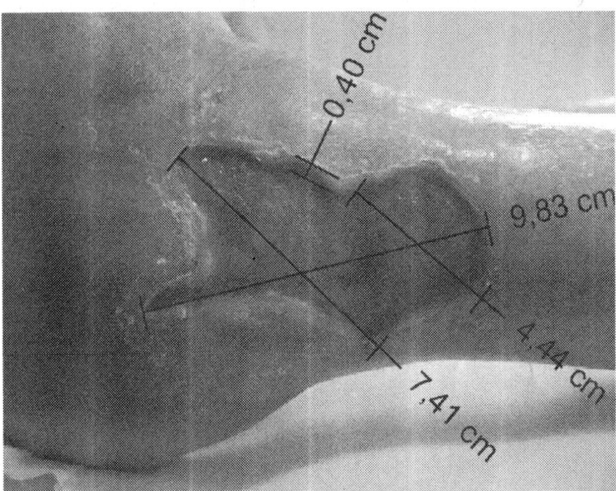

Fig. 13. Patient with left foot injury in the malleolar region before of therapy.

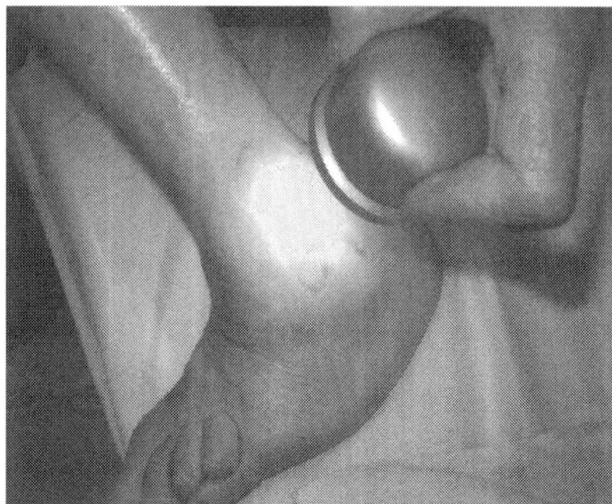

Fig. 14. Application of the array of LEDs during treatment.

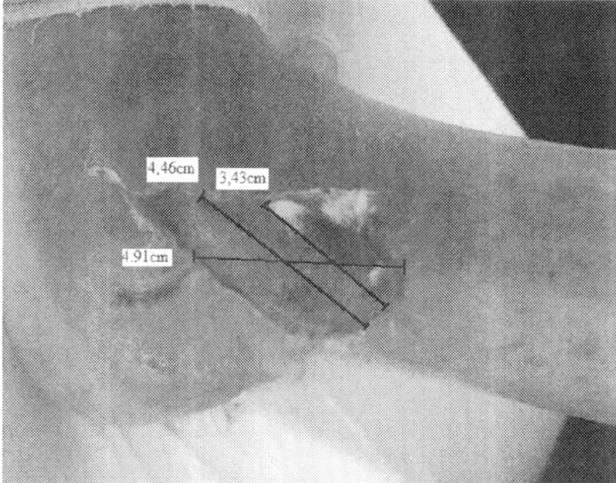

Fig. 15. Accentuated reduction of the ulcer injury.

The third case was a male patient, 27 years who had an accident with a tractor during their work activities where his left leg and right ankle suffered multiple fractures.

The ankle injury suffered a tendon rupture and left leg suffered several breakdowns and crushing bone and muscle. Performed three surgeries and the insertion of pins in order to restructure his leg.

He remained with sequelae such as disparity in length between your legs, swelling and deformity in her left leg and severe stasis ulcer that has formed around the medial malleolus and spread to leg edema presenting with dermatosclerosis. The ankle injury has healed.

The lesion of the left leg showed a great extent with the appearance of the ulcer, which reduced with time due to parallel treatments, but was not cured becoming chronic for a year and two months.

The patient in a routine consultation was invited by the doctor who attended to participate in therapy with LEDs. Occurring contact and accepted, the researcher and medical treatment was started with the issuance LEDterapia red light in the affected region.

In reviewing the case, the group proposed to the patient 20 applications of red light emitted by the array of LEDs, one on each day lasting 40 minutes per session.

Figure 16 shows the lesion in patient. Figure 17 shows the implementation of the arrangement of LEDs. Figure 18 shows the reduction of lesion during treatment. Figure 19 shows the healing of the lesion.

In this procedure was used the Buck converter who supply the LEDs that emit red light.

As the photos show the patient had complete healing of his injury using and enjoying only the application of red light generated by LEDs. The patient did not use any medication during treatment (Moreira, M. C., 2009).

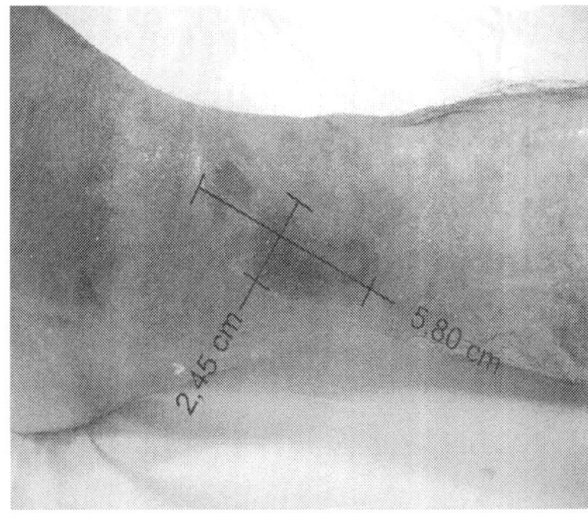

Fig. 16. Initial injury.

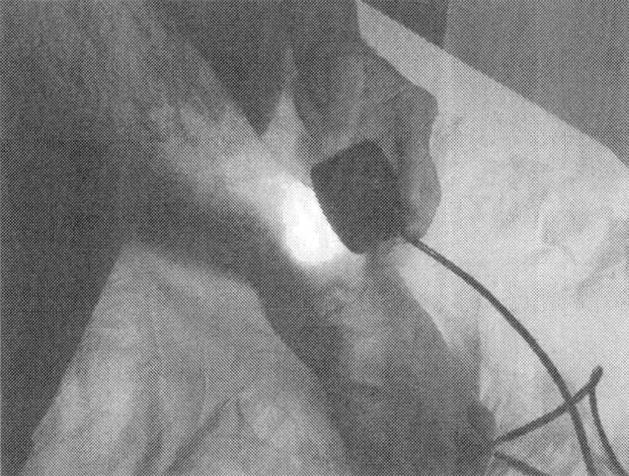

Fig. 17. Application of LEDs.

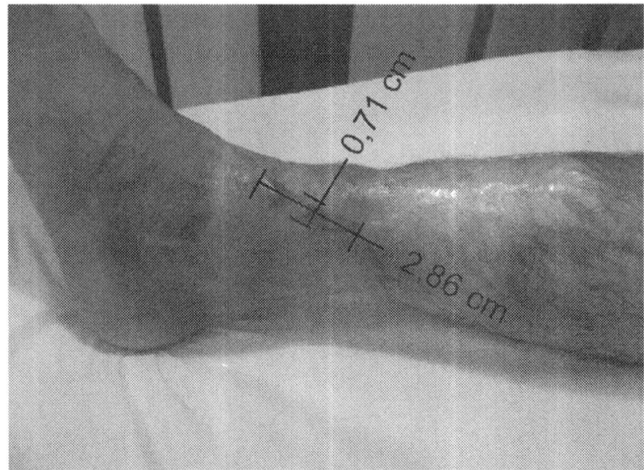

Fig. 18. Reduction of lesion during treatment.

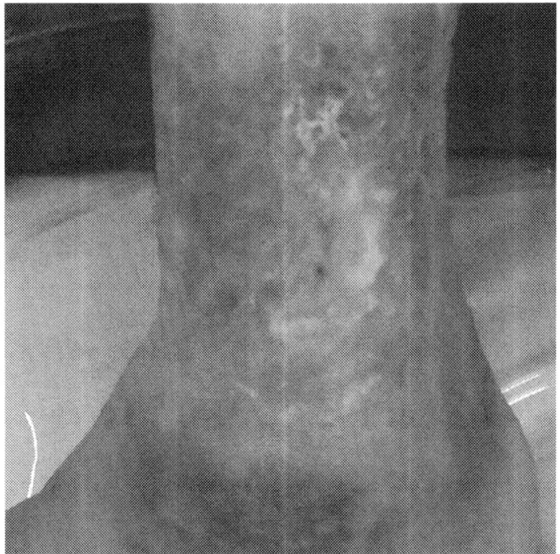

Fig. 19. Healing of the lesion.

The last case presented it is an old lady of 94 years who had a right foot injury. Underwent 20 daily applications of 30 minutes.

The result was the healing of the lesion.

In this procedure was used the Flyback converter who supply the LEDs that emit red light (Moreira, M. C., 2010).

This patient stated that the lesion had existed for over six months and was due to a fall. She complained of pain at the site and had visited a doctor and used several medications.

Figures 20, 21 and 22 show the process of treatment in the patient

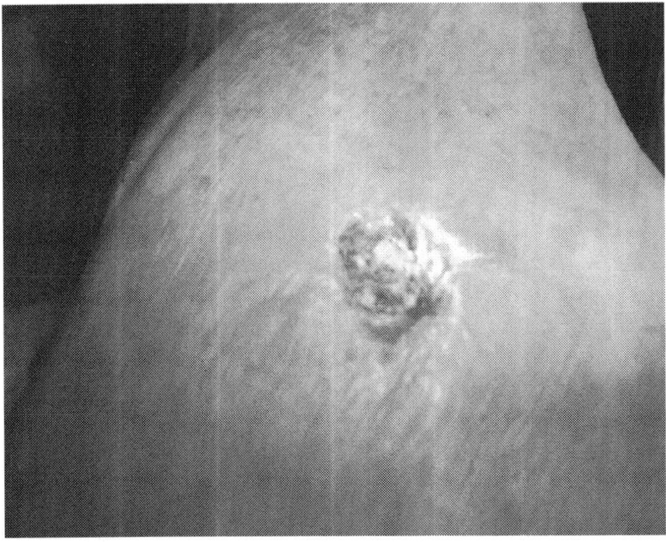

Fig. 20. Initial injury.

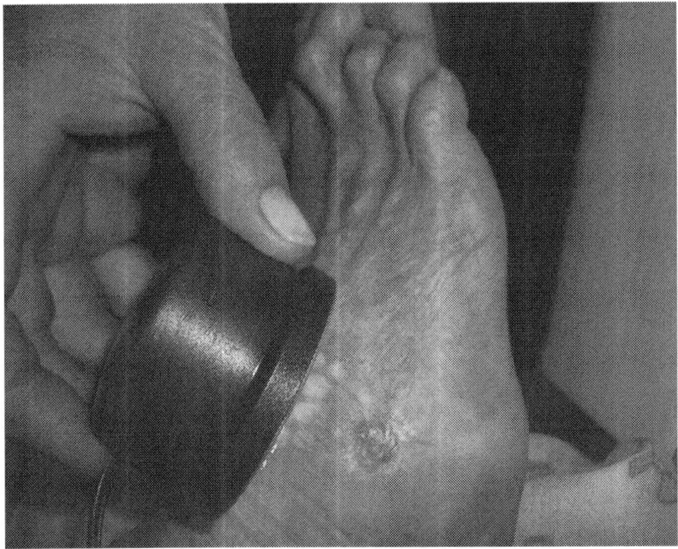

Fig. 21. Application of LEDs.

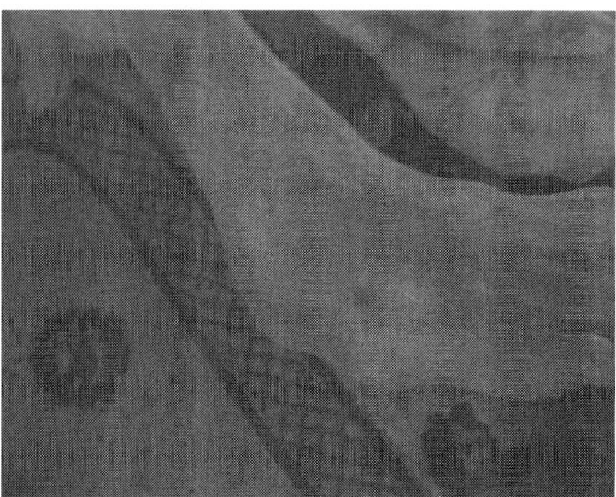

Fig. 22. Final result of treatment.

The arrangement of LED that emits red light contains 30 high intensity LEDs 5mm, with a wavelength in the range of 725 to 730nm. The current in each LED is around 20mA.
The current in each LED is around 20mA.
A total of 30 high-brightness LEDs that emit light in red. The power LEDs, high brightness can be used in LEDtherapy, yet high-gloss generate little heat on human tissue when compared with power LEDs, making high-brightness LEDs longer recommended for use in tissue recovery.
The high-brightness LEDs were used in this research. Well, it requires low power for this purpose and they serve this need in its characteristics, in addition to their low cost.
Buck and Flyback converters had very positive responses. Both presented an optimal control of electrical current that is fundamental to get the desired wavelength (Moreira, M. C., 2009).

8. The future of LED therapy

The application of high-brightness LEDs in human tissue to increases every day. Several scientific institutions have explored this theme.
Much research is underway on the use of therapy with the LED to determine if there are other applications for light therapy. The survey is being conducted on the effects of different spectra of light different in living tissues. The visible red spectrum, which is roughly in the range of 600-700 nanometers, is effective between the cornea to the subcutaneous tissue, such as care of wounds and sores, the wavelengths higher, including infrared, are more penetrating, can reach the bone. Studies also suggest that the spectrum down to 400 or 500 nanometers, which is light blue, can be effective in treating skin diseases, including acne, stretch marks, cellulite and scars.
Probably in the coming years, LEDtherapy is the main treatment for wounds, such as post-surgical wounds and not cured as diabetic ulcers.
Researchers seek to test the technology LEDtherapy in other clinical situations such as spinal cord injuries and for the treatment of Parkinson's disease, strokes, brain tumors and tissue and organ regeneration.

With the advancement and development of new applications for LEDs in health, the manufacturers of these devices have a solid improvement in all parameters of interest for their applicability to the evolution of performance in maintaining lumen (photometric unit), several categories of electric power, availability and reliability of the color spectrum and wavelength.

9. Conclusion

The application of LEDs in interaction with the human tissues shows a great interest of manufacturers and researchers. The correct use of LEDs in this context directly depends on the tissue nature where he wants the light to interact (Moreira, M. C., 2009).

Several parameters are important for satisfactory results, such as wavelength, the kind of color, temperature control of the LED, the characteristics of the used converter, control the brightness, output current, duty cycle and all the observations made in the previous sections of this work.

This is because a small spectral change can lead to a major shift in the lighting characteristics. The LEDs are increasingly becoming a great option to help cure various diseases and to prevent others.

Thus, this work contributed to the development of LED application in human tissues showing that the effect of the emission of light through the high-brightness LEDs offer a new treatment option for opening new ways of therapeutic technique LEDterapia applied to human tissues.

10. Acknowledgment

Thanks to Federal University of Santa Maria (UFSM), Federal Institute of Santa Catarina (IFSC), Coordination for the Improvement of Higher Education Personnel (CAPES), Regional Hospital of Western Chapecó-SC, the doctor Carlos Henrique Mendonça and technicians Ademir Kesterke and Edegar dos Reis Carvalho.

11. References

Elder, D. et al. (2001). "Histopatologia da Pele de Lever". Manual e Atlas. São Paulo: Manole.

Marques C., Martins A., Conrado, L.A. (2004). "The Use of Hyperbaric Oxygen Therapy and Led Therapy in Diabetic Foot. Laser in Surgery: Advanced Characterization, Therapeutics, and System". Proceeding of SPIE 5312, 47-53.

HTM Indústria de Equipamentos Eletro-Eletrônicos Ltda. (2007). Manual do Equipamento Laser HTM, Amparo, São Paulo-SP.

Yoo, B. H.; Park C. M. ; Oh, T. J.; Han, S. H. ; Kang, H. H. (2002). "Investigation of jewelry powders radiating far infrared rays and the biological effects on human skin". Journal of Cosmetic Science, n.53. p. 175-184.

Heelspurs.com (2007), "Led Light Therapy", LLC 3063 Pinehill Road Montgomery, AL 36109.

N. Narendran, Y. Gu, T. Dong and H. Wu (2006) – "Spectral and Luminous Efficacy Change of High-power LEDs Under Different Dimming Methods". Lighting Research Center, Rensselaer Polytechnic Institute, 21 Union St., Troy, NY, 12180 USA.

SÁ JR., E. M. (2007) – "Projeto de Tese de Doutorado: Estudo de Novas Estruturas de Reatores Eletrônicos para LEDs de Iluminação". Programa de Pós-Graduação em Engenharia Elétrica, UFSC, Florianópolis-SC.

Moreira, M. C.; Prado, R. N.; Campos, Alexandre; Marchezan, T. B.; Cervi, M. (2008) "Aplicação de LEDs de Potência nos Tecidos Humanos e sua Interação Terapêutica". In: XVII Congresso Brasileiro de Automática, Juiz de Fora-MG. Anais do XVII Congresso Brasileiro de Automática, p. 1-6.

Moreira, M. C.; "Utilização de Conversores Eletrônicos que Alimentam LEDs de Alto Brilho na Aplicação em Tecido Humano e sua Interação Terapêutica" (2009). Tese de Doutorado, Universidade Federal de Santa Maria, p. 1-165.

Moreira, M. C.; "Utilização de um Conversor Eletrônico que Alimenta LEDs de Alto Brilho na Cor Vermelha em Tecido Humano de Pessoas Idosas" (2010). Artigo publicado na 3ª Semana de Ciência e Tecnologia, IFSC, Chapecó-SC, Brazil, p. 1-6.

A Feasibility of Low Intensity Ultrasound Stimulation for Treatment or Prevention of Osteoporosis and Its-Related Fracture

Dohyung Lim[1], Chang-Yong Ko[2,4], Sung-Jae Lee[3],
Keyoung Jin Chun[1] and Han Sung Kim[2]
[1]Gerontechnology Center, Korea Institute of Industrial Technology,
[2]Department of Biomedical Engineering, Yonsei University,
[3]Department of Biomedical Engineering, Inje University,
[4]Department of Structural and Medical Health Monitoring,
Fraunhofer Institute for Non-destructive Testing Dresden,
[1,2,3]Republic of Korea
[4]Germany

1. Introduction

Osteoporosis is characterized by low bone mass and deterioration of bone architecture, resulting in increased bone fragility and risk for bone fracture. This disease is associated with significant morbidity and mortality and has become a major public health concern. Osteoporosis and its-related fractures are an important public health concern; increasing in physical and/or psychological problems (depression, chronic disabling pain, fear and anxiety) as well as difficulty of the activities of daily life (NIH Consensus Development Panel on Osteoporosis Prevention Diagnosis and Therapy, 2001; Totosy de Zepetnek et al., 2009; WHO (World Health Organization), 2004). In addition, they cause increase in morbidity and mortality, and decrease in functional mobility and thereby reduction in quality of life (QOL) (Tosteson et al., 2008). Also, directly/indirectly financial expenditures for treating and caring of osteoporosis and its-related fracture are increasing over time.

Pharmacological interventions are widely used to treat and prevent osteoporosis and its-related fracture clinically. However, such interventions can be accompanied with undesirable side effects. The long-term estrogen replacement therapy may increase in a risk of breast or ovarian cancer or venous thromboembolism (Grady et al., 2004; Nelson et al., 2002; Noller, 2002; Schairer et al., 2000). The bisphosphonates may cause osteonecrosis of the jaw, a syndrome of myalgias and arthralgias, and gastrointestinal intolerance (Khosla et al., 2007; Lewiecki, 2010; Wysowski,Chang, 2005), and induce osteopetrosis in a child (Marini, 2003; Whyte et al., 2003; Whyte et al., 2008). Calcium and vitamin D supplementation might not be effective for reduction of osteoporotic bone fracture (Porthouse et al., 2005). Furthermore, inadequate vitamin D supplementation may increase in vascular calcification (Tang et al., 2006;Zittermann et al., 2007). Therefore, alternatives to pharmacological interventions are required for reduction of the adverse side effects.

Mechanical signals are the most important one of extrinsic factors for regulating bone homeostasis (Dufour et al., 2007;Judex et al., 2009). The relation between mechanical signal and bone homeostasis is elucidated by the mechanostat theory and the daily stress stimulus theory (Frost, 1987, 2003, 2004;Qin et al., 1996;Qin et al., 1998). The former describes that a net bone is regulated by the strain or deformation applied to the skeleton. In the latter theory, a net bone is modulated by a daily stress stimulus (considering both the magnitude as well as the number of cycles on loading) applied to the skeleton. Therefore, when strain applied on skeleton is bigger than target strain, the daily stress stimulus is bigger than some target stimulus, or a low magnitude and high cycle number, a net bone can be increased. Based on these rationales, external biophysical stimuli have been suggested as alternatives to pharmacological therapies. Ultrasound stimulation is one such promising stimulus (Monici et al., 2007;Perry et al., 2009;Rubin et al., 2001b).

Ultrasound is a high-frequency non-audible acoustic pressure wave with mechanical energy and can be transmitted at osteoporotic sites through biological tissues. It has been applied clinically for diagnosis or operation (Rubin et al., 2001a). Several *in-vivo* studies showed its therapeutic potential. LIUS could improve the defective or damaged bone healing; enhancement of the mechanical properties on the healing callus, bone bridging, nonunion fractures healing and distraction osteogenesis and reduction of healing time (Eberson, 2003;Pilla et al., 1990). Furthermore, in vitro cellular studies supported these in-vivo results (Kokubu et al., 1999;Li et al., 2003;Monici et al., 2007;Naruse et al., 2000;Unsworth et al., 2007;Yang et al., 2005) . LIUS could regulate bone cells; enhancing osteoblast formation and function and suppressing osteoclast formation and function.

Thus, LIUS may be useful for treatment or prevention of osteoporosis and its-related fracture. However, there are arguments about the effects of LIUS on osteoporotic bone. Carvalho and Cliquet (Carvalho,Cliquet Jr, 2004) and Perry et al. (Perry et al., 2009) suggested that LIUS might be beneficial in osteoporotic bone, but not in Warden *et al.*(Warden et al., 2001). The reasons of differences in the effects of osteoporotic bone were unclear. These arguments may be attributable to the several intrinsic and extrinsic limitations of experimental and analytic methodologies. For examples, bone architecture is heterogeneous and variable individually, but the previous studies did not consider those. For evaluation of the effects of LIUS on osteoporotic bones, histomorphometric analysis was widely performed. However, it has several limitations such as analysis of a few fields of view and impossibility of longitudinal analysis of identical specimen, but there were lacks of longitudinal studies j23. Moreover, bone adaptation with an identical bone is variable from location to location24, but there was no study on the effects of LIUS application considering irradiation location/direction of LIUS. Recently, *in-vivo* micro computed tomography (micro-CT) technique is widely used to investigate the longitudinal changes in 3D bone microarchitecture with overcoming these limitations. Finally, there was no study on longitudinal changes in mechanical strength of osteoporotic bone and on prediction of bone fracture risks after LIUS treatment. Finite element (FE) analysis is widely used to evaluate longitudinal changes in bone mechanical or behavior characteristics and predict bone fracture risks.

This study aimed to address such limitations in the previous studies and determine whether LIUS therapy cans effective for treatment or prevention of osteoporosis and its-related fracture based on in-vivo micro-CT technology and FE analysis.

2. Materials and method

2.1 Animal preparation

Eight 14-week-old virginal ICR mice (weighing approximately 24.0 ± 0.7 g) were ovariectomized (OVX) to induce osteoporosis. Osteoporosis was confirmed at 3 weeks after

OVX by changes in the bone biomechanical characteristics (52.2% decrease in bone volume fraction (BV/TV, Fig. 1) (van der Jagt et al., 2009) and 16.8% decreased in effective structural modulus relative to before OVX). All procedures were performed under a protocol approved by the Yonsei University Animal Care Committee (YWC-P107).

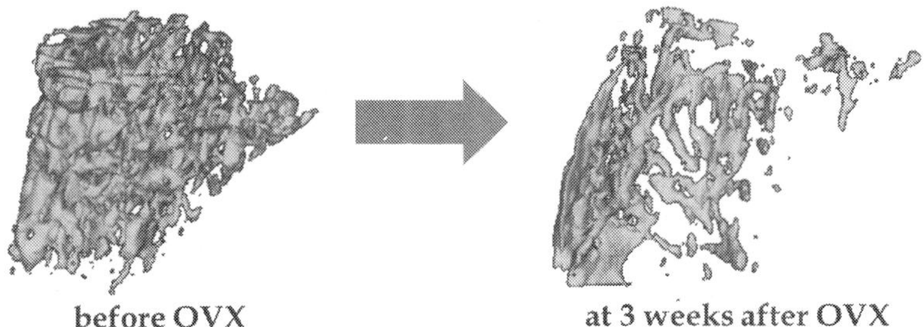

Fig. 1. Changes in trabecular bone structure over time induced by OVX

2.2 Application of LIUS

The right tibiae of each mouse were treated using LIUS (US group), whereas the left tibiae were not treated and served as an internal control (CON group). LIUS was composed of a pulse width of 200 µs containing 1.5MHz sine waves, with a repeated frequency of 1.0 kHz with a spatial-averaged temporal-averaged intensity of 30 mW/cm^2 (Warden, 2001;Warden et al., 2001). Application of LIUS was continued for 6 weeks and consisted of 20min/day and 5days/week. Before the application of LIUS, its output characteristics were measured by hydrophonic scanning. The mice were immobilized using a customized restrainer (David et al., 2003) and both tibiae were submerged in warm (35–40°C) water in a customized tank for the application of LIUS (Fig. 2) (Warden et al., 2001).

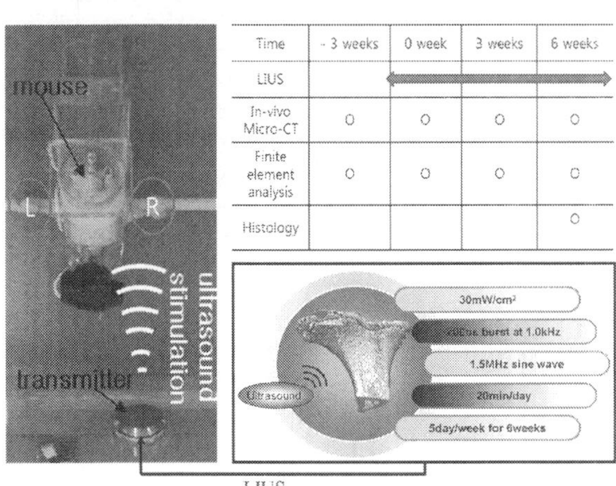

Time	- 3 weeks	0 week	3 weeks	6 weeks
LIUS				
In-vivo Micro-CT	O	O	O	O
Finite element analysis	O	O	O	O
Histology				O

Fig. 2. Experiment setup, LIUS application, in vivo micro-CT scanning, finite element analysis, histology

2.3 Bone structural parameters analysis

Both tibiae of each mouse were scanned at 0, 3 and 6 weeks after application of LIUS, as shown in Fig.1, using an in vivo micro-computed tomography (CT; Skyscan 1076, SKYSCAN N.V., Aartselaar, Belgium) at a voxel resolution with 18 µm in each axis under anesthesia induced by ketamine (1.5 ml/kg, Huons, Seoul, Korea) and xylazine (0.5 ml/kg, Bayer Korea, Seoul, Korea). The volume of interest (VOI) was determined as following; trabecular bone corresponding to the proximal tibia was selected from a 1.8-mm length of bone, located 0.54 mm below the growth plate, and cortical bone corresponding to the diaphyseal tibia was selected from a 0.9 mm length of bone, located 2.88 mm below the growth plate (Fig. 3). To investigate changes in 3D structural characteristics, structural parameters for the trabecular and cortical bone of both tibiae were measured and calculated by using micro-CT images and CT-AN 1.8 software (Skyscan). For the entire trabecular bone, the BV/TV (%), trabecular thickness (Tb.Th, mm), trabecular number (Tb.N, mm-1), trabecular separation (Tb.Sp, mm), structure model index (SMI), and trabecular bone pattern factor (Tb.Pf, mm-1) were measured and calculated. Additionally, to determine whether the LIUS irradiation location/direction affected in detail, the two-dimensional (2D) cross-sectional images of the trabecular bone were subdivided into five regions of interest (ROIs, Fig. 3). The ROIs as they correspond to the maximum selectable diameter in the medullary cavity were 0.5 mm in diameter. The ROI locations are shown in Fig. 3, corresponding to the direction of LIUS application. For the entire cortical bone, cross-section thickness (Cs.Th, mm) and mean polar moment inertia (MMI, mm⁴) were measured and calculated. Additionally, the 2D cross-sectional micro-CT images of the cortical bone were subdivided into four ROIs, to determine whether the LIUS irradiation location/direction affected in detail, as described above (Fig. 3).

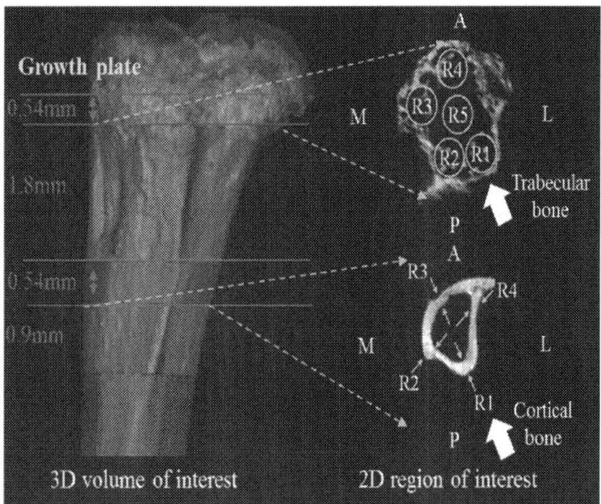

Fig. 3. Location of the 3 dimensional (3D) volume of interest (VOI) and the 2D regions of interests, R1: region 1, R2: region 2, R3: region 3, R4: region 4, R5: region 5, A: anterior, P: posterior, M: medial, L: lateral, white arrow: LIUS. (Figure was modified in Journal of Orthopaedic Research, 29(2011), 116-125)

2.4 Elastic tissue modulus analysis

The elastic tissue modulus, which are related to bone quality, was determined form Hounsfield units, for each element calculated by equation (1) (Rho et al., 1995) using Mimics 12.3 software (Materialise, Leuven, Belgium). To quantitatively evaluate the degree of improvement in bone quality achieved using LIUS, its distributions were used.

$$E = 5.54 \times \rho - 326$$
$$(\rho = 0.916 \times HU + 114)$$

(1)

where ρ is the density, HU is Hounsfield Unit, and E is elastic tissue modulus.

2.5 Effective structural modulus analysis

Binary images of the tibia in each mouse were converted from μ-CT images using BIONIX (CANTIBio, Suwon, Korea). Then 3D tetrahedral FE models with 18 μm mesh size were generated using a mass-compensated thresholding technique (Ulrich et al., 1998). Material property of bone (Young's modulus: 12.5 GPa and Poisson's ratio: 0.3) (Kinney et al., 2000;Woo et al., 2009), which was assumed to be isotropic and perfectly elastic, was assigned into the FE models. To analyze FE models, a compressive displacement of an uniaxial 0.5% strain as displacement boundary conditions was applied to the FE models (Woo et al., 2009). All FE analyses were performed using the commercial FE software package ABAQUS 6.4 (HKS, Pawtucket, RI, USA).

2.6 Histomorphometric analysis

At the end of experiment, mice were sacrificed through cervical dislocation. Both tibiae were extracted, and surrounding tissues (skin, muscle, and tendons) were removed. To perform histology, routine procedures were followed. The first, the tibiae were fixed for 3 days in 10% neutral buffered formalin, treated with 10% formic acid for 1 h. The second, the fixed tibiae were decalcified with a 10% ethylenediaminetetraacetic acid solution and then embedded in paraffin. Then, each tibia was cut at a 4 micrometer sections (4-μm-thick) through the long axis in the sagittal plane with a microtome (Microm, Walldorf, Germany). Finally, Masson's trichrome (MT) stain was performed to visualize. Analyses were performed using a microscope (Olympus BX50, Tokyo, Japan) to evaluate new bone formation (blue: mature mineralization, red: uncompleted mineralization (osteoid)) and osteocytes. To quantity osteocyte, the number of osteocytes in a square (200 $\times$ 200 μm) was counted.

2.7 Statistical analysis

The structural parameters and effective structural modulus were compared using ANOVA with a mixed factorial design and repeated measures. A paired t-test was performed to compare the number of osteocytes and elastic tissue modulus between the US and CON groups. All descriptive data are represented as mean±standard error. All statistical analyses were performed with the SPSS 12.0 (Chicago, IL, USA). p Values <0.05 were considered significant.

3. Results

3.1 Structural changes

During experiment, there were no significant differences in the structural parameters of the trabecular and cortical bone in the US group over time (Fig. 4 ~ 7, p<0.05). However, in the

CON group, the BV/TVs and Tb.Ns significantly decreased over time, whereas the SMIs and Tb.Pfs significantly increased (p<0.05, Fig. 4). The BV/TVs on R1, R4 and R5 in trabecular bone and the Cs.Ths of all regions in cortical bone did not significantly change over time in both the US and CON groups (Fig. 5 and Fig. 7, p>0.05).

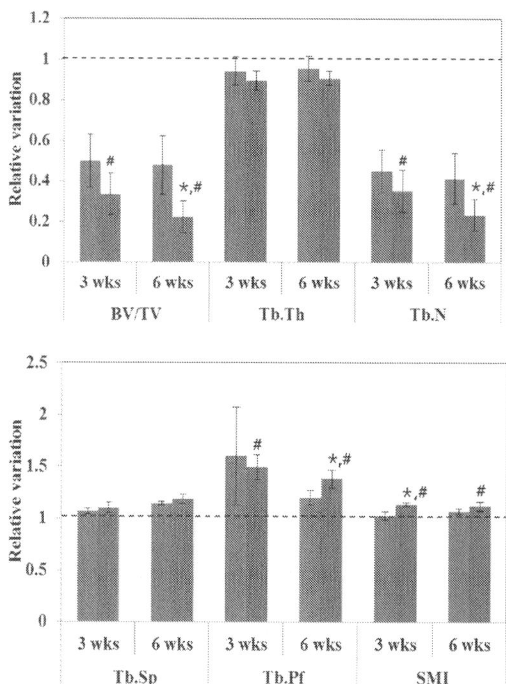

Fig. 4. Results of the structural parameter analysis for trabecular bone (mean ± standard error of relative variations), *significant difference between the US and CON groups (p<0.05), # significant difference in each group over time (p<0.05), blue bar: US group, red bar: CON group, dashed line: 1 at 0 week (Figures were modified in Journal of Orthopaedic Research, 29(2011), 116-125)

The relative variations were determined by calculating the degree of changes relative to the base line value, at 0 week (1 at 0 week). At week 3, the relative variation of the SMI in the US group was significantly smaller than that in the CON group (Fig. 4, p<0.05). However, there were no significant differences between the US and CON group for the other structural parameters (Fig.4, p>0.05). The relative variations of BV/TV, Tb.N and Tb.Pf in the US group were significantly bigger at 6 weeks after LIUS treatment than those in the CON group (Fig.4, p<0.05). However, there were no significant differences of the other structural parameters, Tb.Th, Tb.Sp and SMI, between the two groups (Fig.4, p>0.05). At week 3, the relative variation of the BV/TV in any of the five ROIs between groups did not shown significant differences (Fig.5, p>0.05). However, after 6 weeks of LIUS treatment, the relative variation of BV/TV in R1 was significantly bigger than those in the CON group (Fig.5, p<0.05), whereas there were no significant differences between groups in other regions, R2, R3, R4 and R5 (Fig.5, p>0.05).

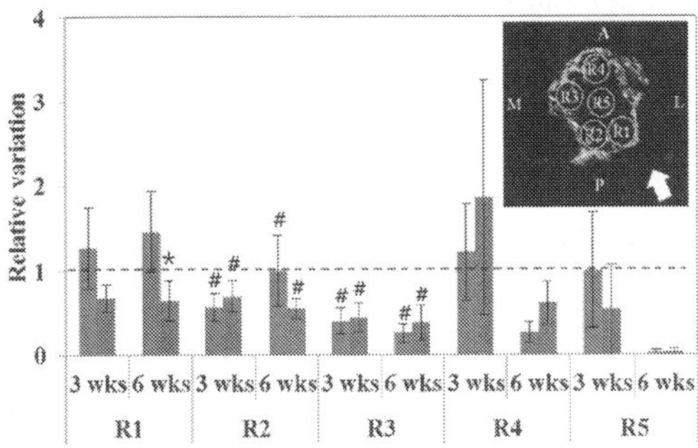

Fig. 5. Results of the BV/TV in five regions of interest for trabecular bone (mean ± standard error of relative variations), *significant difference between the US and CON groups (p<0.05), # significant difference in each group over time (p<0.05), blue bar: US group, red bar: CON group, dashed line: 1 at 0 week, A: anterior, P: posterior, M: medial, L: lateral, white arrow: LIUS (Figure was modified in Journal of Orthopaedic Research, 29(2011), 116-125)

The relative variations of the Cs.Th and MMI for cortical bone were significant differences between the US and CON groups following 3 weeks of treatment (Fig.6, p>0.05). However, in the US group after 6 weeks of LIUS treatment, the relative variation in the MMI was significantly higher than that in the CON group (Fig.6, p<0.05), whereas there were no differences of the relative variation in the Cs.Th between groups (Fig.6, p>0.05). In the regional analysis, at 3 weeks after LIUS, the relative variation in Cs.Th in R2 was significantly increased compared with the CON group (Fig. 7, p<0.05). However, there were no significant differences of Cs.Th in the other regions between groups (Fig. 7, p>0.05). At 6 weeks after LIUS, the relative variations in Cs.Th in R1 and R2 were higher in US group than CON group (Fig. 7, p>0.05), whereas no differences of Cs.Th in the R3 and R4 were observed between groups (Fig. 7, p>0.05). In the US group, the structure of tibia tends to maintain over time, and new bone formation was observed relative to in the CON group as shown in Fig. 8.

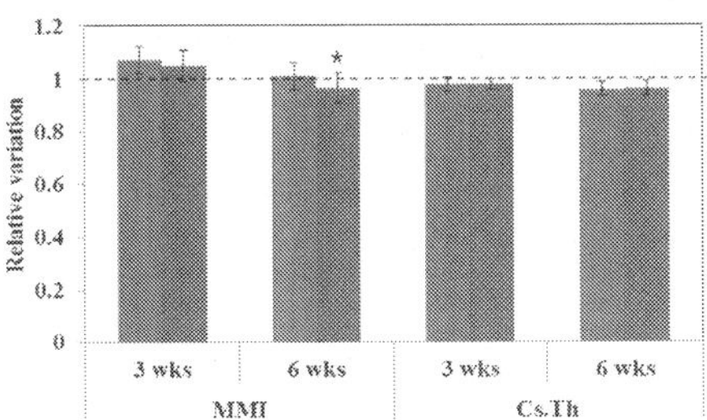

Fig. 6. Results of the structural parameter analysis for cortical bone (mean ± standard error of relative variations), *significant difference between the US and CON groups (p<0.05), blue bar: US group, red bar: CON group, dashed line: 1 at 0 week (Figure was modified in Journal of Orthopaedic Research, 29(2011), 116-125)

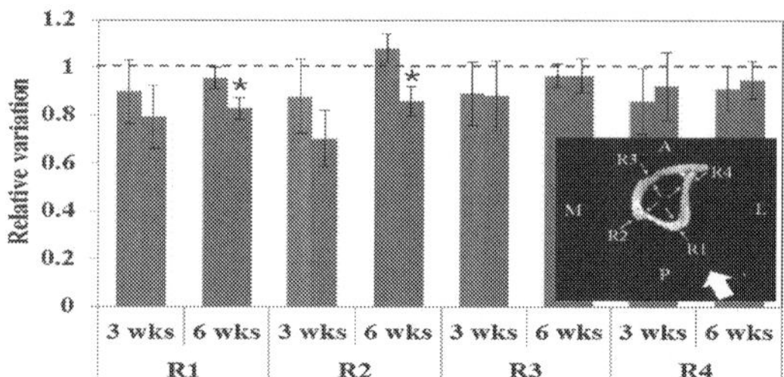

Fig. 7. Results of the Cs.Th in four regions of interest for trabecular bone (mean ± standard error of relative variations), *significant difference between the US and CON groups (p<0.05), # significant difference in each group over time (p<0.05), blue bar: US group, red bar: CON group, dashed line: 1 at 0 week, A: anterior, P: posterior, M: medial, L: lateral, white arrow: LIUS (Figure was modified in Journal of Orthopaedic Research, 29(2011), 116-125)

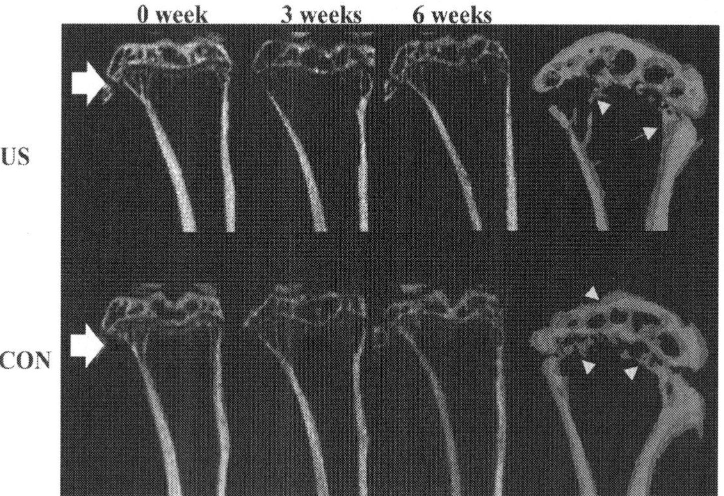

Fig. 8. Representative the changes in bone structure over time in the US and CON groups, overlaid images; 0 week (white) and 6 weeks (red), white arrow: LIUS, yellow arrow head: bone resoprtion, yellow arrow: bone maintaining (Figure was modified in Journal of Orthopaedic Research, 29(2011), 116-125).

3.2 Elastic tissue modulus changes

The volumes of the higher elastic tissue modulus (3046 and 3723 MPa) in the US group were significantly increased relative to those in the CON group (Fig. 9, p<0.05). However, the volume of lower elastic tissue modulus (2369 MPa) in the US group was less than that in the CON group (Fig. 9, p<0.05). Fig. 10 shows the changes of 3D structure of tibia mapped by elastic tissue moduli. The distribution or volume of high values tends to increase in the US group over time, but it tends to decrease in the CON group.

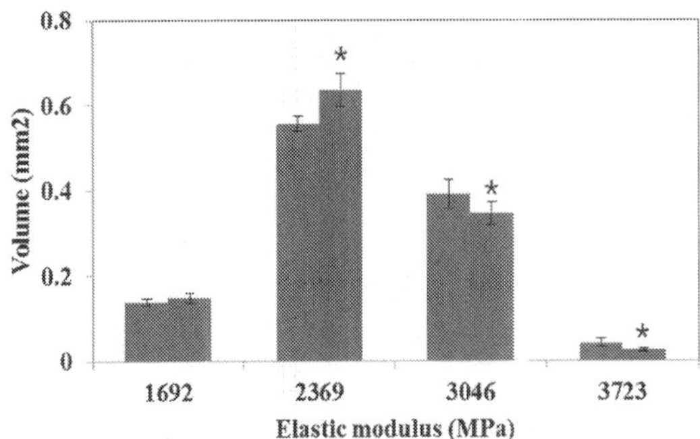

Fig. 9. Results of the elastic tissue modulus (mean ± standard error of relative variations), *significant difference between the US and CON groups (p<0.05), blue bar: US group, red bar: CON group (Figure was modified in Annals of Biomedical Engineering, 38 (2010), 2438-2446)

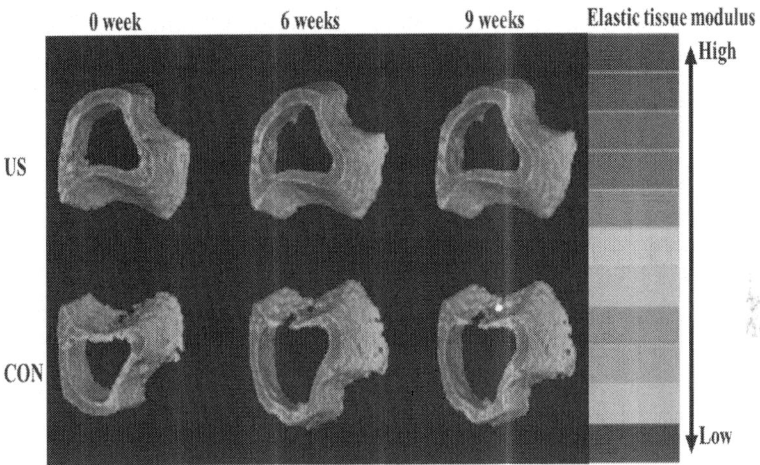

Fig. 10. Representative distributions of the elastic modulus in the CON and US over time (Figure was modified in Annals of Biomedical Engineering, 38 (2010), 2438-2446)

3.3 Effective structural modulus changes

During experiment, the effective moduli were significant differences over time in the US and CON group (Fig. 11, p<0.05). The effective modulus was gradually increased in the US group over time, whereas it was increased at 3 weeks and was decreased at 6 weeks at the CON group. At 3 weeks after LIUS, there was no significant difference of the relative variation in the effective structural modulus between groups (Fig. 11, p>0.05). However, the relative variation in structural modulus in the US group was significantly bigger than that in the CON group (Fig. 11, p<0.05)

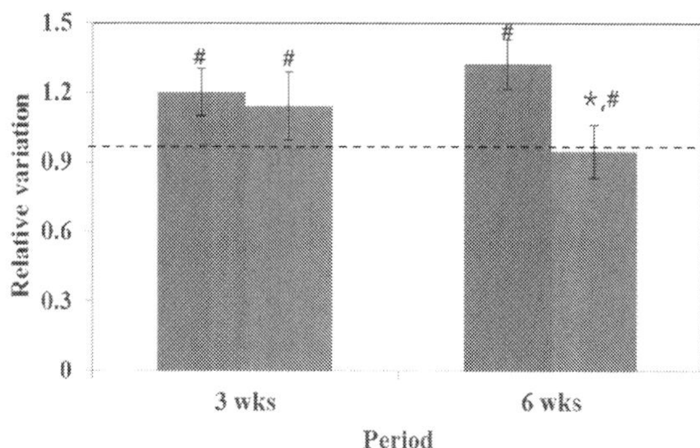

Fig. 11. Results of the effective structural modulus (mean ± standard error of relative variations), *significant difference between the US and CON groups (p<0.05), blue bar: US group, red bar: CON group, dashed line: 1 at 0 week (Figure was modified in Annals of Biomedical Engineering, 38 (2010), 2438-2446)

3.4 Histomorphometric analysis

More osteoid, incomplete bone mineralization, in the US group was observed relative to that the CON group (Fig. 12). Also, the trabeculae and the endosteal cortical bone, which is the near region directly treated with LIUS, in the US group were thicker than those in the CON group. These structural improvements are consistent with the results of structural parameter analysis as well as the micro-CT images, as mentioned above. Moreover, the number of osteocyte in the US group was significantly higher than that in the CON group (Fig. 13, p<0.05).

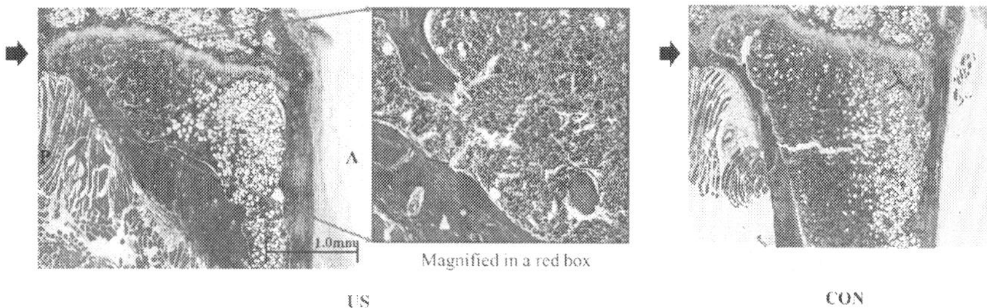

Fig. 12. Representative histology in the US and CON group, yellow arrow head: osteocyte, yellow arrow: osteoid, black arrow: LIUS (Figure was modified in Journal of Orthopaedic Research, 29(2011), 116-125).

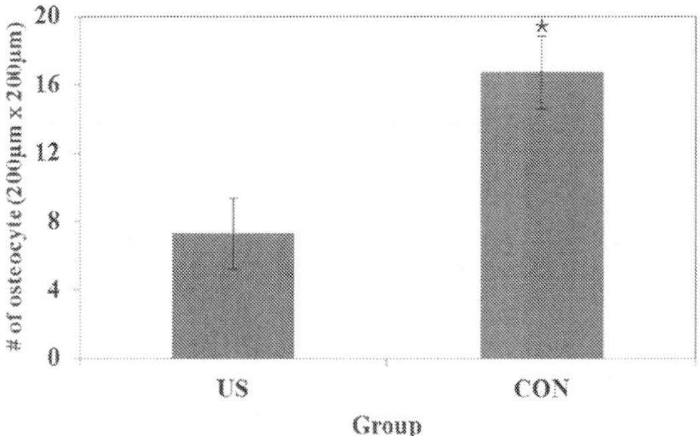

Fig. 13. Comparison of the number of osteocyte, *significant difference between the US and CON groups (p<0.05)

4. Discussion

We evaluated the feasibility of LIUS for treatment or prevention of osteoporosis induced by estrogen deficiency through an analysis of biomechanical characteristics, bone structural characteristics and mechanical characteristics. Bone quality and quantity are regulated by external mechanical loading, because it is a sensitive tissue responding to external mechanical loading. The relationship between bone and mechanical loading is supported by mechanosensory mechanisms, including mechanoreception and mechanotransduction (Chen et al., 2003;Cowin, 2000). These factors suggested that LIUS can enhance bone healing and regeneration. However, the effects of LIUS for treatment or prevention of osteoporosis are controversial (Carvalho,Cliquet Jr, 2004;Perry et al., 2009;Warden et al., 2001). These controversial results may be contributed to the limitations of conventional experimental and analytic methods, lack of longitudinal study and ignoring individual differences, bone heterogeneity and partial effects of LIUS considering irradiation location and direction. It is widely known that in-vivo micro-CT can detect and track longitudinal changes in 3D bone structure of identical small animals without sacrificing them. Moreover, micro FEA is also widely used to evaluate longitudinal changes in bone mechanical strength and predict bone fracture risks. Therefore, we attempted to overcome these limitations using in-vivo micro-CT and micro FEA.

After 6 weeks of LIUS treatment, the relative variations of BV/TV and Tb.N were increased and the relative variation of Tb.Pf was decreased for trabecular bone compared to the non-LIUS treatment group. Moreover, the relative variation in MMI for the cortical bone was increased. These results indicated that 6 weeks of LIUS treatment might prevent bone loss and disconnection, suggesting suppression of the continuous progress of osteoporosis-associated bone loss in both trabecula and cortical bones.

To determine whether irradiation direction/location of LIUS affects bone adaptation site-specifically, BV/TV in five ROIs for trabecular bone and Cs.Th in four ROIs for cortical bone were measured and calculated. In the site of direct LIUS irradiation (R1), the relative variation of BV/TV and Cs.Th were significantly increased in the US group compared to the non-US group. However, in the furthest site of direct LIUS irradiation (R3 and R4), the relative variations of BV/TV and Cs.Th were different between groups. These data indicated that irradiation location/direction of LIUS application might induce site-specific bone adaptation and thereby cause treatment outcome. These results are consistent with previous studies that Responses in bone cell corresponding to the local stimuli, such as strain-energy density and deformation of the bone matrix, may be temporal and positional (Henderson,Carter, 2002;Huiskes et al., 2000;Waarsing et al., 2004;Wolpert, 1989).

From the results of histological analysis, on near the region stimulated directly by LIUS, new bone formation in the endosteal cortical bone was observed in the US group. Moreover, thicker cortical bone and new bone formation in trabecular bone were also observed in the US group. These results show that LIUS stimulation for 6 weeks might enhance new bone formation or suppress bone resorption, consistent with previous studies (Carvalho,Cliquet Jr, 2004;Perry et al., 2009;Pilla et al., 1990). Furthermore, the number of osteocytes in the US group were higher than that in the CON group. Osteocyte regulates activity of bone forming cell (osteoblast) and bone resoprtion cell (osteoclast) and play an important role in mechanotransduction responding to mechanical loading (Skerry, 2008). Moreover, the estrogen deficiency-induced osteocyte apoptosis increased bone fragility and thereby fracture risks (Tatsumi et al., 2007). These results showed that LIUS may prevent estrogen deficiency-induced osteocyte apoptosis and bone fragility, suggesting increase in bone strength and decrease in bone fracture risks. Moreover, LIUS might affect mechanotransduction.

At 6 weeks after LIUS, the volume of higher tissue elastic moduli were increased compared with non-LIUS treatment group. This result showed that LIUS might not only increase bone volume enhance but also tissue material properties. Thus, LIUS might improve bone quantity, which was consistent with the results of structural parameters and histological analysis mentioned above, as well as bone quality, leading to increase in bone strength and thereby decrease in osteoporotic bone fracture risks.

The results of structural, histological and material analysis suggested that LIUS could reduce bone fracture risk. We verified the improvement of bone mechanical characteristics via performing micro FEA. At 6 weeks after LIUS, the effective structural modulus was significantly increased compared with non-LIUS treatment group. This data showed that LIUS improve bone structural strength. Therefore, LIUS could suppress the progressive bone weakening induced by estrogen deficiency, thereby would be effective in preventing or decreasing osteoporotic bone fracture risk.

However, the magnitude of the effects of LIUS for preventing/treating osteoporotic bone loss and weakening seemed to be small. This contributed to an inability of the US to reach osteoporotic bone due to absorption, scattering and reflection during transmitting soft tissues (Malizos et al., 2006;Warden, 2001). Moreover, local site-specific stimuli in partial bone can be contributed to systemic bone adaptation in others bone by neuronal regulation (Sample et al., 2008). Therefore, bones in the CON group have adapted via neuronal regulation despite indirect LIUS stimulation to them. This hypothesis might be supported by temporary increase in the effective structural modulus in the CON group at 3 weeks after LIUS.

In summary, our data show that LIUS may improve the osteoporotic bone microarchitectural characteristics, and bone material properties by regulation of bone homeostasis, enhancing bone formation and suppressing bone resorption, and mecahnostraduction, preventing osteocyte apoptosis caused by estrogen deficiency. Also, LIUS may prevent bone weakening and thereby decrease bone fracture risks. Therefore, the QOL of patients with osteoporosis can improve.

5. Conclusion

LIUS may improve the microarchitectural characteristics, material properties and mechanical strength in the osteoporotic bone, leading to decrease in bone fracture risks. Thus, LIUS may be effective to prevent and treat osteoporosis and thereby contribute to improve the QOL of patients with osteoporosis.

6. Acknowledgment

This research was supported by a grant from Leading Foreign Research Institute Recruitment Program, the National Research Foundation of Korea, Ministry of Education, Science and Technology and a grant from the Korea Healthcare Technology R&D Project, Ministry for Health & Welfare, Republic of Korea (A100023).

7. References

Carvalho, DCL, Cliquet Jr, A. 2004. The action of low-intensity pulsed ultrasound in bones of osteopenic rats. *Artif Organs*, No. 28, pp. 114-118.

Chen, YJ, Wang, CJ, Yang, KD, et al. 2003. Pertussis toxin-sensitive Galphai protein and ERK-dependent pathways mediate ultrasound promotion of osteogenic transcription in human osteoblasts. *FEBS Lett*, No. 554, pp. 154-158.

Cowin, SC. 2000. *Bone mechanics handbook*, CRC pressBoca Raton.

David, V, Laroche, N, Boudignon, B, et al. 2003. Noninvasive in vivo monitoring of bone architecture alterations in hindlimb-unloaded female rats using novel three-dimensional microcomputed tomography. *J Bone Miner Res*, No. 18, pp. 1622-1631.

Dufour, C, Holy, X, Marie, PJ. 2007. Skeletal unloading induces osteoblast apoptosis and targets alpha5beta1-PI3K-Bcl-2 signaling in rat bone. *Exp Cell Res*, No. 313, pp. 394-403.

Eberson, C, Hogan, KA, Moore, DC, Ehrlich, MG. 2003. Effect of Low-Intensity Ultrasound Stimulation on Consolidation of the Regenerate Zone in a Rat Model of Distraction Osteogenesis. *J Pediatr Orthop*, No. 23, pp. 46-51.

Frost, HM. 1987. Bone "mass" and the "mechanostat": a proposal. *Anat Rec*, No. 219, pp. 1-9.

Frost, HM. 2003. Bone's mechanostat: a 2003 update. *Anat Rec A Discov Mol Cell Evol Biol*, No. 275, pp. 1081-1101.

Frost, HM. 2004. A 2003 update of bone physiology and Wolff's Law for clinicians. *Angle Orthod*, No. 74, pp. 3-15.

Grady, D, Ettinger, B, Moscarelli, E, et al. 2004. Safety and adverse effects associated with raloxifene: multiple outcomes of raloxifene evaluation. *Obstet Gynecol*, No. 104, pp. 837-844.

Henderson, JH, Carter, DR. 2002. Mechanical induction in limb morphogenesis: the role of growth-generated strains and pressures. *Bone*, No. 31, pp. 645-653.

Huiskes, R, Ruimerman, R, van Lenthe, GH, Janssen, JD. 2000. Effects of mechanical forces on maintenance and adaptation of form in trabecular bone. *Nature*, No. 405, pp. 704-706.

Judex, S, Gupta, S, Rubin, C. 2009. Regulation of mechanical signals in bone. *Orthod Craniofac Res*, No. 12, pp. 94-104.

Khosla, S, Burr, D, Cauley, J, et al. 2007. Bisphosphonate-associated osteonecrosis of the jaw: report of a task force of the American Society for Bone and Mineral Research. *J Bone Miner Res*, No. 22, pp. 1479-1491.

Kinney, JH, Haupt, DL, Balooch, M, et al. 2000. Three-dimensional morphometry of the L6 vertebra in the ovariectomized rat model of osteoporosis: biomechanical implications. *J Bone Miner Res*, No. 15, pp. 1981-1991.

Kokubu, T, Matsui, N, Fujioka, H, et al. 1999. Low Intensity Pulsed Ultrasound Exposure Increases Prostaglandin E2Production via the Induction of Cyclooxygenase-2 mRNA in Mouse Osteoblasts. *Biochem Biophys Res Commun*, No. 256, pp. 284-287.

Lewiecki, EM. 2010. Intravenous zoledronic acid for the treatment of osteoporosis: The evidence of its therapeutic effect. *Core Evid*, No. 4, pp. 13-23.

Li, JK, Chang, WH, Lin, JC, et al. 2003. Cytokine release from osteoblasts in response to ultrasound stimulation. *Biomaterials*, No. 24, pp. 2379-2385.

Lim, D, Ko, CY, Seo, DH, Woo, DG, Kim, JM, Chun, KJ, Kim, HS. 2011. Low-intensity ultrasound stimulation prevents osteoporotic bone loss in young adult ovariectomized mice. J Orhop Res, No. 29, pp. 116-125.

Malizos, KN, Papachristos, AA, Protopappas, VC, Fotiadis, DI. 2006. Transosseous application of low-intensity ultrasound for the enhancement and monitoring of fracture healing process in a sheep osteotomy model. *Bone*, No. 38, pp. 530-539.

Marini, JC. 2003. Do bisphosphonates make children's bones better or brittle? *N Engl J Med*, No. 349, pp. 423-426.

Monici, M, Bernabeib, PA, Basilec, V, et al. 2007. Can ultrasound counteract bone loss? Effect of low-intensity ultrasound stimulation on a model of osteoclastic precursor. *Acta astronautica*, No. 60, pp. 383-390.

Naruse, K, Mikuni-Takagaki, Y, Azuma, Y, et al. 2000. Anabolic Response of Mouse Bone-Marrow-Derived Stromal Cell Clone ST2 Cells to Low-Intensity Pulsed Ultrasound. *Biochem Biophys Res Commun*, No. 268, pp. 216-220.

Nelson, HD, Humphrey, LL, Nygren, P, et al. 2002. Postmenopausal hormone replacement therapy: scientific review. *JAMA*, No. 288, pp. 872-881.

NIH Consensus Development Panel on Osteoporosis Prevention Diagnosis and Therapy. 2001. Osteoporosis prevention, diagnosis, and therapy. *JAMA*, No. 285, pp. 785-795.

Noller, KL. 2002. Estrogen replacement therapy and risk of ovarian cancer. *JAMA*, No. 288, pp. 368-369.

Perry, MJ, Parry, LK, Burton, VJ, et al. 2009. Ultrasound mimics the effect of mechanical loading on bone formation in vivo on rat ulnae. *Med Eng Phys*, No. 31, pp. 42-47.

Pilla, AA, Mont, MA, Nasser, PR, et al. 1990. Non-invasive low-intensity pulsed ultrasound accelerates bone healing in the rabbit. *J Orthop Trauma*, No. 4, pp. 246-253.

Porthouse, J, Cockayne, S, King, C, et al. 2005. Randomised controlled trial of calcium and supplementation with cholecalciferol (vitamin D3) for prevention of fractures in primary care. *BMJ*, No. 330, pp. 1003.

Qin, YX, McLeod, KJ, Guilak, F, et al. 1996. Correlation of bony ingrowth to the distribution of stress and strain parameters surrounding a porous-coated implant. *J Orthop Res*, No. 14, pp. 862-870.

Qin, YX, Rubin, CT, McLeod, KJ. 1998. Nonlinear dependence of loading intensity and cycle number in the maintenance of bone mass and morphology. *J Orthop Res*, No. 16, pp. 482-489.

Rho, JY, Hobatho, MC, Ashman, RB. 1995. Relations of mechanical properties to density and CT numbers in human bone. *Medical Engineering & Physics*, No. 17, pp. 347-355.

Rubin, C, Bolander, M, Ryaby, JP, Hadjiargyrou, M. 2001a. The Use of Low-Intensity Ultrasound to Accelerate the Healing of Fractures *J Bone Joint Surg Am*, No. 83, pp. 259-270.

Rubin, C, Sommerfeldt, D, Judex, S, Qin, YX. 2001b. Inhibition of osteopenia by low magnitude, high-frequency mechanical stimuli. *Drug Discov Today*, No. 6, pp. 848-858.

Sample, SJ, Behan, M, Smith, L, et al. 2008. Functional adaptation to loading of a single bone is neuronally regulated and involves multiple bones. *J Bone Miner Res*, No. 23, pp. 1372-1381.

Schairer, C, Lubin, J, Troisi, R, et al. 2000. Menopausal estrogen and estrogen-progestin replacement therapy and breast cancer risk. *JAMA*, No. 283, pp. 485-491.

Skerry, TM. 2008. The response of bone to mechanical loading and disuse: fundamental principles and influences on osteoblast/osteocyte homeostasis. *Arch Biochem Biophys*, No. 473, pp. 117-123.

Tang, FT, Chen, SR, Wu, XQ, et al. 2006. Hypercholesterolemia accelerates vascular calcification induced by excessive vitamin D via oxidative stress. *Calcif Tissue Int*, No. 79, pp. 326-339.

Tatsumi, S, Ishii, K, Amizuka, N, et al. 2007. Targeted ablation of osteocytes induces osteoporosis with defective mechanotransduction. *Cell Metab*, No. 5, pp. 464-475.

Tosteson, AN, Melton, LJ, 3rd, Dawson-Hughes, B, et al. 2008. Cost-effective osteoporosis treatment thresholds: the United States perspective. *Osteoporos Int*, No. 19, pp. 437-447.

Totosy de Zepetnek, JO, Giangregorio, LM, Craven, BC. 2009. Whole-body vibration as potential intervention for people with low bone mineral density and osteoporosis: a review. *J Rehabil Res Dev*, No. 46, pp. 529-542.

Ulrich, D, van Rietbergen, B, Weinans, H, Ruegsegger, P. 1998. Finite element analysis of trabecular bone structure: a comparison of image-based meshing techniques. *J Biomech*, No. 31, pp. 1187-1192.

Unsworth, J, Kaneez, S, Harris, S, et al. 2007. Pulsed Low Intensity Ultrasound Enhances Mineralisation in Preosteoblast Cells. *Ultrasound Med Biol*, No. 33, pp. 1468-1474.

van der Jagt, OP, van der Linden, JC, Schaden, W, et al. 2009. Unfocused extracorporeal shock wave therapy as potential treatment for osteoporosis. *J Orthop Res*, No. 27, pp. 1528-1533.

Waarsing, J, Day, J, van der Linden, J, et al. 2004. Detecting and tracking local changes in the tibiae of individual rats: a novel method to analyse longitudinal in vivo micro-CT data. *Bone*, No. 34, pp. 163-169.

Warden, SJ. 2001. Efficacy of low-intensity pulsed ultrasound in the prevention of osteoporosis following spinal cord injury. *Bone*, No. 29, pp. 431-436.

Warden, SJ, Bennell, KL, Forwood, MR, et al. 2001. Skeletal effects of low-intensity pulsed ultrasound on the ovariectomized rodent. *Ultrasound in Medicine and Biology*, No. 27, pp. 989-998.

WHO (World Health Organization). 2004. *Who Scientific Group on the Assessment of Osteoporosis at Primary Health Care Level*, WHO Press.

Whyte, MP, Wenkert, D, Clements, KL, et al. 2003. Bisphosphonate-induced osteopetrosis. *N Engl J Med*, No. 349, pp. 457-463.

Whyte, MP, McAlister, WH, Novack, DV, et al. 2008. Bisphosphonate-induced osteopetrosis: novel bone modeling defects, metaphyseal osteopenia, and osteosclerosis fractures after drug exposure ceases. *J Bone Miner Res*, No. 23, pp. 1698-1707.

Wolpert, L. 1989. Positional information revisited. *Development*, No. 107 Suppl, pp. 3-12.

Woo, DG, Ko, CY, Kim, HS, Seo, JB, Lim, D. 2010. Evaluation of the potential clinical application of low-intensity ultrasound stimulation for preventing osteoporotic bone fracture. Ann Biomed Eng. No. 38, 2438-2446.

Woo, DG, Lee, BY, Lim, D, Kim, HS. 2009. Relationship between nutrition factors and osteopenia: Effects of experimental diets on immature bone quality. *J Biomech*, No. 42, pp. 1102-1107.

Wysowski, DK, Chang, JT. 2005. Alendronate and risedronate: reports of severe bone, joint, and muscle pain. *Arch Intern Med*, No. 165, pp. 346-347.

Yang, RS, Lin, WL, Chen, YZ, et al. 2005. Regulation by ultrasound treatment on the integrin expression and differentiation of osteoblasts. *Bone*, No. 36, pp. 276-283.

Zittermann, A, Schleithoff, SS, Koerfer, R. 2007. Vitamin D and vascular calcification. *Curr Opin Lipidol*, No. 18, pp. 41-46.

3

Electrical Stimulation in Tissue Regeneration

Shiyun Meng[1,2], Mahmoud Rouabhia[2] and Ze Zhang[1]
*[1]Département de chirurgie, Faculté de médecine, Université Laval,
Centre de recherche de l'Hôpital Saint-François d'Assise, CHUQ, Québec,
[2]Groupe de Recherche en Écologie Buccale, Faculté de médecine dentaire,
Université Laval, Québec,
Canada*

1. Introduction

That human body generates biological electric field and current is a well-known natural phenomenon. In 1983, electrical potentials ranging between 10 and 60 mV at various locations of the human body were measured by Barker (Foulds & Barker, 1983), who also located the so-called epidermal or skin "battery" inside the living layer of the epidermis. Naturally occurred electrical field in human body was also reviewed in 1993 (Zipse, 1993). Bioelectricity is inherent in wound healing. An injury potential occurs in the form of a steady direct current (DC) electric field (EF) when a wound is created. This endogenous EF has been shown to guide cell migration to sprout directly toward the wound edge. On the other hand, wound healing is compromised when the EF is inhibited. McCaig et al. (McCaig et al., 2005) revealed that electrical events induced by injury potential could persist for a long time and present across hundreds of microns rather than be confined to the immediate vicinity of the cell membrane. Moreover, a voltage gradient called "action potential" across cell membrane is known to trigger cells to transmit signals and secrete hormones.

The electrical resistivity of biological tissues obviously varies due to the variation in tissue composition, such as tissue type and density, cell membrane permeability, and electrolyte content. The resistivity of these biological tissues has been measured by means of bioelectrical impedance analysis (BIA). When nutritional and metabolic disorders occur, the electrical properties of certain tissues become abnormal. BIA has therefore been used to diagnose human organ malfunctions. However, it remains difficult to delineate living tissue, such as bone tissue, because this tissue is a composite material that is anisotropic in structure and inhomogeneous in composition. For example, in 1975, Liboff (Liboff et al., 1975) reported a resistance ranging widely from 0.7 to 1×10^5 ohm/cm in human tibia. Recent advances in computed three-dimensional microtomography (microCT) now enable us to clarify the interrelationships between the electrical properties and the microstructures of human bone. The electrical property of bones varies widely caused by many factors such as the unevenly distributed and electrolyte-filled pores, moisture content, pH and conductivity of the immersing fluid. Nevertheless, it remains both essential and possible to normalize the resistance and the capacitance of different bone types. Electrical measurements provide a tool for the rapid quantitative diagnosis of bone grafts or bone quality during such procedures as total joint replacement surgery. For example, high bone conductivity is associated with high marrow content, while low conductivity is related to high porosity, low bone mineral density (BMD), and low bone volume to total tissue volume (BV/TV) ratio (Sierpowska et al., 2006). Combined with the microCT technique, microstructural changes, such as the reduction of trabecular thickness and number, can be revealed by electrical and dielectric parameters (Sierpowska et al., 2006).

At cellular level, cells are responsive to the exogenous electric field. The discovery regarding the response of yeast (Mehedintu & Berg, 1997) and diatoms (Smith et al., 1987) to electromagnetic field (EMF) stimulation was such a milestone, as both yeast and diatoms are single cell organisms, which implies that the EMF effects occur at the cellular level. These studies also suggested that the control of cellular behaviours is feasible through a manipulation of the cytoskeleton proteins using external physical stimuli such as EF. Various biological systems respond to endogenous or exogenous ES, suggesting that physiologically relevant EF may serve as an efficient tool to control and to adjust cellular and tissue homeostasis. To date, a variety of cells have been used to study their responses to ES, including mesenchymal stem cells, bone and cartilage cells, neuronal cells, and cardiac cells. Numerous in vitro experiments have shown that EF affects important cellular behaviours such as adhesion, proliferation, differentiation, directional migration, as well as division.

2. How cells respond to ES: Possible mechanisms

The biochemical and biophysical mechanisms of how cells respond to ES are very complex and remain largely unknown. For example, how do cells sense ES? How and at what level do cellular behaviours begin to change in an EF? For now, these questions remain unanswered, as cell response to ES is not only complicated by the complexity of the cell signalling pathways, but also by the complex nature of EF in biological medium. However, despite the lack of knowledge regarding the effect of EF on cell properties, we are not completely in the dark, as important experimental evidences support the following possible mechanisms of electrical signal recognition and signal transduction, as well as the regulation of gene expression.

2.1 Recognition of electrical signals and signal transduction within individual cells

The sophisticated cell membrane is the first point of contact with the environment. The 4 to 10-nm-thick lipid bilayer membrane separates the interior of a cell from the drastically different external medium. Cell membrane surface is negatively charged due to the predominance of negatively charged chemical groups (e.g., carboxylates, phosphates) in membrane proteins and glycans. An electrical potential gradient in the order of -100 mV (negative inside the cell) (Bezanilla, 2008), namely, transmembrane potential, exists across the cell membrane and is generated by the uneven distribution of ions – in particular potassium – on both sides of the membrane.

Cellular activity is regulated by the distribution of soluble ions through various ion channels, pumps and transporters, which are mostly membrane proteins subjected to external stimuli, including electricity. Several membrane proteins, referred to as voltage-sensing proteins, such as ion channels, transporters, pumps, and enzymes not only sense but use external electric field to regulate cellular functions (Bezanilla, 2008). The movement of the charge or the dipole within these proteins, i.e., the transient or gating current, may also be affected by external EF. Although physiological-level EF in the range of mV and μA is too weak to depolarize the lipid bilayer cell membrane, it is strong enough to activate transmembrane channels and transmembrane receptors (Aaron et al., 2004a). An ion flux caused due to the difference in ion concentration across the membrane triggers signalling pathways. The potential difference, in the order of 100 mV between the two sides of the membrane, plays an important role in signal transduction processes. For example, Aaron (Aaron et al., 2004a) observed that cellular response to ES may involve the calcium/calmodulin pathway. The change in transmembrane potential may rearrange the charged groups or dipoles within the membrane; thus, channel-mediated ions such as Na$^+$, and K$^+$ may conduct through the membrane. The charge movement, or gating current (I_g), has been detected by Armstrong (Armstrong & Bezanilla,1973). EF may also alter ligand binding as result of the modification of the density and distribution of receptors through polarizing membrane components, moving receptors, or alternating receptor conformation. For instance, a DC EF adjusted the assembly and distribution of actin filaments within the cytoplasm of endothelial cells (Li & Kolega, 2002). As part of the complex intracellular signalling pathways, cytoskeleton provides structural stability and elasticity to the cell undergoing multiple deformations without losing its integrity. The physical attachment between membrane and cytoskeleton actin takes place through linker proteins such as spectrin and ezrin/radixin/moesin (ERM). EF induced intracellular ATP depletion and consequently inhibited ERM function, resulting in altered membrane characteristics such as endo- and exocytosis, signalling, adhesion, and motility (Orr et al., 2006). This suggests that the ATP depletion may occur as a result of increased ATP transport to the exterior cell membrane and of increased ATP consumption because of the EF-stimulated high metabolic activity.

2.2 Gap junction intercellular communication

Gap junctions are specialized regions of the plasma membrane where protein oligomers establish contact between adjacent cells. The gap junctions in osteoblasts derived from newborn rat calvaria in culture measured between 0.10 and 0.91 μm, with a mean length of 0.43 ± 0.23 μm, and a distance of 2-4 nm between the neighbouring membranes. Gap junctions enable the rapid and efficient propagation of ions, nutrients, metabolites, secondary messengers, and small molecules under ~ 1,000 Da between adjoining cells ("coupling"). In bone cells, the gap junction enables different preosteoblastic cells to progress in a coordinated manner toward a mature phenotype and to maintain the expression of the phenotypic functions associated with differentiated bone tissue. For example, signalling molecules (~ kDa) such as calcium, cyclic nucleotides, and inositol phosphates, exchange through gap junction channels. Moreover, much evidence indicates that gap junction communication is necessary for the development and maintenance of a differentiated osteoblast phenotype, including the production of alkaline phosphatase, osteocalcin, bone sialoprotein, and collagen, as well as decreased mineralization (Stains & Civitelli, 2005). The junctional conductance between coupled cells revealed a high degree of voltage dependence through electrophysiological studies. Two regulation mechanisms were confirmed to respond to the voltage difference between two cells (transjunctional voltage, Vj), i.e., Vj-gating (fast) and loop-gating (slow). The connection composition of gap junction channels defines their unique properties, such as their selectivity for small molecules and voltage-dependent gating. For example, Nakagawa et al. (Nakagawa et al. 2010) reported that the displayed potential in the Cx26 gap junction channel was in the range of $-20kTe^{-1}$ to $20kTe^{-1}$, therefore, gap junctions can even be gated by membrane voltage (Vm), termed Vm-gating. In another study, the boundaries of intercellular communication were altered by applied current, and the current applied to one cell revealed a voltage-current (V-I) relationship (Harris et al., 1983). Lohmann reported that the levels of connection of Cx43 protein were reduced in both MLO-Y4 cells and ROS 17/2.8 cells under low frequency EMF (Lohmann et al., 2003). When applying ES (interval 1 s, duration 100 ms, amplitude 10 mA) to myocytes, Nishizawa et al. (Nishizawa et al., 2007) used a high-speed confocal microscope to analyze cellular communication within the myocytes and discovered that cytosolic Ca^{2+} concentration had been upregulated, which indicates that gap junctions largely contributed to the propagation of intracellular signals. Gap junctions also play a crucial role in the response of cellular networks to extracellular signals through the integration and amplification of the signals.

2.3 The role of extracellular matrix (ECM)
ECM, an intricate 3D network of fibrillar proteins, proteoglycans, and glycosaminoglycans (GAGs), provides an electrochemical environment surrounding cells and conveying signals from the exterior of the cell to the interior and vice versa. Many ECM components can be affected by EF, including soluble ions and charged groups in GAGs and proteins. It was reported that proteins moved along EF to reach the binding sites on cell membrane receptors (Adey, 1993). ES also reportedly influenced the adsorption of serum proteins, specifically fibronectin (FN), onto electrodes (Kotwal & Schmidt, 2001).

2.4 Regulation of gene expression
Numerous studies have investigated how cell gene expression and protein production respond to electrical signals of varying amplitude and frequency. However, little is known regarding the signal transduction cascade that consequently alters many cellular events during/after exposure of bone cells to physiological ES. The release of growth factors and cytokines from bone cells is critical to both bone formation and turnover. Several studies (Zhuang et al., 1997) have suggested direct or indirect effect of ES on the gene expression and protein production of bone cells. For example, ES increased the gene expression of transforming growth factor-β (TGF-β), collagen type-I, alkaline phosphatase (ALP), bone morphogenetic proteins (BMPs), and chondrocyte matrix. According to Aaron (Aaron et al., 1997), an increase in TGF-β1 may cause phenotype autocrine and paracrine signalling that consequently regulates osteochondral cells to proliferate and to differentiate, followed by an increase in extracellular matrix deposition. Meng et al. (Meng et al., 2010) reported that following osteoblast stimulation with 200mV/mm for 6h, osteocalcin (OC) and ALP increased 20% compare to the non-ES control. It is of interest that following a multiple 6h ES at 200mV/mm intensity every two days over a period of 6 days, the gene expression of OC, ALP, Runx-2 and BMP2 increased more than two folds compare with the non-ES controls.

3. ES in bone healing and bone tissue engineering

3.1 ES in bone healing and clinical application
While the first report of a successful use of ES appeared as early as 1841, ES treatment on bone did not occur until 1953 when Yasuda et al. applied continuous electrical current to a

rabbit femur for three weeks and demonstrated new bone formation in the vicinity of the cathode (Ryaby, 1998). Their milestone research launched the age of ES treatment in bone healing applications. It appears that the adjunctive noninvasive or extracorporeal ES therapy could be beneficial for those with bone fractures or osteotomies by speeding up the healing of bone.

3.1.1 Animal experiment

The benefits of ES include increased fracture callus, faster fracture consolidation, increased resistance to refracture, cortical thickening, periosteal or endosteal bone proliferation, reduced incidence of disuse osteoporosis and joint ankylosis. An early review published in 1977 (Spadaro, 1977) showed that 71% of animal experiment involved direct current (DC) stimulation in the 0.1-100 microampere (μA) range, 15% used pulsed DC with frequencies from 0.5 to 500 Hz, pulse widths from 1-500 milliseconds, and peak amplitudes from 0.5-1000 μA, 9% used alternative current (AC) stimulation with frequencies from 5-50 Hz, and only 5% reportedly used EMF with frequencies from 0-60 Hz. The animals involved in the ES experiments included rabbit, rat, sheep, horse, deer, cat, mouse, chick and frog. Capacitive coupling electric field (CCEF) and inductive coupling EMF are used more frequently in recent years. Continuous DC stimulation has also been used. The most frequently used animal models are rabbit, dog, and rat. The principal endpoints include bone mineral content/density, and the content of calcium, phosphorus, and carbon, as well as mechanical properties. (Manjhi et al., 2009).

3.1.2 Clinical application

Electrical bone growth stimulators are categorized as invasive, semi-invasive, or noninvasive. Invasive and semi-invasive DC stimulators deliver DC internally via surgically implanted electrodes, whereby the cathode delivering energy to the bone is placed around the area requiring treatment. The power source of an invasive system is implanted in nearby soft tissue and is removed at the end of treatment. In the semi-invasive system, the cathodes are inserted percutaneously under fluoroscopic guidance, and the power source is attached with anodes placed anywhere on the surface of the skin. Osteogenesis is stimulated at the cathode with a current of 5-100 μA (Aaron et al., 2004b). Current below certain threshold was found to lead to bone formation, while that above the threshold caused cell necrosis. Noninvasive stimulators are based on either capacitive coupling (CC) or inductive coupling (IC). CC stimulators use the CC device to apply an electrical potential of 1-10 V at frequencies of 20-200 kHz. The EF strength generated in the tissue is in the range of 1-100 mV/cm. These stimulators are noninvasive and the electrodes are placed on the skin at the opposite side of the fracture site. IC stimulators use EMF. Noninvasive devices can use DC or AC, either constant or pulsed, and low frequency electromagnetic fields. The ES is delivered to the target site via externally mounted cathodes (in the case of DC or AC) or coils (in the case of EMFs). Most systems are equipped with monitors to assess system function and patient compliance. The applied electromagnetic fields vary in amplitude, frequency, and wave form. The order of magnitude of the magnetic field is in the range of 10 μT to 2 mT and the produced electric field strength is in the range of 1 to 100 mV/cm (Aaron et al., 2004b). Clinically, CCEF has been shown to induce osteogenesis, facilitate the consolidation of recalcitrant nonunions, and modify primary spine fusion (Goodwin et al., 1999) especially for the patients with posterolateral fusion and those with internal fixation.

One study showed that treating nonunions with CCEF achieved a success rate of 60-77% (Beck et al., 2008). Implantable DC/AC stimulators have the advantage of providing stimulation directly at the fracture site. Drawbacks include the risk of infection, tissue reaction, and superficial soft tissue discomfort caused by the protrusion of the device, possible pain caused by the electrode implant, and the stress associated with the operative procedures (Haddad et al., 2007a). No pain or surgery is involved with the noninvasive device which may even be conveniently used by the patient at home. The disadvantages of the capacitive and inductive coupled methods include skin irritation from the electrode disc, the relatively long treatment regimen, and the probability of promoting tumour jeopardy in unexpected regions.

Studies on electrical and electromagnetic stimulation to promote bone union have showed promising results in clinic, showing the significant effect of various types of ES on bone healing. However, a 2008 meta-analysis and systematic review found that evidence from the randomly controlled trials failed to conclude that EMF improves the rate of union in patients with a fresh fracture, osteotomy, delayed union, or non-union (Mollon et al., 2008). Although multiple randomised trials exist to support the various bone stimulation modalities, they are small and are limited primarily to radiological endpoints. Therefore, the universal acceptance of ES in clinical applications will require greater support from larger, more definitive trials. Nonetheless, in a 2008 survey of 268 tibial shaft fracture management cases, 16% of 450 Canadian orthopaedic surgeons reported using electrical bone growth stimulators to manage uncomplicated open and closed tibial shaft fractures, while 45% used them for complicated tibial shaft fractures (Busse et al., 2008).

3.2 Important factors in bone tissue engineering

There are major clinical reasons to develop tissue engineering strategies for bone regeneration. In bone tissue engineering, to summarize, all of the factors can be channelled into three essential elements: (1) osteoblasts or their precursors, (2) an osteo-compatible

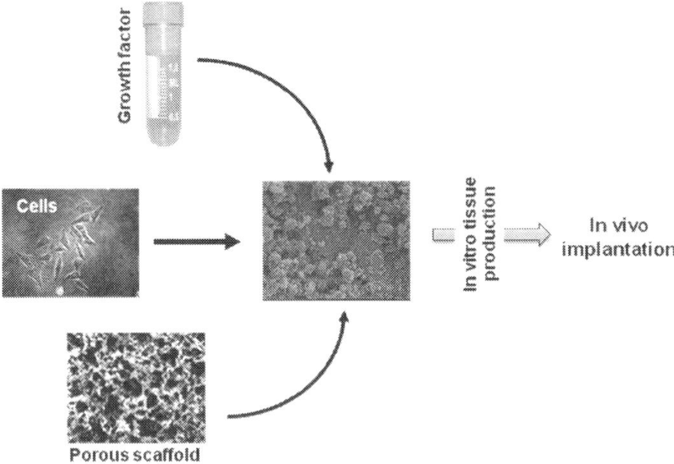

Fig. 1. Basic concept of tissue engineering

scaffold, and (3) biological cues such as growth factors. The functions of various cell types and their interactions with ECM during tissue repair and regeneration have been extensively explored, yet much remains to be investigated. It is apparently accepted that scaffolds with appropriate chemistry and morphological design and assisted by stimulation factors are able to promote cell adhesion, proliferation, and the formation of ECM. When these three essential factors are appropriately assembled together, living bone tissue is hopefully generated in culture and then transplanted into animal models in the hopes of integrating with the host and finally growing into functional tissue or organs, as showing in Figure 1. Because of the directional feature of EF and various biological systems responding to endogenous or exogenous ES, ES contributes to a supportive environment for tissue repair and regeneration.

3.2.1 Osteoblasts and their precursors

Four progenitor cells are commonly used for bone engineering. These include whole freshly collected bone marrow cells, purified and in vitro propagated mesenchymal stem cells (MSCs), embryonic stem cells (ESCs), and stem cell differentiated osteoblasts. Bone marrow possesses a limited number of osteoprogenitor stem cells and the mean prevalence of colony-forming units with osteoblast phenotype is very low (Heliotis et al., 2009). The MSC approach relies on identifying and isolating adult stem cells with a sufficient quantity. This can be a lengthy process, especially with old patients, as cell numbers and proliferative capacities may be low. As for ESCs, ethics remains a major issue, particularly when embryos are used solely for research purposes. In addition, while stem cells may have the potential to be used to generate entire skeletal tissues, the long-term biological consequence of stem cells at the implant site, as well as issues of cell plasticity, remains largely unknown (Heliotis et al., 2009). Osteoblasts, which are active in bone development and bone remodelling as bone-forming cells, have the ability to synthesize and secrete collagen type I and glycoproteins (osteopontin, osteocalcin), cytokines, and growth factors into the unmineralized matrix (osteoid) between cell body and mineralized regions. Furthermore, they are rich in alkaline phosphatase activity (Kartsogiannis & Ng, 2004). Compared to marrow and stem cells, osteoblasts are plentiful and can be harvested from new bone lamellae which they have just secreted.

3.2.2 Scaffolds

The "ideal" scaffold, whether permanent or biodegradable, naturally occurred or synthetic, should firstly be biocompatible, then be osteoinductive or at least osteoconductive, and finally, mechanically compatible with native bone. Various currently available synthetic materials have served for the design of bone implants, including bioresorbable polymers such as polylactide, polyglycolide, copolymers based on lactide, glycolide and ε-caprolactone, trimethylene carbonate, or tyrosine carbonate. In order to gain the desired mechanical and biological properties, these synthetic polymers are often combined with bone components such as hydroxyapatite (HA). The porous 3D scaffold (> 100 micron diameter) provides sufficient opportunity for cell migration and expansion as well as enables the transport of nutrients and metabolic wastes. The porous structure can be generated through various techniques including temperature-induced phase inversion, salt leaching, and prototyping (Hutmacher, 2000). A wide range of porosity and pore size reportedly promotes cell growth and bone formation; for example, 70 to 95% porosity was achieved by adjusting the polymer–to-salt ratio, and the pore size was controlled independently by varying the leachable particle size with standard testing sieves (Hou et al., 2003). 3D scaffolds displaying a high porosity and large pore size often weaken their mechanical properties. Nevertheless, a 3D silk biomaterial matrix prepared by salt leaching achieved a compressive strength up to 175 ± 3 KPa while maintaining porosity between 84 and 98%. , A compressive strength up to 280 ± 4 KPa was achieved at porosity between 87 and 97% when the silk scaffold was fabricated by gas foaming. When the porosity approached 99%, its maximum compressive strength was shown to be only 30 ± 2 KPa (Nazarov et al., 2004).

3.2.3 Growth factors

Tissue regeneration involves many promoters/factors. Cytokines are secreted by many cell types and function as signalling molecules. They also promote and/or prevent cell adhesion, proliferation, migration, and differentiation by up- or down-regulating the synthesis of proteins, growth factors, and receptors. The important signalling molecules in bone healing and development include TGF-β and BMPs. The use of growth factors in bone regeneration is becoming increasingly promising, as this strategy is direct, relatively simple, and highly efficient. These proteins are easily available yet are costly. Of interest is the fact that some of these proteins can be regulated through physical stimulation. Cultured cells and tissues subjected to different biophysical stimuli of varying intensities in both in vitro and in vivo settings have been reviewed (Chao & Inoue, 2003; Wiesmann et al., 2004). These stimuli include mechanical force, electrical and electromagnetic field, laser irradiation, heat shock, and ultrasound. Some of them are already applied in the clinical setting to treat tissue defects (Barrere et al., 2008). Studies have shown that osteoprogenitor cells and osteoblasts increased their proliferation and differentiation, as well as the production of ECM and growth and differentiation factors including TGF-β and BMPs by EMFs (Chao & Inoue, 2003; Dimitriou & Babis, 2007). Therefore, growth factors regulating bone formation can be endogenously induced through the appropriate extrinsic biophysical stimulation to bone cells. Due to the intrinsic instability of the growth factors toward chemical and physical inactivation, and the relatively long contact time between the growth factors and the target cells required to obtain the desired effect, direct injection of growth factors into the regeneration site or their simple dispersion into the porous scaffold may prove to be less effective. Consequently, endogenously induced bone-forming growth factors may provide a solution because of their steady secretion from cells.

3.3 ES methodology and cellular reactions

ES methods vary according to the type of ES used. There is no standardized methodology or setup. According to the methodologies reported in literatures, ES methods can be categorized into the following three groups: 1) DC/AC EF, 2) capacitive coupling-induced EF (CCEF), and 3) electromagnetic field (EMF). Various cell types have been studied and found to be responsive to ES under different experimental settings.

3.3.1 DC/AC EF

Following the discovery of ossification enhancement by DC EF in 1964 (Berg & Zhang, 1993), ES was viewed as a new therapeutic alternative and thus investigated using both DC and AC EF. DC and AC EFs in medical literatures often indiscriminately refer to either electrical potential gradient or electrical current established between two points of different electrical potentials generated by either a DC or an AC power source. Electrical potential gradient and electrical current are related but two very different things, of which the biological consequences can be quite different. Nevertheless, potential gradient and current intensity of DC or AC electricity are probably the most frequently used ES approaches in research. DC/AC EF can be created between two electrodes immersed in electrolytes such as culture medium or tissue fluid. In such circumstances, the charge carriers are the ions in the electrolytes. DC/AC EF can also be established across a solid electrical conductor, such as by directly connecting a conductive polymer into an electrical circuit. Here, polarons/bipolarons serve as the charge carriers.

A variety of experimental setups are used in different labs, as described below.

3.3.1.1 Metallic electrode

Metallic electrodes are easily modified into different forms, connected with a power source, and inserted into culture medium or tissue. However, in order to convert ionic conductivity in the electrolyte into electron conductivity in metal, electrochemical reactions are known to occur on the electrode surface which generates chemical species often referred to as faradic products. The most common irreversible processes encountered with electrodes are water electrolysis and the resulting pH change and gas formation, electrode dissolution due to the oxidative formation of soluble metal complexes (typical of platinum (Pt) electrodes) over 320 μA, and the breakdown of passivity with subsequent pitting or transpassive corrosion (typical of stainless steel electrodes). Compared to salt bridges, the direct exposure of a titanium cathode and its faradic products led to a further lowering of the media calcium levels and also significantly increased the pH in culture medium (Bodamyali et al., 1999). Based on animal experiments and clinical studies, it is believed that electrical current can be injected as a constant or a pulsatile electric energy to treat fresh fractures and osteotomies, spine fusions, as well as delayed and nonunion fractures. A wide range of materials have been used as invasive electrodes, including stainless steel, tungsten, platinum, platinum-iridium alloys, iridium oxide, and titanium nitride in both animal and clinical experiments (Cogan, 2008). Experiments investigating the response of bone cells to ES based on metallic electrodes are rare. Kim et al. (Kim et al., 2006) found that the proliferation of rat calvarial osteoblasts on an Au anode increased 31% after 2 days under an ES of 1.5μA/cm^2.

When electrodes are used as implants in the clinical setting, reliability is crucial. In order to find ways to prevent electrode-related injuries, it is equally important to understand them. In 2007, Netherton (Stecker et al., 2006) discussed four factors that may influence the likelihood of electrode-related injury. The first factor is the heat generated by electrical current passing through resistive tissue, which consequently elevates the temperature of the surrounding tissue. Thus, the denaturation of cellular components, such as proteins, possibly appears. In addition, localized temperature increase due to the current may be significant near the edges of electrodes, near small electrodes, or near the regions where electrical conductivity changes rapidly. The second factor is electroporation, by which pores formed on cell membrane allow charged ions or large molecules to pass. Lee (Lee et al., 2000) suggested that electric fields as low as 60 V/cm may cause electroporation injury to muscle or nerve. Clinically, however, electroporation happens when the electric field is in the order of 500 to 3000 V/cm (Hofmann et al., 1996). The third factor is called electroconformational denaturation of cellular proteins. Because many proteins contain charged groups, their structure can be affected by a strong electric field which can denature proteins and subsequently cause cell damage. The last factor is overstimulation, such as, for example, a phenomenon called excitatory neurotoxicity. Electrochemical injury can be prevented by selecting the appropriate electrode type and by minimizing and maintaining the total level of stimulation below a certain threshold (Stecker et al., 2006).

3.3.1.2 Salt bridge

A salt bridge contains a saturated solution of inert salt, usually $NaClO_4$, KCl, or KNO_3. The term inert refers to the reactivity relative to the reaction under study. When the circuit is closed, the cations (such as K^+) flow out of the salt bridge at the cathode, and the anions (such as Cl^-) flow out at the anode due to the electric field created by the potential gradient. Salt bridges are used to isolate metallic electrodes from direct contact with the cell culture medium during in vitro experiments. With these bridges, the electrolyte composition (culture medium) remains undisturbed when electrical potential is applied and current passes. The primary function of the salt bridge is maintaining the culture medium electroneutrality and avoiding electrochemical or redox product contamination from the metal electrode as it allows the current to flow.

Using a salt bridge system, Sun (Sun et al., 2006) reported that a small fraction (less than 10%) of rat MSCs responded to ES and became contracted, reoriented, and demonstrated changes in cellular morphology in a 3D collagen scaffold. A DC electric field of 2 V/cm affected the actin reorganization and morphology of hMSCs and osteoblasts. A reduced ATP level led to an inhibition of the linker proteins which are known to physically couple the cell membrane and cytoskeleton, causing cell membrane separation from the cytoskeleton. However, in Sun's study, the strong electrical strength (7 V/cm and 10 V/cm) failed to induce any significant MSC reorientation. Curtze et al. (Curtze et al., 2004) used agar bridges to induce ES to cells cultured on either cover slips or collagen-coated polyacrylamide gels. They observed that primary bovine osteoblasts and human osteosarcoma cells exposed to a DC EF of 10 V/cm realigned themselves with their long axis perpendicular to the EF. In short, the cells lost approximately 46% (12 of 26 µm) of their length along the electric field lines. Perpendicular to the electric field lines, the cells lost 16% (4 of 24 µm) in the first 20 minutes and grew 35% (from 20 µm to 27 µm) within 100 minutes. The cells reacted to the electric field in two phases: retraction, followed by elongation. The authors also noticed that when ES was turned off after 10, 30, or 60 minutes, the cells did not continue their process but rather spread in all directions. The cells in this study responded to EF sequentially in opposite ways, namely, retraction followed by elongation. As far as how the ES signal induced the cytoskeletal reorganization to be large enough to cause significant change in cell shape, the authors attributed it to the change of intracellular free calcium levels. In another study, Ferrier et al. (Ferrier et al., 1986) cultured rabbit osteoclasts and rat osteoblast-like cells on glass coverslips in field strengths of 0.1 and 1 V/mm and found that the osteoclasts migrated rapidly toward the positive electrode, while the osteoblast-like cells migrated in the opposite direction toward the negative electrode, showing that different types of bone cells respond differently to the same electrical signal. When salt bridges are used, the so-called faradic products, including hydrogen peroxide, hydroxyl and oxygen ions, free radicals, and other intermediates, are excluded from the culture medium. However, using agarose salt bridges may decrease calcium levels in the media. The authors (Bodamyali et al., 1999) did not look at the calcium on the salt bridge but rather measured the calcium concentration in the media with a spectrophotometer by examining the calcium's reaction with o-cresolphthalein, which forms a red complex at pH 10-12 with an absorbance maximum at 575 nm. Calcium uptake by mouse calvaria was suspected due to the acceleration of the intracellular transport of calcium, as previously reported (Wang et al., 1998), and may increase the activation of the calcium/calmodulin signalling pathway (Lorich et al., 1998; Zhuang et al., 1997).

While the salt bridge technique has been extensively used to study the effect of ES on cultured cells, this approach can be problematic when applied for tissue engineering purposes. Because salt bridges are suspended in cell culture medium, the electrical current primarily passes through the medium rather than the non-conductive substrate. This may constitute a major concern when porous 3D scaffold is used in culture. As most scaffolding materials are not electrically conductive (dielectric), cells inside the porous scaffold or on its surface are not exposed to the same degree of electric field and current. Secondly, through Fickian diffusion, the salt simply escapes from the salt bridges into the culture medium whenever the circuit is open or closed. As a result, when salt bridges are used, the cell culture medium is not homogeneous. Furthermore, salt bridges as electrodes are not easily implanted in animals or used in clinical trials.

3.3.1.3 Carbon nanotube (CNT) electrode

CNTs possess high tensile strength, formidable thermal and chemical stability, and excellent electrical properties. The conductivity of a CNT bundle approaches 1×10^4 S/cm. Despite the non-homogeneous distribution of CNTs with respect to length, diameter, and doping level, CNT networks maintain a conductivity ranging from 10-10^3 S/cm. Their superior physical properties make them ideal for the manufacture of conductive composites at very low concentrations (Sandler et al., 2003). Implantable CNTs may prove useful in bone tissue engineering applications. For instance, CNTs showed a powerful ability to absorb various proteins, including adhesion factors, growth factors, and differentiation-inducing factors. In cell culture, CNTs were found to increase osteonectin, osteopontin, and osteocalcin gene expression. ALP/DNA and total protein/DNA levels on carbon nanotubes were also found to increase. These results indicate that CNTs may facilitate cell adhesion and induce osteogenic maturation of osteoblasts by adsorbing specific proteins (Akasaka et al., 2009). CNTs were also shown to display the ability to inhibit osteoclastic differentiation, suppress a transcription factor essential for osteoclastogenesis in vitro, and inhibit osteoclastic bone resorption in vivo (Narita et al., 2009). Khang et al. cultured human chondrocytes on a film made of CNT/polycarbonate urethane composite. An ES of 3 and 6 h at a frequency of 10 Hz and a current of 10 μA was applied after seeding and was found to significantly enhance chondrocyte functions. Initial fibronectin adsorption, chondrocyte adhesion, and long-term cell density were enhanced by more than 50% (Khang et al., 2008). With polylactic acid/carbon nanotube (PLA/CNT) as the substrate, ES was also reported to promote various important osteoblast functions, notably cell proliferation, collagenous and noncollagenous protein gene expression, and calcium deposition in the extracellular matrix. Specifically, when osteoblasts cultured on the surface of PLA/CNT were exposed to an AC ES with a 10 μA current, cell proliferation increased 46% after 2 days, while extracellular calcium increased 307% after 21 days, and collagen type-I mRNA expression upregulated after both 1 and 21 consecutive days. In the experiments mentioned above, the electrodes were set parallel in either the horizontal or vertical position, and in both cases, the electrodes were in culture medium and produced ionic current.

CNTs are, however, non-biodegradable in nature and may be inherently cytotoxic. Since 2003, studies have shown CNTs to display cytotoxicity. An in vitro evaluation of the inflammatory potential of CNT on peritoneal and alveolar macrophages was reported by Jia (Jia et al., 2005).

At the threshold dose of cytotoxicity, single-walled carbon nanotubes (SWNTs) induced serious damage to alveolar macrophages at a low exposure dose of 0.38 µg/cm²(Zhu & Li, 2008). Cheng et al. (Cheng et al., 2009) found that MWNTs entered the macrophages through the plasma membrane into the cytoplasm and the nucleus, which may result in necrosis and degeneration. Apoptotic cell death was found with a higher dose at 3.06 µg/cm². The mechanisms responsible for CNT cytotoxicity are not yet fully understood. Cells exposed to CNTs resulted in accelerated oxidative stress (increased free radical and peroxide generation as well as depleted total antioxidant reserves), loss in cell viability, and morphological alterations to the cellular structure. CNTs have also been shown to block potassium channel activities in heterologous mammalian cell systems when applied externally to the cell surface, which also suggests a degree of cytotoxicity. A variety of factors are involved in CNT cytotoxicity, including species, impurities, length, aspect ratio, and chemical modification (Zhu & Li, 2008). In general, as long as the CNTs structures are hydrophilically modified, contain no trace metals, as well as do not form fibrous aggregates that frustrate the phagocytic cells, CNTs should show less or mild cytotoxicity. A recent study reported about the toxicity and biodistribution of hydrophilic CNTs showed that PEGylation-CNTs were not acutely toxic and primarily accumulated in the liver and spleen (Berlin et al., 2010).

3.3.1.4 Conducting polymers

Conductive polymers are softer and more compliant than metals or other inorganic conducting materials, such as silicon and carbon fibre. Hence, they represent a unique and useful way to improve the intimate bioelectronics/tissue connection. In addition, conducting polymers may hopefully improve the performance of implantable medical devices by facilitating mechanical compliance, electrical conductance, and the biological affinity between devices and cells. It has indeed been suggested that the inflammation caused by the tissue/conducting material stiffness mismatch will be alleviated.

PPy is the most widely researched conducting material to interact with mammalian cells since the first study in Langer's lab in 1994 when Wong et al. (Wong et al., 1994) demonstrated the effect of EF on cell growth and differentiation through PPy. The biocompatibility of PPy can be improved by choosing different dopants (such as dodecylbenzenesulfonate sodium or heparin (Meng et al., 2008)) and by immobilizing biologically active molecules including enzymes, antibodies, receptors, and even whole living cells to manifest its biological affinity (Ateh et al., 2006). Conducting polymers such as polyaniline (PANi), polythiophene (PT), and their derivatives also have shown sufficient stability and biocompatibility. However, the applications using polyaniline (PANi) in tissue engineering are not as numerous as those with PPy. It was reported that the electrochemical degradation of PANi may occur at a potential greater than 0.6 V in an aqueous solvent and 0.7 V in organic solvents (Mazeikiene & Malinauskas, 2001). The conductivity of PT is too low (10^{-3}-10^{-2} S/cm) to enable the manufacture of a conductive composite with a low PT content (Guimard et al., 2007). By manipulating external electrical potential, the electrical property of the PPy devices can be modified through dopant in- and out-flux. Moreover, PPy is an excellent substrate for the attachment, proliferation, and differentiation of bovine bone marrow stromal cells (BMSC). With a PPy film as substrate and a working electrode, and Au and Ag wires as reference and counter electrodes respectively, a constant EF of 20 V/m ES for 1 hour induced a statistically significant increase in the osteogenic differentiation of BMSC on the thin PPy film substrates. Compared to a conductive indium tin oxide (ITO) glass control, the authors (Shastri et al., 1999) claimed that the increased osteogenic differentiation of BMSC on PPy was attributed to the chemistry of the underlying PPy substrate rather than the electrochemical byproducts formed in solution by the ES. The conducting polymer films may be used to manipulate physiologically relevant ionic interactions with living cells. The chromic transition of conductive polymer caused by the reaction between immobilized ligands and biomolecules has been observed in real time (Englebienne, 1999).

However, the highly conjugative chain structures render genuine conducting polymers generally insoluble and non-fusible, signifying very poor processibility. Conductive polymer composites were thus blended with other processable polymers in order to address this processability issue (Meng et al., 2008). It takes as low as 5wt% of conductive polymer in the composite to reach a percolation threshold at which the conductive phase disperses in the non-conductive matrix and becomes continuous, resulting in a surface conductivity in the range of 0.3-5.3×10³ Ω/square when different amount of heparin was used as dopants. Although the presence of heparin reduced the PPy conductivity, it promoted cell adhesion to PPy (Figure 2) and enhanced its electrical stability as well. When these conductive composites are used as scaffolding materials, the cells cultured on it can receive electrical signals directly from the substrate rather than from the culture medium.

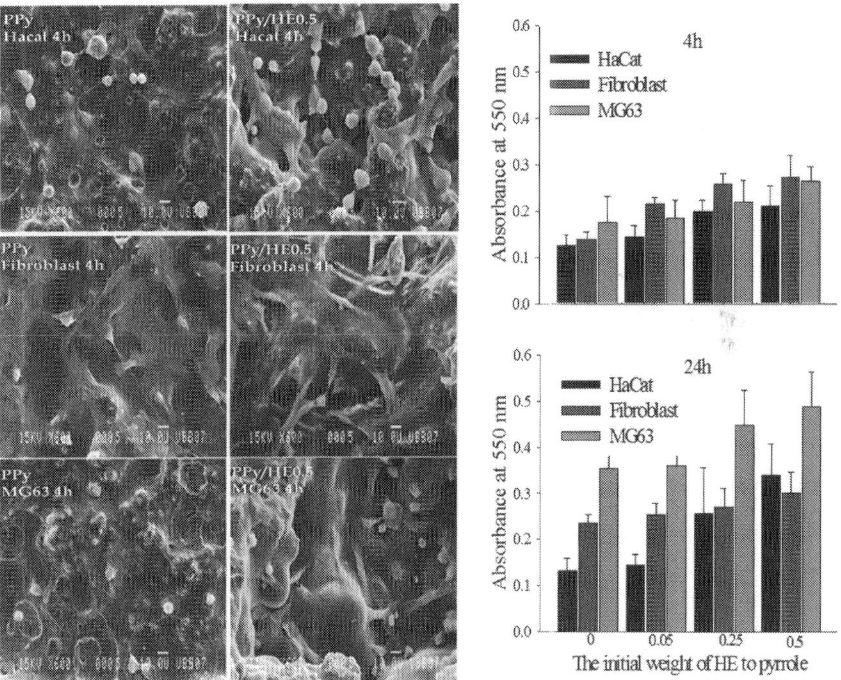

Fig. 2. The morphology of HaCat, fibroblasts and MG63 cells on PPy/PLLA membranes with or without heparin as dopant to PPy after 4h cell culture (left); and the cell viability after 4 and 24h culture on PPy/PLLA membranes with different amount of heparin in PPy (right).

One of the major issues in electrically stimulated cell cultures is to determine the optimal ES parameters including intensity, duration, frequency, and form. These parameters are likely cell type and indicator specific. For example, an effective ES "window" to osteoblasts-like cells Saos-2 was determined to be 6 h of ES at 200 mV/mm (manuscript to be published). When the potential gradient increased to as high as 300 and 400 mV/mm, Saos-2 cell proliferation was suppressed, regardless of the duration of the ES. On the other hand, a weak ES, such as 100 mV/mm, showed insignificant impact on cells. When an EF of 200mV/mm was applied across the surface of the PPy/PLLA membranes, a µA level current was generated. This model barely disturbs the culture medium by avoiding electrode reactions and ionic current, as shown in Figure 3. After an initial multiple ES (merely 3 times) to the osteoblast-like cells, Saos-2, followed by 4 additional weeks of culture, the deposited Ca and P ratio became 1:1.54, comparing the 1:1.46 for the control. The Ca/P ratio in polycrystalline HA varies between 1.5 and 1.71. Thus, the Ca/P ratio in the minerals of the ES group agrees well with the Ca/P ratio in the standard HA. WAXD, a gold-standard method used to identify the mineral phase, demonstrated that the crystalline structure of the mineral deposits on the conductive substrate was almost identical to that of the HA standard, meaning that ES indeed accelerated the formation of bone-like mineralization on the PLLA/PPy/HE substrate. Using these conductive composites, 2D or 3D conductive scaffolds of various shapes and sizes may thus be manufactured.

In summary, the invasive DC ES with an electrode implant provides intimate contact between electrode and cells/tissues, whereby the cells directly respond to the stimulation from the embedded electrodes. When ES signals in the range of 1.0-1.5 mV and 5-20 µA are applied, the electric field is highly localised and decays rapidly as a function of the distance from the electrode. Biochemical reactions, such as decreased local oxygen tension, hydroxyl radical production, corrosion, and electrolysis, occur close to the electrode, even in the presence of the salt bridge. These limitations become even more significant when a large area electrode is required.

3.3.2 Capacitively coupled electric field (CCEF)

As a noninvasive modality, the two capacitor plates of a CCEF are electrically insulated from the culture medium or tissue. No potential problems such as electrochemical reactions or electrode injuries are associated with the capacitors. When a voltage is applied across the two capacitors, the potential gradient between them generates an electric field. When an alternating potential is applied, the polarity of the plates continuously reverses, thereby generating an alternating EF between the plates. In vitro, CCEF has been shown to significantly enhance osteoblast proliferation, maturation, and ECM protein synthesis. For example, in 1984, Dannon et al. cultured rat embryo calvarial bone cells with medium containing radioactively labelled calcium and observed an increase in calcium uptake by counting the ^{45}Ca following stimulation with a CCEF of 12-54 V/cm and 3-100 Hz (Danon & Korenstein, 1984). In 1988, Brighton et al. cultured rat calvarial bone cells under a CCEF of 2.62 mV/cm for 2.5-30 min and found a 59% increase in cAMP (Brighton & McCluskey, 1988). Other experiments showed that CCEF signal transduction induced an increase in cytosolic Ca^{2+} via voltage-gated calcium channels, resulting in activated calmodulin, as well as an increase in TGF-β1 mRNA (Brighton et al., 2001; Zhuang et al., 1997). Lorich (Lorich et al., 1998) explored the mechanisms behind enhanced cell proliferation, showing that Ca^{2+} translocation through voltage-gated calcium channels (inhibited by verapamil) resulted in elevated intracellular Ca^{2+} levels and concomitantly increased phospholipase A_2 (PLA2) activity (blocked by bromophenacyl bromide, BPB). The latter increase led to cyclooxygenase (COX)-dependent prostaglandin E2 (PGE2) synthesis (blocked by indomethacin), which in turn brought on an activation of calmodulin (blocked by N-(6-aminohexyl)-5-chloro-1-naphthalenesulfonamide hydrochloride, W-7). Brighton's group reported that CCEF significantly upregulated BMP-2 mRNA expression, BMP-2 protein production, and alkaline phosphatase activity (Wang et al., 2006). In 2001, Wiesmann et al. reported that an electric field of 6-21kV/m with a saw-tooth shape signal, 63 ms width and 16 Hz frequency, affected the formation of newly formed mineral crystals of osteoblast-like cells in vitro (Wiesmann et al., 2001). A study on chondrocytes showed an upregulation of aggrecan and type II collagen mRNAs of bovine articular chondrocytes following a 30-min stimulation of 60 kHz sine wave signal with an output of 44.81 V (Wang et al., 2004).

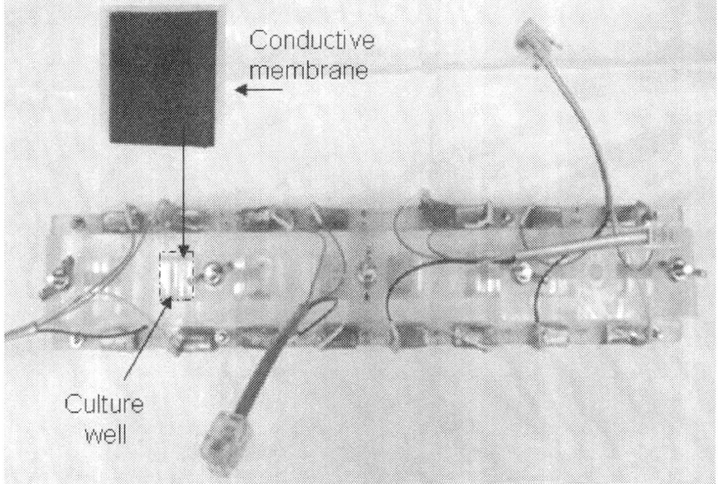

Fig. 3. Home-made multi-well electrical cell culture plate designed for ES

A major disadvantage of CCEF is the need for a high voltage power source (> 1000 V), as this EF energy decays quickly along the EF direction. Because the electrical resistance of an air gap and a cell culture Petri dish is much higher than that of the medium and the cell membrane, the external electric field produces a major voltage drop across the air gap and the culture dish so that only weak electric field acts on the cells. For example, peak-to-peak amplitude of 100 V at the capacitor only led to a 100 µV voltage drop across a cell monolayer. Brighton (Armstrong et al., 1988) calculated that for a peak-to-peak amplitude of 500-1000 V between the capacitors, and using relative dielectric constants of 1.0, 2.25, and 6.0 for air, plastic, and water, respectively, the electric field was only 1.5 to 3.0 × 10^{-2} V/cm (1.5-3.0 mV/mm), which is very weak compared to most values reported in the literature. In addition, in their device the distance between two opposite capacitor plates was only 1 cm. Another issue is that the EF generated in culture medium disturbs the homogeneity of the medium composition, e.g., the calcium migrated toward the anode under CCEF (Danon and Korenstein, 1984).

3.3.3 Electromagnetic field (EMF)

This technique is characterized by its low frequency electric and magnetic fields, and its noninvasive nature. The interaction of low frequency (< 1 MHz) and low magnetic field intensity (< 10 mT) electromagnetic field with human tissue has generated considerable interest. Based on calculations, an external 50-60 Hz EF in the order of kV/m induces an EF in situ in the order of mV/m or less. And, an external 50-60 Hz magnetic field of μT induces an EF in situ of a few tens of μV/m or less (Foster, 2003). At the cellular level, EMF reportedly promotes bone mineralization, osteoblast proliferation and differentiation, and cytokine gene expression and production. EMF was shown to stimulate osteoblast growth, cytokine release (prostaglandin E2 (PGE_2) and transforming growth factor β1 (TGFβ1)), as well as increase in ALP activity. The EMF signal can also enhance short-term NO production, with a concentration and time pattern consistent with chondrocyte proliferation. EMF-stimulated chondrocyte proliferation also involved calcium/calmodulin, nitric oxide synthase, nitric oxide, and cGMP (Fitzsimmons et al., 2008). In addition, Schnoke reported that EMF may be involved in bone anabolism, in part through the activation of proteins such as insulin receptor substrate-1 (IRS-1), S6 ribosomal subunit kinase, and endothelial nitric oxide synthase (eNOS) (Schnoke & Midura, 2007). Fitzsimmons reported a maximum potential gradient of 10^{-5} V/m capable of increasing the net calcium flux in human osteoblast-like cells (Fitzsimmons et al., 1994).

One major issue in EMF-related medical research is the contradictory results reported. For example, regarding gene expression, Berg reviewed that no less than 7 laboratories reported discrepancies with regard to *c-myc, c-fos* histone 2B, α-actin, and URA-3. This review focused on experiments using frequency < 100Hz, amplitude < 12mT and treatment time < 2h, and found the reproducibility of the results to be unsatisfactory (Berg, 1999). The parameters most often mentioned in EMF are frequency, amplitude, and treatment time. One would expect that changing one of these parameters would result in altered bone cell activity. However, Hannay et al. (Hannay et al., 2005) reported that the duration of EMF stimulation did not affect Saos-2 cells (rat osteoblast-like cell line) following four treatments at 15 Hz and < 1.3mT. In order to avoid such discrepancies, measurements using well-defined physical and physiological conditions and experimental parameters must be carefully performed. Another challenge to understand the effect of EMF is that it is difficult to link the biological effect of EMF exposure to the low power density of the EMF signal that is even lower than the power associated with the electromagnetic radiation of home electronics at radiofrequency, microwave, and visible light frequencies. It is also much lower than the power density of EMF used for other medical applications such as neurostimulation. In addition, the frequency-dependent Gauss rate of change is too weak to drive a useful current through the tissues of high impedance. It is unlikely that the mechanism of EMF therapy is solely the impact on transmembrane potentials, as the potentials generated by EMF are much lower than those of the cell membrane (Haddad et al., 2007b). Compared to CCEF, EMF also produces much lower EF strength and lower electric-to-magnetic field ratio.

4. ES, PPy-based scaffolds and other tissues

4.1 Nerves

Due to the intrinsic ability of neurons to transmit electrical signals within the nervous system, they are highly responsive to electrical stimuli. Neurons also grow well on conductive polymers such as PPy. PPy-mediated ES and electrical recording are therefore unique approaches in nerve tissue engineering, including neural probes, nerve conduits, and scaffolds to support neurons for nerve regeneration. Under cell culture conditions, Schmidt et al. (Schmidt et al., 1997) reported a significant increase in neurite length of rat pheochromocytoma 12 (PC-12) cells cultured on PPy films following a steady potential of 100 mV stimulation for 2 h. The median neurite length for the electrically stimulated PC-12 cells was almost twice that recorded in the non-ES controls. ES has also dramatically enhanced the expression and secretion of the NGF and BDNF of Schwann cells compared to the control cells without ES.

To maintain an efficient level of electrical communication between nerve cells and an electronic element, such as neural probes, it is crucial that the PPy-based interface successfully connects to neurons. To take advantage of the anionic dopants in PPy, negatively charged glycosaminoglycans (GAGs) such as hyaluronic acid, heparin, and chitosan were incorporated into PPy as dopant ions. Because GAGs are involved in a number of complex cell signalling events, including migration, attachment, and neuronal sprouting (Serra Moreno et al., 2009), doping with GAGs is expected to increase the bioaffinity of the PPy-coated neural probes. To improve cell attachment and migration and to enhance neurite growth, synthetic peptides and silk-like polymers containing fibronectin fragments (SLPF), laminin fragment p31(CDPGYIGSR), p20(RNIAEIIKDI), and YIGSR sequences (DCDPGYIGSR) (Cui et al., 2003) were also successfully doped into PPy. Other methods include chemical modification such as immobilization of nerve growth factors (NGFs) or neurotrophin-3 (NT-3) (Richardson et al., 2007) on the surface of PPy. All of these strategies have reportedly increased affinity and therefore the communication efficiency between neural probes and neurons. Since substrate morphology regulates cellular behaviours, PPy has been manufactured into various structures to facilitate electrical communication between neurons and neural probes. For example, PPy nanotubes in a narrow range of conductivity was found to promote the outgrowth of neuritis, resulting in a decrease in the number of growth cones and an increase in cell body area (Zheng et al, 2003). The longitudinally implanted electrodes were shown to have stable stimulating and recording characteristics as well as good electrical response (Zheng et al, 2003). When cultured on aligned electrospun poly(lactic-co-glycolic acid) (PLGA) nanofibres, PC-12 stimulated by a 10 mV/cm potential gradient exhibited 40-50% longer neurites and 40-90% more neurite formation than those generated by the non-stimulated cells on the same scaffolds (Lee et al., 2009). Scaffolds to guide nerve regeneration are often tubular in shape. PPy tubes ranging from 25 µm to 1.6 mm of inner diameter as well as multichannel tubes were fabricated by electrodeposition. One- and 2-µm-wide PPy microchannels were fabricated using patterning technology (Gomez et al., 2007). Commercially available patterned junctions of conducting PPy have microelectrode arrays displaying typical dimensions of 200 µm between the electrodes, with each electrode measuring 30 µm in diameter (Simon & Carter, 2006). A low impedance electrode/tissue interface is important to signal transfer quality. Martin et al. (Abidian & Martin, 2008) fabricated nanostructure-conducting polymers that decreased the impedance of microelectrodes typically by two orders of magnitude and increased the charge transfer capacity by three orders of magnitude.

An important issue is mechanical property compliance, i.e., matching the elastic module or stiffness of the PPy implant with the surrounding tissues. In situ PPy polymerization in biodegradable PLLA, hydrogel, or elastomeric silicone may reduce the mechanical mismatch between implant and tissue, resulting in enhanced biocompatibility and long-term performance.

4.2 Cardiac tissues

Coordinated excitation-contraction coupling activation of the ventricular myocardium from apex to base is an electrical stimulated chemical-mechanical behaviour. The ventricular myocardium has long been recognized as an anisotropic tissue with tensile mechanical properties strongly affected by cardiac muscle fibre orientation. Although micropatterning and microabrasion technologies may engineer precise cardiac patch anisotropy to match that of the surrounding host tissue, ES is also considered as an important stimulatory factor. ES to myocardium may progressively enhance the excitation-contraction coupling and improve cell function. For example, Radisic (Radisic et al., 2007) reported that ES to native heart tissue resulted in the progressive development of conductive and contractile characteristics of cardiac tissue, including cell alignment and coupling, which increased the amplitude of synchronous construct contractions and achieved a remarkable ultrastructural organization. At molecular level, ES raised the levels of all of the measured cardiac proteins and enhanced the expression of the corresponding genes. Radisic (Radisic et, 2007) also found that with increasing culture time, the ratio of mature and immature forms of myosin heavy chain (α-MHC and β-MHC, respectively) decreased in non-stimulated constructs and increased in stimulated ones. Moreover, the electrical stimulated cardiac cells showed modulated ion channel expression (Feld et al., 2002). Despite these and many other observations showing the beneficial effect of ES to myocardium and cardiac muscle cells, the application of conductive polymers in cardiac tissue engineering remains very limited. In 2007, Nishizawa et al. (Nishizawa et al., 2007) applied external ES to cultured cardiac myocytes using a microelectrode made of PPy-coated polyimide substrate. In their experiment, the myocytes were cultured on the PPy-coated anodic electrode, with the cathodic Pt immersed in the culture media over the cells. Through confocal fluorescence Ca^{2+} imaging, the authors observed that the cytosolic Ca^{2+} concentration was evoked by the electrical pulses delivered by the electrode (interval 1 s, duration 100 ms, and amplitude 10 mA) and that the cardiac myocytes were electrically conjugated through gap junctions. Using the same system, this group also obtained the threshold conditions from 0.5 to 10 mA using a different pulse duration for the excitation of the myocytes that showed a synchronized beating upon pulsation. The longer pulsed duration exerted an effective stimulation, regardless of current amplitude.

5. Future developments and challenges

Stem cells have been the focus of cell sourcing for a long time. Theoretically, embryo stem cells can differentiate into every cell lineage and eventually develop into every tissue and organ, including bone marrow, peripheral blood, umbilical cord, and adipose tissue. However, the use of human embryos for research purposes remains a highly sensitive ethical issue. On the other hand, adult stem cells are much easier to obtain from bone marrow or other tissues, such as adipose tissue and dental pulp. Studies have shown that adult stem cells have the potential to develop into various important cell phenotypes, including osteoblasts, under appropriate conditions such as growth factors. Cell differentiation may also be promoted by EF. Indeed, considering the role of EF in embryo development, adult stem cells may represent important candidates to study the potential of ES to differentiate stem cells into osteoblasts and other phenotypes.

Because of its critical role in maintaining the long-term survival of engineered tissue, vascularisation is extremely important in tissue engineering. Therefore another cell lineage, namely, endothelial cells, should be co-cultured with osteoblasts to form viable bone. Different cells may react differently when subjected to the same ES in co-culture. Furthermore, because of the crosstalk between the two cell populations, the ES parameters for the co-cultured cells may differ from those acquired in single cell cultures and must therefore be carefully studied.

ES as a distinct feature may be integrated into the design of bioreactors. Currently available well-designed and versatile bioreactors already provide physical stimuli such as shear stress and mechanical force. Integrating ES into the design may either make the conditions in a bioreactor similar to those in vivo, in the case of embryo or stem cell development, or add another dimension to manipulate cellular behaviour to facilitate tissue regeneration.

While materials science has made significant strides in bone regeneration, the ideal substitute has yet to be developed and large bone defects continue to represent a major challenge for orthopaedic and reconstructive surgeons. PPy-based conductive composites can be made elastic, biodegradable, and electrically conductive. This unique feature thus makes them ideal candidates in the process of engineering bone tissue in bioreactors through both mechanical and electrical stimulations.

In an integral biosystem, how do cells differentiate in the precise location, at the right time, and into the devoted phenotype? Many questions remain unanswered. To large extent, the answers depend on the progress in developmental biology, from which cell genetics and the relationships between cells and their surrounding environment can be better understood. Such knowledge is vital to understand how to simulate the "natural environment" with the appropriate biological and physical cues. The fundamental challenge of the next generation of tissue engineering will be to fully elucidate the molecular energy absorption processes that may explain physical and biochemical changes in cells, and to provide cells with the right cues to predictably form functional tissues in various tissue development steps. ES continues to define its roles and should find its place in this increasingly exciting era.

The fabrication of PPy-based conductive scaffolds must take advantage of the most recent technologies and integrate biological components. These technologies include patterning, self-assembly, and 3D prototyping. Natural materials include collagen, coralline, aminoglucosan, chondroitin-sulfate, and fibrin. The ideal technology must be able to control the composition and distribution of these natural materials within various synthetic biodegradable polymers, such as polylactic acid (PLA), poly-4-hydroxybutgrate (P4HB), and copolymers of PGA and PLA (PGLA). The ideal porous structure of a biomaterial must enhance cell attachment, adhesion, growth, nutrition and metabolic exchange, and neovascularity development.

Because osteoprogenitor cell proliferation, differentiation, and matrix mineralization are heterogeneous, one important area of ES research is the optimization of parameters such as intensity, frequency, direction, and duration of the applied electric field in order to accommodate the various bone formation steps. This work is expected to be significantly extensive yet directly relative to potential clinic applications.

6. Conclusions

Although ES has been attempted in clinic setting for a long time, its official authentication and comprehensive acceptation by physicians still need much support from further academic and clinic research. The mechanism of how the smallest organism unit, cell, responds to ES is still very much to be revealed. A physiological level of ES, in the order several tens to hundreds of mV and µA, is believed appropriate to activate voltage-sensitive proteins like transmembrane channels and transmembrane receptors, to modify gene expression, to affect cellular communication, as well as to affect the adhesion of ECM components. The most frequently reported parameters involved in ES experiments such as potential gradient and current density are probably oversimplified, ignoring frequency, wave form, duration and magnetic field. Various conducting materials like metals, CNTs, polymers have been used to prepare conductive scaffolds. From those conductive scaffolds, the adhered cells sense and respond to ES. Up to now, significant amount literatures have validated the role of ES in tissue regeneration, showing the high promise of using conductive materials and ES in tissue engineering, particular for the repair and regeneration of bone, nerve and cardiac tissues.

7. References

Aaron, RK.; Boyan, BD.; Ciombor, DM.; Schwartz, Z. & Simon, BJ. (2004a) Stimulation of growth factor synthesis by electric and electromagnetic fields. Clin Orthop Relat Res: 30-37

Aaron, RK.; Ciombor, D. & Jones, AR. (1997) Bone induction by decalcified bone matrix and mRNA of TGFβ and IGF-1 are increased by ELF field stimulation. Trans Orthop Res Soc 22: 548-564

Aaron, RK.; Ciombor, DM. & Simon, BJ. (2004b) Treatment of nonunions with electric and electromagnetic fields. Clinical Orthopaedics and Related Research: 21-29

Abidian, MR. & Martin, DC. (2008) Experimental and theoretical characterization of implantable neural microelectrodes modified with conducting polymer nanotubes. Biomaterials 29: 1273-1283

Adey, WR. (1993) Biological effects of electromagnetic fields. J Cell Biochem 51: 410-416

Akasaka, T.; Yokoyama, A.; Matsuoka, M.; Hashimoto, T.; Abe, S.; Uo, M. & Watari, F. (2009) Adhesion of human osteoblast-like cells (Saos-2) to carbon nanotube sheets. Bio-Medical Materials and Engineering 19: 147-153

Armstrong, CM.; Bezanilla, F. (1973) Currents related to movement of the gating particles of the sodium channels. Nature 242(5398): 459-61.

Armstrong, PF.; Brighton, CT. & Star, AM. (1988) Capacitively coupled electrical stimulation of bovine growth plate chondrocytes grown in pellet form. J Orthop Res 6: 265-271

Ateh, DD.; Navsaria, HA & Vadgama, P. (2006) Polypyrrole-based conducting polymers and interactions with biological tissues. J R Soc Interface 3: 741-752

Barrere, F.; Mahmood, TA.; de Groot, K. & van Blitterswijk, CA. (2008) Advanced biomaterials for skeletal tissue regeneration: Instructive and smart functions. Materials Science & Engineering R-Reports 59: 38-71

Beck, BR.; Matheson, GO.; Bergman, G.; Norling, T.; Fredericson, M.; Hoffman, AR. & Marcus, R. (2008) Do capacitively coupled electric fields accelerate tibial stress fracture healing? A randomized controlled trial. American Journal of Sports Medicine 36: 545-553

Berg, H. (1999) Problems of weak electromagnetic field effects in cell biology. Bioelectrochemistry and Bioenergetics 48: 355-360

Berg, H. & Zhang, L. (1993) Electrostimulation in Cell Biology by Low-Frequency Electromagnetic-Fields. Electro- and Magnetobiology 12: 147-163

Berlin, JM.; Leonard, AD.; Pham, TT.; Sano, D.; Marcano, DC.; Yan, SY.; Fiorentino, S.; Milas, ZL.; Kosynkin, DV.; Price, BK.; Lucente-Schultz, RM.; Wen, XX.; Raso, MG.; Craig, SL.; Tran, HT.; Myers, JN. & Tour, JM. (2010) Effective Drug Delivery, In Vitro and In Vivo, by Carbon-Based Nanovectors Noncovalently Loaded with Unmodified Paclitaxel. Acs Nano 4: 4621-4636

Bezanilla, F. (2008) How membrane proteins sense voltage. Nature Reviews Molecular Cell Biology 9: 323-332

Bodamyali, T.; Kanczler, JM.; Simon, B.; Blake, DR. & Stevens, CR. (1999) Effect of faradic products on direct current-stimulated calvarial organ culture calcium levels. Biochem Biophys Res Commun 264: 657-661

Brighton, CT. & McCluskey, WP. (1988) Response of cultured bone cells to a capacitively coupled electric field: inhibition of cAMP response to parathyroid hormone. J Orthop Res 6: 567-571

Brighton, CT.; Wang, W.; Seldes, R.; Zhang, G. & Pollack, SR. (2001) Signal transduction in electrically stimulated bone cells. J Bone Joint Surg Am 83-A: 1514-1523

Busse, JW.; Morton, E.; Lacchetti, C.; Guyatt, GH. & Bhandari, M. (2008) Current management of tibial shaft fractures - A survey of 450 Canadian orthopedic trauma surgeons. Acta Orthopaedica 79: 689-694

Chao, EY. & Inoue, N. (2003) Biophysical stimulation of bone fracture repair, regeneration and remodelling. Eur Cell Mater 6: 72-84; discussion 84-75

Cheng, C.; Muller, KH.; Koziol, KK.; Skepper, JN.; Midgley, PA.; Welland, ME. & Porter, AE. (2009) Toxicity and imaging of multi-walled carbon nanotubes in human macrophage cells. Biomaterials 30: 4152-4160

Cogan, SF. (2008) Neural stimulation and recording electrodes. Annual Review of Biomedical Engineering 10: 275-309

Cui, X.; Wiler, J.; Dzaman, M.; Altschuler, RA. & Martin, DC. (2003) In vivo studies of polypyrrole/peptide coated neural probes. Biomaterials 24: 777-787

Curtze, S.; Dembo, M.; Miron, M. & Jones, DB. (2004) Dynamic changes in traction forces with DC electric field in osteoblast-like cells. J Cell Sci 117: 2721-2729

Danon, A. & Korenstein, R. (1984) Capacitive pulsed electrical stimulation of bone cells: Induction of calcium uptake. Bioelectrochemistry and Bioenergetics 13: 49-54

Dimitriou, R. & Babis, GC. (2007) Biomaterial osseointegration enhancement with biophysical stimulation. J Musculoskelet Neuronal Interact 7: 253-265

Englebienne, P. (1999) Synthetic materials capable of reporting biomolecular recognition events by chromic transition. Journal of Materials Chemistry 9: 1043-1054

Feld, Y.; Melamed-Frank, M.; Kehat, I.; Tal, D.; Marom, S. & Gepstein, L. (2002) Electrophysiological modulation of cardiomyocytic tissue by transfected fibroblasts expressing potassium channels: a novel strategy to manipulate excitability. Circulation 105: 522-529

Ferrier, J.; Ross, SM.; Kanehisa, J. & Aubin, JE. (1986) Osteoclasts and osteoblasts migrate in opposite directions in response to a constant electrical field. J Cell Physiol 129: 283-288

Fitzsimmons, RJ.; Gordon, SL.; Kronberg, J.; Ganey, T. & Pilla, AA. (2008) A pulsing electric field (PEF) increases human chondrocyte proliferation through a transduction pathway involving nitric oxide signaling. J Orthop Res 26: 854-859

Fitzsimmons, RJ.; Ryaby, JT.; Magee, FP. & Baylink, DJ. (1994) Combined magnetic fields increased net calcium flux in bone cells. Calcif Tissue Int 55: 376-380

Foster, KR. (2003) Mechanisms of interaction of extremely low frequency electric fields and biological systems. Radiat Prot Dosimetry 106(4):301-10

Foulds, IS. & Barker, AT. (1983) Human skin battery potentials and their possible role in wound healing. Br J Dermatol 109: 515-522

Gomez, N.; Lee, JY.; Nickels, JD. & Schmidt, CE. (2007) Micropatterned Polypyrrole: A Combination of Electrical and Topographical Characteristics for the Stimulation of Cells. Adv Funct Mater 17: 1645-1653

Goodwin, CB.; Brighton, CT.; Guyer, RD.; Johnson, JR.; Light, KI. & Yuan, HA. (1999) A double-blind study of capacitively coupled electrical stimulation as an adjunct to lumbar spinal fusions. Spine (Phila Pa 1976) 24: 1349-1356; discussion 1357

Guimard, NK.; Gomez, N. & Schmidt, CE. (2007) Conducting polymers in biomedical engineering. Progress in Polymer Science 32: 876-921

Haddad, JB.; Obolensky, AG. & Shinnick, P. (2007a) The biologic effects and the therapeutic mechanism of action of electric and electromagnetic field stimulation on bone and cartilage: New findings and a review of earlier work. Journal of Alternative and Complementary Medicine 13: 485-490

Haddad, JB.; Obolensky, AG. & Shinnick, P. (2007b) The biologic effects and the therapeutic mechanism of action of electric and electromagnetic field stimulation on bone and cartilage: new findings and a review of earlier work. J Altern Complement Med 13: 485-490

Hannay, G.; Leavesley, D. & Pearcy, M. (2005) Timing of pulsed electromagnetic field stimulation does not affect the promotion of bone cell development. Bioelectromagnetics 26: 670-676

Harris, AL.; Spray, DC. & Bennett, MV. (1983) Control of intercellular communication by voltage dependence of gap junctional conductance. J Neurosci 3: 79-100

Heliotis, M.; Ripamonti, U.; Ferretti, C.; Kerawala, C.; Mantalaris, A. & Tsiridis, E. (2009) The basic science of bone induction. Br J Oral Maxillofac Surg

Hofmann, GA.; Dev, SB. & Nanda, GS. (1996) Electrochemotherapy: Transition from laboratory to the clinic. Ieee Engineering in Medicine and Biology Magazine 15: 124-132

Hou, Q.; Grijpma, DW. & Feijen, J. (2003) Porous polymeric structures for tissue engineering prepared by a coagulation, compression moulding and salt leaching technique. Biomaterials 24: 1937-1947

Hutmacher, DW. (2000) Scaffolds in tissue engineering bone and cartilage. Biomaterials 21: 2529-2543

Jia, G.; Wang, HF.; Yan, L.; Wang, X.; Pei, RJ.; Yan, T.; Zhao, YL. & Guo, XB. (2005) Cytotoxicity of carbon nanomaterials: Single-wall nanotube, multi-wall nanotube, and fullerene. Environmental Science & Technology 39: 1378-1383

Kartsogiannis, V. & Ng, KW. (2004) Cell lines and primary cell cultures in the study of bone cell biology. Mol Cell Endocrinol 228: 79-102

Khang, D.; Park, GE. & Webster, TJ. (2008) Enhanced chondrocyte densities on carbon nanotube composites: The combined role of nanosurface roughness and electrical stimulation. Journal of Biomedical Materials Research Part A 86A: 253-260

Kim, IS.; Song, JK.; Zhang, YL.; Lee, TH.; Cho, TH.; Song, YM.; Kim do, K.; Kim, SJ. & Hwang, SJ. (2006) Biphasic electric current stimulates proliferation and induces VEGF production in osteoblasts. Biochim Biophys Acta 1763: 907-916

Kotwal, A. & Schmidt, CE. (2001) Electrical stimulation alters protein adsorption and nerve cell interactions with electrically conducting biomaterials. Biomaterials 22: 1055-1064

Lee, JY.; Bashur, CA.; Goldstein, AS. & Schmidt, CE. (2009) Polypyrrole-coated electrospun PLGA nanofibers for neural tissue applications. Biomaterials 30: 4325-4335

Lee, RC.; Zhang, D. & Hannig, J. (2000) Biophysical injury mechanisms in electrical shock trauma. Annu Rev Biomed Eng 2: 477-509

Li, X.; Kolega, J. (2002) Effects of direct current electric fields on cell migration and actin filament distribution in bovine vascular endothelial cells. J Vasc Res 39(5):391-404

Liboff, AR.; Rinaldi, RA.; Lavine, LS. & Shamos, MH. (1975) Electrical-Conduction in Living Bone. Clinical Orthopaedics and Related Research: 330-335

Lohmann, CH.; Schwartz, Z.; Liu, Y.; Li, Z.; Simon, BJ.; Sylvia, VL.; Dean, DD.; Bonewald, LF.; Donahue, HJ. & Boyan, BD. (2003) Pulsed electromagnetic fields affect phenotype and connexin 43 protein expression in MLO-Y4 osteocyte-like cells and ROS 17/2.8 osteoblast-like cells. J Orthop Res 21: 326-334

Lorich, DG.; Brighton, CT.; Gupta, R.; Corsetti, JR.; Levine, SE.; Gelb, ID.; Seldes, R. & Pollack, SR. (1998) Biochemical pathway mediating the response of bone cells to capacitive coupling. Clin Orthop Relat Res: 246-256

Manjhi, J.; Mathur, R. & Behari, J. (2009) Effect of low level capacitive-coupled pulsed electric field stimulation on mineral profile of weight-bearing bones in ovariectomized rats. J Biomed Mater Res B Appl Biomater

Mazeikiene, R. & Malinauskas, A. (2001) Kinetic study of the electrochemical degradation of polyaniline. Synthetic Metals 123: 349-354

McCaig, CD.; Rajnicek, AM.; Song, B. & Zhao, M. (2005) Controlling cell behavior electrically: current views and future potential. Physiol Rev 85: 943-978

Mehedintu, M. & Berg, H. (1997) Proliferation response of yeast Saccharomyces cerevisiae on electromagnetic field parameters. Bioelectrochemistry and Bioenergetics 43: 67-70

Meng, SY; Rouabhia, M. & Zhang, Z. (2010) Accelerated Osteoblast Mineralization on a Conductive Substrate by Multiple Electrical Stimulation. Journal of Bone and Mineral Metabolism. (Accepted)

Meng, SY.; Rouabhia, M.; Shi, GX., & Zhang, Z. (2008) Heparin dopant increases the electrical stability, cell adhesion, and growth of conducting polypyrrole/poly(L,L-lactide) composites. Journal of Biomedical Materials Research Part A 87A: 332-344

Mollon, B.; da Silva, V.; Busse, JW.; Einhorn, TA. & Bhandari, M. (2008) Electrical Stimulation for Long-Bone Fracture-Healing: A Meta-Analysis of Randomized Controlled Trials. Journal of Bone and Joint Surgery-American Volume 90A: 2322-2330

Nakagawa, S., Maeda, S. & Tsukihara, T. (2010) Structural and functional studies of gap junction channels. Curr Opin Struct Biol 20: 423-430

Narita, N.; Kobayashi, Y.; Nakamura, H.; Maeda, K.; Ishihara, A.; Mizoguchi, T.; Usui, Y.; Aoki, K.; Simizu, M.; Kato, H.; Ozawa, H.; Udagawa, N.; Endo, M.; Takahashi, N. & Saito, N. (2009) Multiwalled carbon nanotubes specifically inhibit osteoclast differentiation and function. Nano Lett 9: 1406-1413

Nazarov, R.; Jin, HJ. & Kaplan, DL. (2004) Porous 3-D scaffolds from regenerated silk fibroin. Biomacromolecules 5: 718-726

Nishizawa, M.; Nozaki, H.; Kaji, H.; Kitazume, T.; Kobayashi, N.; Ishibashi, T. & Abe, T. (2007) Electrodeposition of anchored polypyrrole film on microelectrodes and stimulation of cultured cardiac myocytes. Biomaterials 28: 1480-1485

Orr, AW.; Helmke, BP.; Blackman, BR. & Schwartz, MA. (2006) Mechanisms of mechanotransduction. Developmental Cell 10: 11-20

Radisic, M.; Park, H.; Gerecht, S.; Cannizzaro, C.; Langer, R. & Vunjak-Novakovic, G. (2007) Biomimetic approach to cardiac tissue engineering. Philosophical Transactions of the Royal Society B-Biological Sciences 362: 1357-1368

Richardson, RT.; Thompson, B.; Moulton, S.; Newbold, C.; Lum, MG.; Cameron, A.; Wallace, G.; Kapsa, R.; Clark, G. & O'Leary, S. (2007) The effect of polypyrrole with incorporated neurotrophin-3 on the promotion of neurite outgrowth from auditory neurons. Biomaterials 28: 513-523

Ryaby, JT. (1998) Clinical effects of electromagnetic and electric fields on fracture healing. Clin Orthop Relat Res: S205-215

Sandler, JKW.; Kirk, JE.; Kinloch, IA.; Shaffer, MSP. & Windle, AH. (2003) Ultra-low electrical percolation threshold in carbon-nanotube-epoxy composites. Polymer 44: 5893-5899

Schmidt, CE.; Shastri, VR.; Vacanti, JP. & Langer, R. (1997) Stimulation of neurite outgrowth using an electrically conducting polymer. Proc Natl Acad Sci U S A 94: 8948-8953

Schnoke, M. & Midura, RJ. (2007) Pulsed electromagnetic fields rapidly modulate intracellular signaling events in osteoblastic cells: comparison to parathyroid hormone and insulin. J Orthop Res 25: 933-940

Serra Moreno, J.; Panero, S.; Materazzi, S.; Martinelli, A.; Sabbieti, MG.; Agas, D. & Materazzi, G. (2009) Polypyrrole-polysaccharide thin films characteristics: electrosynthesis and biological properties. J Biomed Mater Res A 88: 832-840

Shastri, VP.; Rahman, N.; Martin, I. & Langer, R. (1999) Application of conductive polymers in bone regeneration. Materials Research Society Symposium - Proceedings 550: 215-219

Sierpowska, J.; Hakulinen, MA.; Toyras, J.; Day, JS.; Weinans, H.; Kiviranta, I.; Jurvelin, JS. & Lappalainen, R. (2006) Interrelationships between electrical properties and microstructure of human trabecular bone. Physics in Medicine and Biology 51: 5289-5303

Simon, DT.; Carter, SA. (2006) Electrosynthetically patterned conducting polymer films for investigation of neural signalling. Journal of Chemical Physics 124(20): 204709-204709-5

Smith, SD.; McLeod, BR.; Liboff, AR. & Cooksey, K. (1987) Calcium cyclotron resonance and diatom mobility. Bioelectromagnetics 8: 215-227

Spadaro, JA. (1977) Electrically stimulated bone growth in animals and man. Review of the literature. Clin Orthop Relat Res: 325-332

Stains, JP. & Civitelli, R. (2005) Cell-to-cell interactions in bone. Biochem Biophys Res Commun 328: 721-727

Stecker, MM.; Patterson, T. & Netherton, BL. (2006) Mechanisms of electrode induced injury. Part 1: Theory. American Journal of Electroneurodiagnostic Technology 46: 315-342

Sun, S.; Titushkin, I. & Cho, M. (2006) Regulation of mesenchymal stem cell adhesion and orientation in 3D collagen scaffold by electrical stimulus. Bioelectrochemistry 69: 133-141

Wang, Q.; Zhong, SZ.; Jun, OY.; Jiang, LX.; Zhang, ZK.; Xie, Y. & Luo, SQ. (1998) Osteogenesis of electrically stimulated bone cells mediated in part by calcium ions. Clinical Orthopaedics and Related Research: 259-268

Wang, W.; Wang, ZY.; Zhang, GH.; Clark, CC. & Brighton, CT. (2004) Up-regulation of chondrocyte matrix genes and products by electric fields. Clinical Orthopaedics and Related Research: S163-S173

Wan, ZY.; Clark, CC. & Brighton, CT. (2006) Up-regulation of bone morphogenetic proteins in cultured murine bone cells with use of specific electric fields. Journal of Bone and Joint Surgery-American Volume 88A: 1053-1065

Wiesmann, H.; Hartig, M.; Stratmann, U.; Meyer, U. & Joos, U. (2001) Electrical stimulation influences mineral formation of osteoblast-like cells in vitro. Biochim Biophys Acta 1538: 28-37

Wiesmann, HP.; Joos, U. & Meyer, U. (2004) Biological and biophysical principles in extracorporal bone tissue engineering. Part II. Int J Oral Maxillofac Surg 33: 523-530

Wong, JY.; Langer, R. & Ingber, DE. (1994) Electrically conducting polymers can noninvasively control the shape and growth of mammalian cells. Proc Natl Acad Sci U S A 91: 3201-3204

Zheng, X.; Zhang, J.; Chen, T.& Chen, Z. (2003) Longitudinally implanted intrafascicular electrodes for stimulating and recording fascicular physioelectrical signals in the sciatic nerve of rabbits. Microsurgery 23(3): 268-273

Zhu, Y. & Li, WX. (2008) Cytotoxicity of carbon nanotubes. Science in China Series B-Chemistry 51: 1021-1029

Zhuang, HM.; Wang, W.; Seldes, RM.; Tahernia, AD.; Fan, HJ. & Brighton, CT. (1997) Electrical stimulation induces the level of TGF-beta 1 mRNA in osteoblastic cells by a mechanism involving calcium/calmodulin pathway. Biochemical and Biophysical Research Communications 237: 225-229

Zipse, DW. (1993) Health-Effects of Extremely Low-Frequency (50-Hz and 60-Hz) Electric and Magnetic-Fields. Ieee Transactions on Industry Applications 29: 447-458

4

The ECSIM Concept *(Environmental Control System for Intestinal Microbiota)* and Its Derivative Versions to Help Better Understand Human Gut Biology

Jean-François Brugère[1], David Féria-Gervasio[1],
Zsolt Popse[2], William Tottey[1] and Monique Alric[1]
[1]Université d'Auvergne, Clermont-Université, Clermont-Ferrand,
[2]Global Process Concept, La Rochelle,
France

1. Introduction

Each meal reminds us of our energy needs. As heterotrophs, we have a whole set of organs for food digestion and conversion into substances usable by our body. The breakdown of food (mainly proteins, carbohydrates and lipids) takes place in the gastrointestinal tract (GIT) which assimilates these elements and transfers them into the bloodstream. In a simplified manner, these digestion and absorption functions are provided by the following organs: the mouth, oesophagus, stomach, the small intestine (including the duodenum, jejunum and ileum), the large intestine or colon (formed from the right, transverse and left colon), ending with the rectum and anus. Various functions are required to facilitate the hydrolysis of food. They include a combination of physical factors (temperature, pH, grinding and friction, ...), chemical factors (acid secretions, bile salts, ...) and enzymes (salivary, gastric or pancreatic enzymes,...). Colonic physiology also benefits in parallel from a real contribution by micro-organisms, specifically bacteria.

Several factors contribute to our interest in the human digestive tract. For example, in Europe colorectal cancer is the second cause of cancer in women and the third in men (Boyle & Ferlay, 2005). Some pathologies can be chronic, infectious or even mortal. The digestive tract is also a simple and practical way of giving chemotherapy treatment, whether the pathology is of digestive origin or not.

Proposing more or less advanced simulation systems of the GIT, therefore, can overcome certain ethical, technical and/or financial difficulties in research. Furthermore, it is interesting to model the way the digestive tract works, in order to test various elements independently and/or concomitantly: such as drugs, food/nutrients, microbial agents, even physiological and physical elements.

Animal models work particularly well if they have a similar anatomical/physiological GIT. Rodent models, however, are used more in the laboratory for practical reasons. In order to enhance the resemblance to humans, "humanized" animal GITs have be developed from germ-free, newborn animals turned into gnotobiotic animals after being seeded by a human microbiota (see for example (Samuel & Gordon, 2006). In a more controlled manner, in vitro models are also alternatives which may answer biological questions, in an easier, more complete and less partial manner. In all cases, however, in vitro-in vivo correlations have to be established.

Our laboratory is particularly involved in the development, elaboration and use of in vitro devices able to reproducibly simulate the behaviour of elements in the digestive tract, with special emphasis on the human digestive tract. This involves the study of food, medicines, prebiotics, probiotics and infectious agents in the digestive tract. In this article we will particularly address the workings of the colon and its metabolic and physiological roles which still remain largely unknown. We will also present a fermentation system called ECSIM (Environmental Control System for Intestinal Microbiota), which is a modular system consisting of three reactors from GPC (Global Process Concept, www.gpcbio.com). It can be used in various configurations to mimic the different functions of a human colon depending on whether a simulation of a portion of the colon (for example, P-ECSIM for a simulation of the proximal part) or the colon in its totality and continuity is needed (for example, 3S-ECSIM for 3-stages-ECSIM, for the proximal, then transverse, then distal part). Figure 1 shows the general principle of the equipment.

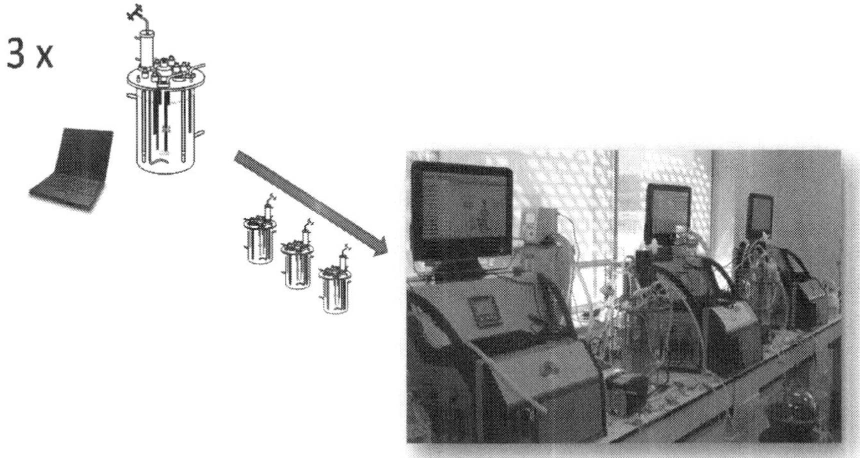

Fig. 1. A general view of the ECSIM platform permitting the simulation of the human gut.

Three computer-controlled bioreactors from Global Process Concept (www.gpcbio.com) are individually or collectively used as one modular system.

2. GIT, colon and gut microbiota

Simulating some or most of the functions of the digestive tract requires an accurate knowledge of the components of the GIT, at both the descriptive and functional levels. This is particularly true for the colon, which is different anatomically and functionally compared to the other parts of the GIT. Water and electrolytes are reabsorbed at this level of the tract, leading gradually to a solidification of faecal matter all along the colon. It also involves an intensive microbial fermentation process: matter which was either only partially digested or not at all digested in the upper parts of the GIT (rapid transfer from the upper part preventing total digestion, absence of necessary enzymes, limiting physicochemical conditions, ...) or finally because these elements do not come from alimentation but from the digestive tract itself (digestive secretions like the epithelial mucins, dead bacterial and human cells,...).

There are 3 distinct parts in the colon: the right (or ascending) side consists of the caecum and proximal colon; the central transverse colon; and the left side (or descending colon) consisting of the distal colon, the sigmoid colon and the rectum.

An important and specific microbial population inhabits each of these levels, whose density is incommensurate with the previous stages (Table 1), reaching values of 10^{12} bacteria per gram of colonic contents (Savage, 1977).

		Length (cm)	pH	Usual transit time (H)	Microbiota abundance per gram	Matter entering the colon (g per day)
Stomach		12	1 – 2.5	2 - 6	$0\text{-}10^{4}$	
Small intestine	Duodenum	25	6-6.5		$10^{4} - 10^{5}$	
	Jejunum	160	6.5	3 - 5	$10^{5} - 10^{7}$	
	Ileon	215	7.5		$10^{7} - 10^{8}$	
Large intestine	caecum	6			$10^{10} - 10^{11}$	Matter entering the colon
	Ascending colon	10 – 15	5.5-6.0		$10^{10} - 10^{11}$	(g per day)
	Transverse colon	50	6.0-6.5	50 - 70	$10^{10} - 10^{11}$	Polysaccharides 10-60g
	Descending colon	25	6.5-7.0		$10^{10} - 10^{11}$	Proteins 6-18g
	Sigmoid colon	40 – 80			$10^{10} - 10^{11}$	Lipids 5-8g
	Rectum	18		1	$10^{10} - 10^{12}$	

Table 1. Some physical, physiological and microbial characteristics of the human GIT.

An estimation of the quantity of matter entering the large intestine is given in the column on the right (adapted from A. Mihajlovski and G. Macfarlane & J. Cummings (G.T. Macfarlane & Cummings, 1991; A. Mihajlovski, 2010)).

The term "microbiota" is used to define this set of micro-organisms living together within our bodies. The genomes of these "indigenous microbes" are known as the "microbiome", the microbial counterpart of our genome. B. Zhu and his colleagues (Zhu et al., 2010) state that this was suggested in 2001 by the Nobel Laureate Joshua Lederberg and by Hooper & Gordon (2001). "Microbiome" can be substituted by the more general term "metagenome" when concerned with environmental genomic studies ("metagenomics" (Handelsman, 2004)). The authors of a recent article did not hesitate to use the terms "human gut microbiome" as "the second genome of human body" in their title (Zhu et al., 2010) and this enthusiasm also accompanies the results of recently obtained gut metagenomics (Qin et al., 2010).

In the early 2000s, once the human genome had been decoded, some scientists called for a collective effort to study global metagenomics to decode all of the bacterial communities inhabiting the human body, from the external communities of the skin, to internal ones, such as oral, intestinal and vaginal flora. The creation of a second "human genome project" (Relman & Falkow, 2001), studying the whole human flora, would complete our knowledge of the human genome. In 2005, the French "National Institute of Agronomic Research" (INRA), initiated an international discussion on the opportunity of structuring an intestinal microbiota research effort. This led to the creation of the project MetaHIT, "Metagenomics of the Human Intestinal Tract", supported by the Seventh Framework Program of the European Union (www.metahit.eu). In parallel, in 2007 the American National Institute of Health created the Human Microbiome Project (HMP, http://nihroadmap.nih.gov/hmp/). Its purpose was to address not only the intestinal tract, but also the skin, mouth and vagina (Peterson et al., 2009). For the intestine, the approach was to directly sequence 1,000 bacterial genomes usually found in this habitat, and in parallel determine the metagenome of 250 human guts. The results are expected in 2014.

2.1 Diversity and repartition of human gut microbiota

If we take a particular look at the microbes in the colon, a great diversity is observed in the part where the microbial density is highest. An overview of the various microbes found shows that planktonic forms predominate in the lumen, and biofilms are principally encountered on the epithelium. In addition, material in transit, in the process of being metabolized, is also colonized by micro-organisms, which move with the matter. Because of the gradual disappearance of oxygen along the digestive tract, and a very negative redox potential (ORP), the main bacterial populations are facultative or strict anaerobic species.

Before the creation and development of molecular microbial ecology tools, studies were based almost entirely on the use of selective or non selective culture media. Such studies were completed by biochemical, metabolic and morphological (microscopic examination and Gram stain) information. There were large discrepancies, however, between the data produced by culture and microbial counts performed by Fluorescent In Situ Hybridization (FISH). In fact, studies with DAPI staining (- 4', 6'-diamidino-2-phenylindole) revealed only 15% of cultured bacteria were found by counting (Langendijk et al., 1995). Since then, numerous molecular methods have been developed to overcome the limitations of microbial culture and assess the number of bacterial species in the digestive tract. The first methods used were based on the development and sequencing of the clone library of bacterial 16S DNA, using techniques that permitted to consider max 50% (even 10%) being cultivated species (Ley et al., 2006; Zoetendal et al., 2004).

It is particularly difficult to precisely define both the concept of species in bacteria and the justification of the rules used for these definitions. Molecular methods are used to define groups of micro-organisms based on their identity for sequences, principally those of 16S RNA considered in part or almost in its entirety. This defines operational taxonomic units (OTUs) on the basis of variations of 1, 2, 3 or 5% among these sequences (or 99%, 98%, 97% or 95% of their identity). It is generally accepted that 98% of the identity used to define phylotypes may be related to the concept of species. On this basis, 500 to more than

1,000 different species have been detected in the gut microbiota of 3 different individuals (Eckburg et al., 2005). M. Rajilić-Stojanović and her colleagues compiled all data available up to 2007 in a meta-analysis and identified 1,200 different phylotypes (Rajilic-Stojanovic et al. 2007). Recent technological advances in sequencing technology, such as the 454 technology of Roche Diagnostics Applied Science or Solexa/Illumina, have facilitated inventorying an even larger number of colonic bacteria (Claesson & O'Toole, 2010; Murphy et al., 2010; Tasse et al., 2010). D.N. Frank and N.R. Pace used metagenomics data to deduce the presence of 15,000 to 36,000 different bacterial species, with variations due to the molecular criteria chosen (Frank & Pace, 2008). It has recently been shown, however, that part of the bacteria are universally shared between individuals (Tap et al., 2009). The work defined a "universal core", more or less large, depending on the degree of sharing among humans. It is important to note that, although the number of non-cultivable species seems very large in these studies, metagenomics enables a "gene catalogue from the human gut microbiome" to be established (Qin et al., 2010). It is theoretically possible, therefore, to extrapolate the activity or the metabolic potential of microbiota.

Unfortunately, a very important part of colonic microbiota remains uncultivable as isolated species. This can be explained by a particularly high sensitivity to O_2, even at low levels of exposure (amount, duration), a high dependence on certain elements not present in the media being used, and a strong dependence on other microbial species providing such elements. It is interesting, therefore, to develop cropping systems which maintain consortia in vitro, and allow the study of biological interactions and ecological and functional relationships between the various members of the colonic ecosystem. Baoli Zhu et al. (2010) indicate that recent results in in vitro systems can detect 50 to 70% of sequences belonging to "uncultivated bacteria". This new data makes current vocabulary inappropriate and requires a rapid evolution and/or a redefinition of the terms being used. For example, one can question the legitimacy of the finality of such terms as "non-cultivable".

The role of the bacterial community should not obscure the importance of other micro-organisms. Two other domains of life which must not be forgotten can be found in this ecosystem: eukaryotic cells (e.g. Blastocystis spp.) and yeasts (e.g. Candida spp.) (Scanlan & Marchesi, 2008), and Archaea, which includes methanogens able to synthesize methane from CO_2 and H_2 from the metabolism of other microbiota microorganisms (Mihajlovski, Doré, Levenez, Alric, & Brugère, 2010; Strocchi, Furne, Ellis, & Levitt, 1991). Some Archaea may also possess other features, closely related, or not, with non-usual methanogens, i.e. potential Thermoplasmatales (Mihajlovski, Alric, & Brugere, 2008; Mihajlovski et al., 2010) or halophilic archaea (Oxley et al., 2010). Furthermore, the presence of a considerable diversity of viral genotypes is also important, as about 1,200 have been described to date (Breitbart et al., 2003). This could have a significant functional and metabolic implication, not per se, but through the role they play in regulating bacterial populations.

2.2 Properties, functions and evolution of gut microbiota

It is important to remember that the contribution of intestinal microbiota is a major, though not essential, factor in the life of the host (germ-free mice are viable but present various alterations). The microbiota acts as a physical barrier to exclude pathogens by coating the mucosa and by inducing antimicrobial peptide production by Paneth cells (Hooper et al., 2003). It also contributes to the maturation, morphology and maintenance of the digestive tract (Hooper et al., 2002), reduces inflammatory response and the number of Peyer's patches, and promotes angiogenesis (Stappenbeck et al., 2002). Furthermore, it is responsible for the production of available vitamins, especially Vit. B9, Vit. B12 and Vit. K (Hill, 1997) and is a source of energy, *per se* and through its metabolism. For example, germ-free mice implanted with a microbiota show a 60% increase in body-fat (Backhed et al., 2004), mainly due to the resulting and excess of energy-release from the fermentation of undigested food residue. Many other research works are being undertaken to understand the relationships linking the microbiota to the regulation of fat storage, or more broadly, how gut microbiota may influence metabolism and body composition (Vrieze et al., 2010).

Microbiota metabolic properties have different functional groups which can be identified according to their metabolic capabilities (including the use of substrate), creating dependencies and mutualistic relationships between organisms. The colon is, therefore, the centre of an intense fermentation activity. The origin of fermented substrates may be due to the non-use, partial-use or total-use of food/nutrients in the upper compartments (right part of Table 1). This may be caused by the transit time being too rapid and not allowing full treatment in the upper parts. Most often though, it is due to the absence of necessary enzyme activities and to unfit physicochemical conditions (especially pH). Other substrates, such as endogenous substrates, may come from the host itself: for example secreted mucopolysaccharides lubricating the digestive tract (mucins), digestive enzymes, cellular debris and even microbial debris.

Less than 100 g of exogenous substrates reaching the colon and available for microbial conversion (Cummings & Macfarlane, 1997) can produce 10% of our energy needs through their metabolism by the colonic microbiota (G.T. Macfarlane & Cummings, 1991). As mentioned in Table 1, these substrates are mostly complex polysaccharides and proteins with some lipids and nucleic acids. Out of the 100 g the complex polysaccharides alone account for 10 to 60 g. These are the substrates for which metabolic pathways are best known. The many different microorganisms and enzymes which provide the first steps of microbial conversion (fibrolytic flora) are still being characterized. The contribution of multiple microbial groups is necessary at this stage (Figure 2). The hydrolysis of polysaccharides by fibrolytic bacteria leads to simple compounds which are, in turn, used by each member of the fermentative microbiota to produce pyruvate. Depending on which microorganism is present, different reactions will then lead to the formation of lactic acid and short chain fatty acids, with over 90% being three major compounds: propionate, butyrate and acetate (the last being in amounts two to three times greater than the other two). Although synthesis takes place mainly in the ascending part of the colon (main area of polysaccharides fermentation), the concentrations observed in humans are nevertheless fairly constant (around 120 mM) in the other parts due to a decreasing absorption along the large bowel (G. T. Macfarlane, Gibson, & Cummings, 1992). Another consequence of this fermentation is the production of gases, particularly CO_2 and H_2. The presence of the latter limits feed-back on the effectiveness of this fermentation. It is necessary, therefore, to eliminate the presence of H_2, which is realised by hydrogenotrophs. This dedicated microbiota is variable among individuals and can eliminate the H_2 in 3 different (sometimes combined) anaerobic reduction processes: sulfate-reduction (synthesis of H_2S from sulfate as acceptor of electrons) realised by sulfate-reducing prokaryotes (SRP), reductive acetogenesis (reduction by a combination of CO_2 and a methyl) realised by acetogens, and hydrogenotrophic methanogenesis (CO_2 reduction to methane) realised by methanogenic archaea.

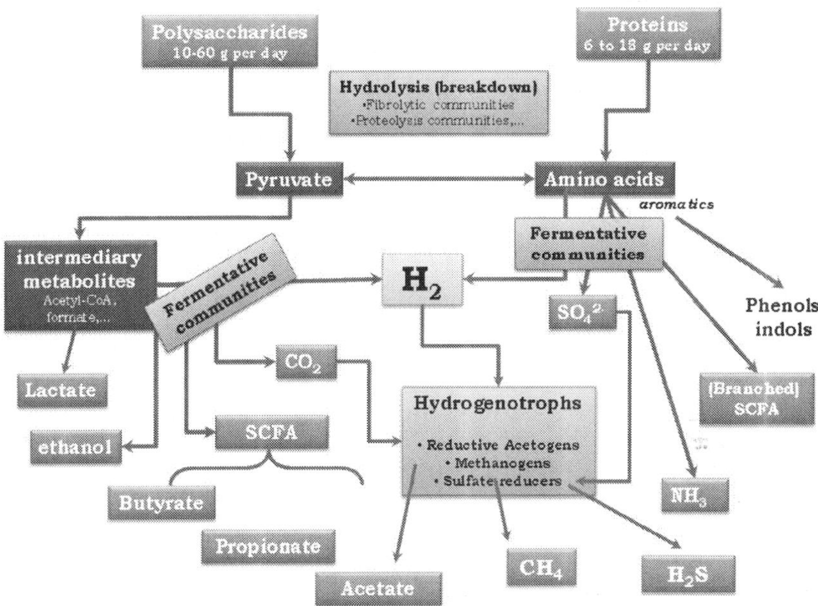

adapted from A. Bernalier-Donadille (2010).

Fig. 2. A schematic overview of the microbial fermentative metabolism in the human colon

The properties and functions of the intestinal microbiota are varied, complex and probably partly unknown. An *in-vitro* system, even with its limitations, could provide a simplified way of addressing various biological questions and problems. There is, therefore, a need to develop *in-vitro* models allowing a controlled approach to physical, chemical and microbiological parameters. As it appears to be extremely difficult to grow a significant part of the microbiota, artificially replicating a colon may provide a solution for growing microbiota as a consortium, and make it easier to determine the impact of environmental factors (*i.e.* all that is external to the microbiota) on its composition and metabolism. This requires a good knowledge of such environmental conditions in order to replicate them *in vitro*, and to have already measured various biological parameters *in vivo* in order to validate the *in vitro* results. Table 1 shows some of the results. The parameters vary with the specificity of nutrition, age and some diseases. The developed model, therefore, should ideally consist of a dynamic, multi-set system, easily adaptable to any simulation requirement, physiological or pathological situation.

3. The ECSIM paradigm

3.1 Simulating gut fermentations: a rapid overview of existing systems

Many *in vitro* systems have been developed to answer biological problems relating to the gastrointestinal tract. For example, there are systems to simulate chewing and to reproduce the size of masticated food in the presence of artificial saliva (Woda et al., 2010). Some tools focus on the digestive kinetics of food and drugs, others are limited to the study of *in-vitro* dissolution [see the various equipments of the pharmacopoeia, USP 1, 2, 3 and 4 (Pharmacopeia, 2011)] or conversely, to replicate kinetic absorption by simple or more complex systems of intestinal cells. In general these systems replicate the different compartments of the GIT anatomically and physico-chemically, with or without a gradual/discontinuous evolution of the conditions encountered along the digestive tract. For example, a simple thermostatic beaker may be sufficient to replicate a basic stomach; a highly acidic pH, controlled/modulated in a liquid medium with ions, bile salts, gastric enzymes, may be sufficient to control the release kinetics of encapsulated active ingredients. The study of colonic fermentation is based on models of varying complexity. George & Sandra Macfarlane (G. T. Macfarlane & Macfarlane, 2007) describe the motivations for using such systems and the essential features found in these models. Generally, these tools range from simple batch cultures to continuous culture systems. The choice of the model is based on the advantages/disadvantages of each to respond to specific biological problems. Various factors must be taken into account and comparisons made relative to the degree of reliability of what actually happens *in vivo* : for example, the ease of experimentation, the amount of experiments (acquisition time and speed), the number of environmental factors which need to be controlled (few/many), the price. This chapter includes, in our opinion, the three systems most likely to replicate the complexity of the colon in a controlled manner.

The SHIME [Simulator of the Human Intestinal Microbial Ecosystem (Molly et al., 1993)], recently available in two identical parallel models (TWIN-SHIME (Van den Abbeele et al., 2010)), is a composite system consisting of five double-jacketed vessels of various volumes, each replicating a particular part of the gastrointestinal microbial ecosystem. It simulates the stomach and the small intestine with two vessels of 0.3 L, and the large intestine with three vessels reproducing three compartments at constant volume and with pH control.

A second system was developed by the TNO in Holland, with several types and two functions. The TIM-1 (TNO Intestinal Model 1) is an *in-vitro* model of the upper part, with compartments replicating the stomach and the three parts of the small intestine (duodenum, jejunum and ileum) (Minekus et al., 1999). This is mainly achieved by a simulation of the saliva flow, gastric and pancreatic juices, and the peristaltic mixing of the chyme. Physical and chemical factors such as the transit time, temperature and pH control, and removal of digested compounds using hollow fibre membranes, are also used. This model seems useful for studying what happens to macro/micro-nutrients and the survival/stability of probiotics in the upper part of the GIT. A second TIM (TIM-2 for TNO Intestinal Model 2) simulates the colon, by controlling pH, anaerobiosis, and the gradual intake of media, as it would be with the upper part metabolism of food (Rajilic-Stojanovic et al., 2010; van der Werf & Venema, 2000).

The final model was also developed in Europe, by the laboratories of George Macfarlane and Glenn Gibson in the United Kingdom (Macfarlane & Gibson, 1998). It is based on a compartmentalized system for simulating the different parts of the human colon (proximal, transverse and distal). An anaerobic continuous culture system is distributed among the different compartments and simulates the continuity of the colon. Our three-stage system (3S-ECSIM) is strongly inspired by this equipment, and is based on the same principles, except for maintaining anaerobic conditions.

These systems, however, do not integrate the epithelial, neuroendocrine and immune host components, but can include means for simulating bacterial biofilms such as those observed on the colonic epithelium or the food in transit (Macfarlane & Macfarlane, 2007).

Core Medium		Trace elements solution 1 mL per L of core medium		Vitamin solution 1 mL per L of core medium	
Elements	g.L^{-1}	Elements	mg.L^{-1}	Elements	mg.L^{-1}
Mucin	4.0	$MnSO_4. 2H_2O$	500	Menadione	1
Starch	5.0	$FeSO_4. 7H_2O$	100	d-biotin	2
Pectin	2.0				
Guar gum	1.0	$CoSO_4$	100	Pantothenate	10
Xylan	2.0	$ZnSO_4$	100	Nicotinamide	5
Arabinogalactan	2.0				
Inulin	1.0	$CuSO_4. 5H_2O$	10	Vitamin B$_{12}$	0.5
Cystein	0.8	$AlK(SO_4)$	10	Thiamin	4
Casein	3.0				
Peptone	5.0	H_3BO_3	10		
Tryptone	5.0	$Na_2MoO_4. 2H_2O$	10	*para*-aminobenzoic	5
Yeast extract	4.5			acid	
Bile salts	0.4	$NiCl_2. 6H_2O$	100		
Tween 80	1.0	Na_2SeO_3	10		
$Fe_2SO_4. 7H_2O$	0.005				
NaCl	4.5				
KCl	4.5				
KH_2PO_4	0.5				
$MgSO_4. 7H_2O$	1.25				
$CaCl_2. 6H_2O$	0.15				
$NaHCO_3$	1.5				
Hemin	0.05				
pH adjusted to 6.0					

Table 2. Composition of the artificial gut medium

This medium is derived from those previously described (Macfarlane et al., 1998; Molly et al., 1993) and is a mix of three solutions: a trace elements solution, a vitamin solution (1 mL of each for 1 L of artificial gut medium) and the core-medium.

3.2 General description of the ECSIM systems

To complete these *in-vitro* systems, we have developed our own infrastructure to simulate the human colon, with the goal of having a modular system for maintaining a human microbiota in similar environmental conditions to those encountered physiologically and pathologically in the human gut. This system was developed with the technical support of Global Process Concept (France, see www.gpcbio.com for more information). It consists of three bioreactors which can operate independently, but also may be associated (see the next chapter 3.3). It is possible to supply each bioreactor with an identical nutritive medium from a unique tank or to supply each with a different medium. The usual medium faithfully replicates the contents of the terminal ileum from an individual with a Western diet, as described by several groups (Macfarlane et al., 1998; Molly et al., 1993). This basal medium is shown in Table 2. If required, it can be modified to simulate other systems or to simulate specific cases, such as the uptake of prebiotics, the excessive presence of protein residues due to poor hydrolysis/absorption in the anterior parts, or an excess of bile acids, ...

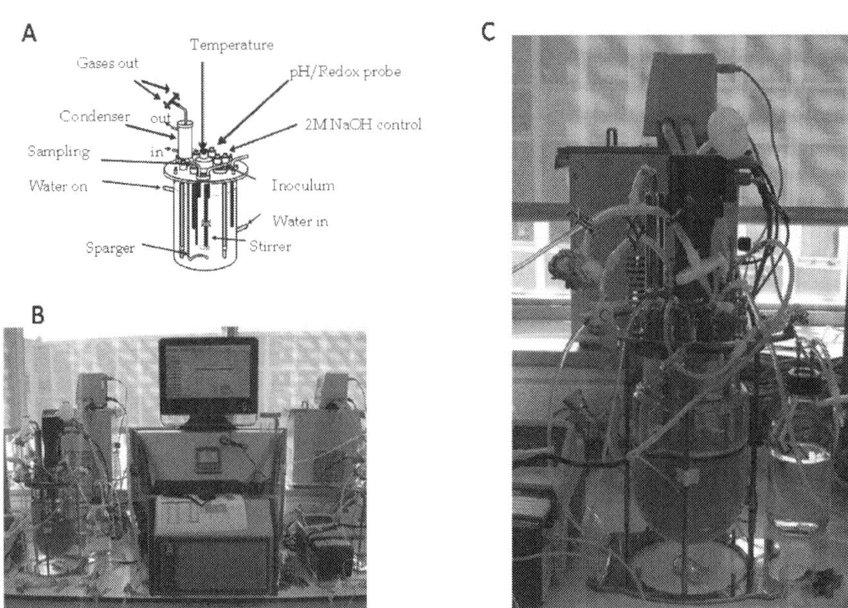

Fig. 3. Description of one module of the ECSIM, a GPC™ bioreactor.
A- Schematic representation of the tank and connections. B- General view of the complete module, command system and the heating/cooling water system (behind).
C- Detailed view of the bioreactor.

Each modular system is based on a bioreactor that can operate autonomously if necessary (Figure 3). Each bioreactor is composed of a tank and an upper plate. The 2-L tank is made from borosilicated glass, mounted on a removable stainless steel frame. Its minimum useful volume is 0.5 L, however, it is used in all our different ECSIM variants with a volume of 1L. The tank has a jacket permitting the circulation of water from its own heating module (tank with electric heater and circulating pump) to maintain the temperature of the culture. The top plate (stainless steel) has various ports and accessories allowing the use of an agitation motor, an aeration at the tank bottom through a removable sparger, and a gas outlet equipped with a stainless steel condenser (for a max flow of 15 L/min) with an expansion chamber and internal coil for circulating cold water. The stirring inside the tank is made in a pendular motion using a Rushton turbine and a marine propeller (each with a diameter of 60 mm) with adjustable height on the stirrer shaft. The system incorporates a temperature sensor, pH electrode, redox electrode, a liquid level or foam (modular) sensor, and an injection input for pH correction (which can be used for the substrate). The plate has a sterile sampling device for sterile medium inoculation, addition and sampling. Each bioreactor has its own control terminal connected to a PC via an Ethernet cable. Dedicated software is used to control the stirring speed (variable from 40 to 1000 rpm), temperature, pH, ORP and the level regulations and measurements. In parallel, the terminal controls four peristaltic pumps (to ensure the addition of nutrient solutions, neutralizing solutions and tests) and valves to automatically control the gas flow. The dedicated software (using Windows™) allows a hierarchical control of experiments (4 levels), ranging from single view measurement tables in real time without the possibility of intervention through access, to full functionality (detailed configuration and complete opportunity to exit the software and turned off the set).

3.3 Coupling/associating ECSIMs to generate other *in vitro* systems

The following describes the use of ECSIM as a chemostat, although sometimes it may be (and is) used for batch cultures. One of the advantages of the ECSIM system is its modularity which allows a variety of different applications using the same components. Our approach consists of three initial modules which can produce three different scenarios depending on their settings (Figure 4). The first case considers these three systems as being totally independent, with each bioreactor having its own experiment controls (left, Figure 4).

This approach provides rapid responses to various issues. If the effect of a component (biotic or abiotic) on the particular microbiota of different individuals has to be addressed, each bioreactor is inoculated with a particular microbiota, and as experimental conditions are identical, the incubation medium is shared between the different systems. If the experiment concerns the dose-effect or formulation of a compound, each bioreactor is started with strictly identical conditions (culture medium, inoculum, pH,…), with each bioreactor pump providing a controlled release of different amounts of the compound from the same stock solution. Other alternatives can be implemented using the same principle. In these cases, the proper control of each bioreactor is provided by a comparison test carried out before, between and after any modification is made. Controls are sampled after obtaining stability, which is considered acceptable after at least 5-times the retention time of the medium in the bioreactor. The experimental measurements are then retrieved either kinetically, during the addition (progressive or not) of the compound, or after re-obtaining a new state of equilibrium, or both. The results can be complementary and depend on the desired information, the disruption of the system itself (specific metabolites of this phase, responsible mechanisms, …) or the final long-term effect of waiting for the new induced equilibrium.

It is possible that the extreme sensitivity of these systems limits the comparisons which can be made between the different bioreactors and experiments. The apparatus, however, is designed to severely limit any technical disruption when working on the bioreactor (especially sampling). Another possible problem is confirming that the observed effect in a test does not result from a deviation of the system over time, independently from the test being performed. The realisation of a witness test and two bioreactor tests (see Figure 4, centre diagram) overcomes this problem by performing a co-inoculation of the three systems at T0, and by comparing these different samples for each bioreactor at different times (during the supposed equilibrium phase in the control, during the disturbance conducted in parallel on two bioreactors, during the equilibrium phase resulting from the disturbance, …).

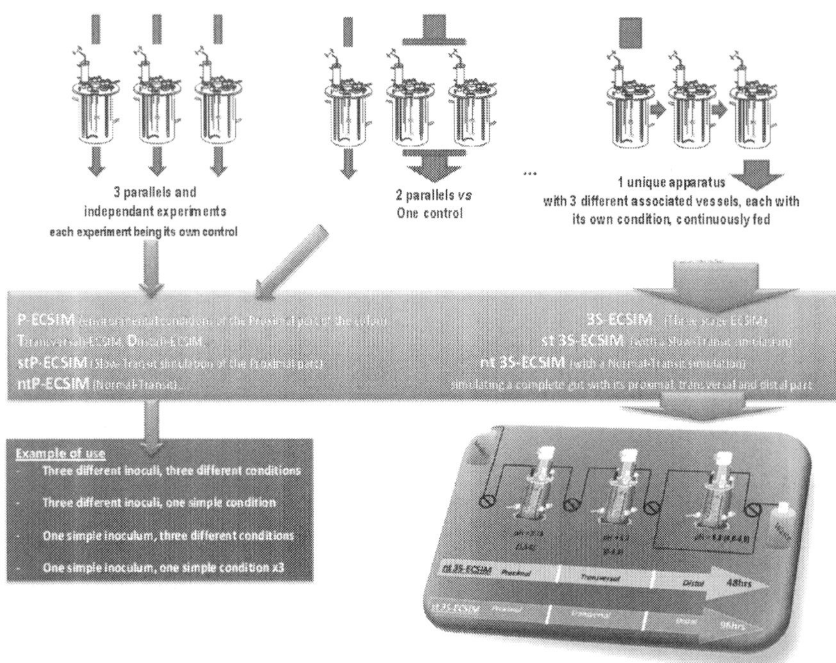

Fig. 4. The ECSIM paradigm: the modular components allow various organizations and various applications with identical elements from Global Process Concept.

Finally, the modularity of the system can be broken down as a grouping of bioreactors, ensuring continuity in the transition from a medium (and microbiota) from a medium stock, to a first bioreactor, then to a second, up to a third. The advantage of this system is the ability to modify the experimental conditions in each of the bioreactors. In all cases the experimental periods are long, extending up to several days in the last case presented. The duration time of a system disruption, therefore, is usually limited to a few seconds for a single injection, or a few hours for an incremental change. The need to obtain a steady state requiring incubation times equal at least to 5 residence times, however, may lead to long experiment times. For example, if we consider that a basic transit-time in the colon is 48 hours (nt, normal transit), and the length of the proximal colon being about 26% of the entire colon (vs 37% for each other of transverse and distal parts), we obtain around 13 hours of transit, only in the proximal part (Table 3). Therefore, a delay of 65 hours (nearly 3 days) is needed to reach a stabilised state. Furthermore, the transit time should be increased to nearly 18 hours in a transverse or a distal compartment, leading to a delay of 90 hours (almost four days) to obtain a steady state. Finally, the delay for two steady states separated by a disturbance (obtaining the first steady state/disturbance/result at stabilization) is, therefore, about a week for an experiment conducted in ntP-ECSIM (normal transit Proximal-ECSIM) and is two weeks for an experiment conducted in stP-ECSIM (slow transit Proximal-ECSIM, simulating a slow transit time of 96 hours for the colon).

When placed in a continuous 3-stage system (3S-ECSIM) to replicate the entire colon in these three functional parts, the completion time of the experiment increases accordingly, each state is expected to be stabilized individually and progressively. For example to simulate a 48-hours transit time, 10 days are needed to get a steady state in the last compartment (the distal part), and, as previously mentioned, the system was already stable in the first bioreactor (simulated proximal part) after 3 days. Therefore, if the effect of a disturbance is studied on the balance of the microbiota, the experiment will take approximately 20 days.

Another consequence would be the minimum doubling time that any microorganism must have to be kept in the reactor. If the time is greater than this minimal value, the microorganism will not be kept in the bioreactor but will be lost through the dilution effect. Table 3 indicates these values for of our system for various cases.

The working volume of each reactor is maintained at 1 L in order to lower the disturbance of the system by the sample intake itself. This means, however, that about 2 L of medium is needed to feed one chemostat bioreactor per day for a normal transit time simulation: either a P-ECSIM alone or a 3S-ECSIM composed of three vessels. This volume is naturally reduced twice while increasing the simulated transit time to a 96-hour simulation (Table 3).

Residence Time (h)	Dilution Rate[1] (h⁻¹)	Feed rate[2] (vol=1L) (mL.min⁻¹)	Medium (L per days)	Minimum doubling time[3] (h)
A-Simulation of a 48-h transit time (nt)				
12.48	0.0801	1.3355	1.9231	8.65
17.76	0.0563	0.9384	1.3514	12.31
17.76	0.0563	0.9384	1.3514	12.31
B-Simulation of a 96-h transit time (st)				
24.96	0.0401	0.6677	0.9615	17.30
35.52	0.0282	0.4692	0.6757	24.62
35.52	0.0282	0.4692	0.6757	24.62

[1]the dilution rate is calculated as the inverse of the residence time.
[2]in this case, the feed rate corresponds directly to the dilution rate, due to the 1-L volume.
[3]the minimum doubling time corresponds to the minimum period in which a microorganism should divide, in order to not be washed by dilution effect: obtained by dividing ln2 by the dilution rate.

Table 3. Characteristics of the dilution rate, feed rate, volume of media needed and the minimal doubling time for simulating the indicated residence time. A working volume of 1L in each vessel, in order to simulate a normal transit time (A, 48h) or a slow transit time (B, 96h).

3.4 Coupling/associating analytical systems

The ECSIM system is actually a very powerful sample generator because of the different controls it can perform. It can test the metabolic activity of microbiota in realistic terms, influenced by typical environmental constraints which may be encountered in humans, whether physiological or pathological or concerning functional, nutritional or other situations. It provides *in vitro* testing of the impact of a living, or an abiotic element, on the constitution and metabolism of a microbiota. It is a valuable tool, but has little or no interest if it is not coupled with an analytical infrastructure, particularly concerning the microbial, biochemical and molecular fields. Figure 5 shows what we feel to be the most important analyses.

Firstly, the analytical platform has to establish a quick inventory of the main microbiological and biochemical components. Classic microbiology, despite its limitations, especially in this particular anaerobic ecosystem, remains of great help in identifying and enumerating total anaerobes, facultative anaerobes, and functional groups and/or some genus (bifidobacteria, lactobacilli, *Bacteroides* spp,...).

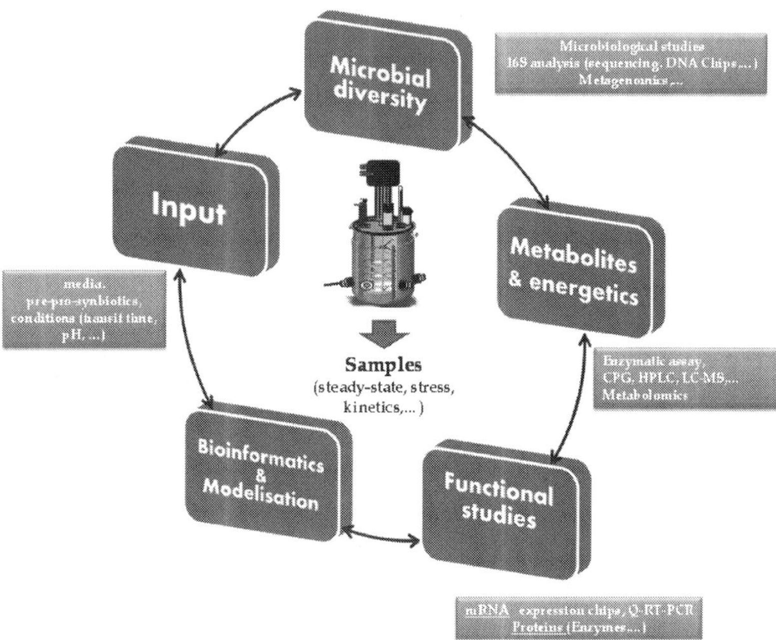

Fig. 5. Example of some analyses and their use to address questions about the gut biology from experiments developed from the ECSIM.

Anaerobic microbiology is technically easier when an anaerobic chamber is used. From a biochemical point of view, special importance is given to nutritional compounds (sugars, lipid and total proteins assays) and also to the major metabolites, such as those issuing from the fermentation process: gases (H_2, CO_2 , H_2S, ...), lactic acid and short chain fatty acids. Gases can be detected and quantified using several methodologies, including Gas Chromatography (GC), and the other elements mainly by High Precision Liquid Chromatography (HPLC). If these elements are essentials, however, other more global approaches are now possible which provide a wealth of consistent information about microbial metabolites and microbes. At the metabolic level, therefore, a metabolomic approach will determine real metabolic identity cards before and after the testing, associated clearly with identified microbial populations.

Working with the platform "exploration du metabolism" from the Clermont-Theix INRA centre (the French National Institute for Agronomic Research), we can already identify metabolic fingerprints and compare experiences between two situations (Feria-Gervasio et al., 2010). Using the same principle, global (comprehensive) approaches for determining microbial diversity are also in progress. For reasons of cost and speed, it uses an approach giving a more informational fingerprint. We usually perform the RISA techniques (ribosomal intergenic spacer analysis, (Cardinale et al., 2004)) in order to obtain comparable fingerprint samples: Figure 6 shows an example. When necessary, rather than using pyrosequencing analysis of 16S rDNA banks, we use a phylogenetic DNA microarray called HuITMiCHIP. This biochip, which is presently being validated, was developed in collaboration with the laboratory of Pr Pierre Peyret (GIIM, UMR UBP-CNRS 6023, Clermont-Ferrand). It has about 5,000 specific oligonucleotides probes designed for detecting 67 bacterial families present in the human GIT. Depending on the method used, it provides a thorough determination of diversity associated with a semi-quantitative evaluation of populations (William Tottey, personal communication). The most interesting data can then be verified by quantitative PCR tools. In the near future we hope to be able to associate metabolic and microbial diversity data to expression analysis concerning quantitative changes of bacterial mRNAs expression, when studying an induced metabolic disturbance (Figure 5).

As a general example, Figure 6 shows an experiment conducted with P-ECSIM studying the impact of transit time on the nature and metabolism of the microbiota. The experiment was initiated from a faecal slurry at 20% (w/v) cultured at 37° C in several successive anaerobic batch with the colonic medium (Table 2), and then stored at -20°C as aliquots at 20% glycerol (v/v). One of these aliquots was unfrozen on ice and used to inoculate a preculture of 5 mL of artificial gut medium, grown at 37°C for 10 hours. It was then transferred for 15 hours into a 1L Erlenmeyer flask containing 95 mL of artificial gut medium. This was then transferred into 900 mL of complete artificial gut medium in two stirred 2-L tank bioreactors, previously N_2-flushed, for a 24-hour batch culture. A continuous cultivation was subsequently launched in parallel in the two bioreactors. The initial dilution rate was of D=0.08 h^{-1}, followed by D=0.04 h^{-1} (Figure 6-A). A dilution rate of 0.08 h^{-1} simulates a transit time in the proximal colon equivalent to 12.5 hours, *i.e.* a colonic transit time of about 48 hours, which is considered normal (ntP-ECSIM, normal transit time Proximal-ECSIM) (see Table 3). Conversely, a dilution rate of 0.04 h^{-1} simulates a slow colonic transit time in proximal condition, approximately 25 hours (stP-ECSIM, slow transit time Proximal ECSIM), equivalent to a global gut transit of 96 hours. Controlling the pump allows for deceleration and acceleration (α=0.0025 h^{-1}), providing a gradual change from one state to another in a few hours. The C-BIO (Global Process Concept inc., France) acquisition and control software was used to adjust the stirring rate at 400 rpm, maintain the temperature at 37° C, and the pH at 5.75 by automatic addition of NaOH. The ORP was monitored every 5 minutes using an Argenthal reference probe from Mettler Toledo (3253i/SG/225 Inpro® probe). Samples were taken over each steady state, mimicking either a normal transit (nt, states 1 and 3) or a slow transit (st, state 2). As presented in Figure 6-B and C, the microbial metabolism and its diversity were affected by this modification of retention time (Feria-Gervasio et al., 2010). The part B highlights the variation of the diversity of the microbiota using the RISA (Ribosomal Intergenic Spacer Amplification). This technique (Cardinale et al. 2004) provides a rapid comparison of conserved and modified patterns. In Figure 6-C, a PCA (Principal Components Analysis) is shown, deduced from the metabolomic data retrieved from the LC-MS analysis. It indicates that the samples may all be differentiated by their origins, either the raw artificial gut medium, the ntP or the stP- ECSIM (E Pujos, JF Martin and JL Sebedio, personal communication). These results also indicate that there are fewer differences among samples from the same steady-state, highlighting the real stability of the so-called steady-state. Moreover, they also indicate that results are very similar between reactors used in the same conditions.

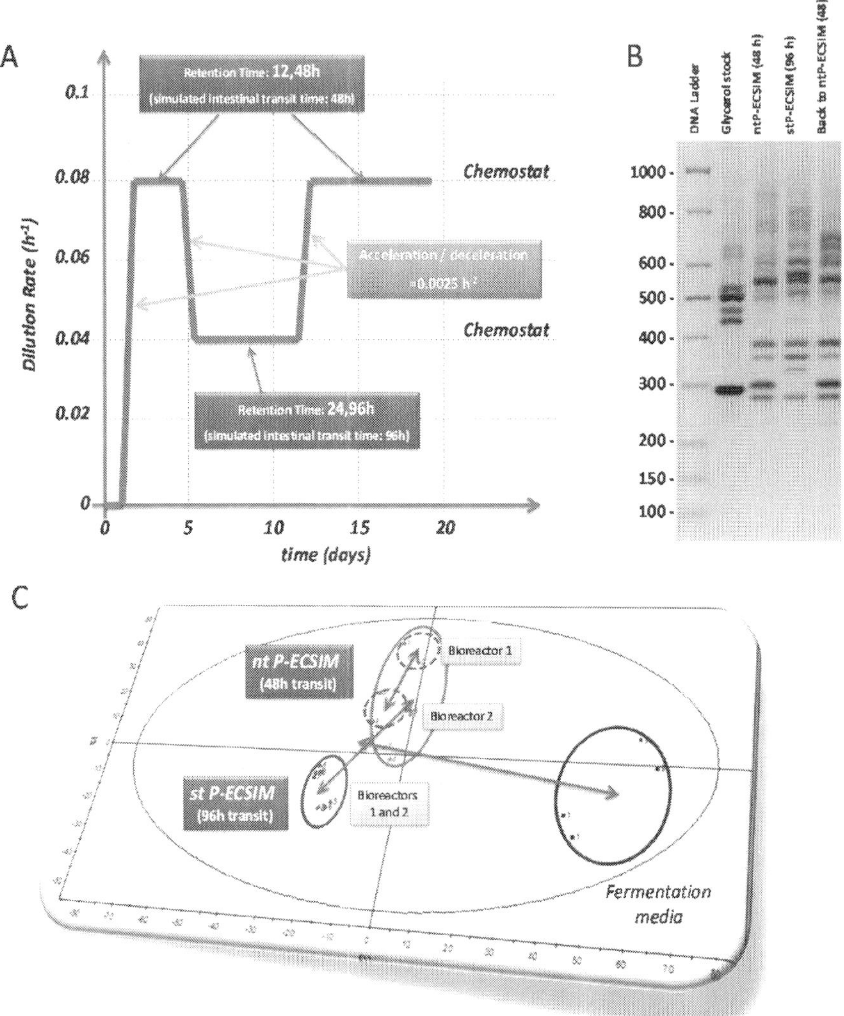

Fig. 6. An example of the use of the ECSIM system: an experiment in P-ECSIM addressing the question of effect of the transit time on the microbial diversity and its metabolism. A- Design of the experiment, with the modulation of the dilution rate in order to simulate a normal (nt P-ECSIM, 48h) or a slow (st P-ECSIM, 96h) transit in the proximal part of the colon.B- Fingerprints obtained from the RISA experiments, showing the impact of the retention time (i.e. the transit time) on the proximal gut microbiota studied in P-ECSIM. C- PCA analysis of the metabolites detected by LC-MS (courtesy of E Pujos, JF Martin and JL Sebedio), highlighting the different metabolic status when changing the residence time, and the similar metabolic fingerprint obtained with two different bioreactors in the same conditions.

4. Conclusion

Studying the role of human microbiota in the digestive tract remains difficult because of various technical and ethical problems, however, in-vitro systems may overcome some of them. We have shown that the ECSIM system proposes a modular and adaptable solution when focusing only on the metabolic behaviour of the microbiota per se, without addressing its cellular and metabolic interaction with the host. The system can be seeded by a faecal microbiota, even to simulate a proximal part, or the whole 3 parts, making it easier technically and ethically throughout the experimentation.

The ECSIM system also helps to mitigate the causes of fluctuations among experiments, due to strict control of parameters. It, therefore, provides an effective means of helping us better understand the role of the human intestinal microbiota, and the role and fate of endogenous and exogenous factors (physico-chemical, nutrients, prebiotics, probiotics, synbiotics, ...). The future development of in-vitro systems, including human intestinal cells (epithelial, immune cells), would be of very great interest, but for the time being remains too technically difficult to undertake. This kind of apparatus, therefore, may also provide a means for safely producing a human microbiota to be reintroduced into a human GIT. This process could be of great interest for several pathologies (for example, Clostridium difficile diarrhoea), using a faecal bacteriotherapy (Bakken, 2009; Borody et al., 2004) provided by a specially designed in vitro production system.

5. Acknowledgement

The authors would like to thank Global Process Concept for their technical help in the development of the ECSIM project, as well as all the people of the ERT-CIDAM laboratory, particularly Claire Ardaens and Céline Vidal for their help with the technical manipulations. Part of this work is supported by a postdoctoral scholarship support to David Féria-Gervasio from the European Union (UE) and the Auvergne Council (FEDER). We also want to thank Pascal Vandekerckove from Lesaffre S.A. for help in the development of some probiotics tests.

6. References

Backhed, F., Ding, H., Wang, T., Hooper, L. V., Koh, G. Y., Nagy, A., et al. (2004). The gut microbiota as an environmental factor that regulates fat storage. *Proc Natl Acad Sci U S A, 101*(44), 15718-15723.

Bakken, J. S. (2009). Fecal bacteriotherapy for recurrent Clostridium difficile infection. *Anaerobe, 15*(6), 285-289.

Bernalier-Donadille, A. (2010). [Fermentative metabolism by the human gut microbiota]. *Gastroenterol Clin Biol, 34 Suppl 1*, S16-22.

Borody, T. J., Warren, E. F., Leis, S. M., Surace, R., Ashman, O., & Siarakas, S. (2004). Bacteriotherapy using fecal flora: toying with human motions. *J Clin Gastroenterol, 38*(6), 475-483.

Boyle, P., & Ferlay, J. (2005). Cancer incidence and mortality in Europe, 2004. *Ann Oncol, 16*(3), 481-488.

Breitbart, M., Hewson, I., Felts, B., Mahaffy, J. M., Nulton, J., Salamon, P., et al. (2003). Metagenomic analyses of an uncultured viral community from human feces. *J Bacteriol, 185*(20), 6220-6223.

Cardinale, M., Brusetti, L., Quatrini, P., Borin, S., Puglia, A. M., Rizzi, A., et al. (2004). Comparison of different primer sets for use in automated ribosomal intergenic spacer analysis of complex bacterial communities. *Appl Environ Microbiol, 70*(10), 6147-6156.

Claesson, M. J., & O'Toole, P. W. (2010). Evaluating the latest high-throughput molecular techniques for the exploration of microbial gut communities. *Gut Microbes, 1*(4), 277-278.

Cummings, J. H., & Macfarlane, G. T. (1997). Colonic microflora: nutrition and health. *Nutrition, 13*(5), 476-478.

Eckburg, P. B., Bik, E. M., Bernstein, C. N., Purdom, E., Dethlefsen, L., Sargent, M., et al. (2005). Diversity of the human intestinal microbial flora. *Science, 308*(5728), 1635-1638.

Feria-Gervasio, D., Pujos, E., Mihajlovski, A., Martin, J. F., Sebedio, J. L., Alric, M., et al. (2010, Jun. 22-25, 2010). *A modular continuous fermentation system for simulating the human colon and assessing the metabolic behavior of the microbiota: metabolomic and microbiological validation.* Paper presented at the Gut Microbiology 7th Biennial Meeting, Aberdeen, Scotland.

Frank, D. N., & Pace, N. R. (2008). Gastrointestinal microbiology enters the metagenomics era. *Curr Opin Gastroenterol, 24*(1), 4-10.

Handelsman, J. (2004). Metagenomics: application of genomics to uncultured microorganisms. *Microbiol Mol Biol Rev, 68*(4), 669-685.

Hill, M. J. (1997). Intestinal flora and endogenous vitamin synthesis. *Eur J Cancer Prev, 6 Suppl 1,* S43-45.

Hooper, L. V., & Gordon, J. I. (2001). Commensal host-bacterial relationships in the gut. *Science, 292*(5519), 1115-1118.

Hooper, L. V., Midtvedt, T., & Gordon, J. I. (2002). How host-microbial interactions shape the nutrient environment of the mammalian intestine. *Annu Rev Nutr, 22,* 283-307.

Hooper, L. V., Stappenbeck, T. S., Hong, C. V., & Gordon, J. I. (2003). Angiogenins: a new class of microbicidal proteins involved in innate immunity. *Nat Immunol, 4*(3), 269-273.

Langendijk, P. S., Schut, F., Jansen, G. J., Raangs, G. C., Kamphuis, G. R., Wilkinson, M. H., et al. (1995). Quantitative fluorescence in situ hybridization of Bifidobacterium spp. with genus-specific 16S rRNA-targeted probes and its application in fecal samples. *Appl Environ Microbiol, 61*(8), 3069-3075.

Ley, R. E., Turnbaugh, P. J., Klein, S., & Gordon, J. I. (2006). Microbial ecology: human gut microbes associated with obesity. *Nature, 444*(7122), 1022-1023.

Macfarlane, G. T., & Cummings, J. H. (1991). The colonic flora, fermentation and large bowel digestive function The large intestine: physiology, pathophysiology, disease. In (pp. 51-92). New York: Raven Press.

Macfarlane, G. T., Gibson, G. R., & Cummings, J. H. (1992). Comparison of fermentation reactions in different regions of the human colon. *J Appl Bacteriol, 72*(1), 57-64.

Macfarlane, G. T., & Macfarlane, S. (2007). Models for intestinal fermentation: association between food components, delivery systems, bioavailability and functional interactions in the gut. *Curr Opin Biotechnol, 18*(2), 156-162.

Macfarlane, G. T., Macfarlane, S., & Gibson, G. R. (1998). Validation of a Three-Stage Compound Continuous Culture System for Investigating the Effect of Retention Time on the Ecology and Metabolism of Bacteria in the Human Colon. *Microb Ecol, 35*(2), 180-187.

Mihajlovski, A. (2010). *évaluation de la biodiversité du microbiote méthanogène intestinal humain et influence de l'âge sur sa constitution.* PhD Thesis, Clermont-Université, Clermont-Ferrand.

Mihajlovski, A., Alric, M., & Brugere, J. F. (2008). A putative new order of methanogenic Archaea inhabiting the human gut, as revealed by molecular analyses of the mcrA gene. *Res Microbiol, 159*(7-8), 516-521.

Mihajlovski, A., Doré, J., Levenez, F., Alric, M., & Brugère, J.-F. (2010). Molecular evaluation of the human gut methanogenic archaeal microbiota reveals an age-associated increase of the diversity. *Environ Microbiol Reports, 2*(2), 272-280.

Minekus, M., Smeets-Peeters, M., Bernalier, A., Marol-Bonnin, S., Havenaar, R., Marteau, P., et al. (1999). A computer controlled system to simulate conditions of the large intestine with peristaltic mixing, water absorption and absorption of fermentation products. *Appl. Microb. Biotechn., 53*, 108-114.

Molly, K., Vande Woestyne, M., & Verstraete, W. (1993). Development of a 5-step multi-chamber reactor as a simulation of the human intestinal microbial ecosystem. *Appl Microbiol Biotechnol, 39*(2), 254-258.

Murphy, E. F., Cotter, P. D., Healy, S., Marques, T. M., O'Sullivan, O., Fouhy, F., et al. (2010). Composition and energy harvesting capacity of the gut microbiota: relationship to diet, obesity and time in mouse models. *Gut, 59*(12), 1635-1642.

Oxley, A. P. A., Lanfranconi, M. P., Würdemann, D., Ott, S., Schreiber, S., McGenity, T. J., et al. (2010). Halophilic archaea in the human intestinal mucosa. *Environmental Microbiology, 12*(9), 2398-2410.

Peterson, J., Garges, S., Giovanni, M., McInnes, P., Wang, L., Schloss, J. A., et al. (2009). The NIH Human Microbiome Project. *Genome Res, 19*(12), 2317-2323.

Pharmacopeia, U. S. (2011). < 724 > *Drug release.* Rockville, MD: United States Pharmacopeial Convention, Inc.

Qin, J., Li, R., Raes, J., Arumugam, M., Burgdorf, K. S., Manichanh, C., et al. (2010). A human gut microbial gene catalogue established by metagenomic sequencing. *Nature, 464*(7285), 59-65.

Rajilic-Stojanovic, M., Maathuis, A., Heilig, H. G. H. J., Venema, K., de Vos, W. M., & Smidt, H. (2010). Evaluating the microbial diversity of an in vitro model of the human large intestine by phylogenetic microarray analysis. *Microbiology, 156*(11), 3270-3281.

Rajilic-Stojanovic, M., Smidt, H., & de Vos, W. M. (2007). Diversity of the human gastrointestinal tract microbiota revisited. *Environ Microbiol, 9*(9), 2125-2136.

Relman, D. A., & Falkow, S. (2001). The meaning and impact of the human genome sequence for microbiology. *Trends Microbiol, 9*(5), 206-208.

Samuel, B. S., & Gordon, J. I. (2006). A humanized gnotobiotic mouse model of host-archaeal-bacterial mutualism. *Proc Natl Acad Sci U S A, 103*(26), 10011-10016.

Savage, D. C. (1977). Microbial ecology of the gastrointestinal tract. *Annu Rev Microbiol, 31*, 107-133.

Scanlan, P. D., & Marchesi, J. R. (2008). Micro-eukaryotic diversity of the human distal gut microbiota: qualitative assessment using culture-dependent and -independent analysis of faeces. *ISME J, 2*(12), 1183-1193.

Stappenbeck, T. S., Hooper, L. V., & Gordon, J. I. (2002). Developmental regulation of intestinal angiogenesis by indigenous microbes via Paneth cells. *Proc Natl Acad Sci U S A, 99*(24), 15451-15455.

Strocchi, A., Furne, J. K., Ellis, C. J., & Levitt, M. D. (1991). Competition for hydrogen by human faecal bacteria: evidence for the predominance of methane producing bacteria. *Gut, 32*(12), 1498-1501.

Tap, J., Mondot, S., Levenez, F., Pelletier, E., Caron, C., Furet, J. P., et al. (2009). Towards the human intestinal microbiota phylogenetic core. *Environ Microbiol, 11*(10), 2574-2584.

Tasse, L., Bercovici, J., Pizzut-Serin, S., Robe, P., Tap, J., Klopp, C., et al. (2010). Functional metagenomics to mine the human gut microbiome for dietary fiber catabolic enzymes. *Genome Res, 20*(11), 1605-1612.

Van den Abbeele, P., Grootaert, C., Marzorati, M., Possemiers, S., Verstraete, W., Gerard, P., et al. (2010). Microbial Community Development in a Dynamic Gut Model Is Reproducible, Colon Region Specific, and Selective for Bacteroidetes and Clostridium Cluster IX. *Appl. Environ. Microbiol., 76*(15), 5237-5246.

van der Werf, M. J., & Venema, K. (2000). Bifidobacteria: Genetic Modification and the Study of Their Role in the Colon. *Journal of Agricultural and Food Chemistry, 49*(1), 378-383.

Vrieze, A., Holleman, F., Zoetendal, E. G., de Vos, W. M., Hoekstra, J. B., & Nieuwdorp, M. (2010). The environment within: how gut microbiota may influence metabolism and body composition. *Diabetologia, 53*(4), 606-613.

Woda, A., Mishellany-Dutour, A., Batier, L., Francois, O., Meunier, J. P., Reynaud, B., et al. (2010). Development and validation of a mastication simulator. *J Biomech, 43*(9), 1667-1673.

Zhu, B., Wang, X., & Li, L. (2010). Human gut microbiome: the second genome of human body. *Protein Cell, 1*(8), 718-725.

Zoetendal, E. G., Cheng, B., Koike, S., & Mackie, R. I. (2004). Molecular microbial ecology of the gastrointestinal tract: from phylogeny to function. *Curr Issues Intest Microbiol, 5*(2), 31-47.

5

Prospects for Neuroprosthetics: Flexible Microelectrode Arrays with Polymer Conductors

Axel Blau
Department of Neuroscience and Brain Technologies,
Italian Institute of Technology, Genoa,
Italy

1. Introduction

Neural prostheses are devices that interface with the central or peripheral nervous system. They target at the capture, modulation or elicitation of neural activity, in most cases to record the information flow within a neural pathway for its online or later decoding, or to mimic or replace neural functionality that has been compromised or lost. While in theory any information carrying modality of the neuron could be tapped into (*e.g.*, concentrations of neurotransmitters in the synaptic cleft, of energy carriers such as ATP or glucose, or of ions or oxygen; optical properties; ionic currents; membrane potential), most devices sample or alter the membrane potential (or a proportional quantity[1] thereto). Since the discovery and description of 'body electricity' by Luigi Galvani and Alessandro Volta in their studies on voltage-induced muscle contraction (Volta, 1793), metal electrodes have been used for establishing a bidirectional communication link between electrically excitable cells[2] and stimulation or recording apparatuses. From an engineering point of view, this has always been the least challenging and technologically least demanding approach. It just requires bringing a locally deinsulated conductor into close vicinity of a neuron to capture or induce fluctuations in its surrounding electrical field. Given the multitude of conductive materials to choose from and the ever growing number of technological possibilities for their structuring and processing into any desired shape and arrangement, historically, the interface of choice for neuroprosthetics has become the electrode array despite some of its fundamental conceptional shortcomings[3]. It has evolved into other clinically relevant

---

[1] Theoretically, any physical variable correlated to the membrane potential may be measured or altered. In a static scenario (*e.g.*, resting potential) it could be the electrical field, in a dynamic scenario (*e.g.*, upon de- or repolarization) its fluctuations, the (ionic) current(s) or even changes in the local magnetic field.

[2] Electrogenic cells in animals are neurons, muscle cells, pancreatic α- and β-cells, kidney fibroblasts or electroplaques. Besides the light-induced electron separation process during photosynthesis in plants, some microorganisms and algae are capable of electrogenesis as well (Logan, 2009; Rabaey & Rozendal, 2010).

[3] The electrical field at an electrode site is usually quite distorted due to the non-homogeneity of the biological environment in its vicinity. This does not only complicate signal source analysis in neural recordings, but it also limits the spatial precision with which neurons can be stimulated electrically. Even worse, if an electrical stimulus triggers an action potential in an axon, it may spread in both directions (towards the synaptic arbor and the soma), which is not observed in natural neural activity propagation.

readout derivatives such as electroencephalography (EEG), electromyography (EMG), electrocorticography (ECoG), and electroretinography (ERG). And it is still competitive with technologies making use of different recording or stimulation principles such as magnetic resonance imaging (MRI), magnetoencephalography (MEG), positron emission tomography (PET) or transcranial magnetic stimulation (TMS) (Clark, 1998; Lapitska *et al.*, 2009).

This chapter will review recent design trends for microelectrode arrays (MEAs) with an emphasis on flexible polymer devices, which may be exploited for neuroprosthetics. A brief synopsis on the history of *in vitro* and *in vivo* interfacing concepts with electrogenic cells introduces the chapter, followed by a discussion on their performance and limitations, to then take a look at latest strategies to overcome these limitations by resorting to new concepts, materials, and fabrication and modification processes. The chapter will conclude with the presentation and discussion of an innovative, versatile, and easy fabrication route for turning microchannel scaffolds into all-polymer neuroprosthetic electrode arrays. This strategy bears the potential of implementing a variety of secondary functionalities such as microfluidics, drug release schemes and optical stimulation paradigms, which may be operated in parallel to electrical recording and stimulation.

1.1 *In vitro* microelectrode arrays

To better understand the events at the cell-electrode interface, a variety of MEAs for the *in vitro* study of electrogenic cells have been developed over the past 40 years (Pine, 2006). Because they do not penetrate the cell membrane, they are considered 'noninvasive'. They sample local fluctuations of the electrical field generated by the membrane potential. Thus, any change in membrane potential due to a local and selective flux of specific ions (mostly Na^+ and K^+) across the cell membrane will lead to a capacitively mediated shift of charges in a nearby conductor (Butt *et al.*, 2003) or at the gate of a field effect transistors (FET) (Fromherz *et al.*, 1991; Fromherz, 2006; Poghossian *et al.*, 2009; Lambacher *et al.*, 2011). While FETs are restricted to the sampling of these events, metals or semiconductors can also be used for actively modifying them. By charging the electrodes (or more

---

Abbreviations: A/D, analog-to-digital; AP, action potential; APS, active pixel sensor; ASIC, application specific integrated circuit; CMOS, complementary metal oxide semiconductor; CNT, carbon nanotube; CP, conducting polymer; CPFET, cell-potential field-effect transistor; CSC, charge storage capacity; CT, computer tomography; CV, cyclic voltammetry; D/A, digital-to-analog; DIV, days in vitro; DRIE, deep reactive ion etching; ECoG, electrocorticography; EEG, electroencephalography; EGEFET, extended gate electrode field-effect transistor; EMG, electromyography; EOSFET, electrolyte oxide semiconductor field-effect transistor; ERG, electroretinography; FET, field-effect transistor; GND, ground (electrode); HMDS, hexamethyldisilazane; ITO, indium tin oxide; ISFET, ion-sensitive field-effect transistor; LCP, liquid crystal polymer; LFP, local field potential; LIGA, Lithographie, Galvanoformung, Abformung; MEA, microelectrode array; MEG, magnetoencephalography; MOSFET, metal-oxide-semiconductor field-effect transistor; MRI, magnetic resonance imaging; MTM, metal transfer micromolding; NCAM, neural cell adhesion molecule; NGF, nerve growth factor; NW, nanowire; PDMS, poly(dimethylsiloxane); PEDOT, poly(3,4-ethylenedioxythiophene); PFOCTS, trichloro(1H,1H,2H,2H-perfluorooctyl)silane; PET, positron emission tomography; PI, polyimide, PMMA, poly(methyl methacrylate); PPX, poly(p-xylylenes); PPy, poly(pyrrole); PS, poly(styrene); PTFE, poly(tetrafluoroethylene); PU, poly(urethane); PVA, poly(vinyl alcohol); S/N, signal-to-noise ratio; SAM, self-assembling monolayer; TMS, transcranial magnetic stimulation; VLSI, very-large-scale integration.

generally speaking, the interface), such capacitive shift can thus be imposed onto the cell membrane[5], which leads to a shift in its membrane potential and may result in the opening of voltage-gated ion channels (Bear *et al.*, 2007). Such arrays are used to find physiologically 'meaningful' electrical communication parameters, to study the influence of electrode topography or (bio-)chemical functionalization on cellular events, and to characterize the physiologically induced changes of such interface over time. In most cases, they are compatible with a majority of microscopy techniques for simultaneous morphology studies or the optical screening of membrane potential-associated variables (*e.g.*, by potential sensitive dyes or by imaging intrinsic changes of the optical properties of a cell, *e.g.*, its refractive index) or activity-associated events (*e.g.*, by calcium imaging). They are furthermore accessible to manipulation techniques such as drug delivery in pharmacological and toxicity assays (Gross *et al.*, 1997; Johnstone *et al.*, 2010), mechanical or laser microdissection in regeneration studies, or optical tweezers for biomechanical manipulation and force spectroscopy (Difato *et al.*, 2011). While an *in vitro* system may not truthfully reproduce the conditions of an *in vivo* environment and the events therein, MEAs have nevertheless been widely adopted for screening studies. They have become a tool and test bed for better understanding the design requirements (*e.g.*, material properties, coatings) of neural probes. Table 1 lists pioneering works and currently active groups or companies that have developed or commercialized key MEA technologies. Light-addressable devices were omitted (Bucher *et al.*, 2001; Stein *et al.*, 2004; Starovoytov *et al.*, 2005; Suzurikawa *et al.*, 2006). The terminology 'passive devices' refers to substrates with microelectrodes, tracks and connection pads that need to be connected to external amplification and signal processing hardware. 'Active devices' carry some of these electronics on-chip (Hierlemann *et al.*, 2011). In 'hybrid' devices, MEAs and signal conditioning electronics are produced separately but packaged together into a standalone device. They can furthermore include other types of electrochemical sensors on-chip (*e.g.*, for temperature, oxygen, pH, impedance, ...).

'Passive' MEAs	# of electr. R: recording S: stimulation	Device type and electrode materials
C.A. Thomas et al.	30	Two rows of 7 μm^2 electroplated Pt on Au/Ni electrodes on glass, insulated by photoresist (Thomas *et al.*, 1972)
G. Gross et al.	36 R,S 64 R,S	Ø 10 μm Au-coated ITO tracks on glass, insulated with a thermosetting polymer (Gross *et al.*, 1977; Gross *et al.*, 1985)
J. Pine	32 R,S	Two rows of sixteen 10 μm^2 electrodeposited Pt electrodes on Au tracks on glass, insulated by SiO_2 (Pine, 1980)

---

[5] The lipid double layer, which constitutes the cell membrane, can be considered a dielectric. The membrane thus acts as a capacitor that has no metal plates. Nevertheless, ions from the intra- and extracellular environments just accumulate at the (at physiological pH) negatively charged hydrophilic headgroups of the phospholipids at both sides of the membrane. If, as for most cells, the intra- and extracellular ionic compositions are different, a potential will build up across the membrane. As with any interface, the distribution of ions will very likely not be homogeneous but, to a first approximation, resemble a Helmholtz layer (Butt *et al.*, 2003). Thus, any additional charges (such as those at the surface of a metal electrode), which create an electrical field gradient in the vicinity of the membrane, will lead to a reorganization of these two electric double layers. Due to the difference in their distances from the electrode, this reorganization will affect the intracellular membrane interface less strongly than the extracellular membrane interface.

'Passive' MEAs (continued)	# of electr. R: recording S: stimulation	Device type and electrode materials
D.A. Israel D.J. Edell R.G. Mark et al.	25 R + 6 S	15 x 15 µm^2 electroplatinized, e-beam evaporated Au on Cr recording electrodes and 40 x 40 to 120 x 120 µm^2 stimulation electrodes on a Ø 40 mm glass coverslip, insulated by photoresist. Ultrasonically welded Au wires Ø 76 µm connection to miniature connector (Israel *et al.*, 1984)
J. Novac S.A. Boppart K. Musick B.C. Wheeler et al.	32 R,S 32 R,(S) 58 R,S	Ø 10 (25) µm Au/Ti on glass electrodes insulated by polyimide (Novak & Wheeler, 1986; Novak & Wheeler, 1988; Musick *et al.*, 2009) Ø 13 and 15 µm electroplatinized Au/Ti electrodes on perforated polyimide, insulated by polyimide (Boppart *et al.*, 1992) Ø 25 µm Au/Ti electrodes on SU-8 above microfluidic PDMS channels on glass (Musick *et al.*, 2009)
P. Connolly L.J. Breckenridge R.J. Wilson M. Sandison A. Curtis C.D.W. Wilkinson et al.	64 R,S	10 x 10 µm^2 or Ø 25 - 30 µm electroplatinized Au on NiCr electrodes on 125 µm thick polyimide insulated by polyimide (Connolly *et al.*, 1990; Breckenridge *et al.*, 1995; Sandison *et al.*, 2002)
Multi Channel Systems & NMI H. Hämmerle M. Janders J. Held A. Stett W. Nisch et al.	24, 36, 72 R,S flex 54, 60 R,S 32 R+12 S 256 R,S 60 R,S (3D)	Ti (or Au/Cr) tracks with TiN- or Pt- coated electrodes (usually Ø 10 or 30 µm) on glass or Au or Ti tracks with Au or TiN electrodes on (perforated) polyimide insulated by Si$_3$N$_4$ or polyimide (Haemmerle *et al.*, 1994; Nisch *et al.*, 1994; Janders *et al.*, 1996; Fejtl *et al.*, 2006) TiN-coated Ø 30 µm, 10 – 50 µm high electrodeposited Au/Ti pillar electrodes on glass insulated by Si$_3$N$_4$ (Held, Heynen, *et al.*, 2010)
P. Thiébaud Y. Dupont L. Stoppini et al.	6 R 34 R,(S) (3D)	10 x 10 µm^2 Pt on Ta electrodes with electroplated Pt (Ø 35 µm) on a perforated Si/SiO$_2$/Si$_3$N$_4$ substrate insulated by Si$_3$N$_4$ (Thiébaud *et al.*, 1997) 47 µm high, 15 µm exposed vapor-deposited Pt-tip on Ta electrodes on a porous (35%) Si substrate insulated by Si$_3$N$_4$ (Thiebaud *et al.*, 1999)
D. Hakkoum S. Duport D. Muller P. Corrèges L. Stoppini et al.	30 R,S 28 R,S	1.3 – 3.2 mm long, 15 µm wide Au/Cu on perforated polyimide (Upilex/Kapton) film (Stoppini *et al.*, 1997) 50 x 100 µm^2 electroplated Au on Cu/Ni on polyimide (Kapton$^®$) with 5 perfusion holes (Duport *et al.*, 1999)
Y. Jimbo A. Kawana	64 R,S	Electroplated Pt-black on 50 x 50 µm^2 ITO tracks on glass insulated by a silicone photoresist (Kawana & Jimbo, 1999)
Alpha MED Scientific H. Oka M. Taketani et al.	64 R,S	50 x 50 µm^2 Au/Ni or 20 x 20 µm^2, 50 x 50 µm^2 or Ø 50 to 70 µm electrodeposited Pt-black electrodes on ITO tracks on a glass carrier insulated by polyimide or polyacrylamide (Oka *et al.*, 1999)
Ayanda Biosystems M. Heuschkel et al.	60 R,S (3D)	Pt, Au or ITO tracks with Pt or Au electrodes on glass; spike-shaped electrodes are available; SU-8 insulator (Heuschkel *et al.*, 2002; Heuschkel *et al.*, 2006)
C.D. James J.N. Turner et al.	124 R	24 x 5 + 4 electroplatinized Au/Ti electrodes (Ø < 10 µm) on fused silica wafer with SiO$_2$/Si$_3$N$_4$/SiO$_2$ insulation stack (James *et al.*, 2004)
F. Morin Y. Takamura E. Tamiya et al.	64	50 x 50 µm^2 Au/Cr electrodes on glass, insulated by "spin-on-glass" or photopatternable silicone (Morin *et al.*, 2005; Morin *et al.*, 2006)
L. Berdondini et al.	60 R,S	Ø 22 – 30 µm vapor-deposited Pt/Ti on Pyrex glass or Si, insulated by Si$_3$N$_4$; some are spatially partitioned by 5 interconnected clustering wells (Ø 3 mm in SU-8) (Berdondini *et al.*, 2006; Berdondini, Massobrio, *et al.*, 2009)
G. Gholmieh T.W. Berger et al.	39R+49S 60 R 64 R	ITO tracks with Ø 28 - 36 µm or 36 x 36 µm^2 Au- or Pt-coated electrodes on glass in a tissue-"conformal" arrangement, insulated by Si$_3$N$_4$ or SU-8 (Gholmieh *et al.*, 2006)

'Passive' MEAs (continued)	# of electr. R: recording S: stimulation	Device type and electrode materials
L. Giovangrandi G.T.A. Kovacs et al.	36 R,S	Ø 75 or 100 µm electroless Au-plated Ni/Cu electrodes on polyimide (Kapton®) insulated by an acrylic adhesive and polyimide (Giovangrandi et al., 2006)
S. Rajaraman M.G. Allen et al.	12 – 13 R (3D) + 25 R (spike, 3D) + 25 R (planar)	Laser scribed, electroplated Ni/Cu/Pt-black electrodes (Ø < 10 µm) on a SU-8 microtower (fluidic) structure (< 500 µm height) on perforated fused silica insulated by parylene (Rajaraman et al., 2007) 300 – 500 µm high, Ø 50 µm Au/Cr spike-tip or Ø 50 µm Au planar electrodes through metal transfer micromolding (MTM) in PDMS on SU-8, PMMA, or PU carrier with parylene insulator either selectively laser- and globally RIE- (CHF$_3$/O$_2$ plasma) deinsulated at the electrode sites, or applied during "capping protection" of the electrode sites. Pt-black plating (Rajaraman et al., 2011)
J. Held O. Paul et al.	64 S,R	Pt/TiW on < 10 µm high, µm Ø Ag or sub-µm Ø Si (electroporation) microneedles on Si insulated by Si$_3$N$_4$ (Held et al., 2008; Held, Gaspar, et al., 2010)
S. Eick B. Hofmann A. Offenhäusser B. Wolfrum et al.	64 R,(S) 30 R,(S)	Ø 10 – 100 µm Au/Ti electrodes on glass sputtered with IrO$_x$ with SiO$_2$, Si$_3$N$_4$, SiO$_2$ insulation sandwich (Eick et al., 2009) Ø 3-5 µm apertures above Au/Ti electrodes on Si/SiO$_2$ with a SiO$_2$, Si$_3$N$_4$ insulator stack (Hofmann et al., 2011)
G. Gabriel M. Bongard E. Fernandez R. Villa et al.	16 or 54 R,(S) + 2 GND	Drop cast CNT-decorated Ø 30 - 40 µm Pt/Ti recording and 2500 µm x 1000 µm GND electrodes (hexagonally arranged) on glass insulated by SiO$_2$, Si$_3$N$_4$ (Gabriel et al., 2009; Bongard et al., 2010)
A. Hai J. Shappir M. Spira et al.	62 R (3D)	Spine-shaped gold protrusions, electroplated on patterned Cu on glass, insulated by a SiC/Si$_3$N$_4$/SiO$_2$ stack (Hai et al., 2009; Hai et al., 2010)
F.T. Jaber F.H. Labeeda M.P. Hughes	16	40 x 40 µm^2 Au/Ti electrodes on glass and 20 x 20 µm^2 SU-8 microwells and interconnecting micro-trenches; SU-8 insulation layer (Jaber et al., 2009)
P. Wei P. Ziaie et al.	4 - 16 (R),S	Ø 250 µm Au-coated nail-head pins and liquid Ga/In (75.5/24.5) tracks in PDMS microchannels (Wei et al., 2009; Ziaie, 2009)
Axion BioSystems J. Ross M.G. Allen B. Wheeler et al.	64 R,S + 2 S (6 - 768 R,S)	Ø 30 µm Pt-black or Au/Ti electrodes on glass insulated by SU-8 or SiO$_2$ (Ross et al., 2010)
P.J. Koester S.M. Buehler W. Baumann J. Gimsa et al.	52 R + 2 GND	Ø 35 µm Pt electrodes with interdigitated electrodes and PT1000 T sensor on glass insulated by Si$_3$N$_4$ (Koester et al., 2010)
S.P. Lacour E. Tarte B. Morrison III et al.	20 R,S	30-75 x 100 µm^2 Au/Cr electrodes on deformable polyimide or PDMS with photo-patternable polyimide or PDMS insulator (Lacour et al., 2010)
T. Ryynänen J. Lekkala et al.	60 R,(S)	Ø 30 µm Ti electrodes on glass insulated by polystyrene (PS) on hexamethyldisilazane (HMDS) (Ryynänen et al., 2010)
W. Tonomura Y. Jimbo S. Konishi et al.	64 R	Electroplated Pt-black on Ø 30 µm Pt/Ti electrodes with Ø 5 or 10 µm substrate through-holes on backside-thinned Si/SiO$_2$ carrier with microchannels insulated by parylene-C (Tonomura et al., 2010)
'Active' MEAs	# of electr. R: recording S: stimulation	Device type and electrode materials
A. Offenhäusser W. Knoll et al.	16 R 64 R	28 x 12 µm^2 and 10 x 4 µm^2 p-channel electrolyte oxide semiconductor FETs (EOSFETs) or Ø 30 - 60 µm extended gate electrode FETs (EGEFETs) insulated by Si$_3$N$_4$ (Offenhäusser et al., 1997; Offenhäusser & Knoll, 2001)

'Active' MEAs (continued)	# of electr. R: recording S: stimulation	Device type and electrode materials
B.D. DeBusschere G.T.A. Kovacs	128 R	2 x 4 arrays of 16 Ø 10 µm Au/TiW/Al electrodes on CMOS IC, insulated by Si_3N_4 (Debusschere & Kovacs, 2001)
P. Bonifazi M. Hutzler A. Lambacher P. Fromherz et al.	4 - 16,384 R	Electrolyte-oxide semiconductor field-effect transistors (EOSFETs) with Ø 4.5 µm charge-sensitive spots at a density of $16000/mm^2$ on silicon chips or multitransistor arrays (MTAs) based on metal-oxide-semiconductor field-effect transistor (MOSFET) technology (Bonifazi & Fromherz, 2002; Hutzler et al., 2006; Lambacher et al., 2011)
F. Patolskiy B. Timko B. Tian T. Cohen-Karni C. Lieber et al.	≤ 150 R,(S)	Straight or kinked, oriented p- and/or n-type Ø 20 nm silicon nanowires (SiNW) spanning about 2-5 µm between Ni (source and drain) or Cr/Pd/Cr metal interconnects insulated by Si_3N_4 or PMMA (Patolsky et al., 2006; Tian et al., 2010)
3Brain K. Imfeld A. Maccione L. Berdondini et al.	4096 R	CMOS APS with 21 x 21 $µm^2$ Al electrodes with optional Au-coating (electroless deposition) (Imfeld et al., 2007; Berdondini, Imfeld, et al., 2009)
F. Heer U. Frey A. Hierlemann et al.	128 R,S 126 R,S out of 11,011	8 x 16 array in CMOS technology with shifted Ø 10 - 40 (30) µm Pt-black (electrodeposited) on Pt (sputtered) electrodes insulated by an alternating Si_3N_4/SiO_2 stack (Heer et al., 2007) 128 x 128 array of Ø 7 µm shifted Pt (sputtered) electrodes at a density of $3150/mm^2$ on switch-matrix array in CMOS technology insulated by an alternating Si_3N_4/SiO_2 stack (Frey et al., 2010)
J.F. Eschermann S. Ingebrandt A. Offenhäusser et al.	16 R	4 x 4 recording sites each with 6 parallel silicon nanowire (SiNW) FETs with widths of 500 nm and pitch of 200 µm on metalized, doped Si source/drain contacts insulated by SiO_2 (Eschermann et al., 2009)
T. Pui P. Chen et al.	100 R	100 µm long silicon nanowires (SiNWs) with 30 x 40 nm^2 rectangular cross section attached to Al on Si contact pads insulated by Si_3N_4 (Pui et al., 2009)
Z&L Creative Corp.	24 R	CMOS with Au-coated Al electrodes (Xin et al., 2009)
'Hybrid' MEAs		
J.J. Pancrazio G.T.A. Kovaces A. Stenger et al.	32 R,S + 4 GND	Electrochemically platinized Ø 14 µm Au/Cr electrodes on Si/SiO_2 carrier connected to a CMOS/VLSI amplifier chip, insulated by Si_3N_4 (Pancrazio et al., 1998)
Bionas GmbH W. Baumann R. Ehret M. Brischwein B. Wolf et al.		Multiparametric sensor with 6 $µm^2$ CPFET and Ø 10 µm Pd or Pt electrodes, ISFET pH electrode, interdigitated impedance electrodes, photodiodes, oxygen and T sensor (Baumann et al., 1999; Ehret et al., 2001; Baumann et al., 2002)
W. Cunningham D. Gunning K. Mathieson A.M. Litke M. Rahman et al.	61 R,S 512 R,S 519 R,S 61 R,S (3D)	Ø 2 - 5 µm electroplated Pt electrodes on ITO on glass, insulated by Si_3N_4, wire-bonded to ASIC readout & stimulation circuitry (Cunningham et al., 2001; Mathieson et al., 2004) Hexagonally arranged, ≤ 200 µm high, partially hollow W needles with electroplated Pt-tips, insulated by SiO_2 and back-side connected to Al tracks, wire-bonded to ASIC readout & stimulation circuitry (Gunning et al., 2010)

Table 1. List of groups and companies that have developed a particular MEA technology[6] sorted by first publication date, then author. Apologies go to any group or technology accidentally omitted or cited wrongly. Consult second page of chapter for abbreviations.

1.2 From *in vitro* to *in vivo*

From a conceptual point of view, the readout and stimulation physics of *in vitro* electrode systems are identical to electrode-based *in vivo* probes. Also, the needs for amplification,

---

[6] News on technological developments may be found on the continuously updated publication list on Multi Channel Systems' website.

filtering, analog-to-digital (A/D) signal conversion and signal (post-) processing electronics are almost the same. This holds for signal readout circuitry on the one hand, and for signal generators and digital-to-analog (D/A) converters for modulating neural activity with electrical stimuli on the other hand. It does not matter whether they are placed in direct vicinity of the electrodes as in recent 'active' MEA designs, or classically connected as modular hardware at the end of the electrode tracks of 'passive' MEAs. A comprehensive review by Jochum *et al.* surveys neural amplifiers with an emphasis on integrated circuit designs (Jochum *et al.*, 2009).

Yet, *in vivo*, new challenges arise. The electrode array encounters a rather different and more complex environment when compared to *in vitro* scenarios. Any array cannot longer be considered 'noninvasive', even if it will not penetrate the cell membrane. This is because a MEA has to be brought first into its recording position, which involves the opening and partial removal of the skull and of any protective encapsulation of the brain. Deep brain implants need to be furthermore inserted into the soft, yet densely packed brain tissue, thereby, in the best case, just displacing, and in the worst case, even destroying neurons, connections and glia cells along the penetration path. This may lead to a partial destruction of the tissue architecture, which the brain needs to compensate for. Apart from the insertion damage, a rigid neural implant may get repositioned upon a sudden movement of the head due to the inertial forces acting on the quasi-floating brain. Furthermore, the immune system may become activated and attack the implanted portion of a device. The implant materials are thereby exposed to a variety of compounds not found in *in vitro* systems that they may chemically react with. In bad scenarios, the reaction products may be toxic, thereby triggering a temporary if not chronic immune response[7]. Any change of the device material may furthermore be categorized as 'degradation', which could compromise device stability and performance over time. The latter may also be simply lowered by device encapsulation in tissue scars, thereby electrically insulating the recording and stimulation sites. This scarring is considered as one of the most common reasons for device failure. Stimulation electrodes carry additional risks of tissue damage by their electrochemical erosion or overheating (Dowling, 2008; Marin & Fernandez, 2010). In summary, implant materials should be chosen that are sufficiently biostable against alterations or degradation by the physiological environment. They should furthermore not trigger any immune response or alter cell physiology in an uncontrolled and undesirable fashion[8]. In other words, a neuroprosthetic recording device should behave as if it were not present, and a stimulation device should in addition induce a neural response as similar to neural signaling mechanisms as possible.

Another critical issue is the actual interconnection of the devices to the outside world. Signals are commonly transferred to extracorporeal signal conditioning and processing electronics by cables. Not only are the connection points between cable and device a source of failure due to the detachment of the cable ends to the device by chemical degradation or mechanical forces. Once passing through the skin or skull, the pass-through hole has to be well sealed and stabilized to not let contaminants pass and become a site of chronic infection, and to not let the cables move and thereby exert mechanical stress onto the surrounding tissue. Recent trends therefore target at the transmission of signals through the

---

[7] Apart from reaction products stemming from device degradation, exposed implant materials may also have catalytic properties.

[8] This statement does not exclude the temporary or permanent chemical and/or topographical device functionalization for manipulating or triggering a cell or tissue response in a controlled way (*e.g.*, to support device – tissue integration or tissue regeneration).

skull by telemetric technologies, which, however, pose new challenges with respect to miniaturization, circuit protection against humidity, and energy transfer for powering the telemetric electronics. And it does not provide a solution for stabilizing the internal circuit-to-MEA connection, which may still be exposed to movement-related stress.

1.3 Electrode arrays for *in vivo* electrophysiology

For getting a general overview on *in vivo* neuroprosthetic[9] implants and brain-machine interfaces including the diverse types of microelectrode arrays, their specific applications and main vendors, the reader shall be referred to recent overview articles and reviews (Hetke & Anderson, 2002; Rutten, 2002; Navarro *et al.*, 2005; Cheung, 2007; Winter *et al.*, 2007; Dowling, 2008; Hajjhassan *et al.*, 2008; Lebedev *et al.*, 2008; Wise *et al.*, 2008; Stieglitz *et al.*, 2009; Graimann *et al.*, 2010; Mussa-Ivaldi *et al.*, 2010; Rothschild, 2010; Hassler *et al.*, 2011). This paragraph will just summarize some of the basic design concepts, general fabrication approaches and the limitations they impose on the performance of chronically implanted devices.

1.3.1 Design and fabrication aspects

In the 80's of the last century, the boom in microfabrication technologies opened the door for designing elaborate multi-microelectrode arrays with spatially distributed recording or stimulation sites. However, the choice of carrier, conductor and insulator materials depends on (and is thereby limited by) the often harsh fabrication and processing conditions. Given that materials in tissue-contact also need to fulfill the condition of being biocompatible (that is foremost, not being cytotoxic) and biostable (that is, not become degraded by the physiological environment), the number of suitable materials is quite low. Almost all of them are considerably more rigid than soft tissue, and the devices made from them tend to have sharp edges. Anyone ever having experienced a splinter in the thumb will remember how painful[10] it is each time the splinter moves only the tiniest bit. The simple reason is: the splinter is rigid and edgy whereas the tissue of the thumb is not. Thus, despite the tremendous research investments into diverse neuroprosthetic technologies, intracortical probes still lack functional stability during chronic use due to the large discrepancy between their biomechanical and chemical properties and those of the tissue environment (Marin & Fernandez, 2010).

The need for designing more flexible electrode arrays was already addressed in the 60's of the last century (Rutledge & Duncan, 1966). Various strategies have been suggested since then to overcome some of the above mentioned limitations, particularly in the context of designing cochlear, retinal and deep brain implants. Today, the most commonly used flexible carrier and track insulation materials are polyimides (PIs), poly(p-xylylene) (PPX, and in particular poly(chloro-p-xylylene) (Parylene®-C)), poly(dimethylsiloxane) (PDMS), poly(tetrafluoroethylene) (PTFE), and occasionally less flexible liquid crystal polymers (LCPs) or photoresists (*e.g.*, SU-8) (Navarro *et al.*, 2005; Cheung, 2007; Myllymaa *et al.*, 2009; Hassler *et al.*, 2011). Noble metals[11] such as Pt, Ir, W and Au are sputter- or vapor-deposited, often requiring other metals (*e.g.*, Ti, Cr) as adhesion promoters. They are structured into electrodes, tracks and connection pads by etching through a sacrificial mask of photoresist, glass or metals

---

[9] The most well-known neuroprosthetic devices are cochlear implants, retinal implants, spinal cord stimulators, deep brain implants and bladder control implants.

[10] While the brain processes information on pain in other body parts, it does not feel pain itself.

[11] Sometimes less noble metals like Ni or Cu are used as track and connection pad conductors. If the insulation layer of the probe has defects, they may partially dissolve into cytotoxic ionic species.

(Patrick *et al.*, 2006; Wang *et al.*, 2007; Mercanzini *et al.*, 2008; Rodger *et al.*, 2008). With few exceptions, each device needs to be fabricated in a clean room environment. Only recently, new strategies have been proposed to microstructure conductors under normal laboratory conditions that allow their transfer onto or embedding into polymer carriers that do not withstand high temperatures or vacuum. Hu *et al.* first sintered metal nanopowders within micropatterned, temperature-resistant multilevel microchannel quartz molds, which were then embedded into PDMS, parylene or polyimide. This allowed the generation of high-aspect (10:1) 3D conductors with, depending on the chosen mold generation process (ion milling, laser milling, deep reactive-ion etching (DRIE)), a wide variety of arbitrary shapes. A volume reduction between 5 % and 25% during sintering led to gaps between the conductor and the mold, which were filled with PDMS, thereby automatically insulating the tracks (Hu *et al.*, 2006). A different approach was chosen by Dupas-Bruzek and coworkers, which was based on the UV (248 nm) laser-assisted activation of PDMS followed by the electroless deposition of Pt onto the laser-treated and thereby chemically modified surface areas (Dupas-Bruzek, Drean, *et al.*, 2009; Dupas-Bruzek, Robbe, *et al.*, 2009). Henle *et al.* created a PDMS-Pt-PDMS sandwich by placing a 12.5 µm thin Pt film directly onto a partially cured PDMS carrier substrate, structuring it by an IR (1064 nm) laser, manually discarding excess material and spin-coating a second PDMS layer on top (Henle *et al.*, 2011). All of these fabrication approaches have in common that pads and electrodes get insulated during device fabrication and need to be reexposed in a post-processing step (*e.g.*, by laser deinsulation or etching). Furthermore, tracks, pads and electrodes are always made from metals. Often, their long-term performance is limited due to the delamination of insulation layers or material fatigue over time. And finally, even such flexible neural implants still contain parts that are either more rigid than the surrounding tissue or lack the arbitrary deformability to follow its shape.

We therefore decided to deviate from common microelectrode array fabrication paradigms by resorting to a microchannel replication strategy with conductive polymers (CPs) completely replacing metals. This does not only allow the implementation of one and the same electrode layout in different types of insulating polymer backbones (*e.g.*, of different shore hardness). It also gives more freedom in the choice of conductive materials that have biomechanical properties more similar to the embedding substrate. Fundamental proof-of-principle results have been published recently (Blau *et al.*, 2011). The concept is sketched out in Fig. 1. It exemplarily illustrates the master fabrication and the replica-molding routes for *in vitro polyMEAs* with or without spike electrodes on the one hand, and copies of the master on the other hand. The initial **master** with bi-level microstructures for electrodes, conductor tracks and contact pads can be made out of two SU-8 layers following standard photolithography recipes[12]. A silicon wafer (m1) is spin-coated with SU-8 (m2), which is then soft-baked and illuminated through a photo mask (m3) to create the features of all three elements, the electrodes, tracks and pads. After a post-exposure bake (m4), a second SU-8 layer is spun on top of the first and soft-baked (m5), then exposed through the carefully aligned second photo mask with electrode and pad features only (m6). Thereafter follows a standard post-exposure bake (m7) and the development of both layers (m8). The individual layer thicknesses can be controlled by the spin coating parameters to define separate heights for buried track channels and for scaffold-penetrating electrodes and pad wells, respectively. Although the one-time fabrication of the molding master may still

---

[12] Alternatively, arbitrary 3D shapes could be inscribed into a photo-patternable polymer when resorting to UV laser or multi-photon lithography. One of the advantages would be the direct generation of non-vertical (*e.g.*, conical) structures (Li & Fourkas, 2007; Thiel *et al.*, 2010).

require a clean room infrastructure[13], devices can be fabricated in a normal laboratory environment. In addition, a master can be replicated at negligible cost by the very same replica-molding procedure that is used to manufacture individual devices.

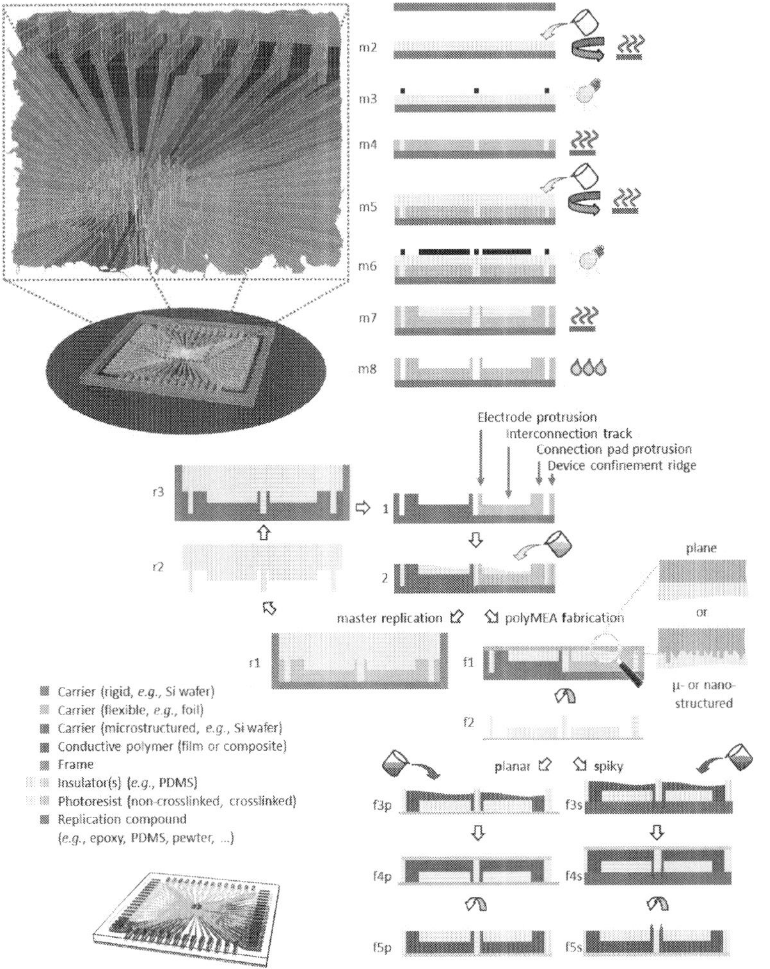

Fig. 1. Summary of the eight steps (**m1-m8**) for fabricating a bi-level replication master in SU-8 on a Si-wafer (upper left sketch with zoom onto the electrode columns), the three master-replication steps (**r1-r3**) and the five steps (**f1-f5**) for fabricating a *polyMEA* (lower left sketch). See text for details. Legend: **f**, device fabrication route; **m**, master production; **r**, master replication route; **p**, plane electrodes; **s**, spike electrodes.

---

[13] If device geometries are simple and dimensions stay above a few tens of microns, even the master can be fabricated in the laboratory, as demonstrated by several groups (*e.g.*, (Mensing *et al.*, 2005)).

The bi-level master (1, grey, orange) (*e.g.,* made of a high aspect ratio photoresist) is usually coated by an anti-adhesive film[14] before being filled with a curable polymer gel (2, sky blue) (*e.g.,* PDMS). Alternatively, the master (or a sturdier copy thereof) can be used for hot-embossing into a thermomoldable polymer. A plane or micro-/nanostructured (zoom in) sacrificial carrier foil (green) levels the polymer with the highest protrusions of the master (f1). This ensures the complete penetration of the polymer by the elevated structural features of the master. After the curing of the thin polymer microchannel scaffold, such carrier helps in scaffold removal from the master without running the risk of tearing it apart. It furthermore allows the purposeful imprinting of a topofunctional texture into the PDMS surface and/or the electrodes of a *polyMEA* (*e.g.,* for steering neural differentiation or guiding neurites). After flip over (f2), the carrier also temporarily supports the scaffold during the subsequent processing steps for generating a *polyMEA* with **plane** electrodes (route **p**). To create the electrodes, tracks and pads, the microchannels and cavities of the scaffold are filled with the CP (f3p). If the CP wets the channel-separating plateaus in this step, it can be rather easily scraped off after partial evaporation of the solvent. After curing, the scaffold is backside-insulated by a second polymer layer (f4p). If a foil or panel is chosen as the insulator and a film-forming CP as the conductor, the channels stay hollow and can serve for microfluidic or optical add-on applications. In this case, the sizes of the electrodes are less well defined. On the top-side of the *polyMEA*, they will have ring shapes with a through-hole diameter and wall thickness equaling the film thickness of the CP rather than being planar. However, a neuron could partially get into contact with the CP-coated channel sidewalls upon entering the channel or sending any of its processes into the channel. Thus, theoretically, the entire channel surface will serve as an electrode. Alternatively, all cavities are filled with the same or a similar curable polymer gel from which the scaffold was made of. Depending on the stickiness of the temporary carrier foil, the disk-like CP depositions on the carrier at the electrode sites and contact pads are more likely to be transferred to the polymer rather than sticking to the carrier. This is because a dried CP film usually has a nano-structured surface that gets physically entrapped by the polymer-gel insulator. This issue is discussed in the next paragraph in more detail. After removing the carrier[15], the *polyMEA* with planar electrodes (f5p) is ready for use. No other deinsulation step is required. If spike electrodes shall be generated instead (route **s**), the scaffold is transferred onto a carrier with cone-like indentations (red), which can be generated by *e.g.,* anisotropic etching of Si (Jansen *et al.*, 1996; Williams & Muller, 1996) or multidirectional UV lithography in photoresist (Yong-Kyu *et al.*, 2006). After aligning those with the electrode through-holes of the scaffold, the CP can be filled into the cavities and cured (f3s). Rajaraman *et al.* recently presented a similar approach for pyramid-shaped metal electrodes

---

[14] To generate a Teflon®-like, fluorine-terminated anti-stick film, the wafer with the SU-8 microstructure or its epoxy copy can be either exposed for 5 minutes to C_4F_8 in a reactive ion etcher or to trichloro(1H,1H,2H,2H-perfluorooctyl)silane (PFOCTS) for one hour in a desiccator.

[15] One strategy to pull 50 - 200 µm thin PDMS microchannel scaffolds from their molding masters without tearing them apart was to place coated overhead or inkjet transparencies with their coated sides onto the uncured PDMS. In most cases, the water-soluble coating had a texture, which seemed to physically entrap the PDMS. After curing, the PDMS thus stuck to the sacrificial support transparency. It would detach from it automatically upon dissolution of the coating during immersion into water or ethanol for a few hours, leaving the texture topographies imprinted in the PDMS surface. As already briefly mentioned earlier, the transparency or its coating can be purposefully micro- or nanostructured to permanently transfer topographical cues into the PDMS and/or the CP electrodes.

(Rajaraman *et al.*, 2011). As before, a backside insulation layer is applied (f4s) to give a *polyMEA* with spike electrodes after its peeling from the microstructured carrier. The spikes can either be used as such or, if a small recording/stimulation site is desired, be insulated by a thin coat of PDMS and then be clipped at their tops (*e.g.*, by a razor-blade through a mask with holes) to expose the CP.

During the *polyMEA* fabrication steps sketched out in Fig. 1, the CP will always get into contact with the transfer carrier foil (green) at the pad and electrode openings in the scaffold. Depending on the surface structure and chemistry of the foil, film-forming CPs like PEDOT:PSS from aqueous dispersion might stick more or less well to it (Fig. 2, a1 & a2). Upon peeling the foil from hollow channels, the sub-µm-thick CP membrane spanning the electrode through-hole may get partially or completely torn off and/or stay stuck to the carrier foil (Fig. 2, a2, left channel). If, instead, CP-coated channels are backfilled with a polymer gel like PDMS, the gel will get mechanically entrapped in the CP film due to its roughness (on the nm scale) thereby acting as a mechanical support for the membrane after curing (Fig. 2, a2, right channel).

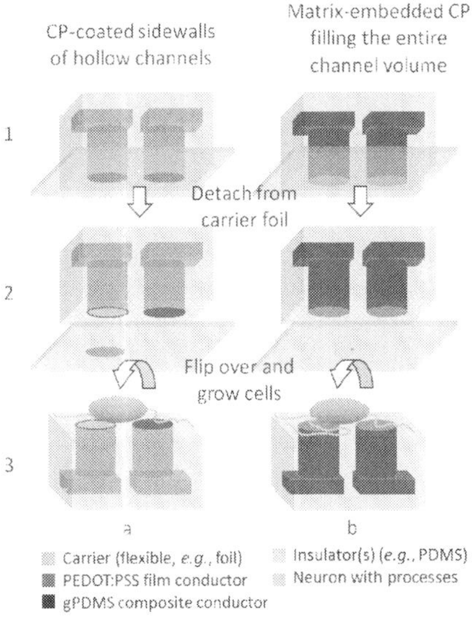

Fig. 2. Zoom onto a sketch of two electrode channels in contact with a transfer carrier to illustrate how different CPs give different types of electrodes.

Both scenarios give useful devices for different application needs. A neuron may just grow its processes into a CP-coated channel without electrode membrane (Fig. 2, a3, left channel). Thus, the recorded signal can be easily attributed to that very neuron. Alternatively, if the well diameter were reduced to a few µm, a planar-patch-like recording array could be created. As recently reported by Klemic *et al.* (Klemic *et al.*, 2005), Chen and Folch (Chen & Folch, 2006), Tonomura *et al.* (Tonomura *et al.*, 2010), and Hofmann *et al.* (Hofmann *et al.*, 2011), neurons tend to seal such microapertures to result in high signal-to-noise (S/N) ratios and selectivity. A back-filled channel with an intact electrode membrane (Fig. 2, a3, right channel) or a gPDMS composite (Fig. 2, b1-3) will act like a classical electrode instead. Even if the CP membrane were missing, the electrode would be defined by the nm-thick ring-shaped CP coating at the end of a channel. It is still an open question whether the impedance of these ring electrodes is sufficiently low to capture or induce neural signals.

1.3.2 PDMS as a soft and flexible substrate material

The platinum-catalyzed addition-crosslinking of vinyl-endblocked silicone polymers and silicone polymers with SiH functionality gives medical grade polydimethylsiloxane (PDMS) (*e.g.*, Dow Corning, Sylgard 184; Wacker, Elastosil RT 601), a rubberlike polymer with particular properties (Colas & Curtis, 2004). Not only can a wide variety of different hardness and tear resistances be chosen from. It is furthermore dimensionally stable and will not shrink or expand upon curing. If not chemically activated (*e.g.*, by plasma oxygenation or other types of surface functionalization (Donzel *et al.*, 2001)), it reversibly adsorbs to almost any smooth surface but will not react with it. It demonstrates outstanding bioperformance and has a favorable toxicological profile in diverse medical contexts (Briquet *et al.*, 1996). It is therefore FDA-approved and part of common implants that are in direct tissue contact (*e.g.*, breast implants, contact lenses, tubing in heart surgery, catheters) (Colas, 2001; Curtis & Colas, 2004). It can furthermore be used as a molding material to cast itself[16] or various other materials such as plasters, concrete, wax, low-melt metal alloys (tin, pewter) or resins (urethane, epoxy or polyester) for master replication purposes (Smoothon, 2008). After depositing a conductive seed layer, it can also be electroplated to give LIGA-type master replicas (Jung *et al.*, 2008).

1.3.3 Flexible, polymer-based electrode materials

The desire of incorporating electronics into bendable and stretchable lightweight consumer devices (*e.g.*, rollable displays, garment, conformal solar panels) has driven the research and development of unconventional elastomeric conductors (Rogers *et al.*, 2010) including inks based on single-walled carbon nanotubes (Sekitani *et al.*, 2009) or silver nanoparticles (Ahn *et al.*, 2009). Despite their lower electrical conductivity (Kahol *et al.*, 2005), conductive polymers promise to become a low-cost alternative to metals for their flexibility and easier processability (Inganäs, 2010). Currently, PEDOT:PSS is one of the CPs with the highest conductivity, is transparent, forms bendable films, is chemically inert and non-cytotoxic. It has therefore found its way into the biosciences as a selective sensing layer in biosensors (Janata & Josowicz, 2003; Lange *et al.*, 2008; Rozlosnik, 2009) and more recently as a feature enhancer of metal microelectrodes (Guimard *et al.*, 2007; Widge *et al.*, 2007). Besides the two conductivity modes (electron-hole and ionic) of CPs, their biophysical properties and process-dependent micro- and nano-topographies seem to enhance their bio-acceptance and tissue integration (Ateh *et al.*, 2006; Guimard *et al.*, 2007; Owens & Malliaras, 2010).

While graphite and, in particular, carbon black are usually not categorized as polymers, they share some of their properties with respect to their extended carbon backbone. For their high electrical conductivity, biological inertness, low price and easy handling, they are excellent filler materials for creating flexible, voluminous conductor tracks or coatings with

---

[16] PDMS adheres strongly to itself. For a successful PDMS replication from a PDMS master, the master surface needs to be coated with an anti-stick layer. The one-hour exposure to trichloro(1H,1H,2H,2H-perfluorooctyl)silane (PFOCTS) in a desiccator results in a reusable Teflon®-like transferring layer (Zhang *et al.*, 2010).

silicones or polyurethanes as the matrix (Calixto *et al.*, 2007; Huang *et al.*, 2011). As with any conductive filler (*e.g.*, antimony- or indium-doped tin oxide, silver (Ahn *et al.*, 2009; Gong & Wen, 2009; Larmagnac *et al.*, 2010; Zhang *et al.*, 2011), carbon, or any form of their nanoparticle derivatives (Sekitani *et al.*, 2009; Pavesi *et al.*, 2011)), a conductive polymer can be generated when the percolation threshold[17] of the filler has been surpassed (Kirkpatrick, 1973; Milliken and Company, 1997). Rather than being a thin film conductor[18] such as PEDOT:PSS or most of the vapor-deposited metal electrodes, the composite fills the entire volume of the microchannel, thus being less prone to dramatic changes in its conductivity upon deformation[19]. As shown for other flexible wire composites (Ahn *et al.*, 2009), it is hypothesized that the main reason for the stability in conductivity of such flexible wires is the disperse distribution of graphite flakes in the PDMS. Upon shifting these flakes against each other, the current will just follow an alternative or even newly established conductive pathway between different flakes being or getting into contact with each other. Thus, by filling channels of extended dimensions with gPDMS, the shortcoming of its lower conductivity compared to metals can be partially compensated by its bulk-like distribution.

1.3.4 Electrode functionalization and post-processing strategies

The postprocessing of devices serves two main goals: i) the improvement of the electrical characteristics of the electrodes (mainly with respect to the decrease of their electrical impedances and/or the increase of their reversible charge delivery capacity (CDC)[20], and ii) the enhancement of their biocompatibility for their better tissue integration. The electrical impedance is a more general concept of electrical resistance; it describes the frequency-dependent resistance of an electrical conductor. At '0 Hz', the alternating current (AC) impedance of an electrode is identical to its direct current (DC) resistance. Over the physiologically relevant frequency range between 0.5 - 100 Hz (relevant for slow oscillations as in local field potentials (LFPs)) and 1 - 5 kHz (for the capture of individual action potentials (APs) of neurons[21]), the impedance of conductors can decrease by 2-3 orders of magnitude. In general, it can be stated that the smaller the geometrical electrode area (*e.g.*, πr^2 for disk-like electrodes with radius r), the higher the impedance. The impedance of a

---

[17] Percolation as a mathematical concept refers to the long-range connectivity and its nature in random systems. The percolation threshold is the critical value of the (volume) occupation probability where infinite connectivity, in this case between conductive particles, first occurs.

[18] The resistance of thin-film electrodes may considerably deviate by two to three orders of magnitude from that of the bulk conductor material (Hu *et al.*, 2006).

[19] Nevertheless, any wire deformation will alter the resistance of a wire. This phenomenon is exploited in strain gauge sensors. However, while the working principle of a strain gauge sensor relies on the mechanically induced changes in the cross-section geometry of the conductor, the resistivity of a composite material such as gPDMS seems to be dominated by the number of parallel conductive pathways. While the resistance in a strain gauge sensor increases with strain, the resistance of carbon- or silver-blended PDMS was actually found to decrease upon stretching for the better contact of the conductive particles (Niu *et al.*, 2007).

[20] Often, the reversible CDC is also referred to as the reversible charge storage capacity (CSC) or the save/reversible/capacitive charge injection limit (CIL).

[21] The reasoning is as follows: During the firing of an action potential, the depolarization of the cell membrane lasts for about 1-2 ms. The temporal width of the extracellularly recorded component of such action potential is usually 1 ms (or less). This translates into a theoretical frequency of 1 kHz (or above) because 1000 (or more) such components will fit into 1 s.

small-diameter electrode can be lowered by increasing its real (or effective) surface area, *e.g.*, by adding a microtopography to the electrode (*e.g.*, by increasing its roughness). Depending on the structure of that surface topography (*e.g.*, fractal or columnar) and the type and electrical properties of the material that creates it, the capacitance[22] C of the electrode may be affected as well. Decreasing the impedance will increase the signal-to-noise ratio and decrease the required voltage U to charge the electrode-electrolyte interface. Increasing the capacitance of the electrode gives room for more charges Q to accumulate on the electrode surface at a given voltage ($Q = C \cdot U$), thereby increasing the number of separated ionic charges at the electrode-electrolyte-tissue interface. Consequently, the increase in the locally generated electrical field may increase the likelihood of sufficiently shifting the membrane potential over its depolarization threshold in stimulation experiments[23]. The effect of decreasing electrode impedances by depositing non-planar metal layers (*e.g.*, porous Pt-black, columnar TiN or fine-grained IrO_x) has been exploited for a long time. A new trend is the deposition of carbon nanotubes (CNTs), which have favorable electrical and biophysical properties. They not only improve the impedance and the charge transfer capacity by more than one order of magnitude, but provide nano-textured anchoring points that cells can make use of (Keefer *et al.*, 2008; Park *et al.*, 2009; Malarkey & Parpura, 2010). Recent studies show the same effect for CPs. Ludwig *et al.* reported on an about 10-fold decrease in impedance at 1 kHz for electrochemically deposited PEDOT coatings on $\varnothing$ 15 µm Au recording electrodes, which reduced noise levels by about half (Ludwig *et al.*, 2011). In earlier studies, the same effect was demonstrated for polypyrrole (PPy) (Cui *et al.*, 2001). Kotov *et al.* and Beattie *et al.* recently summarized the potential of nanomaterials for neural interfaces (Beattie *et al.*, 2009; Kotov *et al.*, 2009).

Many works have addressed the issue of providing signaling cues on electrode and substrate surfaces to mask the non-biological properties of a material, and to alleviate the acute and chronic disturbances imposed by a neuroprosthetic device onto its surrounding biological environment (Leach *et al.*, 2010). By adsorbing polycations onto ready-made CP layers (Collazos-Castro *et al.*, 2010) or by entrapping or intermingling cell adhesion and differentiation promoting proteins or their fragments (*e.g.*, neural cell adhesion molecules (NCAMs), nerve growth factor (NGF), laminin and fibronectin) into the CP during its

---

[22] In a first approximation, the electrode can be considered the plate of a parallel-plate capacitor. Its electrical capacitance C is then directly proportional to the real electrode surface area A, which is equal or bigger than the geometrical electrode area. ($C = \varepsilon \cdot A / d$, with the permittivity ε of the dielectric and the distance d between the plates). While the proportionality holds, the situation at the electrode-cell interface is certainly more complex: The second plate is not of the same type as the electrode but the cell membrane with a different surface area. Furthermore, the dielectric, the medium between electrode and cell membrane, is not static, and thus its permittivity is not a constant.

[23] Two types of currents are distinguished: Capacitive currents just charge the electrode; electrons will accumulate on the outer electrode surface without being injected into the electrolyte. Most stimulation electrodes are designed to be capacitive. In contrast, Faradaic currents pass the electrode-electrolyte interface. Because free electrons cannot be dissolved in aqueous environments, they become immediately involved in a redox-reaction. The occurrence of such undesirable reactions leads to chemical products that alter the composition of the physiological environment. To avoid any Faradaic currents, stimulation electrodes can be sealed by dielectric films (*e.g.*, TiO_2, Ta_2O_5 and $BaTiO_3$). They are generated by oxidizing the respective metal electrodes, sputtering, sol-gel deposition or precipitation from organic or water-based dispersions. For an in-depth discussion see (Merrill *et al.*, 2005; Cogan, 2008; Zhou & Greenberg, 2009; Merrill, 2010).

electrochemical or self-assembled monolayer (SAM) formation, it could be shown that brain-derived cells attached preferentially to the CP (Cui *et al.*, 2001; Widge *et al.*, 2007; Asplund *et al.*, 2010; Green *et al.*, 2010; Thompson *et al.*, 2010). Recent studies indicate that, apart from its overall geometry and surface chemistry, the nano and micro surface texture of a substrate may have considerable impact on cell adhesion, differentiation, cell morphology and gene expression as well (Wilkinson, 2004; Barr *et al.*, 2010). Depending on the type of starting material, the deposition parameters (temperature, pH, U, Q, time) and the choice of solvents and auxiliary components (such as surfactants), the form, texture and order of CPs can be fine-tuned (George *et al.*, 2005; Yang *et al.*, 2005; Abidian *et al.*, 2010). And since Wong *et al.* observed that the shape and growth of (endothelial) cells could be noninvasively controlled by just switching the oxidation state of fibronectin-coated PPy (Wong *et al.*, 1994), and that current flow through PPy would promote protein synthesis and neurite outgrowth (Schmidt *et al.*, 1997), later works exploited this combination of conductivity and particular geometries of CPs for the programmable control of *e.g.*, neurite extension, protein adsorption and cell adhesion, or for the spatially defined release of ions, antibiotics, anti-inflammatories, neurotransmitters and other signaling factors (Abidian *et al.*, 2010; Ravichandran *et al.*, 2010; Sirivisoot *et al.*, 2011; Svennersten *et al.*, 2011). While the roughening of electrodes and the incorporation of biofunctional cues in all cases provide mechanical and biochemical anchoring points for cells, CP coatings are lightweight and usually less brittle than metal deposits. Furthermore, unlike metals, both CNTs and CPs are chemically accessible to covalent pre- or post-modification with bioactive molecules (Ravichandran *et al.*, 2010).

1.3.5 Performance of *polyMEA* devices

The electrical, mechanical and optical characteristics as well as the recording performance of *in vitro polyMEAs* and epidural *in vivo* probes derived therefrom have been presented in a recent proof-of-concept study (Blau *et al.*, 2011). The main characteristics are summarized below. *polyMEAs* for *in vitro* applications were designed to fit the pin-layout of a commercial 60-channel amplifier system (Multi Channel Systems). Their overall dimensions of 4.9 x 4.9 cm² matched commercial MEAs. Their minimal thickness could not stay below the height of the bilayer master features, which were between 200 and 500 μm. To reach the standard height of 1 mm of commercial MEAs, either temporary spacers or a permanently fused PDMS backside insulation coat were used. Device flexibility depended on device thickness. With increasing thickness above 200 μm, the PDMS still stayed flexible but slowly lost its surface conformability. A *polyMEA* with gPDMS electrodes, tracks and pads of approximate thickness of 300 μm is depicted in Fig. 3a. Electrode diameters of the 8 x 8 (- 4 corner electrodes) electrode matrix were nominally 80 μm. Electrode spacing was 400 μm with the exception of an 800 μm cross-shaped gap in the center of the electrode matrix. Device transparency of a *polyMEA* with PEDOT:PSS conductive films and PDMS-flooded cavities is demonstrated in Fig. 3b & c. At the edge of a cortico-hippocampal cell carpet, individual neurons and connections can be identified on top of electrodes and buried connection tracks alike. Between 1 Hz and 5 kHz, *polyMEAs* with PEDOT:PSS electrodes (Ø below 100 μm) had almost flat impedances of about 1.2 MΩ on average (Fig. 3d, blue dotted line). In contrast, gPDMS composite electrodes of same dimensions had significantly lower impedances of about 35 kΩ at 1 kHz with a logarithmic increase to about 15 MΩ at 1 Hz (Fig. 3d, black dashed line), which is typical for plain metal electrodes (Fig. 3d, orange line for Ø 30 μm TiN on Ti or on ITO electrodes). Despite their rather large electrode diameters and high impedances, PEDOT:PSS electrodes were able to capture action potentials and local field fluctuations alike. And despite of the larger noise floor between ~ 20 µV (with gPDMS counter electrode or Pt wire GND) and 50 - 80 µV (with internal PEDOT:PSS counter electrode), signal-to-noise ratios (S/N) were typically 5 for neural recordings and up to 100 for cardiomyocyte recordings. This was confirmed with cortico-hippocampal co-cultures (Fig. 3f), retinal whole mounts and acute cardiac tissue preparations (both not shown). Local field responses to visual stimuli in epicortical recordings from the visual cortex of mice were clearly visible after 59x averaging (Fig. 3g).

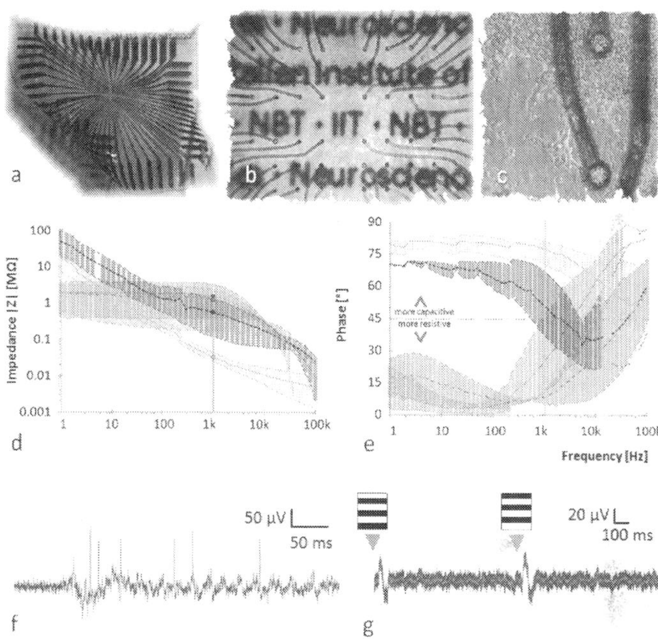

Fig. 3. **a)** *polyMEA* flexibility (~ 300 µm thick, with gPDMS composite conductor). **b)** Transparency of the PDMS substrate and of the PEDOT:PSS thin-film electrodes and buried tracks at the center of a *polyMEA* on top of a printout with letters of point 3 font size. **c)** Neurons of a cortico-hippocampal network (38 DIV) can be imaged and individually distinguished through the Ø 80 µm PEDOT:PSS electrodes and buried tracks. **d)** Impedance of Ø 80 µm PEDOT:PSS (blue) or gPDMS (black) electrodes, or of PEDOT:PSS electrodes with gPDMS pad fillings (green) compared to that of Ø 30 µm TiN-coated Ti or ITO electrodes of commercial MEAs (yellow). Dashed lines indicate averages, dotted borders extreme values. All spectra were recorded in saturated KCl. **e)** Phases for the electrode types and configurations mentioned in d). **f)** Simultaneous recording of action potentials on top of local field fluctuations from cortico-hippocampal co-cultures (rat E18, 38 DIV) on top of a PEDOT:PSS film electrode. **g)** Stimulus-induced local field potentials (after 59x averaging) captured by one out of 16 PEDOT:PSS film electrodes in epicortical recordings from the visual cortex of an anesthetized rat upon pattern reversal (arrows) of a grating as the visual cue. Blue trace: no filter; red trace: 200 Hz low pass filter. In both cases, a Pt wire served as a counter electrode. (Blau *et al.*, 2011).

Judging from the low phase of the impedance at low frequencies, the electrodes of the *polyMEA* devices show mostly resistive behavior. As discussed above, stimulation electrodes are usually designed to have a highly capacitive character (Cogan, 2008). Theoretically, the polymer electrodes therefore may need to be altered in postprocessing steps to increase their capacitance. However, impedance spectra were taken in a non-physiological scenario. Several groups have already demonstrated that PEDOT-decorated electrodes are good and sufficiently stable performers in neural stimulation experiments with a CSC of 2.3 - 15 mC/cm^2, which is already close to the 25 mC/cm^2 reported for IrO_x stimulation electrodes (Merrill *et al.*, 2005; Cui & Zhou, 2007; Cogan, 2008; Wilks *et al.*, 2009; Boretius *et al.*, 2011).

We tested 80 μm PEDOT:PSS and gPDMS electrodes on dense carpets of cortical and hippocampal neurons from rats in cultured neural networks for their suitability as voltage-controlled stimulation electrodes without success[24]. It may very well be that polymer electrodes of same or different diameters will nevertheless perform sufficiently well as stimulation electrodes when resorting to charge-controlled stimulation protocols or different stimulation waveforms. It is furthermore likely that, apart from the dimensional and electrical properties of an electrode and the medium composition, the distance and the capacitive and dielectric properties of the lipid double layer of the cell membrane have a larger than thought impact on the CSC[25]. If true, the stimulation performance of an electrode should depend on the type of cellular environment it is tested in.

1.3.6 Interconnection technologies

Connecting a microelectrode array to any kind of electronics is a critical issue. The mechanical clamping of contact pads requires a mechanism that is difficult to miniaturize and which might simply detach. Classical (wire) bonding introduces materials with limited flexibility that, due to stress and/or the contact chemistry between the different materials (including the humidity absorbed by a packaging compound), become the location of corrosion and break. By design, *polyMEA* arrays may alleviate the bonding issue. When the microchannel tracks are filled with elastomeric gPDMS (or alternatively with hydrogel conductors (Guiseppi-Elie, 2010)), they may be bent and twisted to a large degree. This property, together with the liberty to shape channels with increasing volumes downstream of the electrodes, allows for integrating ribbon cable-type wiring to external electronics as part of the electrode array. Thus, the point of connection may be placed wherever the mechanical stress onto the connector may be least. In one experimental approach, the gPDMS connection pads at the end of a supracortical prototype array were simply slipped into a standard dual row connector during their temporary depression (Fig. 4). Upon pressure release, the rubbery gPDMS was wedged by the pins, thus ensuring proper seating and electrical connectivity. And because the thickness of the back insulation layer of an *in vivo polyMEA* can be applied non-uniformly[26] (*e.g.*, thin at the recording site, thick at the

---

[24] Stimulation was based on charge-balanced biphasic voltage pulses not exceeding ±900 mV and 100 μs duration. Both polarity sequences (+, then -; -, then +) were tried.

[25] For a circular section of the cell membrane with a diameter matching that of commonly used electrodes (10 - 50 μm), the separated charge Q on the intracellular and extracellular side of the membrane during the resting (~ - 60 mV) or the action potential (~ 100 mV) is on the order of the CSC (several mC/cm^2) of above mentioned stimulation electrodes.

[26] Non-uniform, wedge-like shaping of a device only requires the covering of the non-cured PDMS backside insulation by a sheet positioned in a ramp-like configuration during its curing. For acute ramp angles, adhesion forces between the PDMS and the sheet will prevent PDMS efflux.

connector site), the contact pressure can be tuned to fit different connector types. The concept resembles that of zebra strip connectors. After insertion, probe and connector can be fixated by sewing and be encapsulated by PDMS or epoxies.

1.3.7 Shielding

Because long, and in particular, high-impedance wires may act like antennas which tend to pick up noise from the environment, they are usually avoided. Instead, high-to-low impedance conversion electronics are placed as closely to the electrodes as possible (as in 'active' MEA devices). However, today, the rigidity of any type of conversion electronics would still compromise device flexibility. Therefore, proper shielding (like in coaxial cables) remains the only alternative. Also in this case, PEDOT:PSS or gPDMS may substitute graphite-based conductive lacquers to create a mechanically more flexible, tightly device-wrapping shielding. When graphite is mixed into non-cured PDMS, the viscosity of the paste, once it has reached the desired conductivity, can be decreased temporarily with solvents such as iso-propanol. The external surface[27] of a device can thus be painted with such slurry gPDMS mix, which is then cured at elevated temperatures (80 °C – 150 °C). During the curing, the solvent will evaporate, resulting in a homogeneous conductive coating. It can be insulated by an upper coat of non-conductive PDMS. If a spot of the conductive gPDMS is kept deinsulated, it can serve as a counter electrode as part of the gPDMS shield. And, if necessary, the impedance of the gPDMS spot can be further tuned by electrochemical deposition of other conductors.

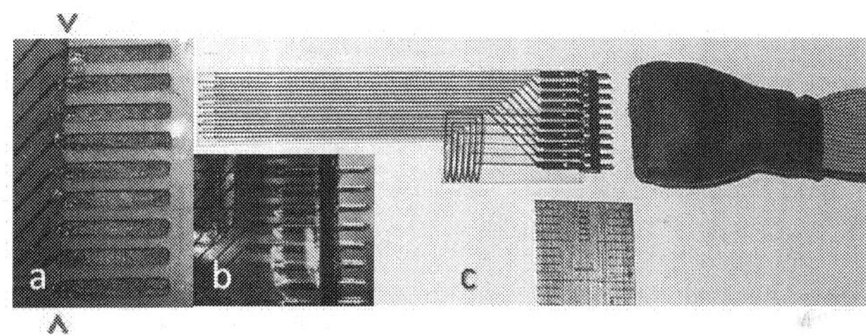

Fig. 4. **a)** gPDMS pads and tracks embedded in a 200 μm thick, still unfolded PDMS scaffold. Tracks had been topside-insulated by a thin film of PDMS. Pads (and electrodes, not shown) had been protected by scotch tape (red arrows indicate ridge after tape removal). **b)** Zoom onto pads slipped in between and squeezed by the pins of a standard 1.27 mm pitch, dual row, double pin connector, encapsulated by PDMS. **c)** Folded supracortical dummy probe demonstrating the slip-in concept. The flexibility of the PDMS scaffold and gPDMS tracks allows probe bending by 180° without compromising conductivity.

1.3.8 Other observations

For some not-yet understood and investigated reasons, PDMS seems to provide a more favorable surface for cell and tissue adhesion than other common culture substrates. In two acute slice experiments (retinal whole mounts) it was observed that, after an initial weigh-

---

[27] After a brief exposure of PDMS to oxygen plasma, PDMS can be permanently bonded to itself. In this case, a short oxygen-plasma treatment of the device will enhance the adhesion of the shielding layer to the PDMS surface. Such plasma exposure did not have any detrimental effect on PEDOT:PSS electrodes.

down by a nylon-stocking ensheathed platinum U-wire for enhancing the tissue electrode contact, the weight could be removed after 30 minutes without compromising the signal quality. While the PDMS and the electrodes had been coated with poly-D-lysine and laminin in a standard procedure for enhancing cell adhesion on MEAs, this type of stickiness had never been observed in our lab with insulation layers made of silicon nitride, silicon dioxide (glass) or polymer (photo-) resists such as SU-8 or polyimide. A similar observation has been reported by Guo *et al.* (Guo *et al.*, 2010). There, however, the improved contact to the tissue surface was mainly attributed to the geometries of the conical well encasing of the electrodes. At this point, it is not yet clear to what degree the short O_2 plasma hydrophilization[28] of the PDMS (for the better wetting with the adhesion mediators) contributed to its enhanced tissue interaction by not only altering the surface chemistry but also its morphology (Cvelbar *et al.*, 2003). A process-related micro- or nano-texturing of the PDMS surface may have played a role as well (Barr *et al.*, 2010). However, the most likely cause may be the tendency of silicones to absorb lipids (*e.g.*, from the cell membrane) resulting in partial cell or debris fusion with the PDMS surface and its dimensional swelling (Mchenry *et al.*, 1970; Colas & Curtis, 2004).

Preliminary results indicate that PEDOT:PSS can be embedded into a polymer matrix made of polyvinyl alcohol (PVA), glycerin and a di- or tricarboxylic acid as a crosslinker to render the PVA insoluble. However, this composite of high transparency and largely uncompromised conductivity will slightly swell in an aqueous environment. While a change in device geometries within the body is generally undesirable, a slight swelling of a polymer and/or its (hydrogel) electrodes may actually be favorable to enhance the electrode-tissue contact after device insertion. The water-uptake of PDMS itself is very low (below 1%). However, this might be just sufficient to stabilize device position within the tissue.

1.3.9 Open issues

As mentioned before, PDMS is very hydrophobic. Therefore, it is not wettable by aqueous or polar dispersions of organic conductors. Oxygen plasma treatment will render the PDMS surface hydrophilic by creating and exposing hydroxyl, carboxyl and peroxide groups on its surface, though. Depending on the storage conditions, this hydrophilicity is temporally more or less stable (Donzel *et al.*, 2001). Under ambient conditions, it will usually degrade rapidly after the first 30 minutes. It can be anticipated that with shrinking channel feature sizes, the presented method of filling these channels (by coating the entire scaffold backside with the CP dispersion and then scraping it from the plateaus after the partial evaporation of the solvent) may not necessarily work well anymore. However, by playing with the two extremes of wettability, a channel-only plasma treatment may solve the problem. By temporarily covering the *polyMEA* with two adhesive sheets on both sides during plasma exposure, only the channel walls will be hydrophilized. After sheet removal and upon spreading the dispersion onto the scaffold, it will self-distribute within the channels only. For each channel geometry, finding the proper plasma parameters (power, frequency, pressure, temperature, time) might not be trivial, though.

While the softness and flexibility of all-polymer MEAs is one of their main assets, they have one major drawback: a MEA will not be easy to insert into dense tissue. A removable insertion device may alleviate this problem, though. During device fabrication, stiffer insertion and guidance aids could be embedded into the polymer microchannel scaffold

---

[28] Plasma surface activation parameters for all types of MEAs stayed in the following ranges: One to three minutes at 30 – 60 W at 2.45 GHz in a 0.2 – 0.4 mbar pure oxygen atmosphere.

such as anti-stick-coated polymer or glass fibers, which would then be withdrawn once the *polyMEA* is in its final position.

The used type of PDMS already breaks after 100% tear. Softer and more stretchable polyurethanes or silicones are available that would render the devices even more flexible and tear-resistant. However, most of them have still to be tested for their biocompatibility. And some of them are only milky translucent, which make them less suitable for concurrent cell imaging studies.

1.3.10 Optional strategies and future directions

The flexibility of PDMS can be exploited for fabricating spherically bent neural probes that may become useful as retinal implants or for electroretinogram recordings as described *e.g.*, by Rodger *et al.* for parylene-based platinum electrode arrays (Rodger *et al.*, 2008). While the current master production gives microstructures on a plane, a copy thereof may take on any shape. It only requires the placing of a PDMS scaffold onto the inverted shape of the desired topography during master reproduction in epoxy. The bending of the PDMS slab will certainly distort some of the microchannel features. But as long as the curvatures are not too sharp, electrode geometries will not be compromised. The concept is sketched out in Fig. 5.

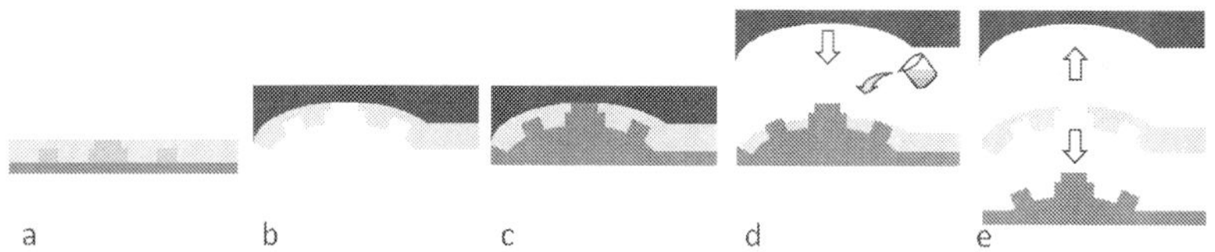

Fig. 5. Concept of fabricating non-planar *polyMEAs*. **a**) Replica-molding of a PDMS *polyMEA* microchannel scaffold (light blue) from planar master (orange). **b**) Fitting of the planar *polyMEA* scaffold into a non-planar template (black). **c**) Filling of shaped *polyMEA* microcavities with epoxy (green). **d**) After lifting off the template and removing the curved *polyMEA* from the cured epoxy, the non-planar epoxy master copy is coated with uncured PDMS and covered by the curved template. e) Removal of epoxy master copy and template after curing of PDMS gives a non-planar *polyMEA* microchannel scaffold.

Similar to classical soft-lithography, the microchannels could also serve for the assisted transfer of conductive patterns onto other carrier substrates (Fig. 6). When placed onto a (nano-porous) carrier (*e.g.*, a (filter) membrane) (Fig. 6-1), the channels may be filled with any kind of colloidal conductor material (Fig. 6-2). Upon applying a vacuum (underneath the membrane), the solvent will evaporate thereby leaving a conductor pattern on the membrane (Fig. 6-3). By filling the electrode and pad cavities with a sacrificial paste (*e.g.*, wax) (Fig. 6-4), removing the microchannel scaffold (Fig. 6-5), spin coating an insulation layer on the top (and bottom) side of the carrier (Fig. 6-6) and removing the sacrificial plugs from electrodes and pads in a final step (Fig. 6-7), a CP electrode array with design features similar to that reported by Guo *et al.* can be generated in the most straightforward and cost-efficient fashion (Guo *et al.*, 2010).

PEDOT:PSS can be purchased as an inkjet-compatible formulation. Thus, the filling of the microchannels with the conductor could not only be further automated, but different thicknesses or blends be deposited in different regions.

Alternatively, after the local laser-assisted alteration of the PDMS channel surfaces and the autocatalytic deposition of a Pt priming layer (Dupas-Bruzek, Drean, *et al.*, 2009), EDOT or other precursors could be polymerized electrochemically to give electroconductive electrodes and tracks. The microchannels and the PDMS itself could be furthermore exploited in controlled drug-release strategies (Fig. 7b) (Colas, 2001; Musick *et al.*, 2009). Various neural implant design studies with included microfluidics have already been reported (*e.g.*, (Metz *et al.*, 2004; Suzuki *et al.*, 2004; Seidl & *Et al.*, 2010)) and their benefit been discussed recently (Musienko *et al.*, 2009). Although the stable coupling of the microchannels to outside fluidics might be possible (*e.g.*, by making use of multilayer bonding concepts (Zhang *et al.*, 2010) or reversible mechanical, pressure- or vacuum-assisted interconnection strategies (Chen & Pan, 2011)), without doubt it will be even more challenging than the design of fail-proof electrical connectors as discussed above.

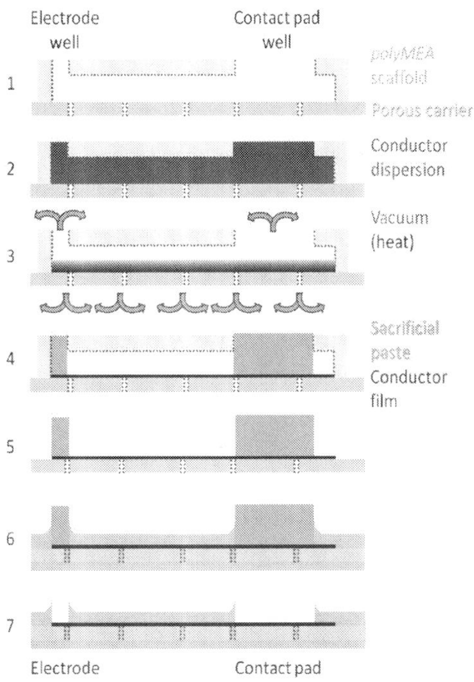

Fig. 6. *polyMEA* scaffold-assisted microelectrode patterning of thin-film carrier substrates. **1)** Placing of scaffold onto carrier and **2)** filling of microchannel cavities with conductor dispersion. **3)** Solvent evaporation leaves micropatterned conductor traces on the carrier. **4)** Temporary protection of electrodes and pads by application of a sacrificial paste through electrode and pad through-holes, **5)** removal of scaffold and **6)** application of top-side insulation layer (*e.g.*, by spin- or dip-coating) and **7)** removal of paste to deinsulate electrodes and pads.

With or without taking advantage of microfluidic connectors, neural processes could grow into the microchannels (Fig. 7b, left) as demonstrated by various groups (Morin *et al.*, 2005; Claverol-Tinture *et al.*, 2007; Benmerah *et al.*, 2009; Lacour *et al.*, 2010). This would increase the likelihood of identifying the actual origin of the bioelectrical signals. Alternatively, the preloading of empty or CP-coated microchannels with slow-release (electroconductive) hydrogels carrying diverse drugs could be pursued (Fig. 7a), thereby steering neural differentiation, regeneration and activity with growth or signaling factors, alleviating probe insertion damage by antibiotics and anti-inflammatory drugs, or attenuating the formation of glial scars by mitotic inhibitors (Peppas *et al.*, 2006; Guiseppi-Elie, 2010). In that case, the electrical conductivity of the gel should be sufficiently high to warrant the coupling between the neuron and the conductive PEDOT:PSS film covering the microchannel walls. Alternatively or in combination, the PDMS itself could be loaded with drugs that are either soluble in PDMS or stored in porous cavities in a local silicone co-formulation. Delivering organic drugs through polymeric microchannels bears the risk of undesirable dissolution and accumulation of the compounds within the polymer over time, though. PDMS is particular prone to absorb *e.g.*, organic solvents (Lee *et al.*, 2003). In consequence, the absorption and release kinetics would have to be tested for each substance. While this absorption behavior could be a disadvantage in acute studies, it may become advantageous for chronic drug delivery where a slow and constant release of a drug is desired. In combination with the local deposition of photoelectric polymers, light-mediated electrical stimulation sites could be created (Fig. 7c) (Antognazza *et al.*, 2009; Facchetti, 2010; Ghezzi *et al.*, 2011). On a similar line, optical fibers or waveguides could be embedded into these channels for the light stimulation of optogenetic probes (Fig. 7d) (Im *et al.*, 2011). Neural activity from light-responsive neurons could thus be recorded from the PEDOT:PSS electrodes at the end of PEDOT:PSS-coated channels upon their optical stimulation through the very same channel.

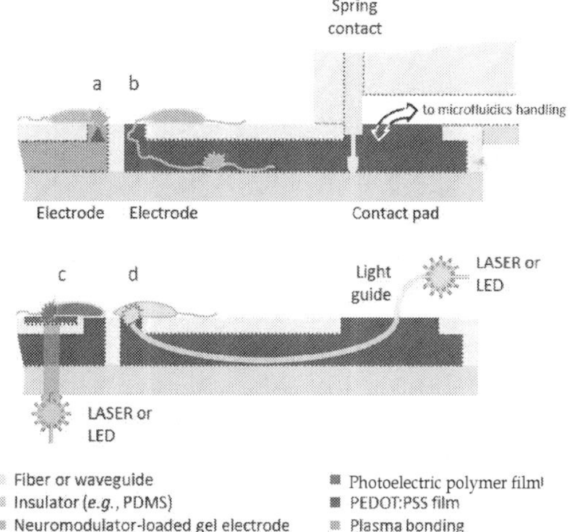

Fig. 7. Conceptual device enhancements. Delivering drugs **a)** passively through microchannel-embedded gel electrodes or **b)** actively by resorting to multilayer bonding concepts reported *e.g.* by Zhang *et al.* (Zhang *et al.*, 2010) or reversible mechanical, pressure- or vacuum-assisted interconnection strategies (*e.g.*, "fit-2-flow" (Chen & Pan, 2011)). Recording from neural processes after their ingrowth into PEDOT:PSS coated electrode microchannels. **c)** Photo stimulation of neurons through patterned photoelectric polymer films. **d)** Optical stimulation of optogenetically engineered neurons through channel-embedded waveguides or fiber optics.

2. Conclusions

Neuroprosthetic devices should mimic as best as possible the tissue they are placed into. The tissue would then accept them as its own or just ignore them. They should furthermore be chemically, mechanically and functionally time-invariant for uncompromised performance. Fabricating electrode arrays exclusively from soft polymeric materials may be one step into that direction. The innovative concept of filling bi- or multi-level microchannel electrode array scaffolds with polymer conductors opens several new routes for designing and fabricating neuroprosthetic devices not only on the laboratory bench, but also through existing replica mass production schemes (*e.g.*, mold-injection, hot-embossing). In contrast to metal MEAs (Sadleir *et al.*, 2005), polymer conductors may turn out to be compatible with computer tomography (CT) and magnetic resonance imaging (MRI), minimizing or avoiding image artifacts (Chen & Wiscombe, 1998; Flanders & Schwartz, 2008). Given the vast choice of insulation and conductor materials, device properties and performance can be tuned in a multitude of ways. While thin coatings of the microchannel walls with PEDOT:PSS lead to largely transparent devices suitable for combined electrophysiological and microscopy *in vitro* studies, currently, film stability with respect to bending and stretching is still limited. Nevertheless, depending on the fabrication approach, electrodes can be shaped as ring electrodes or classical area electrodes. Alternatively, channels can be filled entirely with rubber-like gPDMS or other conductive PDMS or PU composites, rendering the devices excellently stable to bending and stretching. If both transparency and flexibility are required, a hybrid strategy of combining PEDOT:PSS electrodes with gPDMS tracks and connector pads may be chosen. While the presented results refer to proof-of-concept studies with *polyMEAs* still having rather large electrode and track dimensions, there is no conceptual hurdle that prevents their further miniaturization. It can thus be foreseen that the presented *polyMEA* concept heralds a new generation of implantable neuroprosthetic electrode arrays.

3. Acknowledgements

Several talented students and researchers contributed to the development and evolution of the various *polyMEA* devices. Their enthusiasm, help and dedication is greatly appreciated. In particular, I would like to thank Angelika Murr, Sandra Wolff, Christian Dautermann, Stefan Trellenkamp, Jens Wüsten and Mario Cerino for their support in exploring diverse device designs including their fabrication and testing, Tanja Neumann, Simone Riedel, Marina Nanni, Francesca Succol, and Maria Teresa Tedesco for their assistance in cell culture preparation and maintenance, Evelyne Sernagor for the preparation of retinal whole mounts, Paolo Medini and Giuliano Iurilli for epicortical recordings, Laura Gasparini and Francesco Difato for support in microscopy, Giacomo Pruzzo for his advice and assistance in developing various electronic gadgets, Tommaso Fellin for insightful discussions on future *polyMEA* exploitation pathways, Christiane Ziegler for providing the startup infrastructure and research environment, Sergio Martinoia and the Dept. of Biophysical and Electronic Engineering at the University of Genoa for temporary lab access, and Fabio Benfenati for subsequent support in shaping the *polyMEA* research line. A generous PDMS sample provided by Wacker Chemie AG is highly appreciated. This work is supported by the Italian Institute of Technology Foundation.

4. References

Abidian, M.R., Corey, J.M., Kipke, D.R. & Martin, D.C. (2010). Conducting-polymer nanotubes improve electrical properties, mechanical adhesion, neural attachment, and neurite outgrowth of neural electrodes, *Small*, Vol. 6 No. 3, pp. 421-429.

Ahn, B.Y., Duoss, E.B., Motala, M.J., Guo, X., Park, S.I., Xiong, Y., Yoon, J., Nuzzo, R.G., Rogers, J.A. & Lewis, J.A. (2009). Omnidirectional printing of flexible, stretchable, and spanning silver microelectrodes, *Science*, Vol. 323 No. 5921, pp. 1590-1593.

Antognazza, M.R., Ghezzi, D., Musitelli, D., Garbugli, M. & Lanzani, G. (2009). A hybrid solid-liquid polymer photodiode for the bioenvironment, *Applied Physics Letters*, Vol. 94 No. 24, pp. 243501.

Asplund, M., Nyberg, T. & Inganas, O. (2010). Electroactive polymers for neural interfaces, *Polymer Chemistry*, Vol. 1 No. 9, pp. 1374-1391.

Ateh, D.D., Navsaria, H.A. & Vadgama, P. (2006). Polypyrrole-based conducting polymers and interactions with biological tissues, *J R Soc Interface*, Vol. 3 No. 11, pp. 741-752.

Barr, S., Hill, E. & Bayat, A. (2010). Patterning of novel breast implant surfaces by enhancing silicone biocompatibility, using biomimetic topographies, *Eplasty*, Vol. 10, pp. e31.

Baumann, W., Schreiber, E., Krause, G., Stüwe, S., Podssun, A., Homma, S., Anlauf, H., Freund, I. & Lehmann, M. (2002). Multiparametric neurosensor microchip, in *Eurosensors XVI* ISBN, Prag, pp. 1169-1172

Baumann, W.H., Lehmann, M., Schwinde, A., Ehret, R., Brischwein, M. & Wolf, B. (1999). Microelectronic sensor system for microphysiological application on living cells, *Sensors and Actuators B: Chemical*, Vol. 55 No. 1, pp. 77-89.

Bear, M.F., Connors, B.W. & Paradiso, M.A. (2007). *Neuroscience: Exploring the brain*, Lippincott Williams & Wilkins, Baltimore.

Beattie, A.J., Curtis, A.S.G., Wilkinson, C.D.W. & Riehle, M. (2009). Nanomaterials for neural interfaces: Emerging new function and potential applications, in Offenhäusser, A. & Rinaldi, R. (Eds.), *Nanobioelectronics - for electronics, biology, and medicine*. Springer New York, 978-0-387-09459-5, pp. 277-286.

Benmerah, S., Lacour, S.P. & Tarte, E. (2009). Design and fabrication of neural implant with thick microchannels based on flexible polymeric materials, *Conference Proceedings, Annual International Conference of the IEEE Engineering in Medicine and Biology Society*, Vol. 2009, pp. 6400-6403.

Berdondini, L., Chippalone, M., Van Der Wal, P.D., Imfeld, K., De Rooij, N.F., Koudelka-Hep, M., Tedesco, M., Martinoia, S., Van Pelt, J., Le Masson, G. & Garenne, A. (2006). A microelectrode array (mea) integrated with clustering structures for investigating in vitro neurodynamics in confined interconnected sub-populations of neurons, *Sensors and Actuators B*, Vol. 114, pp. 530-541.

Berdondini, L., Imfeld, K., Maccione, A., Tedesco, M., Neukom, S., Koudelka-Hep, M. & Martinoia, S. (2009). Active pixel sensor array for high spatio-temporal resolution electrophysiological recordings from single cell to large scale neuronal networks, *Lab on a Chip*, Vol. 9 No. 18, pp. 2644-2651.

Berdondini, L., Massobrio, P., Chiappalone, M., Tedesco, M., Imfeld, K., Maccione, A., Gandolfo, M., Koudelka-Hep, M. & Martinoia, S. (2009). Extracellular recordings from locally dense microelectrode arrays coupled to dissociated cortical cultures, *J Neurosci Methods,* Vol. 177 No. 2, pp. 386-396.

Blau, A., Murr, A., Wolff, S., Sernagor, E., Medini, P., Iurilli, G., Ziegler, C. & Benfenati, F. (2011). Flexible, all-polymer microelectrode arrays for the capture of cardiac and neuronal signals, *Biomaterials,* Vol. 32 No. 7, pp. 1778-1786.

Bongard, M., Gabriel, G., Villa, R., Gomez, R., Benito, N. & Fernandez, E. (2010). Spike recordings from ganglion cell populations using a new type of carbon nanotubes surface multielectrodes, in Stett, A. (Ed.), *Proceedings of the 7th Int. Meeting on Substrate-Integrated Microelectrode Arrays, June 29 – July 2.* BIOPRO Baden-Württemberg GmbH, ISBN, Reutlingen, pp. 259-260.

Bonifazi, P. & Fromherz, P. (2002). Silicon chip for electronic communication between nerve cells by non-invasive interfacing and analog–digital processing, *Advanced Materials,* Vol. 14 No. 17, pp. 1190-1193.

Boppart, S.A., Wheeler, B.C. & Wallace, C.S. (1992). A flexible perforated microelectrode array for extended neural recordings, *IEEE Transactions on Biomedical Engineering,* Vol. 39 No. 1, pp. 37-42.

Boretius, T., Schuettler, M. & Stieglitz, T. (2011). On the stability of poly-ethylenedioxythiopene as coating material for active neural implants, *Artificial Organs,* Vol. 35 No. 3, pp. 245-248.

Breckenridge, L.J., Wilson, R.J., Connolly, P., Curtis, A.S., Dow, J.A., Blackshaw, S.E. & Wilkinson, C.D. (1995). Advantages of using microfabricated extracellular electrodes for in vitro neuronal recording, *Journal of Neuroscience Research,* Vol. 42 No. 2, pp. 266-276.

Briquet, F., Colas, A. & Thomas, X. (1996). Silicones for medical use, in, ISBN, pp. 10.

Bucher, V., Brunner, B., Leibrock, C., Schubert, M. & Nisch, W. (2001). Electrical properties of a light-addressable microelectrode chip with high electrode density for extracellular stimulation and recording of excitable cells, *Biosensors & Bioelectronics,* Vol. 16 No. 3, pp. 205-210.

Butt, H.-J., Graf, K. & Kappl, M. (2003). *Physics and chemistry of interfaces,* Wiley, 3-527-40413-9, Weinheim.

Calixto, C.M.F., Mendes, R.K., Oliveira, A.C.D., Ramos, L.A., Cervini, P. & Cavalheiro, É.T.G. (2007). Development of graphite-polymer composites as electrode materials, *Materials Research,* Vol. 10, pp. 109-114.

Chen, A. & Pan, T. (2011). Fit-to-flow (f2f) interconnects: Universal reversible adhesive-free microfluidic adaptors for lab-on-a-chip systems, *Lab on a Chip,* Vol. 11 No. 4, pp. 727-732.

Chen, C. & Folch, A. (2006). A high-performance elastomeric patch clamp chip, *Lab on a Chip,* Vol. 6 No. 10, pp. 1338-1345.

Chen, J.C. & Wiscombe, B. (1998). Method and pdt probe for minimizing ct and mri image artifacts, in. Light Sciences Limited Partnership (Issaquah, WA), ISBN, pp. 15.

Cheung, K.C. (2007). Implantable microscale neural interfaces, *Biomed Microdevices,* Vol. 9 No. 6, pp. 923-938.

Clark, J.W. (1998). The origin of biopotentials, in Webster, J.G. (Ed.), *Medical instrumentation: Application and design* John Wiley and Sons, Inc., NY, pp. 121-182.

Claverol-Tinture, E., Cabestany, J. & Rosell, X. (2007). Multisite recording of extracellular potentials produced by microchannel-confined neurons in-vitro, *IEEE Transactions on Bio-medical Engineering,* Vol. 54 No. 2, pp. 331-335.

Cogan, S.F. (2008). Neural stimulation and recording electrodes, *Annual Review of Biomedical Engineering,* Vol. 10, pp. 275-309.

Colas, A. (2001). Silicones in pharmaceutical applications, in, ISBN, pp. 24.

Colas, A. & Curtis, J. (2004). Silicone biomaterials: History and chemistry, in Ratner, B.D., Hoffman, A.S., Schoen, F.J. & Lemans, J.E. (Eds.), *Biomaterials science - an introduction to materials in medicine.* Academic Press, 978-0-12-582463-7, pp. 80-86.

Collazos-Castro, J.E., Polo, J.L., Hernandez-Labrado, G.R., Padial-Canete, V. & Garcia-Rama, C. (2010). Bioelectrochemical control of neural cell development on conducting polymers, *Biomaterials,* Vol. 31 No. 35, pp. 9244-9255.

Connolly, P., Clark, P., Curtis, A.S.G., Dow, J.a.T. & Wilkinson, C.D. (1990). An extracellular microelectrode array for monitoring electrogenic cells in culture, *Biosensors & Biolelectronics,* Vol. 5, pp. 223-234.

Cui, X., Lee, V.A., Raphael, Y., Wiler, J.A., Hetke, J.F., Anderson, D.J. & Martin, D.C. (2001). Surface modification of neural recording electrodes with conducting polymer/biomolecule blends, *Journal of Biomedical Materials Research,* Vol. 56 No. 2, pp. 261-272.

Cui, X.T. & Zhou, D.D. (2007). Poly (3,4-ethylenedioxythiophene) for chronic neural stimulation, *Neural Systems and Rehabilitation Engineering, IEEE Transactions on,* Vol. 15 No. 4, pp. 502-508.

Cunningham, W., Mathieson, K., Mcewan, F.A., Blue, A., Mcgeachy, R., Mcleod, J.A., Morris-Ellis, C., O'shea, V., Smith, K.M., Litke, A. & Rahman, M. (2001). Fabrication of microelectrode arrays for neural measurements from retinal tissue, *Journal of Physics D: Applied Physics* No. 18, pp. 2804.

Curtis, J. & Colas, A. (2004). Medical applications of silicones, in Ratner, B.D., Hoffman, A.S., Schoen, F.J. & Lemans, J.E. (Eds.), *Biomaterials science - an introduction to materials in medicine.* Academic Press, 978-0-12-582463-7, pp. 697-707.

Cvelbar, U., Pejovnik, S., Mozetiè, M. & Zalar, A. (2003). Increased surface roughness by oxygen plasma treatment of graphite/polymer composite, *Applied Surface Science,* Vol. 210 No. 3-4, pp. 255-261.

Debusschere, B.D. & Kovacs, G.T.A. (2001). Portable cell-based biosensor system using integrated cmos cell-cartridges, *Biosensors and Bioelectronics,* Vol. 16 No. 7-8, pp. 543-556.

Difato, F., Maschio, M.D., Marconi, E., Ronzitti, G., Maccione, A., Fellin, T., Berdondini, L., Chieregatti, E., Benfenati, F. & Blau, A. (2011). Combined optical tweezers and laser dissector for controlled ablation of functional connections in neural networks, *Journal of Biomedical Optics,* Vol. 16 No. 5, pp. 051306-051309

Donzel, C., Geissler, M., Bernard, A., Wolf, H., Michel, B., Hilborn, J. & Delamarche, E. (2001). Hydrophilic poly(dimethylsiloxane) stamps for microcontact printing, *Advanced Materials*, Vol. 13 No. 15, pp. 1164-1167.

Dowling, J. (2008). Current and future prospects for optoelectronic retinal prostheses, *Eye*, Vol. 23 No. 10, pp. 1999-2005.

Dupas-Bruzek, C., Drean, P. & Derozier, D. (2009). Pt metallization of laser transformed medical grade silicone rubber: Last step toward a miniaturized nerve electrode fabrication process, *Journal of Applied Physics*, Vol. 106 No. 7, pp. 074913:074911-074915.

Dupas-Bruzek, C., Robbe, O., Addad, A., Turrell, S. & Derozier, D. (2009). Transformation of medical grade silicone rubber under nd:Yag and excimer laser irradiation: First step towards a new miniaturized nerve electrode fabrication process, *Applied Surface Science*, Vol. 255 No. 21, pp. 8715-8721.

Duport, S., Millerin, C., Muller, D. & Correges, P. (1999). A metallic multisite recording system designed for continuous long-term monitoring of electrophysiological activity in slice cultures, *Biosensors & Bioelectronics*, Vol. 14 No. 4, pp. 369-376.

Ehret, R., Baumann, W., Brischwein, M., Lehmann, M., Henning, T., Freund, I., Drechsler, S., Friedrich, U., Hubert, M.L., Motrescu, E., Kob, A., Palzer, H., Grothe, H. & Wolf, B. (2001). Multiparametric microsensor chips for screening applications, *Fresenius' Journal of Analytical Chemistry*, Vol. 369 No. 1, pp. 30-35.

Eick, S., Wallys, J., Hofmann, B., Van Ooyen, A., Schnakenberg, U., Ingebrandt, S. & Offenhäusser, A. (2009). Iridium oxide microelectrode arrays for in vitro stimulation of individual rat neurons from dissociated cultures, *Frontiers in Neuroengineering*, Vol. 2 No. 16, pp. 1-12.

Eschermann, J.F., Stockmann, R., Hueske, M., Vu, X.T., Ingebrandt, S. & Offenhausser, A. (2009). Action potentials of hl-1 cells recorded with silicon nanowire transistors, *Applied Physics Letters*, Vol. 95 No. 8, pp. 083703-083703.

Facchetti, A. (2010). Π-conjugated polymers for organic electronics and photovoltaic cell applications†, *Chemistry of Materials*, Vol. 23 No. 3, pp. 733-758.

Fejtl, M., Stett, A., Nisch, W., Boven, K.-H. & Möller, A. (2006). On micro-eletrode array revival: Its development, sophistication of recording and stimulation, in Taketani, M. & Baudry, M. (Eds.), *Advances in network electrophysiology. Using multi-electrode arrays*. Springer, 978-0-387-25857-7 (Print) 978-0-387-25858-4 (Online), New York, pp. 24-37.

Flanders, A., E. & Schwartz, E.D. (2008). Spinal trauma, in Atlas, S.W. (Ed.), *Magnetic resonance imaging of the brain and spine*. Wolters Kluwer Health, pp. 1564-1623.

Frey, U., Sedivy, J., Heer, F., Pedron, R., Ballini, M., Mueller, J., Bakkum, D., Hafizovic, S., Faraci, F.D., Greve, F., Kirstein, K.U. & Hierlemann, A. (2010). Switch-matrix-based high-density microelectrode array in cmos technology, *Solid-State Circuits, IEEE Journal of*, Vol. 45 No. 2, pp. 467-482.

Fromherz, P. (2006). Three levels of neuroelectronic interfacing, *Annals of the New York Academy of Sciences*, Vol. 1093 No. 1, pp. 143-160.

Fromherz, P., Offenhausser, A., Vetter, T. & Weiss, J.A. (1991). Neuron-silicon junction: A retzius cell of the leech on an insulated-gate field-effect transistor, *Science*, Vol. 252, pp. 1290-1293.

Gabriel, G., Gómez, R., Bongard, M., Benito, N., Fernández, E. & Villa, R. (2009). Easily made single-walled carbon nanotube surface microelectrodes for neuronal applications, *Biosensors and Bioelectronics*, Vol. 24 No. 7, pp. 1942-1948.

George, P.M., Lyckman, A.W., Lavan, D.A., Hegde, A., Leung, Y., Avasare, R., Testa, C., Alexander, P.M., Langer, R. & Sur, M. (2005). Fabrication and biocompatibility of polypyrrole implants suitable for neural prosthetics, *Biomaterials*, Vol. 26 No. 17, pp. 3511-3519.

Ghezzi, D., Antognazza, M.R., Dal Maschio, M., Lanzarini, E., Benfenati, F. & Lanzani, G. (2011). A hybrid bioorganic interface for neuronal photoactivation, *Nat Commun*, Vol. 2, pp. 166.

Gholmieh, G., Soussou, W., Han, M., Ahuja, A., Hsiao, M.C., Song, D., Tanguay, A.R., Jr. & Berger, T.W. (2006). Custom-designed high-density conformal planar multielectrode arrays for brain slice electrophysiology, *Journal of Neuroscience Methods*, Vol. 152 No. 1-2, pp. 116-129.

Giovangrandi, L., Gilchrist, K.H., Whittington, R.H. & T.A. Kovacs, G. (2006). Low-cost microelectrode array with integrated heater for extracellular recording of cardiomyocyte cultures using commercial flexible printed circuit technology, *Sensors and Actuators B: Chemical*, Vol. 113 No. 1, pp. 545-554.

Gong, X. & Wen, W. (2009). Polydimethylsiloxane-based conducting composites and their applications in microfluidic chip fabrication, *Biomicrofluidics*, Vol. 3 No. 1, pp. 12007.

Graimann, B., Allison, B. & Pfurtscheller, G. (2010). Brain-computer interfaces, in. Springer, ISBN, Berlin, pp. 300.

Green, R.A., Lovell, N.H. & Poole-Warren, L.A. (2010). Impact of co-incorporating laminin peptide dopants and neurotrophic growth factors on conducting polymer properties, *Acta Biomaterialia*, Vol. 6 No. 1, pp. 63-71.

Gross, G.W., Harsch, A., Rhoades, B.K. & Gopel, W. (1997). Odor, drug and toxin analysis with neuronal networks in vitro: Extracellular array recording of network responses, *Biosensors & Bioelectronics*, Vol. 12 No. 5, pp. 373-393.

Gross, G.W., Rieske, E., Kreutzberg, G.W. & Meyer, A. (1977). A new fixed-array multimicroelectrode system designed for long-term monitoring of extracellular single unit neuronal activity in vitro, *Neuroscience Letters* No. 6, pp. 101-105.

Gross, G.W., Wen, W.Y. & Lin, J.W. (1985). Transparent indium-tin oxide electrode patterns for extracellular, multisite recording in neuronal cultures, *Journal of Neuroscience Methods*, Vol. 15 No. 3, pp. 243-252.

Guimard, N.K., Gomez, N. & Schmidt, C.E. (2007). Conducting polymers in biomedical engineering, *Progress in Polymer Science*, Vol. 32 No. 8-9, pp. 876-921.

Guiseppi-Elie, A. (2010). Electroconductive hydrogels: Synthesis, characterization and biomedical applications, *Biomaterials*, Vol. 31 No. 10, pp. 2701-2716.

Gunning, D.E., Hottowy, P., Dabrowski, W., Hobbs, J.P., Beggs, J.M., Sher, A., Litke, A.M., Kenney, C.J. & Mathieson, K. (2010). High-density micro-needles for in vitro neural studies, in Stett, A. (Ed.), *Proceedings of the 7th Int. Meeting on Substrate-Integrated Microelectrode Arrays, June 29 – July 2*. BIOPRO Baden-Württemberg GmbH, ISBN, Reutlingen, pp. 275-275.

Guo, L., Meacham, K.W., Hochman, S. & Deweerth, S.P. (2010). A pdms-based conical-well microelectrode array for surface stimulation and recording of neural tissues, *IEEE Transactions on Bio-medical Engineering*, Vol. 57 No. 10, pp. 2485-2494.

Haemmerle, H., Egert, U., Mohr, A. & Nisch, W. (1994). Extracellular recording in neuronal networks with substrate integrated microelectrode arrays, *Biosensors & Biolelectronics*, Vol. 9 No. 9-10, pp. 691-696.

Hai, A., Dormann, A., Shappir, J., Yitzchaik, S., Bartic, C., Borghs, G., Langedijk, J.P.M. & Spira, M.E. (2009). Spine-shaped gold protrusions improve the adherence and electrical coupling of neurons with the surface of micro-electronic devices, *Journal of the Royal Society Interface*, Vol. 6 No. 41, pp. 1153-1165.

Hai, A., Shappir, J. & Spira, M.E. (2010). In-cell recordings by extracellular microelectrodes, *Nat Meth*, Vol. 7 No. 3, pp. 200-202.

Hajjhassan, M., Chodavarapu, V. & Musallam, S. (2008). Neuromems: Neural probe microtechnologies, *Sensors*, Vol. 8 No. 10, pp. 6704-6726.

Hassler, C., Boretius, T. & Stieglitz, T. (2011). Polymers for neural implants, *Journal of Polymer Science Part B: Polymer Physics*, Vol. 49 No. 1, pp. 18-33.

Heer, F., Hafizovic, S., Ugniwenko, T., Frey, U., Franks, W., Perriard, E., Perriard, J.C., Blau, A., Ziegler, C. & Hierlemann, A. (2007). Single-chip microelectronic system to interface with living cells, *Biosensors & Bioelectronics*, Vol. 22 No. 11, pp. 2546-2553.

Held, J., Gaspar, J., Koester, P.J., Tautorat, C., Cismak, A., Heilmann, A., Baumann, W., Trautmann, A., Ruther, P. & Paul, O. (2008). Microneedle arrays for intracellular recording applications, in *Micro Electro Mechanical Systems, 2008. MEMS 2008. IEEE 21st International Conference on*, ISBN, pp. 268-271.

Held, J., Gaspar, J., Ruther, P., Hagner, M., Cismak, A., Heilmann, A. & Paul, O. (2010). Solid silver microneedle electrode arrays for intracellular recording applications, in Stett, A. (Ed.), *Proceedings of the 7th Int. Meeting on Substrate-Integrated Microelectrode Arrays, June 29 – July 2*. BIOPRO Baden-Württemberg GmbH, ISBN, Reutlingen, pp. 247-248.

Held, J., Heynen, J., Stumpf, A., Nisch, W., Burkhardt, C. & Stett, A. (2010). Micro pillar electrodes on meas for tissue stimulation, in Stett, A. (Ed.), *Proceedings of the 7th Int. Meeting on Substrate-Integrated Microelectrode Arrays, June 29 – July 2*. BIOPRO Baden-Württemberg GmbH, ISBN, Reutlingen, pp. 241-242.

Henle, C., Raab, M., Cordeiro, J., Doostkam, S., Schulze-Bonhage, A., Stieglitz, T. & Rickert, J. (2011). First long term in vivo study on subdurally implanted micro-ecog electrodes, manufactured with a novel laser technology, *Biomedical Microdevices*, Vol. 13 No. 1, pp. 59-68.

Hetke, J. & Anderson, D. (2002). Silicon microelectrodes for extracellular recording, in *Handbook of neuroprosthetic methods*. CRC Press, 978-0-8493-1100-0, pp. 29.

Heuschkel, M.O., Fejtl, M., Raggenbass, M., Bertrand, D. & Renaud, P. (2002). A three-dimensional multi-electrode array for multi-site stimulation and recording in acute brain slices, *J Neurosci Methods,* Vol. 114 No. 2, pp. 135-148.

Heuschkel, M.O., Wirth, C., Steidl, E.-M. & Buisson, B. (2006). Development of 3d multi electrode arrays for use with acute tussue slices, in Taketani, M. & Baudry, M. (Eds.), *Advances in network electrophysiology. Using multi-electrode arrays.* Springer, 978-0-387-25857-7 (Print) 978-0-387-25858-4 (Online), New York, pp. 69-111.

Hierlemann, A., Frey, U., Hafizovic, S. & Heer, F. (2011). Growing cells atop microelectronic chips: Interfacing electrogenic cells in vitro with cmos-based microelectrode arrays, *Proceedings of the IEEE,* Vol. 99 No. 2, pp. 252-284.

Hofmann, B., Katelhon, E., Schottdorf, M., Offenhausser, A. & Wolfrum, B. (2011). Nanocavity electrode array for recording from electrogenic cells, *Lab on a Chip.*

Hu, Z., Zhou, D.M., Greenberg, R. & Thundat, T. (2006). Nanopowder molding method for creating implantable high-aspect-ratio electrodes on thin flexible substrates, *Biomaterials,* Vol. 27 No. 9, pp. 2009-2017.

Huang, J.-R., Lin, W.-T., Huang, R., Lin, C.-Y. & Wu, J.-K. (2011). Conductive coating method to inhibit marine biofouling, in, ISBN.

Hutzler, M., Lambacher, A., Eversmann, B., Jenkner, M., Thewes, R. & Fromherz, P. (2006). High-resolution multi-transistor array recording of electrical field potentials in cultured brain slices, *Journal of Neurophysiology,* Vol. 96, pp. 1638--1645.

Im, M., Cho, I.-J., Wu, F., Wise, K.D. & Yoon, E. (2011). Neural probes integrated with optical mixer/splitter waveguides and multiple stimulation sites, in *24th IEEE International Conference on Micro Electro Mechanical Systems (MEMS),* ISBN, Cancun, Mexico, pp. 1051-1054.

Imfeld, K., Garenne, A., Neukom, S., Maccione, A., Martinoia, S., Koudelka-Hep, M. & Berdondini, L. (2007). High-resolution mea platform for in-vitro electrogenic cell networks imaging, in *Engineering in Medicine and Biology Society, 2007. EMBS 2007. 29th Annual International Conference of the IEEE,* ISBN, pp. 6085-6088.

Inganäs, O. (2010). Hybrid electronics and electrochemistry with conjugated polymers, *Chemical Society Reviews,* Vol. 39 No. 7, pp. 2633-2642.

Israel, D.A., Barry, W.H., Edell, D.J. & Mark, R.G. (1984). An array of microelectrodes to stimulate and record from cardiac cells in culture, *American Journal of Physiology - Heart and Circulatory Physiology,* Vol. 247 No. 4, pp. H669-H674.

Jaber, F.T., Labeed, F.H. & Hughes, M.P. (2009). Action potential recording from dielectrophoretically positioned neurons inside micro-wells of a planar microelectrode array, *Journal of Neuroscience Methods,* Vol. 182 No. 2, pp. 225-235.

James, C.D., Spence, A.J., Dowell-Mesfin, N.M., Hussain, R.J., Smith, K.L., Craighead, H.G., Isaacson, M.S., Shain, W. & Turner, J.N. (2004). Extracellular recordings from patterned neuronal networks using planar microelectrode arrays, *IEEE Trans Biomed Eng,* Vol. 51 No. 9, pp. 1640-1648.

Janata, J. & Josowicz, M. (2003). Conducting polymers in electronic chemical sensors, *Nat Mater,* Vol. 2 No. 1, pp. 19-24.

Janders, M., Egert, U., Stelzle, M. & Nisch, W. (1996). Novel thin film titanium nitride micro-electrodes with excellent charge transfer capability for cell stimulation and sensing applications, in Boom, H., Robinson, C., Rutten, W., Neuman, M. & Wijkstra, H. (Eds.), *Proceedings of 18th Annual International Conference of the IEEE Engineering in Medicine and Biology Society*. Naturwissenschaftliches und Med. Inst. Reutlingen Germany

Jansen, H., Gardeniers, H., Boer, M.D., Elwenspoek, M. & Fluitman, J. (1996). A survey on the reactive ion etching of silicon in microtechnology, *Journal of Micromechanics and Microengineering*, Vol. 6 No. 1, pp. 14.

Proceedings of the 18th Annual International Conference of the IEEE Engineering in Medicine and Biology Society. `Bridging Disciplines for Biomedicine' (Cat. No.96CH36036). IEEE New York NY USA, ISBN, Amsterdam, Netherlands, pp. 245-247.

Jochum, T., Denison, T. & Wolf, P. (2009). Integrated circuit amplifiers for multi-electrode intracortical recording, *Journal of Neural Engineering*, Vol. 6 No. 1, pp. 012001.

Johnstone, A.F., Gross, G.W., Weiss, D.G., Schroeder, O.H., Gramowski, A. & Shafer, T.J. (2010). Microelectrode arrays: A physiologically based neurotoxicity testing platform for the 21st century, *Neurotoxicology*, Vol. 31 No. 4, pp. 331-350.

Jung, S., Kang, C., Jung, I., Lee, S., Jung, P. & Ko, J. (2008). Fabrication of curved copper micromesh sheets using flexible pdms molds, *Microsystem Technologies*, Vol. 14 No. 6, pp. 829-833.

Kahol, P.K., Ho, J.C., Chen, Y.Y., Wang, C.R., Neeleshwar, S., Tsai, C.B. & Wessling, B. (2005). On metallic characteristics in some conducting polymers, *Synthetic Metals*, Vol. 151 No. 1, pp. 65-72.

Kawana, A. & Jimbo, Y. (1999). Neurointerface: Interfaces of neuronal networks to electrical circuit, in *Micro Electro Mechanical Systems, 1999. MEMS '99. Twelfth IEEE International Conference on*, ISBN, pp. 14-20.

Keefer, E.W., Botterman, B.R., Romero, M.I., Rossi, A.F. & Gross, G.W. (2008). Carbon nanotube coating improves neuronal recordings, *Nat Nano*, Vol. 3 No. 7, pp. 434-439.

Kirkpatrick, S. (1973). Percolation and conduction, *Reviews of Modern Physics*, Vol. 45 No. 4, pp. 574.

Klemic, K.G., Klemic, J.F. & Sigworth, F.J. (2005). An air-molding technique for fabricating pdms planar patch-clamp electrodes, *Pflügers Archiv European Journal of Physiology*, Vol. 449 No. 6, pp. 564-572.

Koester, P.J., Buehler, S.M., Stubbe, M., Tautorat, C., Niendorf, M., Baumann, W. & Gimsa, J. (2010). Modular glass chip system measuring the electric activity and adhesion of neuronal cells-application and drug testing with sodium valproic acid, *Lab on a Chip*, Vol. 10 No. 12, pp. 1579-1586.

Kotov, N.A., Winter, J.O., Clements, I.P., Jan, E., Timko, B.P., Campidelli, S., Pathak, S., Mazzatenta, A., Lieber, C.M., Prato, M., Bellamkonda, R.V., Silva, G.A., Kam, N.W.S., Patolsky, F. & Ballerini, L. (2009). Nanomaterials for neural interfaces, *Advanced Materials*, Vol. 21 No. 40, pp. 3970-4004.

Lacour, S., Benmerah, S., Tarte, E., Fitzgerald, J., Serra, J., Mcmahon, S., Fawcett, J., Graudejus, O., Yu, Z. & Morrison, B. (2010). Flexible and stretchable micro-electrodes for in vitro and in vivo neural interfaces, *Medical and Biological Engineering and Computing*, Vol. 48 No. 10, pp. 945-954.

Lambacher, A., Vitzthum, V., Zeitler, R., Eickenscheidt, M., Eversmann, B., Thewes, R. & Fromherz, P. (2011). Identifying firing mammalian neurons in networks with high-resolution multi-transistor array (mta), *Applied Physics A: Materials Science & Processing*, Vol. 102 No. 1, pp. 1-11.

Lange, U., Roznyatovskaya, N.V. & Mirsky, V.M. (2008). Conducting polymers in chemical sensors and arrays, *Analytica Chimica Acta*, Vol. 614 No. 1, pp. 1-26.

Lapitska, N., Gosseries, O., Delvaux, V., Overgaard, M., Nielsen, F., Maertens De Noordhout, A., Moonen, G. & Laureys, S. (2009). Transcranial magnetic stimulation in disorders of consciousness, *Rev Neurosci*, Vol. 20 No. 3-4, pp. 235-250.

Larmagnac, A., Musienko, P., Vörös, J. & Courtine, G. (2010). Highly stretchable pdms-based multi-electrode array for epidural electrical stimulation to regain motor function after spinal cord injury, in Stett, A. (Ed.), *Proceedings of the 7th Int. Meeting on Substrate-Integrated Microelectrode Arrays, June 29 – July 2*. BIOPRO Baden-Württemberg GmbH, ISBN, Reutlingen, pp. 229-230.

Leach, J.B., Achyuta, A.K. & Murthy, S.K. (2010). Bridging the divide between neuroprosthetic design, tissue engineering and neurobiology, *Front Neuroengineering*, Vol. 2, pp. 18.

Lebedev, M.A., Crist, R.E. & Nicolelis, M.a.L. (2008). Building brain-machine interfaces to restore neurological functions, in Nicolelis, M.A.L. (Ed.), *Methods for neural ensemble recordings*. CRC Press, Boca Raton.

Lee, J.N., Park, C. & Whitesides, G.M. (2003). Solvent compatibility of poly(dimethylsiloxane)-based microfluidic devices, *Analytical Chemistry*, Vol. 75 No. 23, pp. 6544-6554.

Li, L. & Fourkas, J.T. (2007). Multiphoton polymerization, *Materials Today*, Vol. 10 No. 6, pp. 30-37.

Logan, B.E. (2009). Exoelectrogenic bacteria that power microbial fuel cells, *Nat Rev Microbiol*, Vol. 7 No. 5, pp. 375-381.

Ludwig, K.A., Langhals, N.B., Joseph, M.D., Richardson-Burns, S.M., Hendricks, J.L. & Kipke, D.R. (2011). Poly(3,4-ethylenedioxythiophene) (pedot) polymer coatings facilitate smaller neural recording electrodes, *Journal of Neural Engineering*, Vol. 8 No. 1, pp. 014001.

Malarkey, E.B. & Parpura, V. (2010). Carbon nanotubes in neuroscience, *Acta Neurochir Suppl*, Vol. 106, pp. 337-341.

Marin, C. & Fernandez, E. (2010). Biocompatibility of intracortical microelectrodes: Current status and future prospects, *Frontiers in Neuroengineering*, Vol. 3 No. 8, pp. 5.

Mathieson, K., Kachiguine, S., Adams, C., Cunningham, W., Gunning, D., O'shea, V., Smith, K.M., Chichilnisky, E.J., Litke, A.M., Sher, A. & Rahman, M. (2004). Large-area microelectrode arrays for recording of neural signals, *Nuclear Science, IEEE Transactions on*, Vol. 51 No. 5, pp. 2027-2031.

Mchenry, M., Smeloff, E., Fong, W., Miller, G., Jr & Ryan, P. (1970). Critical obstruction of prosthetic heart valves due to lipid absorption by silastic, *J Thorac Cardiovasc Surg*, Vol. 59 No. 3, pp. 413-425.

Mensing, G., Pearce, T. & Beebe, D.J. (2005). An ultrarapid method of creating 3d channels and microstructures, *Journal of Laboratory Automation*, Vol. 10 No. 1, pp. 24-28.

Mercanzini, A., Cheung, K., Buhl, D.L., Boers, M., Maillard, A., Colin, P., Bensadoun, J.-C., Bertsch, A. & Renaud, P. (2008). Demonstration of cortical recording using novel flexible polymer neural probes, *Sensors and Actuators A: Physical*, Vol. 143 No. 1, pp. 90-96.

Merrill, D.R. (2010). The electrochemistry of charge injection at the electrode/tissue interface, in Zhou, D. & Greenbaum, E. (Eds.), *Implantable neural prostheses 2*. Springer New York, 978-0-387-98120-8, pp. 85-138.

Merrill, D.R., Bikson, M. & Jefferys, J.G.R. (2005). Electrical stimulation of excitable tissue: Design of efficacious and safe protocols, *Journal of Neuroscience Methods*, Vol. 141 No. 2, pp. 171-198.

Metz, S., Bertsch, A., Bertrand, D. & Renaud, P. (2004). Flexible polyimide probes with microelectrodes and embedded microfluidic channels for simultaneous drug delivery and multi-channel monitoring of bioelectric activity, *Biosens Bioelectron*, Vol. 19 No. 10, pp. 1309-1318.

Milliken and Company (1997). Zelec (r) ecp electroconductive powders: Product overview, Available from
http://www.zelec-
ecp.com/domino/milliken/zelec/zelec.nsf/files/ECPoverview.html

Morin, F., Nishimura, N., Griscom, L., Lepioufle, B., Fujita, H., Takamura, Y. & Tamiya, E. (2006). Constraining the connectivity of neuronal networks cultured on microelectrode arrays with microfluidic techniques: A step towards neuron-based functional chips, *Biosensors and Bioelectronics*, Vol. 21 No. 7, pp. 1093-1100.

Morin, F.O., Takamura, Y. & Tamiya, E. (2005). Investigating neuronal activity with planar microelectrode arrays: Achievements and new perspectives, *J Biosci Bioeng*, Vol. 100 No. 2, pp. 131-143.

Musick, K., Khatami, D. & Wheeler, B.C. (2009). Three-dimensional micro-electrode array for recording dissociated neuronal cultures, *Lab on a Chip*, Vol. 9 No. 14, pp. 2036-2042.

Musienko, P., Van Den Brand, R., Maerzendorfer, O., Larmagnac, A. & Courtine, G. (2009). Combinatory electrical and pharmacological neuroprosthetic interfaces to regain motor function after spinal cord injury, *Biomedical Engineering, IEEE Transactions on*, Vol. 56 No. 11, pp. 2707-2711.

Mussa-Ivaldi, S., Alford, S.T., Chiappalone, M., Fadiga, L., Karniel, A., Kositsky, M., Maggiolini, E., Panzeri, S., Sanguineti, V., Semprini, M. & Vato, A. (2010). New perspectives on the dialogue between brains and machines, *Frontiers in Neuroscience*, Vol. 5, pp. 5.

Myllymaa, S., Myllymaa, K. & Lappalainen, R. (2009). Flexible implantable thin film neural electrodes, in Naik, G.R. (Ed.), *Recent advances in biomedical engineering.* InTech, ISBN: 978-953-307-004-9, Available from: http://www.intechopen.com/articles/show/title/flexible-implantable-thin-film-neural-electrodes, pp. 165-190.

Navarro, X., Krueger, T.B., Lago, N., Micera, S., Stieglitz, T. & Dario, P. (2005). A critical review of interfaces with the peripheral nervous system for the control of neuroprostheses and hybrid bionic systems, *Journal of the Peripheral Nervous System,* Vol. 10 No. 3, pp. 229-258.

Nisch, W., Bock, J., Egert, U., Hammerle, H. & Mohr, A. (1994). A thin film microelectrode array for monitoring extracellular neuronal activity in vitro, *Biosensors & Bioelectronics,* Vol. 9 No. 9-10, pp. 737-741.

Niu, X.Z., Peng, S.L., Liu, L.Y., Wen, W.J. & Sheng, P. (2007). Characterizing and patterning of pdms-based conducting composites, *Advanced Materials,* Vol. 19 No. 18, pp. 2682-2682.

Novak, J.L. & Wheeler, B.C. (1986). Recording from the aplysia abdominal ganglion with a planar microelectrode array, *Biomedical Engineering, IEEE Transactions on,* Vol. BME-33 No. 2, pp. 196-202.

Novak, J.L. & Wheeler, B.C. (1988). Multisite hippocampal slice recording and stimulation using a 32 element microelectrode array, *Journal of Neuroscience Methods,* Vol. 23 No. 2, pp. 149-159.

Offenhausser, A. & Knoll, W. (2001). Cell-transistor hybrid systems and their potential applications, *Trends in Biotechnology,* Vol. 19 No. 2, pp. 62-66.

Offenhäusser, A., Sprossler, C., Matsuzawa, M. & Knoll, W. (1997). Field-effect transistor array for monitoring electrical activity from mammalian neurons in culture, *Biosensors & Bioelectronics,* Vol. 12, pp. 819-826.

Oka, H., Shimono, K., Ogawa, R., Sugihara, H. & Taketani, M. (1999). A new planar multielectrode array for extracellular recording: Application to hippocampal acute slice, *Journal of Neuroscience Methods,* Vol. 93 No. 1, pp. 61-67.

Owens, R.M. & Malliaras, G.G. (2010). Organic electronics at the interface with biology, *Mrs Bulletin,* Vol. 35 No. 6, pp. 449-456.

Pancrazio, J.J., Bey, R.P., Jr., Loloee, A., Manne, S., Chao, H.C., Howard, L.L., Milton-Gosney, W., Borkholder, D.A., Kovacs, G.T.A., Manos, P., Cuttino, D.S. & Stenger, D.A. (1998). Description and demonstration of a cmos amplifier-based-system with measurement and stimulation capability for bioelectrical signal transduction, *Biosensors-&-Bioelectronics,* Vol. 13 No. 9, pp. 971-979.

Park, J., Seyeoul, K., Seung Ik, J., Mcknight, T.E., Melechko, A.V., Simpson, M.L., Dhindsa, M., Heikenfeld, J. & Rack, P.D. (2009). Active-matrix microelectrode arrays integrated with vertically aligned carbon nanofibers, *Electron Device Letters, IEEE,* Vol. 30 No. 3, pp. 254-257.

Patrick, E., Ordonez, M., Alba, N., Sanchez, J.C. & Nishida, T. (2006). Design and fabrication of a flexible substrate microelectrode array for brain machine interfaces, *Conference Proceedings, Annual International Conference of the IEEE Engineering in Medicine and Biology Society,* Vol. 1, pp. 2966-2969.

Pavesi, A., Piraino, F., Fiore, G.B., Farino, K.M., Moretti, M. & Rasponi, M. (2011). How to embed three-dimensional flexible electrodes in microfluidic devices for cell culture applications, *Lab on a Chip*, Vol. advance publication.

Patolsky, F., Timko, B.P., Yu, G., Fang, Y., Greytak, A.B., Zheng, G. & Lieber, C.M. (2006). Detection, stimulation, and inhibition of neuronal signals with high-density nanowire transistor arrays, *Science*, Vol. 313 No. 5790, pp. 1100-1104.

Peppas, N.A., Hilt, J.Z., Khademhosseini, A. & Langer, R. (2006). Hydrogels in biology and medicine: From molecular principles to bionanotechnology, *Advanced Materials*, Vol. 18 No. 11, pp. 1345-1360.

Pine, J. (1980). Recording action potentials from cultured neurons with extracellular microcircuit electrodes, *Journal of Neuroscience Methods*, Vol. 2 No. 1, pp. 19-31.

Pine, J. (2006). A history of mea development, in Taketani, M. & Baudry, M. (Eds.), *Advances in network electrophysiology. Using multi-electrode arrays.* Springer, 978-0-387-25857-7 (Print) 978-0-387-25858-4 (Online), New York, pp. 3-23.

Poghossian, A., Ingebrandt, S., Offenhausser, A. & Schoning, M.J. (2009). Field-effect devices for detecting cellular signals, *Seminars in Cell & Developmental Biology*, Vol. 20 No. 1, pp. 41-48.

Pui, T.-S., Agarwal, A., Ye, F., Balasubramanian, N. & Chen, P. (2009). Cmos-compatible nanowire sensor arrays for detection of cellular bioelectricity, *Small*, Vol. 5 No. 2, pp. 208-212.

Rabaey, K. & Rozendal, R.A. (2010). Microbial electrosynthesis — revisiting the electrical route for microbial production, *Nat Rev Micro*, Vol. 8 No. 10, pp. 706-716.

Rajaraman, S., Choi, S.-O., Shafer, R.H., Ross, J.D., Vukasinovic, J., Choi, Y., Deweerth, S.P., Glezer, A. & Allen, M.G. (2007). Microfabrication technologies for a coupled three-dimensional microelectrode, microfluidic array, *J. Micromech. Microeng.*, Vol. 17 No. 1, pp. 163-171.

Rajaraman, S., Choi, S.O., Mcclain, M.A., Ross, J.D., Laplaca, M.C. & Allen, M.G. (2011). Metal-transfer-micromolded three-dimensional microelectrode arrays for in-vitro brain-slice recordings, *Microelectromechanical Systems, Journal of*, Vol. PP No. 99, pp. 1-14.

Ravichandran, R., Sundarrajan, S., Venugopal, J.R., Mukherjee, S. & Ramakrishna, S. (2010). Applications of conducting polymers and their issues in biomedical engineering, *Journal of the Royal Society Interface*, Vol. 7, pp. S559-S579.

Rodger, D.C., Fong, A.J., Li, W., Ameri, H., Ahuja, A.K., Gutierrez, C., Lavrov, I., Zhong, H., Menon, P.R., Meng, E., Burdick, J.W., Roy, R.R., Edgerton, V.R., Weiland, J.D., Humayun, M.S. & Tai, Y.-C. (2008). Flexible parylene-based multielectrode array technology for high-density neural stimulation and recording, *Sensors and Actuators, B: Chemical*, Vol. 132 No. 2, pp. 449-460.

Rogers, J.A., Someya, T. & Huang, Y. (2010). Materials and mechanics for stretchable electronics, *Science*, Vol. 327 No. 5973, pp. 1603-1607.

Ross, J., Brown, E.A., Rajaraman, S., Allen, M.G. & Wheeler, B. (2010). Apparatus and methods for high throughput network electrophysiology and cellular analysis, in, ISBN, USA.

Rothschild, R.M. (2010). Neuroengineering tools/applications for bidirectional interfaces, brain computer interfaces, and neuroprosthetic implants - a review of recent progress, *Frontiers in Neuroengineering,* Vol. 4, pp. 12.

Rozlosnik, N. (2009). New directions in medical biosensors employing poly(3,4-ethylenedioxy thiophene) derivative-based electrodes, *Analytical and Bioanalytical Chemistry,* Vol. 395 No. 3, pp. 637-645.

Rutledge, L.T. & Duncan, J.A. (1966). Extracellular recording of converging input on cortical neurones using a flexible microelectrode, *Nature,* Vol. 210 No. 5037, pp. 737-739.

Rutten, W.L.C. (2002). Selective electrical interfaces with the nervous system, *Annual Review of Biomedical Engineering,* Vol. 4 No. 1, pp. 407-452.

Ryynänen, T., Kujala, V., Ylä-Outinen, L., Kerkelä, E., Narkilahti, S. & Lekkala, J. (2010). Polystyrene coated mea, in Stett, A. (Ed.), *Proceedings of the 7th Int. Meeting on Substrate-Integrated Microelectrode Arrays, June 29 – July 2.* BIOPRO Baden-Württemberg GmbH, ISBN, Reutlingen, pp. 265-266.

Sadleir, R.J., Grant, S.C., Demarse, T.B., Woo, E.J., Lee, S.Y., Kim, T.S., Oh, S.H., Lee, B.I. & Seo, J.K. (2005). Study of mri/mea compatibility at 17.6 tesla, *International Journal of Bioelectromagnetism,* Vol. 7 No. 1, pp. 278-281.

Sandison, M., Curtis, A.S.G. & Wilkinson, C.D.W. (2002). Effective extra-cellular recording from vertebrate neurons in culture using a new type of micro-electrode array, *Journal of Neuroscience Methods,* Vol. 114 No. 1, pp. 63-71.

Schmidt, C.E., Shastri, V.R., Vacanti, J.P. & Langer, R. (1997). Stimulation of neurite outgrowth using an electrically conducting polymer, *Proceedings of the National Academy of Sciences of the United States of America,* Vol. 94 No. 17, pp. 8948-8953.

Seidl, K. & *Et al.* (2010). In-plane silicon probes for simultaneous neural recording and drug delivery, *Journal of Micromechanics and Microengineering,* Vol. 20 No. 10, pp. 105006.

Sekitani, T., Nakajima, H., Maeda, H., Fukushima, T., Aida, T., Hata, K. & Someya, T. (2009). Stretchable active-matrix organic light-emitting diode display using printable elastic conductors, *Nature Materials,* Vol. 8 No. 6, pp. 494-499.

Sirivisoot, S., Pareta, R. & Webster, T.J. (2011). Electrically controlled drug release from nanostructured polypyrrole coated on titanium, *Nanotechnology,* Vol. 22 No. 8, pp. 085101.

Smoothon, I. (2008). Smooth-sil® platinum cure silicone rubber (technical bulletin), in, ISBN.

Starovoytov, A., Choi, J. & Seung, H.S. (2005). Light-directed electrical stimulation of neurons cultured on silicon wafers, *J Neurophysiol,* Vol. 93 No. 2, pp. 1090-1098.

Stein, B., George, M., Gaub, H.E. & Parak, W.J. (2004). Extracellular measurements of averaged ionic currents with the light-addressable potentiometric sensor (laps), *Sensors and Actuators B: Chemical,* Vol. 98 No. 2-3, pp. 299-304.

Stieglitz, T., Rubehn, B., Henle, C., Kisban, S., Herwik, S., Ruther, P. & Schuettler, M. (2009). Brain-computer interfaces: An overview of the hardware to record neural signals from the cortex, in Verhaagen, J., Hol, E.M., Huitenga, I., Wijnholds, J.,

Bergen, A.B., Boer, G.J. & Dick, F.S. (Eds.), *Progress in brain research*. Elsevier, 0079-6123, pp. 297-315.

Stoppini, L., Duport, S. & Correges, P. (1997). A new extracellular multirecording system for electrophysiological studies: Application to hippocampal organotypic cultures, *Journal of Neuroscience Methods*, Vol. 72 No. 1, pp. 23-33.

Suzuki, T., Ziegler, D., Mabuchi, K. & Takeuchi, S. (2004). Flexible neural probes with micro-fluidic channels for stable interface with the nervous system, in *Engineering in Medicine and Biology Society, 2004. IEMBS '04. 26th Annual International Conference of the IEEE*, ISBN, pp. 4057-4058.

Suzurikawa, J., Takahashi, H., Takayama, Y., Warisawa, S., Mitsuishi, M., Nakao, M. & Jimbo, Y. (2006). Light-addressable planar electrode with hydrogenated amorphous silicon and low-conductive passivation layer for stimulation of cultured neurons, in *Engineering in Medicine and Biology Society, 2006. EMBS '06. 28th Annual International Conference of the IEEE*, ISBN, pp. 648-651.

Svennersten, K., Larsson, K.C., Berggren, M. & Richter-Dahlfors, A. (2011). Organic bioelectronics in nanomedicine, *Biochimica et Biophysica Acta (BBA) - General Subjects*, Vol. 1810 No. 3, pp. 276-285.

Thiebaud, P., Beuret, C., Koudelka-Hep, M., Bove, M., Martinoia, S., Grattarola, M., Jahnsen, H., Rebaudo, R., Balestrino, M., Zimmer, J. & Dupont, Y. (1999). An array of pt-tip microelectrodes for extracellular monitoring of activity of brain slices, *Biosensors & Bioelectronics*, Vol. 14 No. 1, pp. 61-65.

Thiébaud, P., De Rooij, N.F., Koudelka-Hepp, M. & Stoppini, L. (1997). Microelectrode arrays for electrophysiological monitoring of hippocampal organotypic slice cultures, *IEEE Transactions on Biomedical Engineering*, Vol. 44 No. 11, pp. 1159-1163.

Thiel, M., Fischer, J., Von Freymann, G. & Wegener, M. (2010). Direct laser writing of three-dimensional submicron structures using a continuous-wave laser at 532 nm, *Applied Physics Letters*, Vol. 97 No. 22, pp. 221102-221103.

Thomas, C.A., Springer, P.A., Loeb, G.E., Berwald-Netter, Y. & Okun, L.M. (1972). A miniature microelectrode array to monitor the bioelectric activity of cultured cells, *Experimental Cell Research*, Vol. 74, pp. 61-66.

Thompson, B.C., Richardson, R.T., Moulton, S.E., Evans, A.J., O'leary, S., Clark, G.M. & Wallace, G.G. (2010). Conducting polymers, dual neurotrophins and pulsed electrical stimulation - dramatic effects on neurite outgrowth, *Journal of Controlled Release*, Vol. 141 No. 2, pp. 161-167.

Tian, B., Cohen-Karni, T., Qing, Q., Duan, X., Xie, P. & Lieber, C.M. (2010). Three-dimensional, flexible nanoscale field-effect transistors as localized bioprobes, *Science*, Vol. 329 No. 5993, pp. 830-834.

Tonomura, W., Moriguchi, H., Jimbo, Y. & Konishi, S. (2010). Parallel multipoint recording of aligned and cultured neurons on micro channel array toward cellular network analysis, *Biomedical Microdevices*, Vol. 12 No. 4, pp. 737-743.

Volta, A. (1793). *Schriften über die thierische elektrizität* Johann Mayer, Prag.

Wang, T., Yang, W., Huang, H. & Fu, C. (2007). A novel fabrication method of flexible micro electrode array for neural recording, in *Micro Electro Mechanical Systems, 2007. MEMS. IEEE 20th International Conference on*, ISBN, pp. 295-300.

Wei, P., Taylor, R., Ding, Z., Higgs, G., Norman, J.J., Pruitt, B.L. & Ziaie, B. (2009). A stretchable cell culture platform with embedded electrode array, in *Micro Electro Mechanical Systems, 2009. MEMS 2009. IEEE 22nd International Conference on*, ISBN, pp. 407-410.

Widge, A.S., Jeffries-El, M., Cui, X., Lagenaur, C.F. & Matsuoka, Y. (2007). Self-assembled monolayers of polythiophene conductive polymers improve biocompatibility and electrical impedance of neural electrodes, *Biosens Bioelectron*, Vol. 22 No. 8, pp. 1723-1732.

Wilkinson, C.D. (2004). Making structures for cell engineering, *Eur Cell Mater*, Vol. 8, pp. 21-25; discussion 25-26.

Wilks, S.J., Richardson-Burns, S.M., Hendricks, J.L., Martin, D.C. & Otto, K.J. (2009). Poly(3,4-ethylene dioxythiophene) (pedot) as a micro-neural interface material for electrostimulation, *Frontiers in Neuroengineering*, Vol. 2, pp. 1-8.

Williams, K.R. & Muller, R.S. (1996). Etch rates for micromachining processing, *Microelectromechanical Systems, Journal of*, Vol. 5 No. 4, pp. 256-269.

Winter, J.O., Cogan, S.F. & Rizzo, J.F. (2007). Retinal prostheses: Current challenges and future outlook, *Journal of Biomaterials Science, Polymer Edition*, Vol. 18, pp. 1031-1055.

Wise, K.D., Sodagar, A.M., Ying, Y., Gulari, M.N., Perlin, G.E. & Najafi, K. (2008). *Microelectrodes, microelectronics, and implantable neural microsystems : Progress in development of tiny electrodes, cables, circuitry, signal processors and wireless interfaces promises to advance understanding of the human nervous system and its disorders*, Institute of Electrical and Electronics Engineers, New York, USA.

Wong, J.Y., Langer, R. & Ingber, D.E. (1994). Electrically conducting polymers can noninvasively control the shape and growth of mammalian cells, *Proceedings of the National Academy of Sciences*, Vol. 91 No. 8, pp. 3201-3204.

Xin, Z., Wai Man, W., Yulong, Z., Yandong, Z., Fei, G., Nelson, R.D. & Larue, J.C. (2009). Design of a cmos-based multichannel integrated biosensor chip for bioelectronic interface with neurons, in *Engineering in Medicine and Biology Society, 2009. EMBC 2009. Annual International Conference of the IEEE*, ISBN, pp. 3814-3817.

Yang, J., Kim, D.H., Hendricks, J.L., Leach, M., Northey, R. & Martin, D.C. (2005). Ordered surfactant-templated poly(3,4-ethylenedioxythiophene) (pedot) conducting polymer on microfabricated neural probes, *Acta Biomaterialia*, Vol. 1 No. 1, pp. 125-136.

Yong-Kyu, Y., Jung-Hwan, P. & Allen, M.G. (2006). Multidirectional uv lithography for complex 3-d mems structures, *Microelectromechanical Systems, Journal of*, Vol. 15 No. 5, pp. 1121-1130.

Zhang, M., Wu, J., Wang, L., Xiao, K. & Wen, W. (2010). A simple method for fabricating multi-layer pdms structures for 3d microfluidic chips, *Lab Chip*, Vol. 10 No. 9, pp. 1199-1203.

Zhang, R., Moon, K.-S., Lin, W., Agar, J.C. & Wong, C.-P. (2011). A simple, low-cost approach to prepare flexible highly conductive polymer composites by in situ reduction of silver carboxylate for flexible electronic applications, *Composites Science and Technology*, Vol. 71 No. 4, pp. 528-534.

Zhou, D.D. & Greenberg, R.J. (2009). Microelectronic visual prostheses, in Greenbaum, E. & Zhou, D. (Eds.), *Implantable neural prostheses 1*. Springer New York, 978-0-387-77261-5, pp. 1-42.

Ziaie, B. (2009). Stretchable bioelectrodes, in *Engineering in Medicine and Biology Society, 2009. EMBC 2009. Annual International Conference of the IEEE*, ISBN, pp. 1049-1052.

6

Contributions to Novel Methods in Electrophysiology Aided by Electronic Devices and Circuits

Cristian Ravariu
"Politehnica" University of Bucharest – Faculty of Electronics, BioNEC group
Romania

1. Introduction

One of the challenges in the biomedical engineering domain is the bio-signal processing with special electronics devices and circuits, (Kutz, 2009). A parallel target is the remote medicine, which need mobile platforms for diagnosis and an internet link to ensure the telemedicine requirements, (Hung & Yuan-Ting, 2003). In this scope, the electronic devices and circuits play a crucial role. For instance, a noisy amplifier involves pseudo-signals, while an active filter can reject the undesired frequencies and adjust the useful signal, (C. Ravariu, 2010a).

The remote diagnosis centers, automate instruments for drug delivery (F. Ravariu et al., 2004) or mobile platforms for domestic applications (Woodward et al., 2001) are common targets accepted by the medical insurance companies form the world wide. The physician-patient remote interaction, so necessary in telemedicine, needs the development of various tools for home analysis, in order to be able to send all the collected tests to a database on Internet, (Fong, 2005). In real labs, more accurate results extracted from the electrophysiological measurements need the development of different hardware or software tools in order to send proper tests, without noise or pseudo-signals, to a medical center, (Babarada, 2010a).

On the other hand, this chapter has the following additional scopes: (i) it offers an alternative circuit for the noise rejection in electromyography and (ii) it represent a starting platform for new others electrophysiological signals recording, starting from cellular origin of the electrical biosignals (Sanmiguel, 2009) and the products can be easily used for learning in bioelectronics platforms, too (C. Ravariu, 2009b).

2. A mobile ECG platform

In this chapter is firstly proposed a simple and cheap platform for the electrocardiogram ECG recording on a Personal Computer PC. Why still ECG? Unfortunately, because the cardiovascular diseases are maintaining their first place in morbidity and mortality too, in many countries, (WHO Reports, 2008). The general electrical circuit for the ECG recording was adapted in order to be available for home applications. The amplified signal is then connected via the microphone muff to PC. A conversion of the input "noise" signal from microphone, into an ECG trace is available on PC. In this way, the ECG becomes available, in the simpler mode directly on the computer screen, without any expensive tracer.

For instance this apparatus can become mobile with a laptop connection or with its own LCD display and can be used by customers without medical knowledge. Therefore, one of the original points of this chapter consists in the practical assembling of the hardware parts into a so called "mobile ECG platform".

Two extreme facts occur in a medical center with the classical ECG equipment: 90% of the daily tests are false alerts. At the opposite extreme are placed the grave cases that don't benefit in time about these kinds of centers. The mobile ECG platform provide in 1-2 minutes the main electrocardiograph shape, at home, and can alert the person if a dangerous situation is recorded, as emergency in cardiovascular diseases, (Drew, 2011).

2.1 The electronic components selection

The prime novelty of the paper isn't a new spectacular circuit, because the standard ECG analog blocks are used, (Popa, 2006). But some distinct theoretical principles were collected together with the own implementation idea, to practically create this particular ECG. As integrated circuit, the TL 084 CN has been used, which possesses four operational amplifiers OP, figure 1.

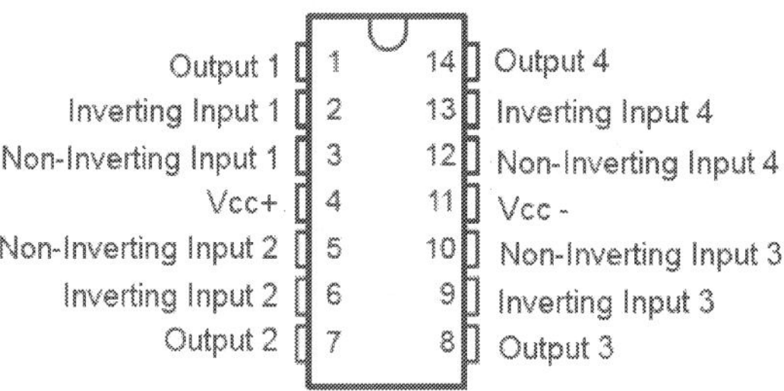

Fig. 1. The internal configuration of the integrated circuit TL 084 CN, (Texas Instruments, 2007)

The internal electronic scheme of each OP amplifier is represented in figure 2, (Texas Instruments, 2007).

The bipolar and JFET technologies combination conffers special performances, useful in biomedical applications. A first demand is the noise immunity , ensured by the JFET input configuration with extremely low gate currents as inputs. Then, the bipolar transistors are the most sensitive components in transconductance term, suitable for the biological signal amplification, as another demand.

The advantages of this circuit are: low power consumption, wide common-mode and differential voltage ranges, low input bias and offset currents, output short-circuit protection, high input impedance due to the JFET-input stage, common-mode input voltage range includes V_{CC}^+, high slew rates. The CN-suffix devices are characterized for operation from 0^0C to 70^0C, suitable for the human environment.

The interconnections among these operational amplifiers, since to produce the input signal amplification, besides to the low pass filter function, are presented in the design paragraph.

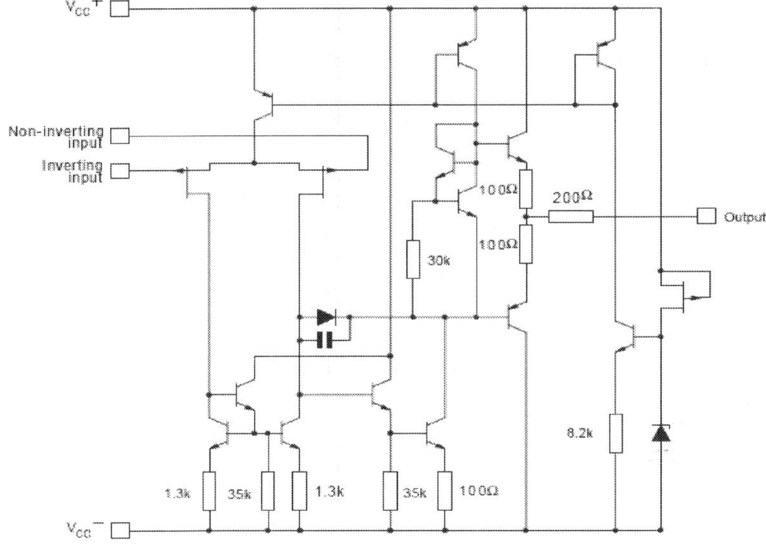

Fig. 2. The internal schema of one operational amplifier

2.2 The electronic circuit design

The work principle is based on the voltage difference measuring between two electrodes applied on the chest skin in respect with a third electrode – the reference electrode applied on the left hand skin. The electrodes are simple metal plates. For a smaller contact resistance, an electrolyte or gel is applied onto the electrode.

In this scope, an instrumentation amplifier function was made up from three previous operational amplifiers, figure 3.

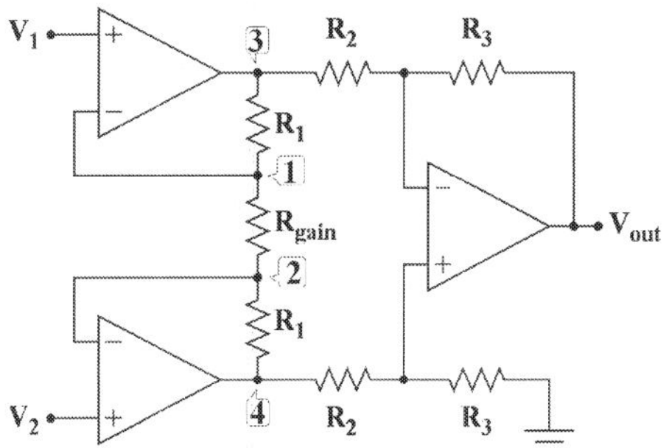

Fig. 3. The design of the amplifier

This circuit is constructed from a buffered differential amplifier stage with three new resistors, linking two buffer circuits together, (Rusu, 2008). All resistors have equal values, excepting for R_{gain}: $R_1=R_2=R_3=R$. The negative feedback of the upper-left operational amplifier causes the voltage in the point 1 to be equal with V_1. Likewise, the voltage in the point 2 is held to a value equal with V_2. This establishes a voltage drop across R_{gain} equal to the voltage difference between V_1 and V_2. That voltage drop causes a current through R_{gain}; since the feedback loops of both operational amplifiers draw no current on inputs, the same amount of current through R_{gain} must be going through two R_1 resistors, above and below it. This produces a voltage drop between the points 3 and 4 equal to:

$$V_3 - V_4 = \left(V_1 - V_2 \right)\left(1 + \frac{R_1 + R_2}{R_{gain}} \right) \tag{1}$$

The regular differential amplifier on the right-hand side of the circuit then takes this voltage drop between points 3 and 4 and amplifies it:

$$V_{out} = \left(V_4 - V_3 \right)\frac{R_3}{R_2} \tag{2}$$

The gain becomes 1, assuming again that all "R" resistors are of the same value. Although this method looks like a cumbersome way to build an instrumentation amplifier, it has the distinct advantages of possessing extremely high input impedances on the V_1 and V_2 inputs, because they connect straight into the non-inverting inputs of their respective operational amplifier and adjustable gain that can be set by a single resistor. The global gain of the amplifier results from eq. (1) and (2), taking into account that $R_1 = R_2 = R_3 = R$:

$$A_v = \left(1 + \frac{2R}{R_{gain}} \right) \tag{3}$$

Because there are very small voltage differences, there is also a low pass filter added in one branch of the instrumentation amplifier, fig. 4.

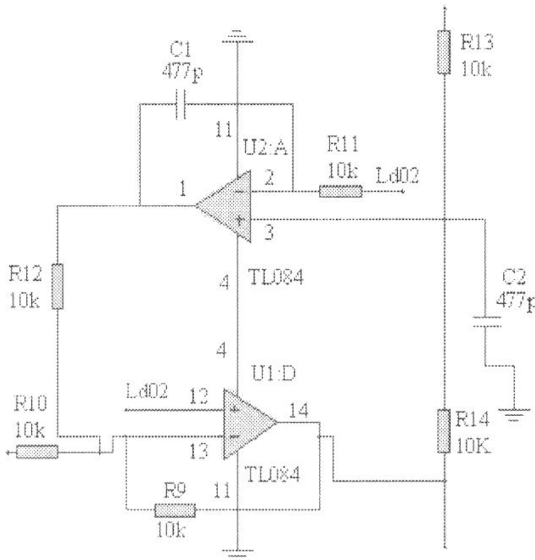

Fig. 4. Low pass active filter with operational amplifiers

The advantage of this circuit is that it is powered from only one 9V battery, the 0 level is at $V_{CC}/2$. The $V_{CC}/2$ level is given by one simple resistor divider, followed by a buffer.
The final schema used for the hardware implementation of the mobile ECG platform is available in figure 5.

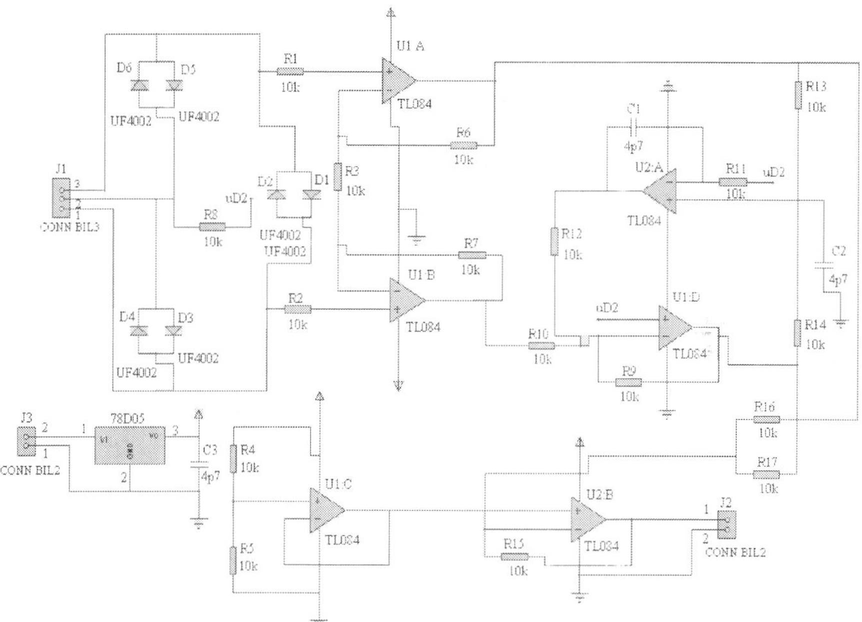

Fig. 5. Final scheme of the ECG circuit

The body potential is firstly recorded at $V_{CC}/2$, connecting the "body electrode" to the left hand. Next, the instrumentation amplifier measures the voltage fluctuations between electrode 1 and 2, amplifies the signal, filtering it and send it to the computer microphone input.
The performances of the proposed circuit, in the case of Varta Superlife9V battery using, are provided in table 1.

The performances of the proposed circuit	Estimated values
Power consumption	max. 15W
Voltage powering	230V AC Univ., 50Hz, 80VA (or 9V DC battery)
Battery life	12 hours
CMRR of amplifier	75-86dB
Circuit bandwidth	0.05-120Hz

Table 1.

The inter-connection of this hardware to a PC or laptop implies some potential hazards for patients and additional noise introducing. Therefore, a main set of algorithms used for the

ECG conditioning with respect to different types of hazards, noise and artifacts in order to extract the basic electrocardiographic signal, is briefly discussed. As the specialty literature notify, the electrical safety should be very careful concerning a home-built circuit connection to something that is running off a significant power source. In principle, one can more safely read out the circuit using a laptop computer that is running off its battery, (Sornmo, 2006). Nevertheless, this leaves the laptop's ground floating, without a good ground connection, with a remarkable amount of noise superposed over the ECG collected signal. Only if the circuit can be connected to a good ground point, then using a battery powered laptop should work well. A solution is to connect the ground of the circuit and the input and output cables to a metal box housing the circuit as carcase, which still fulfils a shield effect. Consequently, the circuit ground will then come from whatever device is looking to the output – either the laptop, PC or oscilloscope. Since these devices are usually powered from the line voltage, the ground from the wall socket often provides a very good ground connection.

Even with the laptop plugged into the mains socket, a significant amount of noise is still found. The best results were obtained by keeping the cables connecting the subject to the circuit close together, thereby reducing the inductive pick-up.

Professionally medical devices are built with significant overvoltage protection, so that line power glitches do not represent a hazard to patients, during the test. To supplementary increase the safety an optically-coupled linear **ISO**lation amplifier can be added to the existing circuit so that the subject is completely isolated from the power supply. In simpler applications, the pair diodes provide limited over-voltage protection.

2.3 Tests and signal processing

The software can process the incoming signal from the ECG output and can offer information about the heart beat, (Rusu, 2008). It is a display software, converting the input analog signal from the microphone muff into a graph. Usually, the program analyses the beat ration, suggesting a normal ECG trace, after the periodicity and beat numbers, or abnormal trace, in terms of P-Q-R-S-T-U waves, (Macfarlane, 2011). The ventricular contraction produces the most clears QRS complex displayed on PC. The P and T waves aren't so consistent in our experiments. Therefore, this mobile ECG system is more recommended for ventricular alerts, especially encountered in the QRS complex deformation.

In absence of a suitable ECG signal generator (e.g. fluke medSim 300B), the circuit was tested directly on a healthy patient, 24 years, as a real ECG signal source. Some output waves recorded with the previous circuit and exposed on PC are presented in fig. 7, 8, 9. Without a 50Hz filter and without a shield additional protection, the dragging signal looks like in fig. 7, due to the antenna behavior of the human body versus the 230V, 50Hz AC signal from laboratory.

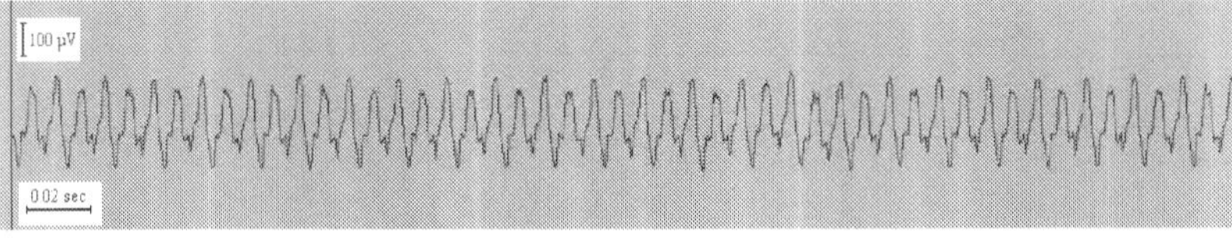

Fig. 7. The output signal without the 50Hz filter

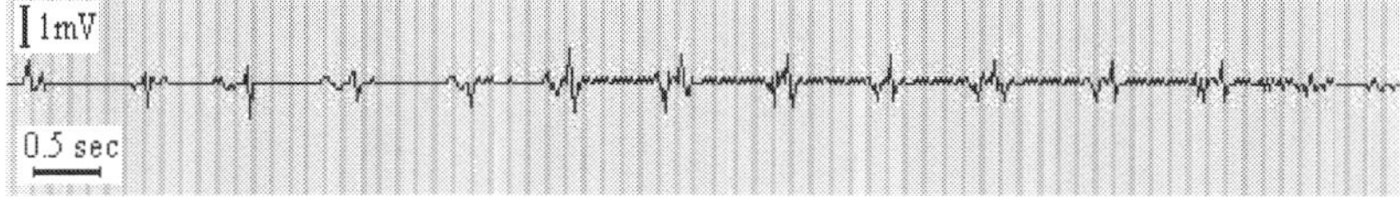

Fig. 8. The output signal with the 50Hz filter

After the 50Hz signal removal, the ECG signal recorded by prior circuit and displayed on PC looks like in fig. 8. Here are obviously the heartbeats, via QRS incipient complex. The output signal from fig. 9 is the best recorded signal, after a low pass filter and choosing different skin sensors with electrolyte solution.

This ECG mobile system has the advantage that it can be connected to a home computer or laptop and it can be used by anyone, not only by the medical staff. The global product is available in fig. 10.

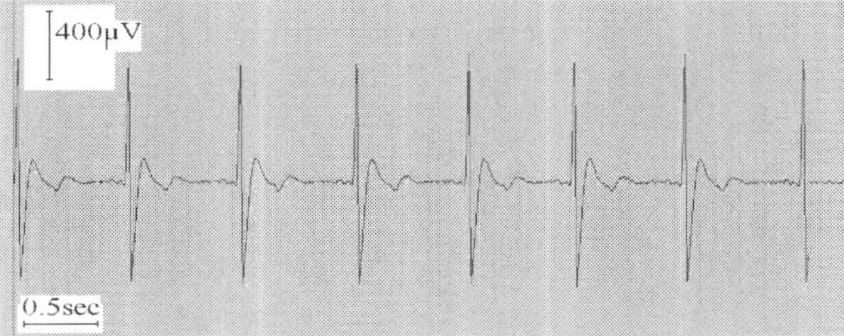

Fig. 9. The final output signal after low pass filter and different skin sensors

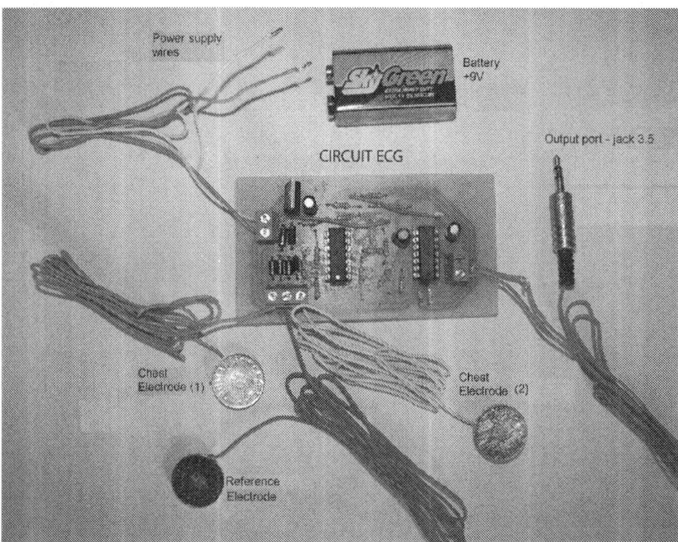

Fig. 10. The circuit, battery, electrodes, connectors and jack output of the circuit

Adding a LCD device to monitor anytime the signal (e.g. at office, walking, running situations), the system can be improved, in order to offer a small, cheap and portable ECG compact device, (Kara, 2006). The power dissipation can be minimized if the circuit is integrated. Some major software improvements could consist in the comparison of the recorded waves within an implemented database, alerting the user if there is a change in the ECG trace and suggesting an initial diagnosis, or normal ECG state.

3. Circuit design for noise rejection in electromyography

In the biomedical engineering domain, the circuits design with high noise immunity for electrophysiology is maintained as a main aim. Besides to the classical ECG, others electro-physiological methods have been developed in order to record the electrical activity of muscles at the skin level. This is the Electro-Myo-Graphy (EMG), (Merletti, 2004). There are two kinds of EMG: surface EMG and intramuscular EMG. A surface electrode may be used to monitor the general picture of the muscle activation, while a few fibers activity can be observed using only an invasive needle, intramuscular applied, (Raez, 2006). The non-invasive EMG method suffers from noise, collected by the surface electrodes.

3.1 Noise in EMG

There are many types of noise to be considered, when EMG is recorded through surface electrodes.

- *Inherent noise in electronics equipment*: It is generated by all electronics equipment and can't be eliminated. It is only reduced by high quality components using. It has a frequency range: 0 – several thousand Hz, (Babarada, 2010b).
- *Ambient noise:* The cause is the electromagnetic radiation, with possible sources: radio transmission, electrical wires, fluorescent lights. It has a dominant frequency of 60Hz and amplitude of 1 – 3 x EMG signal.
- *Motion artifact*: It has two main sources: electrode / skin interface and electrode / cable, having a frequency range of 0 – 20Hz. It is reducible by a proper circuitry and set-up.
- *Inherent instability of signal:* All electronics equipments generate noise and the amplitude is somewhat randomized, being in correlation with the discrete nature of the matter. This noise has a frequency range of 0 – 20Hz and cannot be removed.

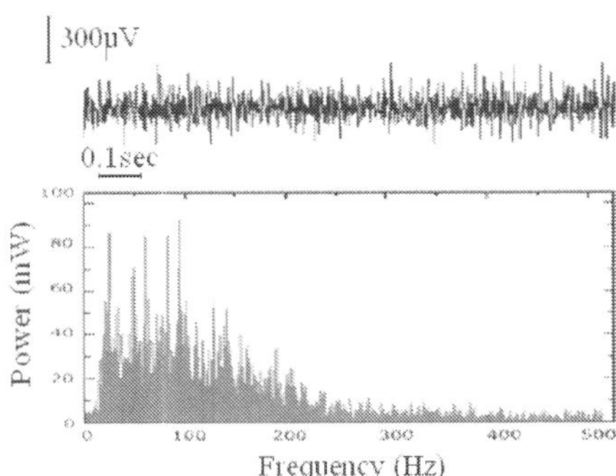

Fig. 11. A noisy signal (black) and power spectrum (red), in typical EMG

The electrical potential measured by non-invasive EMG represents the grouped activity of many muscles fibers firing in varying sequences, at different rates. It has an amplitude range of 0–10 mV peak to peak, prior to amplification and a useable energy for f=0 - 500Hz. The dominant frequency is 50 – 150Hz, fig. 11.

Activity above 500Hz is rather an external electrical artifact and can be hardware eliminated by low-pass filters, with 400-450Hz as cut-off frequency and with a usual roll-off slope of 40dB/dec. Lower frequencies can be contaminated with external noise from the wall power and from biological sources such as ECG and EEG activity - eliminated by the high-pass filters.

3.2 Hardware method in the noise reduction

At the skin level, the entire electrical activity spans a frequency range from several cycles per second through 500Hz. A special attention must be paid to those spectral characteristics of the EMG that dramatically shifts toward lower frequency ranges, when muscles become fatigued. The noise filters must take into account this useful domain.

The first stage of a differential amplifier, frequently used for the EMG acquiring, works also as a high-pass filter, which removes noise caused by the electrode movement on skin. A common-mode feedback is often adopted to reduce the common mode voltage on the subject.

Theoretically, if a biosignal is equally applied on the differential inputs of the operational amplifier, the output should not be affected. In practice, changes in common mode voltage propagate changes to output. The common-mode rejection ratio (CMRR) is the ratio of the common-mode gain to differential-mode gain. The common-mode rejection ratio expressed in decibels, dB, is referred as common-mode rejection (CMR).

In EMG signal acquisition, the amplifier should have the capability to reject the common mode voltages, mainly the power line voltage between subject and ground, which may be thousand times higher then the surface EMG signal. Therefore, a CMR range of 100-120dB is required to limit the equivalent input voltage to a value negligible in respect with EMG, (Bogdan, 2009). Hence, a common mode feedback is often adopted to reduce the common mode voltage. This technique consists in detecting and re-applying of the common mode voltage to the subject, with opposite phase.

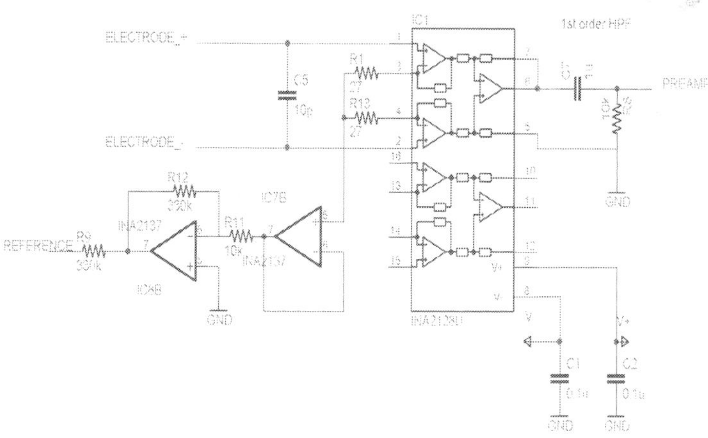

Fig. 12. The proposed active filter for the EMG recording

Figure 12 proposes a circuit based on an amplifier/high-pass filter, with INA2128, INA2137 as instrumentation amplifiers that uses the negative feedback. Due to the INA2128 current-feedback topology, the gate voltage is roughly 0.7V, less than the common-mode input voltage, (Texas Instruments, 2007). This DC offset into the guard potential is satisfactory for many guarding applications.

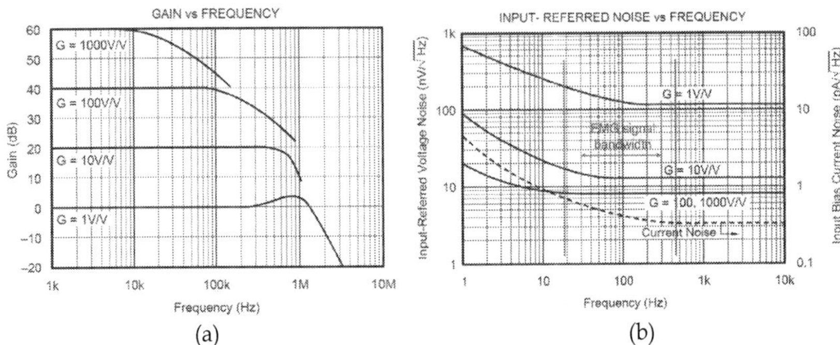

Fig. 13. (a) Gain versus Frequency for the prior filter; (b) the input-referred noise versus frequency

The amplitude of the acquired EMG signals ranges from 10µV to 1000µV. These signals need amplification from 60 to 100dB, so that 1V signal is available for the amplification sub-system. This technique also helps to the EMG signal quality and keeps the distortions as minimal as possible. INA2128 has an adjustable gain, using a single external resistor, R:

$$A_v = \left(1 + \frac{50k\Omega}{2R}\right) \tag{4}$$

where R = R_1 = R_{13}, from fig. 12, are expressed in kΩ. Despite to the quiescent current, the Gain - Frequency curve presents wide bandwidth, even at high gain. This is due to its current-feedback topology, fig. 13.a. The output-referred noise does not allow a fair comparison of the circuits performances because it depends on the gain between the input refereed noise and the input signal - both multiplied by the gain as they are processed by circuit. Thus, the input-referred noise indicates how much the input signal is corrupted by the circuit's noise, fig. 13.b.

3.3 Software processing of EMG signal

Another way to remove the noise from an EMG signal is by software processing of the acquired signal. Some methods that proved their efficiency are:

- *Artificial intelligence*: Some artificial intelligence techniques based on neural networks can be used for the EMG signal processing. This kind of technique is very useful for real-time application like EMG signal recording and analysis.
- *Autoregressive model*: an autoregressive moving average model from neural firing data from motor cortical decoding was studied for the hand motion decoding, (Fisher, 2006).

The autoregressive (AR) time series model can be used in EMG study, too. A surface electrode picks up the EMG activity from all the active muscles in its vicinity, while the intramuscular EMG is highly sensitive, with only minimal crosstalk from adjacent muscles. The EMG signal is represented as an AR model with the delayed intramuscular EMG as input. An artificial neural network combined with an autoregressive model was used to drive the biceps of an arm prosthesis, (Fisher, 2006). The Ag electrodes are placed on biceps at 3cm distance from each other and behind the triceps. The EMG signal obtained from the electrodes is amplified and passed through a low-pass filter to be sent to the level determining circuit.

- *Wavelet analysis*: The wavelet transform (WT) represents a very suitable method for the classification of EMG signals because it has the advantage of being linear, yielding a multi-resolution representation and not being affected by cross terms, (Jahankhani, 2008).

Figure 14 shows the result of wavelet analysis in the EMG processing.

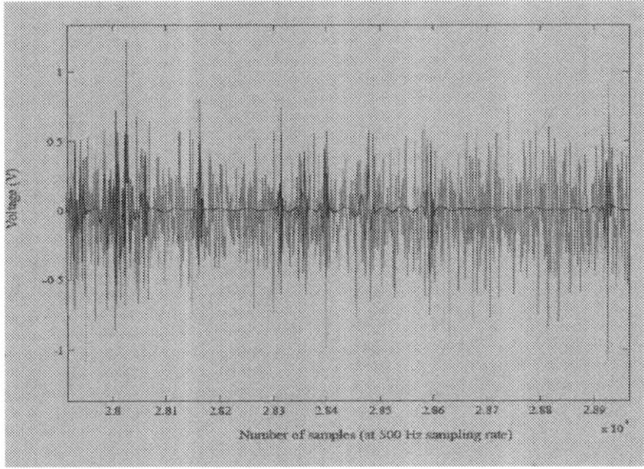

Fig. 14. Comparison of the initial noisy signal (grey) and the denoised signal (black)

4. Toward new electro-grams

In the last years the biology has advanced in the natural pacemakers researching. Although all of the heart's cells possess the ability to generate the electrical impulses or action potentials, only a specialized portion of the heart, called the sinoatrial node, is responsible for the whole heart's beat. The cells that create these rhythmical impulses are called pacemaker cells. Besides to the cord rhythm and brain periodical activity, others and others organs were discovered with a cyclic activity. For instance, the digestive muscles, without any alimentary stimulus, have periodic contractions, from 0.3 up to 12 cycles / minute. In this case, the Interstitial Cajal Cells (ICC), distributed along the gastrointestinal tract, fulfill the pacemaker role, (Sanders & Ward, 2006). Many types of smooth muscle tissues have recently been shown to contain ICC, but with few exceptions, the functions of these cells are a research subject, being still unknown. In this way, the electrophysiological measurements are possible, recording the electrical gastric activity within the electrogastrography, EGG, (Květina, 2010).

Another electrophysiological test is the electroretinography, ERG, relatively recent standardized, (Marmor, 1999), but still a rare clinical test. A related electrophysiological eyes test measures the resting potential of retina, by electro-oculography, EOG, (Brown, 2006). Unlike the electroretinography, the EOG does not represent the response to individual visual stimuli. Also, an electrohepatography, EHG, was possible in a canine model, revealing waves with identical frequency and amplitude from the 3 electrodes, which were sutured to the capsule on the anterior surface of the canine liver. The mean frequency of the waves was 10.6 ± 1.8 cycles/sec and the amplitude 63.7 ± 11.6 µV. The waves were reproducible when the test was repeated in the same animal. Hepatoarrhythmic electric activity was registered in liver insult of the canine model or in liver diseases, (Shafik, 2000).

There are some organs, whose pacemakers were proved, but are not known yet. For instance, the pancreas presents a cyclic insulino-secretion, with or without meals, which prooves the existance of some cells with natural pacemaker role, (Ravariu, 2011). Probably, an electrophysiological activity coud be detected, in the next future, in a same manner as for liver or brain. So, the way toward new electrophysiological methods will be opened in the next years.

4.1 The cellular origin of the electrophysiological signals

The excitable cells, like neurons, myocytes or some secretory cells in glands, like beta cells alpha cells, maintain a negative potential difference across the cellular membrane, due to a gradient of the ionic charges. All these phenomena are caused by specific changes in membrane permeability for potasium, sodium, calcium and chloride, which produces concerted changes in the functional activity of different ion channels, ionic pumps, exchangers and protein transporters. Conventionally, the membrane resting potential, RP, can be defined as the value of the transmembranar voltage from i.c. to e.c. environment in these cells. Any kind of cell posses its own resting potential value, (e.g. RP = -70mV for some neurons, RP = -60mV for beta cells), (Fox et al, 2006).

An action potential, AP, is a self-regenerating wave of electrochemical activity that allows excitable cells to carry a signal over a distance. This feature of the excitable cells is to provide an output reply to an input stimulus. Among the neuronal cells, the stimulus consists in neurotransmitters and the reply is propagating as the action potential, also named nervous impulse. For small incoming stimulus, the potassium current prevails thru the ionic channels and the membranar voltage turns back to its resting value, typically −70mV, (Purves, 2008). For stronger stimulus that overcomes a critical threshold value, typically 15mV, higher than the resting value, the sodium channels are opening. This produces a positive feedback from the sodium current that activates others sodium channels. Thus, the cell fires, producing an action potential, (e.g. AP = +30mV for neurons or AP = -30mV for beta cells).

In the case of muscular activity, the electrical stimulus of myocytes is provided by a motor neuron and electrochemically transmitted by acetylcholine neurotransmitter. For instance, a motor unit is defined as one motor neuron and all of the muscle fibers it innervates. The area where the nerve contacts the muscle is called the neuromuscular junction. After the action stimulus is transmitted across the neuromuscular junction, an action potential is elicited in all of the innervated muscle fibers of that particular motor unit. The sum of all these electrical activities is known as a motor unit action potential (MUAP), (Raez et al, 2006). This electrophysiological activity from multiple motor units is the typical signal evaluated during an EMG.

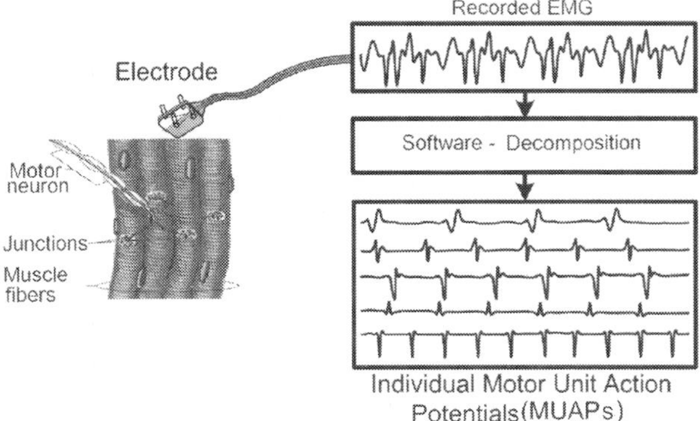

Fig. 15. EMG signal and the decomposition of MUAPs

In figure 15 can be observed in principle the EMG recording signal, the neuromuscular junction and the shapes of the motor unit action potential, after a decomposition of the physical signal.

4.2 A weak signal from non-invasive EGG

The interstitial Cajal cells serve as electrical pacemakers and generate spontaneous electrical slow waves in the gastrointestinal tract. Electrical slow waves spread from ICC to smooth muscle cells and the resulting depolarization initiates the calcium ion entry and contraction. The Cajal cells trigger the gut contractions with different frequencies: 3 per minute for stomach, 12 per minute for duodenum, 10 per minute for ileum, 3 per hour for colon, ensuring the bowel peristalsis. Therefore, the electrical activity recording of the bowels is possible, by electrogastrography. The classical method is invasive, with needle inserted in the stomach during the endoscopy or by surgical act. Nowadays methods try to use a non-invasive recording, with a pair of bipolar electrodes configuration.

In a first experiment, the six electrodes of a standard ECG apparatus, were placed onto the gastric zone, since to observe an electrogastrography trace, fig. 16.a. Unfortunately, the collected signal preserve the heart beat cadence, due to the internal set-up of the dedicated cardiac apparatus, fig. 16.b. In this way, was proved that the cardiac signal is strong enough to cover all surrounding organs. Other experiments are necessary.

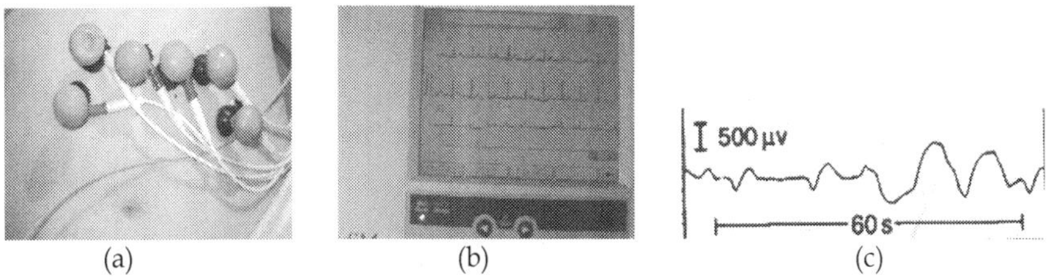

Fig. 16. The electrodes places and the recorded EGG

The prior electrophysiological equipment, designated for the ECG mobile platform, was re-allocated toward the gastric signal detection, by skin electrodes. In this scope, three plat electrodes were placed on skin, on the epigastric zone. The filter resistances were adjusted in order to collect only 1Hz-0.05Hz frequencies, as useful domain for an EGG test. The subject was monitored, after 3 hours post-prandial. Figure 16.c presents the acquired signal. It appears rather as an electromyography signal, probably due to the strong muscular abdominal wall. The interaction among different organs and tissues signals, at skin level, represents the main disadvantage of the remote electrophysiological techniques.

4.3 The remote electrophysiology concept

This paragraph intends to promote a novel term for the medical techniques, in order to be more precise. There are well-known and well-accepted the investigations classifications, after body space or intrusion, as in vivo / in vitro and also intrusive / non-invasive methods. From our experimental tests in electrophysiology, a distinct concept arises in order to proper characterize a measurement. For instance, an electrogastrography is classical recorded by invasive needles. Obviously, this is a strong invasive method, applied in vivo. A less invasive technique is to introduce some plate electrodes, by endoscope, till they contact the internal stomach wall. This last EGG is in vivo recorded, but is almost non-invasive, avoiding the tissue penetration. However, the electrodes touch the gastric mucosa and a special attention has to be paid to the instruments sterilization. It doesn't enter in touch with the blood, as for the needles case, but the danger of diseases transmission still exists. Therefore, both methods are named "*in-touch*" methods.

If the electrogastrography EGG test occurs with some surface electrodes, at skin level, the gastric signal is remotely registered. This is a non-invasive technique, applied in vivo, at a considerable distance from the source electrical signal emitted by the stomach pacemakers. These "*remote*" electrophysiological measurements are crucial in some cases, when any invasive method is forbidden. For instance the liver is inaccessible without a minimum surgical act. Also, for pancreas or brain any invasive or even "in-touch" method, can irreversible damage the tissue, (C. Ravariu, Tirgoviste, 2009).

There are many other medical techniques that can collect signs and tests, either by an immediate contact with the investigated organ, either by remote recording. As much as more biological layers and tissues are interposing between the medical tool terminal and the target organ, the test move from "*in-touch*" to "*remote*". In the last years, due to the sterilizing accidents, non-invasive methods were preferred. Low invasive electrodes with micro-needles, are still dangerous, being in contact with blood capillary, (Gowrishankar et al, 2008). The "in-touch" methods, with surface electrodes in immediate contact with teguments or mucosa suffer form facile microbial transmission. Therefore a more accurate distinction must be made among: invasive, low invasive, in-touch and remote investigation methods.

5. Conclusions

One of the main contributions of this chapter is the global application idea for an ECG mobile platform and its practical implementation. An integrated circuit - TL 084 CN – was used, which posses four operational amplifiers. The advantage of the proposed circuit is that it is powered from only one 9V battery, the 0 level is at $V_{CC}/2$. The $V_{CC}/2$ level is given by one simple resistor divider, followed by a buffer.

The amplified signal is introduced in a PC, by the microphone muff. The incoming signal can be software processed and shown as ECG trace on the computer display. This electronic format of the ECG data avoids the additional expensive mechanics tracer for customer and can be easily transferred to a medical center, via the telemedicine methods.

Secondly, the chapter discussed some hardware and software methods to reduce the noise during the Electromyography. The hardware technique consists in detecting and re-applying of the common mode voltage to the subject with opposite phase via the INA2128 current-feedback topology. The main software contribution is by wavelet transform (WT) that represents a very suitable method for the classification of EMG signals due to its linearity advantage, yielding a multi-resolution representation.

Finally, an incursion into nowadays electrophysiology is exposed, in order to estimate the new challenges. The electrogastrography EGG was intensively investigated in the last ten years in the world wide, but it is a novelty in Europe. This study reveals the interferences among the EGG, ECG and EMG signals, at skin level. The strongest is the cardiac signal and the weakest is the gastric signal. But the low level of the non-invasive EGG collected signal is related to many biological layers and frontiers between the target organ and the skin electrodes. In this way, a novel concept was introduced: remote electrophysiological tests versus in-touch tests. Sometimes, only remote methods can be accepted, in respect with the tissue particularities. The term of "remote medicine" ensure a larger spectrum, taking into account the remote diagnosis centers, coupled with telemedicine. Therefore, the term of remote medicine find a technical sense in electrophysiology, but also a social dimension in the modern medicine.

6. Acknowledgment

The work has been co-funded by the Sectorial Operational Program Human Resources Development of the Romanian Ministry of Labor, Family and Social Protection through the Financial Agreement POSDRU/89/1.5/S/62557 // Partenership PN2 - 62063 - 12095 // contract no. 717/code 449.

7. References

Kutz, M. (2009). *Biomedical Engineering and Design Handbook,* Volume 2, McGraw Hill Publishing Press, 589-816, ISBN 978-007-149-839-5, New York, USA

Hung, K. & Yuan-Ting, Z. (2003). Implementation of a WAP-based telemedicine system for patient monitoring. *International Journal of IEEE Transactions on Information Technology in Biomedicine,* Vol.7, No.2, (June 2003), pp. 101 - 107, ISSN 1089-7771

Ravariu, C. (2010a). *Electronics Biodevices: from nanostructures to medical applications,* Politehnica Press Publisher, ISBN 978-606-515-071-3, Bucharest, Romania

Ravariu, F.; Podaru, C.; Nedelcu, O.; Ravariu, C. & Manea, E. (2004). A Silicon nanoporous membrane used for drug delivery, *Proceedings of IEEE 2004 27th International Annual Conference of Semiconductors,* pp. 101-104, ISBN 0-7803-8499-7, Sinaia, Romania, Oct. 4-6, 2004

Woodward, B.; Istepanian, R.S.H. & Richards, C.I. (2001). Design of a telemedicine system using a mobile telephone. *International Journal of IEEE Transactions on Information Technology in Biomedicine,* Vol.5, No.1, (March 2001), pp. 13-15, ISSN 1089-7771

Fong, B.; Fong, A.C.M. & Hong, G.Y. (2005). On the performance of telemedicine system using 17GHz orthogonally polarized microwave links under the influence of heavy rainfall. *International Journal of IEEE Transactions on Information Technology in Biomedicine,* Vol.9, No.3, (September 2005), pp. 424-429, ISSN 1089-7771

Babarada, F.; Arhip, J. & Ravariu, C. (2010a). The analog processing and digital recording of electrophysiological signals, *Proceedings of* MEDICON 2010, *12th International Conference on Medical and Biological Engineering and Computing IFMBE,* Springer, Vol. 29, pp. 132-135, ISBN 978-3-642-13038-0, Chalkidiki - Porto Cararas, Greece, May 27-30, 2010

Sanmiguel, C.P.; Conklin, J.L.; Cunneen, S.A.; Barnett, P.; Phillips, E.H.; Kipnes, M.; Pilcher, J. & Soffer, E.E. (2009). Gastric Electrical Stimulation with the TANTALUS System in Obese Type 2 Diabetes Patients: Effect on Weight and Glycemic Control. *International Journal on Diabetes Science Technology,* Vol.3, No.4, (July 2009), pp. 964-970, ISSN 1401-1320

Ravariu, C. (2009b). *Advanced Learning,* Chapter Number 25, Learning in Bioelectronics, Edited by Raquel Hijon-Neira, Aleksandar Lazinica, InTech, ISBN 978-953-307-010-0, pp. 381-396, Vienna, Croatia-Austria

WHO Reports. (2008). World Health Organization, Available from http://www.who.int/en/

Drew, B.J.; Sommargren, C.E.; Schindler, D.M.; Benedict, K.; Zegre-Hemsey, J. & Glancy, J.P. (2011). A Simple Strategy Improves Prehospital Electrocardiogram Utilization and Hospital Treatment for Patients with Acute Coronary Syndrome. *American Journal of Cardiology,* Vol.1, No.107, (February 2011), pp. 347-352

Popa, R. (2006). *Medical Electronics,* Matrix Publisher House, ISBN 978-973-755-083-5, Bucharest, Romania

Texas Instruments. (2007). Datasheet Catalog for Integrated Circuits, Available from http://www.datasheetcatalog.com/datasheets_pdf/T/L/0/8/TL084CN.shtml

Rusu, Al.; Golescu, N. & Ravariu, C. (2008). Manufacturing and tests of a mobile ECG platform, *Proceedings of CAS 2008   31th IEEE International Conference of Semiconductors,* pp. 433-436, ISBN 978-1-4244-2004-9, Sinaia, Romania, Oct 13-15, 2008

Sornmo, L.; & Laguna,P. (2006). *Electrocardiogram (ECG) Signal Processing,* Chapter in, Wiley Encyclopedia of Biomedical Engineering, Ed. Webster, Wiley, DOI: 10.1002/9780471740360.ebs1482, http://onlinelibrary.wiley.com

Macfarlane, P.W.; Oosterom, A.V.; Pahlm, O.; Kligfield, P.; Janse, M. & Camm, J. (2011). *Comprehensive Electrocardiology,* 2nd ed. XVIII, Springer-Verlag Publisher, ISBN: 978-1-84882-045-6, ISBN 978-953-7619-34-3, London, UK

Kara, S.; Kemaloglu, S. & Kirbas, S. (2006). Low-Cost Compact ECG With Graphic LCD and Phonocardiogram System Design, *Springer Journal of Medical Systems ,* Vol. 30, Number 3, pp. 205-209, DOI: 10.1007/s10916-005-7989-6

Merletti, R. & Parker, A.P. (2004). *Electromyography: Physiology, Engineering, And Non-invasive Applications,* IEEE Computer Society Press, New York, USA

Raez, M.B.I.; Hussain, M.S. & Mohd-Yasin, F. (2006). Techniques of EMG signal analysis: detection, processing, classification and applications. *International Journal of Biol. Proced.,* Vol.8, No.11, (November 2006), pp. 11-35, DOI 10.1251/bpo115

Babarada, F. (2010b). *Semiconductor Technologies,* Chapter, Semiconductor Processes and Devices Modelling, InTech, ISBN ISBN978-953-7619-X-X, Vienna, Austria

Bogdan, D.; Craciun, M.; Dochia, R.I.; Ionescu, M.A. & Ravariu, C. (2009). Circuit design for noise rejection in electromyography, *Proceedings of INGIMED 2009 2nd National Conference on Biomedical Engineering*, pp. 76-81, Bucharest, Romania, ICPE-CA Publisher, November 12-14, 2009

Texas Instruments. (2007). INA2128 dual low power instrumentation amplifier datasheet, Available from http://focus.ti.com/docs/prod/folders/print/ina2128.html

Fisher, J. & Black, M.J. (2006). Motor Cortical Decoding Using an Autoregressive Moving Average Model, *Proceedings of IEEE-EMBS 2006 27th Annual International Conference of the Engineering in Medicine and Biology*, pp. 2130 – 2133, ISBN: 0-7803-8741-4, Shanghai, Jan 17-18, 2006

Jahankhani, P. & Kodogiannis, V. (2008). Intelligent Decision Support System for Classification of EEG Signals using Wavelet Coefficients, Chapter 2 In: *Data Mining in Medical and Biological Research,* Eugenia G. Giannopoulou, (Ed.), 19-38, InTech, ISBN 978-953-7619-30-5, Vukovar, Croatia

Sanders, K. & Ward, S. (2006). Interstitial cells of Cajal: a new perspective on smooth muscle function. *International Journal of Physiology,* Vol.576, No.3, (March 2006), pp. 721-726, PMID 16873406

Květina, J.; Varayil, J.E.; Ali, S.M.; Kuneš, M.; Bureš, J.; Tachecí, I.; Rejchrt, S. & Kopáčová, M. (2010). Preclinical electrogastrography in experimental pigs. *International Journal of Interdiscip. Toxicol.,* Vol.3, No.2, (June 2010), pp. 53-58, DOI: 10.2478/v10102-010-0011-5, PMC2984130

Marmor, M.F. & Zrenner, E.(1999). Standard for clinical electroretinography. *International Journal of Documenta Ophthalmologica,* Vol.97, No.2, (2009), pp. 143-156, Kluwer Academic Publishers, Printed in the Netherlands

Brown, M.; Marmor, M. & Vaegan, I. (2006). ISCEV Standard for Clinical Electro-oculography (EOG). *International Journal of Documenta Ophthalmologica,* Vol.113, No.3, pp. 205-212, Kluwer Academic Publishers, Printed in the Netherlands

Shafik A. (2000). Electrohepatogram in pathologic liver conditions. *International Journal of Front. Biosci.,* Vol.1, No.5, (June 2000), pp. B1-4, PMID: 10833465

Ravariu, C.; Tirgoviste, C.I. & Dumitrache, O. (2011). The modeling of the insulin exocytosys after a glycemic stimulus, *Proceedings of IASTED 2011 8th International Conference on Biomedical Engineering BioMED*, pp. 144-147, ISBN 978-508-233-3, Innsbruck, Austria, February 16-18, 2011

Fox, J.E.M.; Gyulkhandanyan, A.V.; Satin, L.S. & Wheeler, M.B. (2006). Oscillatory Membrane Potential Response to Glucose in Islet -Cells: A Comparison of Islet-Cell Electrical Activity in Mouse and Rat. *International Journal of Endocrinology,* Vol.147, No.10, (Oct 2006), pp. 4655-4663, DOI: 10.1210/en.2006-0424, ISSN 0013-7227

Purves, D.; Augustine, G.J.; Fitzpatrick, D.; Hall, W.C.; LaMantia, A.S.; McNamara, J.O. & White, L.E. (2008). *Neuroscience. 4th ed,* Sinauer Associates, pp. 7, 27–28, ISBN 978-0-87893-697-7, New York, USA

Ravariu, C.; Tirgoviste, C.I. & Ravariu, F. (2009). Glucose biofuels properties in the bloodstream, in conjunction with the beta cell electro-physiology, *Proceedings of IEEE - ICCEP 2010 2nd International Conference on Clean Electrical Power*, pp. 124-127, ISBN 978-1-4244-2544-0, Capri, Italy, June 9-11, 2009

Gowrishankar, T.R.; Herndon, T. & Weaver, J.C. (2008). Transdermal drug delivery by localized intervention. *International IEEE Journal on Engineering in Medicine and Biology*, Vol.28, No.1, (March 2008), pp. 55-68, DOI: 10.1109/MEMB.2008.918840

7

Towards Affordable Home Health Care Devices Using Reconfigurable System-on-Chip Technology

Mohammed Abdallah and Omar Elkeelany
Tennessee Tech University
USA

1. Introduction

Multi-channel data acquisition (DAQ) is a crucial component in digital instrumentation and control. It typically involves the sampling of multiple analog signals, and converting them into digital formats so that they can be processed either on-board or externally. In either cases, DAQ systems also involve microprocessors, microcontrollers, digital signal processing, and/or storage devices. Multi-channel DAQs, which utilize some sort of processing for simultaneous input channels, are needed in home health care monitoring devices. In this chapter, a low-cost real-time multi-channel Analog Signal Acquisition and Processing (ASAP) system is presented. It is divided into five systems. First, the Multi-channel Analog Signal Acquisition system is used to acquire multi-channel real-time analog signals. Second, Archiving system stores the acquired data into a Flash memory or SDRAM. Third, the Digital Signal Processing Unit performs digital signal processing. Fourth, the Frequency Deviation Monitoring (FREDM) system detects any change in input channels' frequencies. Finally, the Heterogeneous Maximal Service (HMS) Scheduler is presented to be integrated with FREDM system.

In home health care devices, storage is limited and power consumption need to be minimum. Therefore, fixed sampling rate is not the optimal solution for multi-channel human body data acquisition. Hence, heterogeneous sampling rates are identified for each channel, and optimized for best data quality with minimal storage requirement and power consumption. The fidelity of the ASAP system is increased by using reconfigurable chip technology, where flexibility, concurrency and reconfiguration can be achieved in hardware. The proposed ASAP allows for the sampling of up to 32 heterogeneous signals with a single high speed Analog to Digital Converter (ADC) taking into account the performance as well.

In the biomedical field, the first step of diagnose a patient is recording biomedical data. Monitoring the vital signs of the patient in acute life-threatening states or being under surgical procedures or anesthesia conditions requires online analysis and immediate visualization. If the immediate visualization is irrelevant, storage of the acquired data is needed. Electrocardiogram (ECG) devices are the most important diagnostic tools for heart patients. Respiratory problems represent one of the main causes of disease in our world. Most of research papers proposed in this field use computer-based devices to acquire signals from the human body. Moreover, there were no scheduling algorithms used. The proposed ASAP system can be used to acquire human body signals such as the heart beat, pressure and the lung sound at home. Using a varying sampling rate per channel is the optimal solution in terms of scalability, power consumption and memory requirements. It is also considered as a versatile instrument that can be the base of developing a spectroscopic imaging. To date, the complexity associated with constructing a high-fidelity multi-channel, multi-frequency data acquisition instrument has limited widespread development of spectroscopic electrical impedance imaging concepts. To contribute to developing spectroscopic imaging systems, varying sampling rate need to be addressed.

Data acquisition systems (DAQ) are devices and/or software components used to collect information in order to monitor and/or analyze some phenomenon. As electronic technology advances, the data acquisition process has become accurate, versatile, and reliable. Typically, data acquisition devices interface to various sensors that specify the phenomenon under consideration. Most data acquisition systems obtain data from different kinds of transducers that produce analog signals. Many applications require digital signal processing. Therefore, analog signals are converted to a digital form via an Analog to Digital Converter (ADC) to be processed. Existing DAQs, can acquire single channel or multi-channel signals. Many applications require a multi-channel DAQ. Particularly, simultaneous multi-channel DAQs are employed in numerous applications such as medical diagnosis and environmental measurements. If the signals are simultaneously acquired, simultaneous acquisition of additional data can be used to obtain additional information within the same acquisition time. However, exiting computer based multi-channel DAQ systems are cumbersome, expensive, and/or require design redundancy to achieve high reliability and high speed acquisition. Therefore, embedded processing capability must be used to reduce the system size, avoid the design redundancy and reduce the cost and power consumption.

This research is necessary in wide-range applications, particularly demanding heterogeneous and large number of input signals. Therefore, this is the motivation of this research work to try to solve certain problems. One major problem is acquiring high-quality data from large number of input channels simultaneously without the need of computers. This will in turn help the reduction of the cost of the system, and the reduction of the circuit size. Exiting computer-based multi-channel DAQ systems are cumbersome, expensive, and/or require design redundancy to achieve high reliability and high speed acquisition. Contrary to single channel data acquisition, in acquiring multi-channel input signals using a single shared multiplexed ADC, the sampling rate must be much greater than twice the highest frequency component of the input channels. This limits the number of channels being acquired. To increase the number of the input channels, a faster and more expensive ADC must be used in existing technology. In this work, a design of an optimal scheduling module of the ADC with the multiplexer is done. It adaptively selects the proper sampling rate for each channel without affecting the quality of the high frequency input channels or oversampling low frequency spectrum channels. It minimizes the required speed of the single shared ADC, and hence reduces the overall cost of the system, for the same number of heterogeneous input channels. In addition, it minimizes the amount of data being acquired. This leads to minimize the storage requirements. Oversampling low frequency spectrum channels leads to unnecessary data acquisition, which in turn requires extra storage requirements. Hence, an optimization problem is solved in order to compromise between the acquisition quality and amount of data being acquired.

While solving the problem, certain goals will be achieved:

- The total cost of the system should be minimized. The cost can be determined by adding up the cost of every component in the system.

- The circuit size should be minimized. The circuit size will be measured in terms of the number of the gates and logic blocks used in the FPGA chip.

- The system performance should be maximized. For fastest performance, real time operation systems cannot be used. The performance will be measured in terms of:
  - Root Mean Square of errors of the acquired signals
  - The number of channels that can be acquired using the system
  - The required ADC sampling rate for a given set heterogeneous input channels
  - The number of logic elements of FPGA resources
  - The memory requirements

To achieve these goals, one needs to accomplish certain objectives:

1. Heterogeneous multi-channel data acquisition using FPGA-based System-on-Chip

2. Data recording: acquired data has to be stored into Flash Memory for further analysis and/or archiving purposes.

3. Data monitoring: data has to be displayed into an integrated graphical display module.

4. Frequency monitoring: frequency of each channel has to be monitored and any change in frequency should be detected and reported.

5. Optimized sampling: adaptive pre-processing and scheduling techniques are required to sample heterogeneous signals, with adaptive multiplexer scheduling technique.

The efficient implementation of these objectives in FPGA-SoC chip technology has its unique challenges:

- The absence of real time operating system in the desired system leads to the design of all FPGA-SoC to peripheral communication drivers.

- The absence of peripheral drivers (Flash memory, ADC, Graphical display) in FPGA hardware or software. This leads to designing all needed drivers in FPGA. For hardware designed modules, thorough testing must be done for each module independently and collectively after system integration. There are no system simulation tools to guarantee that. Instead, timing simulation is used to verify independent component operation. Each module must be tested and accurate measurements must be verified for fast speed operation. When peripherals are integrated, a reassessment of timing must be done to insure that FPGA-SoC system as a whole performs correctly. Various verification cycles might be needed.

- Synchronization must be maintained between concurrent operating modules. This becomes a challenge when each module operates at different speed. This synchronization has to be implemented in hardware too.

- Adaptive sampling must take place on-the-fly. It needs a continuous monitoring of input channels' frequency.

To eliminate the need of cumbersome hardware, and a personnel computer, one has to map all the functions of a classical data acquisition system inside a single reconfigurable FPGA chip. All needed functions of the computer-based data acquisition and processing system are mapped into the proposed portable multi-functional ASAP system. Note that the FPGA will be designed to manage all the aspects of processing, and storage, as needed. In particular, to make the proposed ASAP a low cost stand-alone reconfigurable system, the following capabilities have to be built: Capability 1: Accept various input signals with different amplitudes and frequencies. It is desired to acquire analog input voltage signals of amplitude range from mV to V range. Also, the desired input signal in the frequency range of Hz to MHz. This allows the system to accommodate for a variety of sensors at the same time (e.g., low frequency electric pulses, acoustic, ultra-sounds, etc). Multi-channel Analog Signal Acquisition (MASA) system is proposed to perform this capability. Capability 2: Perform automatic signal conditioning such as bias addition and removal, and signal scaling. In addition, it has the built-in capability to perform digital signal processing of FFT for one dimensional digital signal. In this research, Digital Signal Pre-processing Unit (DSPU) is proposed to perform this capability. In addition, it detects the input channels' frequencies. Capability 3: Store the acquired signals without the need of an external computer. A Flash memory controller is designed and integrated with other designed modules in the same FPGA to write data directly to a Flash memory card or the SDRAM. Capability 4: Display the acquired signals on real-time. A displaying capability was designed independently. It is integrated with the proposed design. The acquired analog signals are displayed into an integrated display module (Not Presented here). Capability 5: Detect and monitor frequency change of input channels. In addition, an appropriate action should be taken upon change. Frequency Deviation and Monitoring (FREDM) module is proposed to perform this capability. Capability 6: Perform adaptive heterogeneous maximal service scheduling for the ADC multiplexed interface, for variable number of channels. If all channels have the same characteristics, then it will be equivalent to a round-robin sampling technique (i.e. uniform sampling, one sample per channel per cycle). This increases the number of channels being acquired as well as reduces the required ADC sampling rate which in turn, reduces the cost, power consumption and storage requirements. Heterogeneous Maximal Service (HMS) scheduling technique is proposed to achieve these advantages.

Even though some of the above listed capabilities may be achieved by existing Data Acquisition (DAQ) technology for a limited and fixed number of channels, none of the existing DAQs are capable of performing automatic adaptive maximal service scheduling. In addition, existing DAQs have one or more of the disadvantages: cumbersomeness, high cost, and/or limited hardware scalability. The proposed ASAP system is unique, as compared with traditional existing DAQ systems. The uniqueness can be illustrated in different aspects. First, a novel real-time adaptive maximal service scheduling is designed in the proposed ASAP system. In the case of input signals with different bandwidths, it is the best way to optimize the ADC sampling rate. Meanwhile, it also reduces the overall sampling rate required which leads to reduce the cost of the required ADC with large number of channels especially in high frequency inputs as well as reduces the amount of acquired data which reduces the memory requirements. Second, instead of using multiple ADC for simultaneous multi-channel data acquisition, the proposed design uses a single high speed ADC along with a multiplexer to perform quasi-simultaneous data acquisition. A single high speed ADC can be used efficiently with an optimal sampling schedule to acquire multiple channels. Hence, this can reduce the circuit size, the cost, and the power consumption. Third, the proposed research provides a design philosophy that takes full advantage of the capabilities of the FPGA. Full system reconfigurability based on FPGA is the best solution in terms of fault tolerance, portability and the system can be reused with different configurations. In various applications, especially biomedical field, a fixed sampling rate is not the optimal solution. The proposed Heterogeneous Maximal Service (HMS) Scheduler achieves the optimal solution for large number of channels. It also reduces total power consumption and memory requirements. If the input signals have different frequency bandwidths, then the proposed HMS is required to perform adaptive sampling instead of using the highest frequency as a fixed sampling rate for all channels. Oversampling low frequency spectrum channels leads to unnecessary data, which in turn requires extra storage capabilities and more power consumption.

2. Existing data acquisition systems

Many sophisticated data acquisition systems exist in the market. However, they are either expensive, cumbersome or both Arshak et al. (2008); Gray (n.d.); Pimentel et al. (2001); *Technical series on data acquisition* (n.d.). For example, the cost of an ADC board can be as high as $3000. Also, in another example, a computer-based biomedical DAQ system consumes 600 watts of power, and thus requires an isolated power supply unit. That system cost is around $5,500 not including a laptop Inc (n.d.). To make, for example, medical diagnosis affordable, one would want to be able to buy similar sophisticated device and use it at home. In such case, affordability plays a major role in the decision of a patient with chronic disease that requires frequent monitoring of some of his/her body signals.

2.1 Multi-channel data acquisition

Existing multi-channel DAQ systems of heterogeneous input signals either use a super fast ADC with homogeneous sampling rate Jackson et al. (1996); Lan et al. (1998); Luengo-garcia et al. (1997); Nadeemm et al. (1994); Posada & Liou (1991), or dedicated ADC for each channel Chang et al. (2004); Komarek et al. (2006); Morgado et al. (1991); Petrinovic (1998a); Xv et al. (2007). Both of these solutions are inefficient, and/or expensive. In addition, they become infeasible for the acquisition of large number of simultaneous channels. Moreover, they require high storage requirements and power consumption. Researches in Artukh et al. (2007); Artyukh, Bilinskis, Sudars & Vedin (2008); Artyukh et al. (2005); Artyukh, Bilinskis, Sudors & Vedin (2008); Bilinskis (2007); Bilinskis & Sudars (2008a;b); Bilinskis & Sudors (2007); Morgado & Domingues (1991); Sudars & Ziemelis (2007) provided a detailed discussion about the multi-channel DAQ. A special sampling technique, event timing, was employed. A sample value is taken at time instants when the input signal crosses a sinusoidal reference function. A prevailing limitation on the number of input channel was acknowledged. An extended research tried to reduce this limitation. However, there are still some drawbacks in this research. First, the reconfigurability is not achieved due to the use of a computer and only using the FPGA for controlling the time to digital converter (TDC). Second, amplitude, frequency, phase angle of the input channel signals have to be given in advance. Third, the acquisition quality depends on the frequency of the reference sinusoidal signal. Increasing of the reference signal frequency is limited. It was mentioned in these researches that these drawbacks have to be traded off with the low power consumption of their proposed system. The demand for this type of converter is based on the fact that physical processes in many cases directly generate events and their timing data carry valuable information. In other applications, sensors or transducers using voltage-to-frequency converters and pulse width modulators convert slowly varying signals into event streams at their outputs. Nallatech provides a stand-alone FPGA-based DAQ Nallatech (n.d.). Nallatech does utilize the FPGA in their dual 3Gsps ADC board (i.e., all main design modules are performed using FPGA), but they use a dedicated ADC per channel, which in turn increases the power consumption, cost, and the circuit size. The cost of the Nallatech standalone BenADCï£¡-3G is $22,000 Nallatech (n.d.). It also has only dual channels. Therefore, it is not scalable. Some other DAQs such as in Lyrtech, Bittware, Hunt Engineering, and Southwest Research Institute Bittware (n.d.); Engineering (n.d.); Lyrtech (n.d.); Theis & Persyn (2006) only use the FPGA for limited purposes, where the FPGA works as a co-processor for fixed architecture based processing units. This prevents the design from achieving low cost and compact size advantages should the design have been fully integrated in a high capacity FPGA. In Table 1, the literature review on DAQ systems is summarized illustrating the contribution of some research teams and/or affiliations. From Table 1, one can see that the proposed system is unique, as compared with any of research teams appeared in the table.

3. Existing multi-channel data acquisition scheduling algorithms

In real-time single multiplexed ADC systems, input channels scheduling is crucial, because it ensures that input channels meet their requirements. In real-time bad timing can have severe consequences! In heterogeneous real-time systems, each input channel has different restrictions or deadlines. Existing scheduling algorithms can be classified as shown in Figure 1. Dynamic scheduling algorithms are done in run-time, and are more flexible, allowing schedule modifications as inputs change. But dynamic requires computation power that is not needed in static scheduling such as round-robin. In round-robin, processor time (ADC sampling rate) is equally divided among all processes (input channels), before any process is served (input channel is sampled). Each input channel gets equal time slot of the shared single ADC. If heterogeneous multi-rate input channels are scheduled by a single ADC, round-robin scheduling technique assigns the shared ADC to all input channels with a fixed sampling rate Leung & Anderson (2004). In Rate Monotonic (RM), channels are assigned different priorities. Tasks with higher priority will interrupt the current task and replace it. This also means that the system is preemptive. The priorities are assigned to channel based on their frequency. Priorities are assumed to be static, so the channel periods also need to be static. Hence, RM cannot be used if input channels have varying frequency Brucker (2007). Earliest Deadline First (EDF) places input channels in a priority queue. The channel which is closest to its deadline will be scheduled for execution. It has some drawbacks such as situations where deadlines are not known in advance, they are provided but subject to change and/or situations that require uniform sampling spacing Brucker (2007). EDF also does not guarantee equal time spacing between multiple sampling times of periodic signals.

Various research works have been presented in order to achieve adaptive dynamic sampling rate algorithm. Adaptive sampling can be traced back to the research on anti-aliasing in ray tracing Whitted (1980). For example, Painter and Sloan Painter & Sloan (1989) presented adaptively progressive refinement on the entire image plane to locate image features and place more samples along edges. Other research teams proposed different adaptive sampling algorithms in the field of realistic image synthesis. Based on the root mean square signal to noise ratio (RMS SNR), Dippe and Wold Dippe & Wold (1985) proposed an error estimate of the mean to do adaptive sampling. Lee et al. Lee et al. (1985) sampled the pixel adaptively based on the variance of sample values. Purgathofer Purgathofer (1987) used the confidence interval for adaptive sampling. Kirk and Arvo demonstrated a correction scheme to avoid the bias of variance based approaches. Rigau et al. Rigau et al. (2002; 2003a;b) introduced the Shannon entropy and also the f-divergences as the measure to conduct adaptive sampling. Mitchell Mitchell (1987), and later Simmons and Sequin Simmons & Sequin (2000), utilized the contrast to do adaptive sampling. Tamstorf and Jensen Tamstorf & Jensen (1997) refined

Research Work/Affiliations	Multi channel	Multiplexed ADC	Reconfigurability			Adaptive		
			No	Partial	System	No	Manual	Auto
Four-Channel ADC, Nallatech Nallatech (n.d.)	Y	N	-	-	Y	Y	-	-
VHS-ADC Lyrtech Lyrtech (n.d.), Tetra-PMC Bittware Bittware (n.d.), HERON-IO5 Hunt Engineering Engineering (n.d.), HS ADC, Southwest Research Institute Theis & Persyn (2006)	Y	N	-	Y	-	Y	-	-
LabVIEW FPGA, National Instruments Instruments (n.d.)	Y	Y	-	Y	-	-	Y	-
HS ADC / European Atomic Energy Community , CERN in Portugal, Hewlett Packard University of Barcelona in Spain Bautista-Palacios et al. (2005); Cardoso et al. (2004); Loureiro & Correia (2002)	N	N	-	Y	-	Y	-	-
HE ADC/ University of Zagreb in Croatia Meurer & Raulesfs (2000a)	Y	Y	Y	-	-	-	Y	-
100MHz-ADC/ University of EST China Lin & Zhengou (2005) -/Wright State University Lee & Chen (2009)	N	N	-	-	Y	Y	-	-
Four Channel Event Timing Modular Multi-channel DAQ in Latvia Bilinskis (2007)-Artyukh et al. (2005)	Y	N	-	Y	-	Y	-	-
ASAP proposed system at TTU, USA	Y	Y	-	-	Y	-	-	Y

Table 1. Summary of literature review

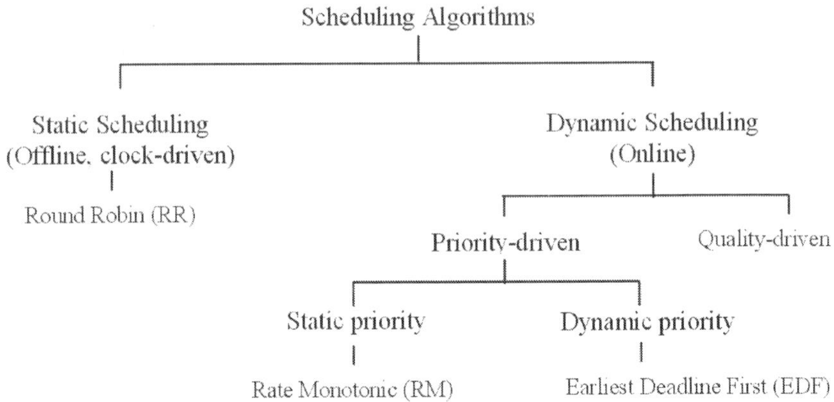

Fig. 1. Classification of existing scheduling algorithms

Purgathofer's approach to propose the tone operated confidence interval. Qing Xu et al. Xu & Sbert (2007) investigated the use of entropy in the domain of information theory to measure pixel quality and to do adaptive sampling based on the nonextensive Tsallis entropy. By utilizing the least-squares design, an entropic index can be obtained systematically to run adaptive sampling effectively.

As signal frequency increases, its corresponding sampling rate has to be increased proportionally in order to have a faithful reconstruction of the signal. It means that more signal samples are to be taken per unit time which means additional storage space is required. Widdershoven et al. Widdershoven & Hiasma (2007) proposed a patent to solve this extra storage issue. They proposed a dynamic shift register which can accommodate to the varying sampling rates in the system. J. Stefan Karlsson Edstrom et al. (2006) proposed a multi-channel modular-based wireless system for medical use. Sampling rate can be individually selected for each channel. The main goal is minimize the total amount of data being acquired to be transmitted. Alex Hartov et al. Hartov et al. (2007) used an under-sampling technique to accelerate data acquisition. Their work was used in developing electrical impedance spectroscopic.

Adaptive sampling is established as a practical method to reduce the sample data volume. Robert Rieger et al. Rieger & Taylor (2009) proposed a low-power analog system, which adjusts the converter clock rate to perform a peak-picking algorithm on the second derivative of the input signal. Their proposed ADC clocking scheme operates the converter at minimum sampling frequency and increases the clock rate only during phases of high curvature (i.e., second derivative) of the signal, essentially performing a peak-picking algorithm on this derivative. The system employs low-power analog circuits to set dynamically the required sample rate without involving the ADC or digital circuitry. Their main application is using this proposed system in the ECG.

From Table 1 and from the literature review, one can see that the proposed system is unique, as compared with any of research teams appeared in the literature review. One can notice that each listed research work has its own advantages. However, the proposed system is unique as related to existing technologies. Instead of using multiple ADC for simultaneous multi-channel data acquisition, the proposed design uses a single high speed ADC along with a multiplexer to perform quasi-simultaneous data acquisition. In the medical field for example, where various biomedical signals are in the low frequency range from 25 Hz to 5 KHz Abdallah et al. (2009), the proposed DAQ can be appropriate without the need of additional hardware or cost. For applications that require very fast simultaneous multi-channel data acquisition, such as in the military field, dedicated ADC per channel will be more appropriate. A single super high speed ADC can be used efficiently with an optimal sampling schedule to acquire multiple channels. Hence, this can reduce the circuit size, the cost, the power consumption, the system scalability and the storage requirements. Second, full system reconfigurability based on FPGA is the best solution in terms of fault tolerance, portability, and the system can be reused with different configurations. Third, hardware real-time adaptive sampling is only available in the proposed system. It leads to the design security where using the hardware design immunes the reverse engineering and secure the design. In the case of input signals with different bandwidths, the hardware real-time adaptive sampling is the best way to optimize the ADC sampling rate. Meanwhile, it also reduce the overall sampling rate required which leads to reduce the cost of the required ADC with large number of channels especially in high frequency inputs.

Our proposed research provides a design philosophy that takes full advantage of the capabilities of the FPGA as well as using a single multiplexed ADC for multi-channel DAQP. This will lead to small size, cost, memory requirements, and power consumption for the DAQP as well as the design hardware scalability (i.e., to add more channels as desired without changing the system board). The optimal sampling capability of the device allows for the sampling of a large number of heterogeneous signals without increasing the size of the ADC.

4. Software acquisition and multiplexing approach

The software acquisition and multiplexing approach is employed using embedded C programming language and Hardware Description Language (HDL). As a rule of thumb, any time-critical task is implemented in hardware, while other functions are developed in software using embedded C programming language. Components of the computer-based data acquisition system are custom designed in the proposed system.

4.1 Archiving implementation in software

In the beginning, a design decision regarding which functions will be accomplished in hardware and which can be done in software has to be taken. In order to get benefit from the simplicity and flexibility of the embedded C programming, two main tasks are assigned to be performed by the NIOS II processor using embedded C programming. Storing the acquired data into the flash memory (SD card) and multiplexing between the multi-input analog channels are performed by the NIOS II processor. Storing the acquired data into the SD card consists of many other subtasks such as store the acquired data in the SDRAM as a temporary location, initialize the SD card, calculating the CRC, check the status of CRC response of a block and put the acquired data in a wave file format.

4.2 Software acquisition and multiplexing approach verification

In this subsection, a comparison study between the proposed MASA system with the archiving module and an existing technology DAQ system is presented. The National Instrument (NI) data acquisition card is chosen because it has the closest similarity to the proposed DAQ (although it is a computer-based, it uses adaptive sampling and a multiplexer). The NI test-bench is a PCI 6024E- 200 kS/s 16 channel DAQ card. National Instruments DAQ

	Sequential Single Channel 100 KSPS	
Input signal	FPGA	NI
1 KHz	rms(e)= 0.0523	rms(e)= 0.016
4 KHz	rms(e)= 0.0754	rms(e)= 0.029
8 KHz	rms(e)= 0.3766	rms(e)= 0.0907
10 KHz	rms(e)= 0.3812	rms(e)= 0.11

Table 2. Root mean square of the error for the proposed software acquisition and multiplexing approach and NI-based DAQ (N= 1000 samples)

has been used as a comparison reference. It is a computer-based DAQ. For the sake of fairness, the sampling rate is fixed for both systems to be 100KSPS. Different signals have been applied to both systems. Acquired signals from both systems have been tested in terms of root mean square of errors.

Different signal generator has been used to generate 1 KHz, 4 KHz, 8 KHz and 10 KHz sine waves. Each signal has been applied into both DAQs. The input signals are applied to the input of the MUX. The proposed FPGA-based DAQ stores the input signal as a wav file into a flash memory. It works as stand-alone without any interfere from the computer. All the processing and control has been done by the FPGA. On the other hand, the NI-based DAQ needs a LabView program which run on a computer in order to store the input signal into a file in the computer attached with the card. Both acquired/stored signals by both systems have been tested by Matlab. The root mean square of errors has been used as an evaluation parameter. In Figure 2, three signals have been presented, the FPGA-based stored signal, NI-based stored signal, and the source signal for 1 KHz and 4 KHz sine waves.

In Table 2, the results of these experiments are listed in terms of the root mean square of errors.

4.3 Software acquisition and multiplexing approach problems

NIOS II processor instructions have a nonuniform execution time. In other words, the time between each acquired sample is not equal. The logic analyzer is used to proof this notice. The logic analyzer is connected to the acquisition clock of the NIOS II processor via one pin of I/O pins of the used FPGA. Figure 3 shows the nonuniformity of the generated acquisition clock of the NIOS II processor. This affects the frequency of the stored signal. So, one can find after some time that the stored signal starts to be slower and deviate from the original signal. It can be noticed from Table 2, the root mean square of errors for the proposed sequential MASA with archiving module system is greater than NI-based DAQ. If the root mean square of error is calculated for less number of samples, the root mean square of errors for the proposed system will be less than the numbers mentioned in Table 2. Figure 4 shows the frequency deviation from the source signal of the stored signal after some time.

This comes from the fact that NIOS II processor is instruction-based which makes the data acquisition nonuniform. In other words, the time between each acquired sample is not equal. This affects the frequency of the stored signal. In addition, the speed of data acquisition, processing and storing is slow. It reaches 100 seconds to process and store 8000 blocks of data where each block is 512 samples. Hence, another design approach will be adopted in the following section. Hardware acquisition and multiplexing design is proposed in order to get fast data acquisition, processing and storing system, as well as maintain an accurate signal reconstruction in terms of its frequency.

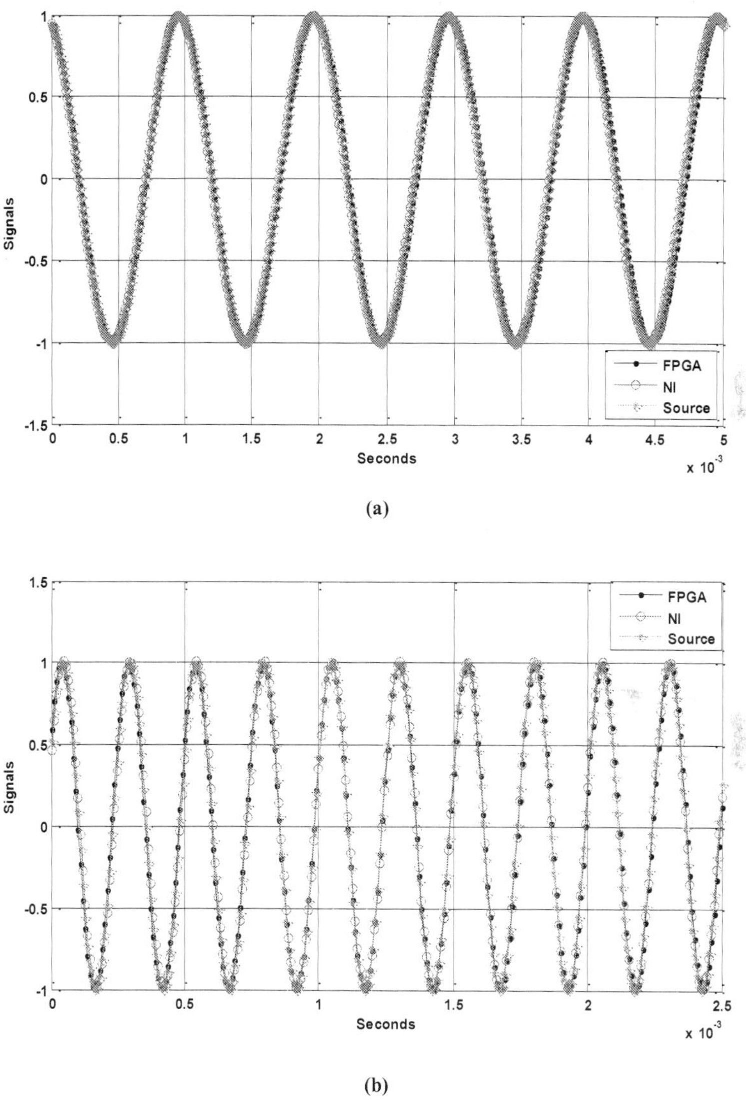

(a)

(b)

Fig. 2. Comparison between FPGA-based, NI-based DAQs (a) 1 KHz sine wave (b) 4 KHz
sine wave in sequential channel DAQ

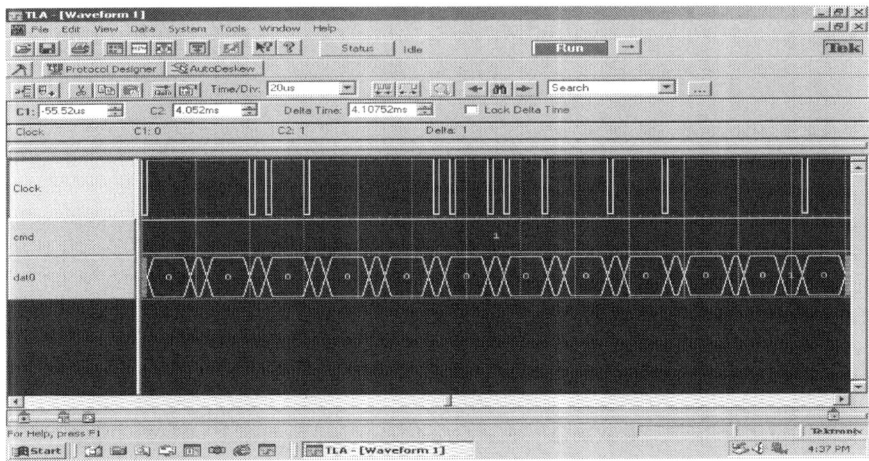

Fig. 3. Logic analyzer shows the nonuniform behavior of the NIOS II processor acquisition rate

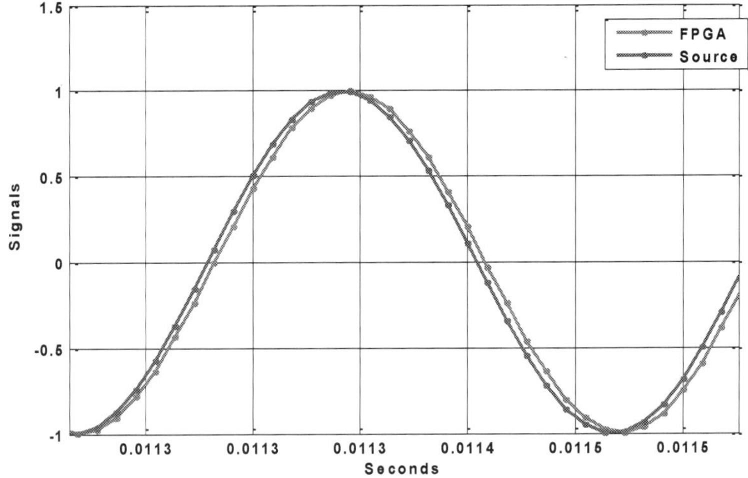

Fig. 4. Frequency deviation problem in the Software Acquisition Approach

		RMSe(proposed system) for(N) Samples			RMSe(NI-DAQ) for(N) Samples			%Improvment N=10000
OSR	Signal	100	1000	10000	100	1000	10000	
500	200Hz	0.009	0.017	0.018	0.013	0.020	0.0202	11
100	1KHz	0.014	0.015	0.015	0.018	0.016	0.0165	9
50	2KHz	0.02	0.027	0.027	0.039	0.04	0.0425	37
25	4KHz	0.02	0.029	0.029	0.029	0.029	0.0334	13
20	5KHz	0.05	0.057	0.057	0.061	0.069	0.06	5
12.5	8KHz	0.083	0.0832	0.082	0.0907	0.0907	0.1	18
6.667	15KHz	0.13	0.13	0.13	0.15	0.155	0.166	22

Table 3. Root mean square of the error for both proposed hardware FPGA-based acquisition and multiplexing design and NI-based DAQs (sequential MASA)

5. Hardware acquisition and multiplexing approach

Due to the previously mentioned problems of the software acquisition and multiplexing, another approach is used to implement the archiving system. All tasks have to be designed and implemented in hardware. No HAL drivers are used. Every peripheral driver and controller is built. The SDRAM controller is designed and implanted in Hardware Description Language. The Avalon fabric and its components are not used in the new approach. In this approach, the acquired data is stored in the SDRAM.

5.1 Hardware acquisition and multiplexing approach verification

The comparison of the acquired data is shown in Table 3. The root mean square of errors (RMS(e)) is used as an evaluating parameter. From Table 3, the performance of MASA with the archiving module is better than the NI-DAQ, although the NI card has two signal conditioning stages. First, adaptive programmable amplitude amplifier is used after the multiplexer and before the ADC inputs. Second, a dithering unit is used to enhance the resolution by 0.5 LSB. As shown from Table 3, seven analog sine waves (200 Hz to 15 kHz) signals are applied into the input of both DAQ systems. Different number of samples (N = 100 to 10,000) is considered. A comparison between the acquired/stored signals via both DAQ systems with respect to the source signal is done. The RMS(e) is calculated for both systems. As the number of samples increases, the RMS(e) is increased (it can be seen if you go right for each system in Table 3). As oversampling ratio (OSR) decreases, RMS(e) is also increased (it can be seen if you go down in a same column). The best performance for sequential MASA with the archiving module has 37% better (smaller) RMS(e) than NI-base DAQ in the case of 10000 sample of 2 KHz input signal. Figure 5 shows the stored signal by NI-based DAQ and the proposed system DAQ as well as the source signal for a 8 KHz sine wave in the case of MASA.

6. Why Heterogeneous Maximal Service (HMS) scheduling?

HMS is needed to sample a large number of heterogeneous signals without increasing the size of the ADC taking into account the performance as well. Sampling rate, resolution and number of channels can be selected and optimized in order to minimize the amount of data being acquired which eventually will be stored or transmitted. Accordingly, storage requirements and power consumption will be reduced. Moreover, a case study is introduced to show the importance of the HMS. In the single multiplexed ADC, it is known that the

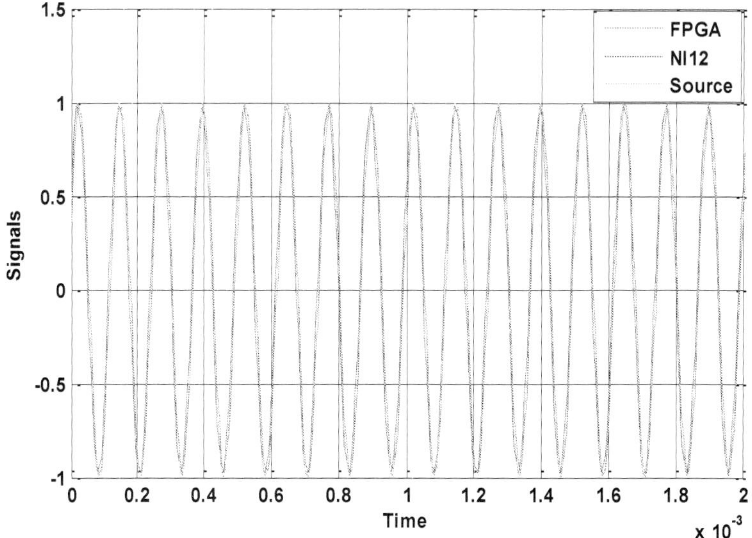

Fig. 5. 8 KHz sine wave acquired by the sequential (proposed FPGA-based system vs. NI-based)DAQ

sampling frequencyF_s must be greater than the Nyquist's sampling frequencyF_x:

$$F_x \geq N \times F_s, F_s \geq 2 \times B_w \tag{1}$$

where N is the total number of channels, and Bw is the highest frequency component of the input channels (widest bandwidth) Meurer & Raulesfs (2000b). This means that the single ADC must be faster than the Nyquist's rate multiplied by the number of channels. If input signals are not in the same frequency range, then an optimized ADC scheduler will be required to perform adaptive sampling, instead of using the highest frequency to set the sampling rate. It is a challenge to achieve the optimal control module of the ADC without affecting the quality of the high frequency input channels or oversampling low frequency spectrum channels. Oversampling low frequency spectrum channels leads to unnecessary data acquisition, which in turn requires extra storage capabilities and more power consumption. According to Equation 2, the dynamic power increases as the activity factor (α) increases, which in turn will increase the total power consumption. If the sampling rate increases, the activity factor will be increased.

$$P_{dynamic} = \alpha C V^2 F \tag{2}$$

where C is capacitance, V is voltage, F is processor clock frequency. Generally speaking, dynamic power can be reduced by using different smaller rates of activity factor for less frequent sampling for channels that require a much smaller minimum service rate as compared to channels with higher service rates.

Second, the determination of optimal maximal service scheduling requires identification of input features, which are generally not known at the design time. Hence, optimal maximal service scheduling cannot be static. A real-time dynamic (optimal) scheduling is proposed in this research. The timing of such scheduler must be accurate to avoid channel skipping or data corruption Petrinovic (1998b). It also has to adapt to changing input features from one application to the other. In addition, each channel will be modulated at the appropriate sampling frequency to maximize the total number of channel acquisition. An optimal ADC scheduler is needed to manage the variable switching time of the ADC multiplexer such that an arbitrary large number of channels can be sampled without loss of signal quality. Moreover, HMS maximizes the quality of rapidly changing channels as well as slow changing channels. On the other hand, round-robin scheduler maximizes the quality of slow changing channels over the rapid ones. In the next section, a comparison between the proposed HMS and round-robin scheduler techniques is introduced.

6.1 Optimization problem

The problem can be formulated as an optimization problem. Given a maximum sampling rate (F_s) of ADC and a total number (N) of channels, an optimized sampling rate (F_{si}) for each channel needs to be assigned.

$$Max \sum_{i=1}^{N} log_2(OSR_i) \tag{3}$$

$$subject\ to\ \sum_{i=1}^{N} f_{si} \leq F_s \qquad ,i = 1, ..., N$$

$$T_{si} \% T_s = 0$$

$$T_{si} \times M1 \neq T_{sj} \times M2 + T_s \times M3$$

where oversampling ratio for channel (i) = OSR_i = F_{si}/F_i ; i, j =1„N; i $\neq$ j; T_{si} = $1/F_{si}$; T_s= $1/F_s$; M1,M2,M3 are integers ($\leq$ 2 Max(T_{si})) ; M3 is the number of time periods (T_s) between channel (j) and channel (i). The objective of this optimization problem is to maximize the assigned sampling rate (or minimize sampling period) for each channel. However, there are various restrictions that limit the OSR_i. First, the summation of assigned sampling rates for all channels must be less than or equal the total sampling rate of the available ADC. Second, the assigned sampling rate for any channel cannot be an arbitrary number. Its inverse (i.e., the time period) must be a multiple of the inverse of the total sampling rate of the available ADC (T_s). Third, at any given time, no more than one channel can be sampled. For example, assume T_s is 0.625 nsec, Ch1 has T_{s1} is equal to 2.5 nsec, and Ch2 has T_{s2} is equal to 1.875 nsec, Figure 6 shows that there is a problem at time T=2.5 nsec. Both Ch1 and Ch2 need to be sampled at the same time. This problem is called Same Time Sampling (STS) Problem. This situation has to be avoided in order to maintain high signal reconstruction.

Therefore, in order to implement the proposed HMS scheduler, two main aspects should be considered. First, the frequency of each channel has to be determined. So, FFT has to be performed for each channel. The DSPU performs this task. Channels' frequencies may be changed overtime. So, adaptive scheduler is needed to monitor any change in frequency. FREDM takes care of this task. Hence, a combination of DSPU and FREDM is a basic tool to achieve the adaptive HMS scheduler.

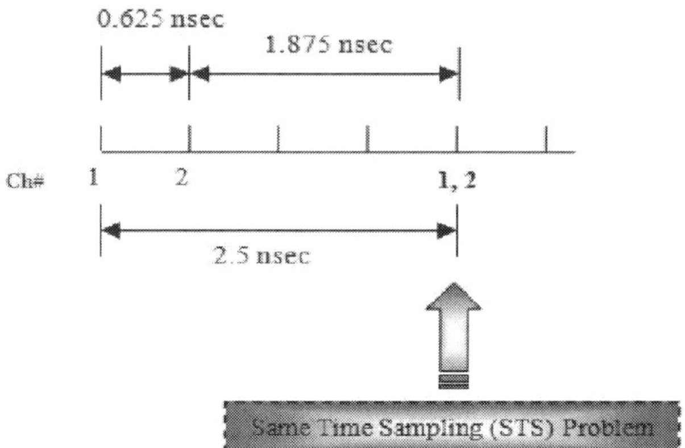

Fig. 6. Same Time Sampling (STS) Problem

7. Optimal sampling Heterogeneous Maximal Service (HMS) scheduler

An array of different analog sensors are connected to the ASAP system. If any channel has a known frequency, this frequency is stored in a lookup table. Otherwise, its frequency is determined by the FFT module in DSPU. The lookup table is updated via FREDM when any frequency change is detected.

7.1 HMS procedure

In Figure 7, HMS flow chart is presented. The inputs to the HMS are frequency bandwidths of input channels. The HMS technique starts with state 0 where each channel has its own sampling rate Fsi which equals to Nyquist's sampling rate. Therefore, each channel sampling period Tsi is calculated by inversing Fsi in state 1. Tsi should be multiples of Ts. If it is, the flow goes to state 2. Otherwise, Tsi should be updated to be multiplies of Ts. In state 2, Brute force search method is used. It is necessary to check the total summation of sampling frequencies of channels. If it exceeds the maximum sapling rate of the available ADC, the task will not be schedulable. Otherwise, the control goes to sate 3. Current sampling frequencies could be a solution. However, the STS problem should be checked before judging on the solution in hand. It comes to state 4 where channels order iterations will take place. In each order, STS problem will be checked. If there is an STS problem, a success rate will be calculated and then the control goes to state 4 again for the next iteration. If there is no STS problem, we have a valid solution and it is needed to be stored as a possible optimal solution. After storing the solution or after the whole iterations are finished without finding a solution, state 5 should be reached. In state 5 for each channel, Tsi will be decremented once by the value of Ts taking into account that Tsi cannot be smaller than Ts. Then, the flow goes again to state 2. One can notice from Figure 7 that there is a flag called start. It is used to determine whether the task in hand is not schedulable or it can be scheduled but there is an STS problem. If start is 0, it

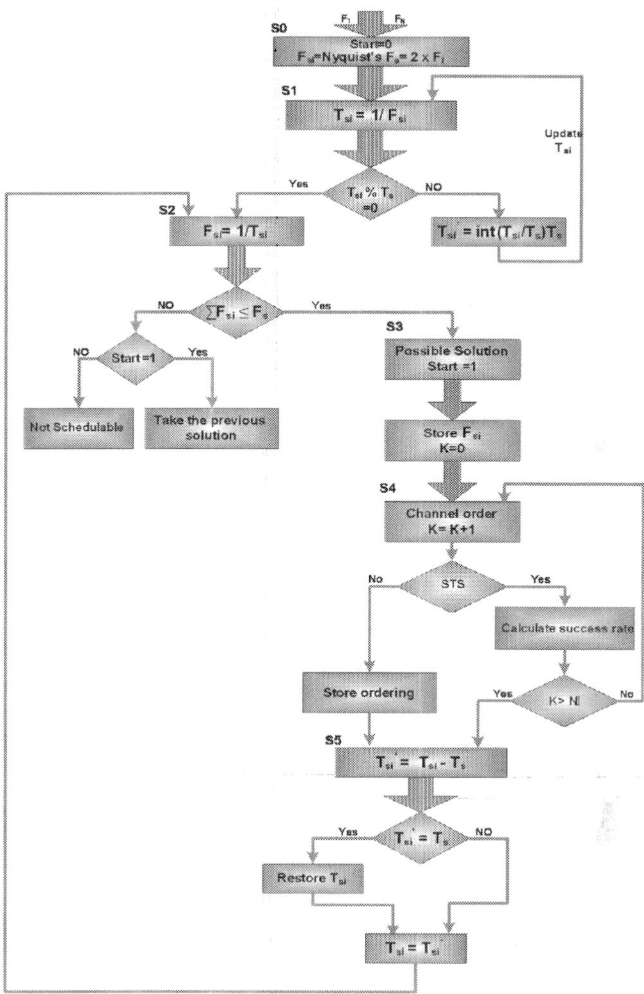

Fig. 7. HMS flowchart

means that no possible solution is achieved. But if start is 1, it means that there is a possible solution that can sample input signals but there is an STS problem. So, if such situation is faced, the previous valid solution should be the optimal solution.

8. Experimental setup

In this section, different experiments are implemented in order to test each subsystem. A multisignal generator (Sony Tektronix AFG310) is used to generate different sine waves as inputs to the proposed system. A Tektronix TLA610 Logic Analyzer is also used in the real-time experiments to verify frequency change of any channel.

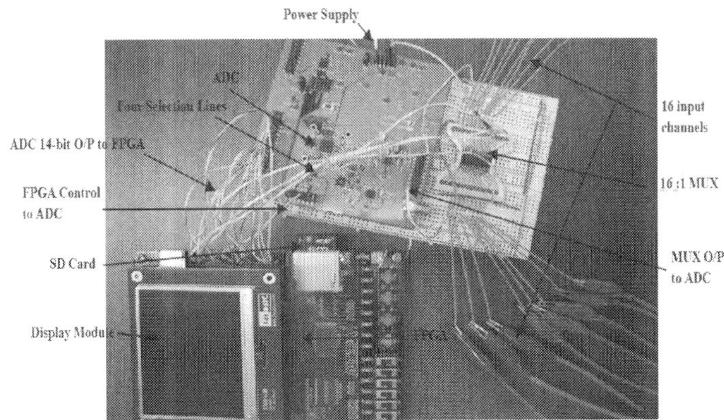

Fig. 8. FPGA Prototype of 16 multiplexed input channels ASAP

8.1 Specification

The designed FPGA ASAP prototype, shown in Figure 8, is set up with a Dual 16:1 Multiplexer/Demultiplexer (Analog Devices ADG506AKRZ), and a Texas Systems ADC (ads7891). This particular low power ADC consumes 85 mW. This ADC operates at clock frequency up to 3MHz. The sampling rate is fixed to be 100 kS/s per channel. This is to have enough data to be displayed and represent the input signal. If high sampling rate such as 3MSPS is chosen, and due to the limited memory in the logic analyzer, the acquired data will represent only a small part of the input signal.

The total number of channels is set via the board switches. The proposed system can handle up to 32 channels. The number of channels can easily be increased by only changing the multiplexer while maintaining everything of the proposed system. The selected FPGA is a Cyclone II (EP2C35F672C6) from Altera, with a main clock of 50 MHz.

9. Verification

The proposed system design is tested and evaluated in terms of signal preprocessing and FFT accuracy done by DSPU, frequency deviation monitoring capability by FREDM, and HMS significance. Each parameter is discussed in more details in this section. Verification using simulation and real-time experiments are considered. A Matlab and Altera simulation tool are used to verify the simulation results of FFT process done by DSPU. A Tektronix Logic Analyzer is used in the real-time experiments to verify frequency change of any channel detected by FREDM. A Matlab program is developed to test and verify the significance of the proposed HMS.

9.1 DSPU evaluation
9.1.1 FFT simulation results

For simulation and verification purposes, the Altera simulation tool is used. Let M= 512 input points. As shown in Figure 9, (*source_real*, *source_imag*) are the real part and the imaginary part of each output point, respectively. The signal (py) is the Power Spectral Density (PSD) of the first 255 points. The signal (*s_pyy_max*) is the highest PSD and (*s_pyy_max_index*) is its index. In other words, (*s_pyy_max_index*) is the location (fci) of the greatest frequency

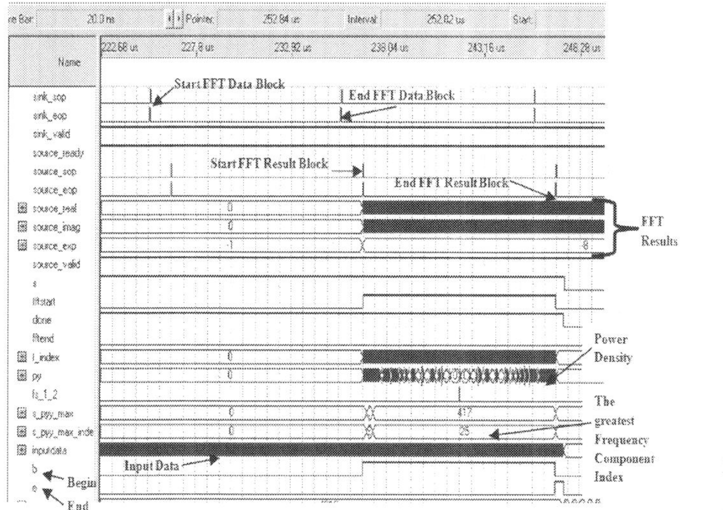

Fig. 9. FFT Simulation Results

component. The greatest frequency component (represents signal frequency) F_i can be easily calculated by

$$F_i = (fci/M) \times F_s, fci = 0, 1, 2, ..., M/2, i = 1, 2, 3, ..., N \tag{4}$$

where N is the number of channels and M is the number of output points of FFT and F_s is the sampling frequency (100 KSPS). A 5 KHz sine wave is the input to the simulation. As shown from Figure 9, ($s\_pyy\_max\_index$) which is the greatest frequency component index (fci) is equal to 25. Substituting in Equation 4 with fci = 25, one can find that the input frequency will be 5 KHz.

9.1.2 FFT Matlab-based merification

A Matlab script was written to generate the required input simulation files. To compare Matlab results with Altera FPGA FFT MegaCore function, one needs first to scale the FPGA output. FPGA scaling is done using the exponent output value:

$$FinalOutput = (MegaCoreFunctionOutput)/(2^{exp}) \tag{5}$$

In other words, FPGA gives a very well scaled output and then it is needed to divide it down. To divide by $2n$ in hardware, it is needed to shift right n bits and extend the sign bit n times. Remember the exponent varies according to FFT block values. In Matlab, results are close but with some rounding difference. Rounding was not done in the hardware module. For verification purposes, the same data set of a maximum frequency component of 5 KHz is considered for both FPGA-based and Matlab-based FFT process. The accuracy of the FPGA-based FFT module is 98% compared to the FFT function in Matlab. Moreover, the proposed FPGA-based FFT module accuracy can be increased via using more FFT points (M). Only 512 points are considered in this work. If M = 2048, the accuracy will be more than 99%. Figure 10 shows a comparison between the Matlab-based FFT and FPGA-based FFT done by DSPU for the same input signal (of a maximum frequency component of 5 KHz). The

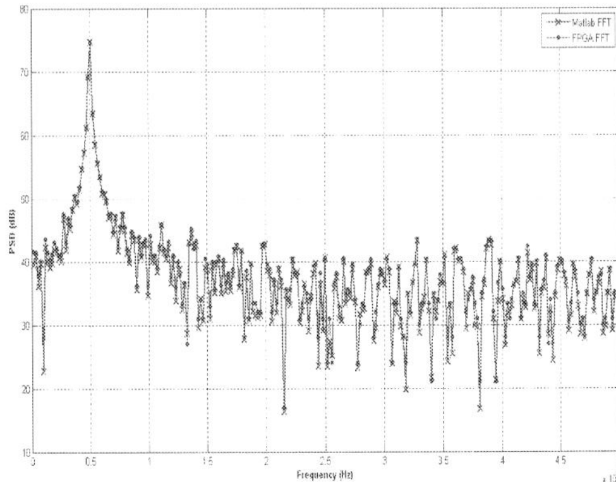

Fig. 10. Matlab FFT verification of a data set of a maximum frequency component of 5 KHz

Frequency	Frequency Component Index (fci)
5 kHz	25
10 kHz	50
15 kHz	76

Table 4. Frequency and the corresponding frequency component index (fci) from Equation 4

horizontal axis is the frequency in Hz and the vertical axis is the power spectrum density in dB. As shown in the figure, the maximum power density exits at frequency of $0.5x10^4$ which is 5 KHz.

9.2 FREDM evaluation

Two experiments are performed here. First, two input signals (15 KHz and 5 KHz) are connected to a multiplexer as inputs to the FREDM. Figure 11 (a) shows a snap shoot of the logic analyzer connected to the FPGA board for verification purposes. As seen in Figure 11, both channel number and its frequency component number are detected (see Equation 4). Table 4 shows both signal frequency and the corresponding frequency component index.

In the second experiment, 16 input channels are applied to the multiplexer. For simplicity, the logic analyzer considers channel 1 only. A 5 KHz sine wave is applied to the channel 1. A change in frequency is taken place to be 10 KHz. Figure 11 (b) illustrates frequency change detector capability of the proposed FREDM system. As seen from the figure, the fci of channel 1 is presented before and after the change. Enable signal is changed from (0 to 1) when frequency change is detected.

9.3 HMS evaluation and significance

A comparison between the proposed HMS and round-robin scheduling technique is presented here. A simulation Matlab program is developed. There are three possible scenarios. First, both techniques cannot schedule a given task (i.e., un-schedulable task). Second, both techniques can schedule it. Third, HMS can schedule it and round-robin cannot. Let's consider

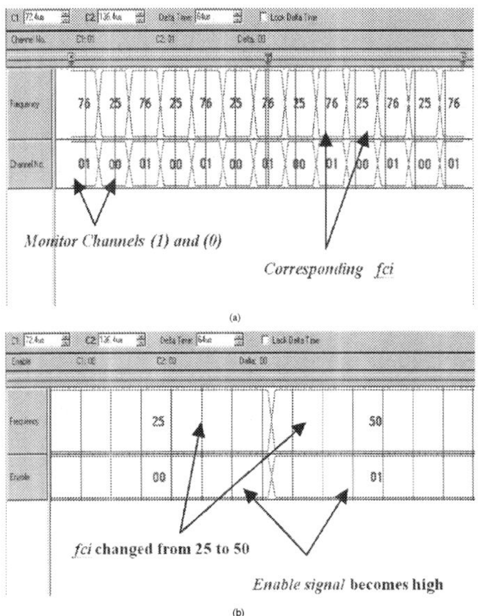

Fig. 11. FREDM verification (a) Real-time frequency monitoring and (b) frequency change/deviation detection

the second scenario where both techniques can give a solution to the given case study. A case study is considered with eight sinusoidal analog signals. The frequencies of the eight input channels are 500kHz, 200 kHz, 190 kHz, 185 kHz, 160 kHz, 100 kHz, 100 kHz, and 100 kHz. Let the maximum sampling rate Fs of the available ADC be 10 MSPS (Ts = 100 nsec). The HMS solution is presented in Figure 12. In this case, round-robin scheduling technique can schedule given signals with a fixed sampling rate for all channels (1/800nsec= 1.25MSPS). This leads to oversampling low frequency signals (such as the 100 kHz), which in turn causes extra memory storage requirements and power consumption as well. On the other hand, the HMS schedules the eight input channels to be sampled at a varying sampling rate. This reduces the amount of data being acquired, which in turn decreases the required memory as well as power consumption according to Equation 2. The total amount of data being acquired using the proposed HMS is less than that acquired by round-robin by 59%.

Now let's consider the third scenario where HMS can schedule the given task and round-robin cannot get a solution for the same task. Let the maximum sampling rate F_s of the given ADC be 100 kS/s. The time period is 10 μ sec. Three analog signals are applied to MASA system, 25 kHz, 10 kHz, and 2 kHz, respectively. In addition, assume that no channel has priority. Applying Nyquist's law, one can find the following. $F_{s1} \geq 50$ KS/s, $F_{s2} \geq 20$ KS/s, $F_{s3} \geq 4$ KS/s; where F_{si} is sampling frequency for channel (i). In other words, $T_{s1} \leq 20$ μsec, $T_{s2} \leq 50$ μsec, $T_{s3} \leq 250$ μsec; where T_{si} is sampling time period for channel (i). If round-robin sampling technique is applied, these three signals cannot be sampled using the available ADC. Applying HMS, these analog signals can be optimally scheduled using the available ADC. As shown in Figure 13, the optimal scheduling is $T_{s1} = 20$ μsec, $T_{s2} = 40$ μsec, $T_{s3} = 240$ μsec ($F_{s1} = 50$ KS/s, $F_{s2} = 25$ KS/s, $F_{s3} = 4.166$ KS/s). The three constraints are satisfied in the optimal maximal service scheduler.

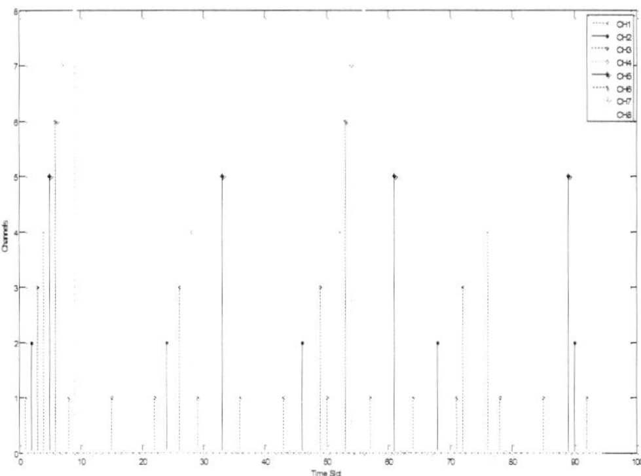

Fig. 12. Eight channels with a varying sampling rate

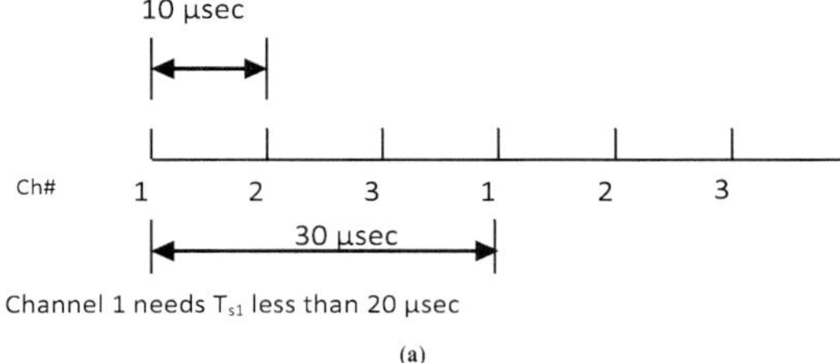

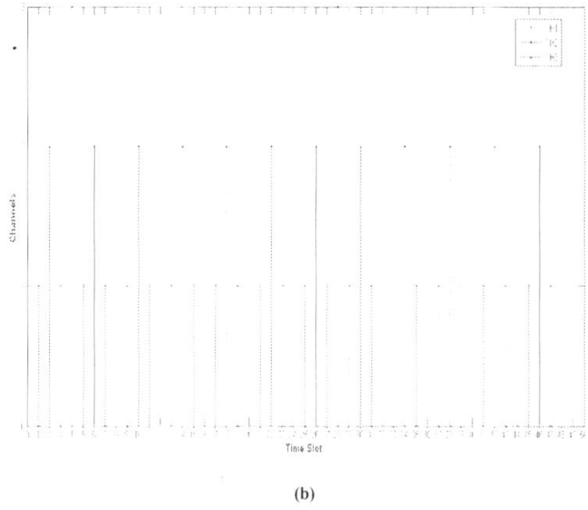

Fig. 13. Comparison between scheduling techniques(a) round-robin (cannot schedule the given signals) and (b) HMS (can optimally schedule them using the available ADC)

The horizontal axis represents the time slots where the period between each consecutive time slots is the (T_s) which is equal to 10 μsec in this example. The vertical axis represents the channel being sampled at a certain time slot. As shown in the figure, three channels are mentioned in the vertical axis. At time slots (1, 3, 5,etc), channel 1 is sampled. At time slots (2, 6, 10,etc), channel 2 is sampled. At time slots (4, 28,etc), channel 3 is sampled.

10. Conclusions

The proposed ASAP system can be used to acquire human body signals such as the heart beat, pressure and the lung sound at home. Using a varying sampling rate per channel is the optimal solution in terms of scalability, power consumption and memory requirements. It is also considered as a versatile instrument that can be the base of developing a spectroscopic imaging. To date, the complexity associated with constructing a high-fidelity multi-channel, multi-frequency data acquisition instrument has limited widespread development of spectroscopic electrical impedance imaging concepts. To contribute to developing spectroscopic imaging systems, varying sampling rate need to be addressed.

Existing computer-based multi-channel DAQ systems are cumbersome, expensive, and/or inefficient when various heterogeneous signals are acquired. Embedded microcontroller-based DAQ systems have some advantages such as low cost, compact size, and low power consumption. However, it is not reconfigurable due to its fixed hardware architecture and can not be used for reconfigurable heterogeneous sampling. So, another DAQs category is needed in order to overcome other categories problems. Reconfigurable FPGA is used in this research as the center piece of the proposed system. In addition, the proposed system is unique as related to existing technologies. It has the maximal service scheduling capability which efficiently utilizes the single ADC to acquire heterogeneous multi-channel input signals. This leads to reduction in the circuit size, cost, power consumption, and storage requirements. In addition, the proposed DAQ is used without the need to computing systems such as a PC. Full system reconfigurability based on FPGA as well as the adaptive sampling is only available in the proposed ASAP system.

Two design methodologies are used to implement the archiving. Software acquisition and multiplexing approach is done via Hardware Description Language (HDL) and embedded C programming language. This approach has some drawbacks. Therefore, a second approach, hardware acquisition and multiplexing, is proposed using only Verilog HDL.

In hardware acquisition and multiplexing approach, different signals were applied to the proposed system and the NI systems. Acquired signals by both DAQ systems were tested in terms of root mean square of errors. It is found that, the best performance for proposed system has 37% better (smaller) RMS(e) than NI-base DAQ in the case of 10000 sample of 2 KHz input signal.

FFT implementation is done to determine each channel frequency. The accuracy of the FPGA-based FFT module implemented inside the DSPU is 98% in the case of using 512 FFT points. It reaches more than 99% in the case of using 2048 FFT points. After detecting frequency bandwidths via DSPU, FREDM detects and monitor any change in frequency values at any input channel.

Finally, to acquire human body multichannel signals, a fixed sampling rate is not the optimal solution. The proposed Heterogeneous Maximal Service Scheduler (HMS) achieves the optimal solution for large number of channels. It also reduces total power consumption and memory requirements. If the input signals have different frequency bandwidths, then the proposed HMS is required to perform adaptive sampling, instead of using the highest frequency as a fixed sampling rate for all channels. That is because oversampling low frequency spectrum channels leads to unnecessary data, which in turn requires extra storage capabilities and more power consumption. Different case studies are studied in this research. As a result, the proposed HMS can schedule given tasks that are not schedulable via round-robin technique. Even in scenarios that both round-robin and proposed HMS can successfully schedule the given task, proposed HMS reduces the amount of data being acquired by 59%, which in turn decreases memory requirements and power consumption as well.

11. References

Abdallah, M., Elkeelany, O. & Alouani, A. (2009). A low cost stand-alone multi-channel data acquisition monitoring and archival system with on-chip signal pre-processing, *IEEE Transaction on Instrumentation and Measurement* 59(4): 1–15.

Arshak, K., Arshak, A., Jafer, E., Waldern, D. & Harris, J. (2008). Low-power wireless smart data acquisition system for monitoring pressure in medical application, *Microelectronics International* 25(1).

Artukh, Y., Bilinskis, I., Rybakov, A. & Stepins, V. (2007). Pseudo-randomization of multiplexer-based data acquisition from multiple signal sources, *DASP Workshop* .

Artyukh, Y., Bilinskis, I., Sudars, K. & Vedin, V. (2008). Alias-free data acquisition from wideband signal sources, *Digital signal processing and its applications* .

Artyukh, Y., Bilinskis, I., Sudors, K. & Vedin, V. (2005). Wideband rf signal digitizing for high purity spectral analysis, *International Workshop on Spectral Methods and Multirate Signal Processing* .

Artyukh, Y., Bilinskis, I., Sudors, K. & Vedin, V. (2008). Multi-channel data acquisition from sensor systems, *Digital Signal Processing and its Applications* .

Bautista-Palacios, M., Baldez, L. & HermsBerenguer, A. (2005). Configurable hardware/software architecture for data acquisition: implementation on fpga, *IEEE Field programmable logic and applications* pp. 241–246.

Bilinskis, I. (2007). *Digital alias-free signal processing*, UK: John Wiley and Sons, Ltd.

Bilinskis, I. & Sudars, K. (2008a). Digital representation of analog signals by timed sequences of events, *Electronics and Electrical Engineering* 83(3).

Bilinskis, I. & Sudars, K. (2008b). Specifics of constant envelope digital signals, electronics and electrical engineering, *Electronics and Electrical Engineering* 84(4).

Bilinskis, I. & Sudors, K. (2007). Processing of signals sampled at sine-wave crossing instants, *Workshop on Digital Alias-free Signal Processing (WDASP'07)* pp. 45–50.

Bittware (n.d.). Tetra-pmc, http://www.bittware.com/products/boards/prod_ desc.cfm?ProdShrtName=TRPM.

Brucker, P. (2007). *Scheduling Algorithms*, Springer.

Cardoso, J., Simoes, J. & Correia, C. (2004). A high performance reconfigurable hardware platform for digital pulse processing, *IEEE transactions on nuclear science* 51(3).

Chang, W., Jeon, C., Park, Y., Yang, S., Ki, S. & Huh, Y. (2004). The design of the multiplexing data acquisition and monitoring system for magnetocardiography (mcg), *TENCON 2004* 3: 585–587.

Dippe, M. & Wold, E. (1985). Antialiasing through stochastic sampling, *Computer graphics, Imaging and visualization jouranl* 19(3).

Edstrom, U., Skonevik, J., Backlund, T. & Karlsson, A. (2006). A flexible measurement system for physiological signals in mobile health care, *27th Annual International Conference of the Engineering in Medicine and Biology Society* pp. 2161–2162.

Engineering, H. (n.d.). Heron-io5 module, http://www.hunteng.co.uk/products/fpga/heron-io5.htm.

Gray, J. (n.d.). Building a risc system in an fpga, http://www.fpgacpu.org/xsoc/cc.html.

Hartov, A., Mazzarese, R., Reiss, F., Kerner, T. & Osterman, K. (2007). A multichannel continuously selectable multifrequency electrical impedance spectroscopy measurementsystem, *IEEE transactions on biomedical engineering* 47(1).

Inc, C. (n.d.). Portable eeg and psg system, http://www.grass-telefactor.com/products/clinsystems/cmeeg1.html.

Instruments, N. (n.d.). Ni labview fpga module, http://sine.ni.com/nips/cds/view/p/lang/en/nid/11834.

Jackson, T., Li, T., Wood, E., O'Neill, P. & Engman, E. (1996). Sir-c/x-sar as a bridge to soil moisture estimation using current and future operational satellite radars, *Geoscience and Remote Sensing Symposium* .

Komarek, M., Novotny, M., Ramos, P. & Pereira, J. (2006). A dsp based prototype for water conductivity measurements, *Instrumentation and Measurement Technology Conference* pp. 2348–2352.

Lan, Y., Jing, J., Delin, Z. & Changwen, T. (1998). A high-speed multi-channel data acquisition and processing system for coherent radar, *Signal Processing Proceedings* 2: 1632–1635.

Lee, M., Redner, R. & Uselton, S. (1985). Statistically optimized sampling for distributed ray tracing, *In SIGGRAPH '85: Proceedings of the 12th annual conference on Computer graphics and interactive techniques* pp. 61–68.

Lee, Y. & Chen, C. (2009). Dynamic kernel function fast fourier transform with variable truncation scheme for wideband coarse frequency detection, *IEEE transactions on instrumentation and measurement* 58(5): 1555–1562.

Leung, J. & Anderson, J. (2004). *Handbook of Scheduling: Algorithms, Models, and Performance Analysis*, CRC Press LLC.

Lin, T. & Zhengou, Z. (2005). The implementation of 100mhz data acquisition based on fpga, *The 3rd IEEE International Workshop on system-on-chip for real-time applications* pp. 241–246.

Loureiro, C. & Correia, C. (2002). Innovative modular high-speed data-acquisition architecture, *IEEE transactions on nuclear science* 49(3).

Luengo-garcia, D., Pantaleon-Peieto, C., Satamaria-Caballero, J. & Gomez-Cosio, E. (1997). Simultaneous sampling by digital phase correction, *IEE instrumentation and measurement technology conference Ottawa* .

Lyrtech (n.d.). Vhs-adc, http://www.lyrtech.com/index.php?act=view&pv=VHS-ADC.

Meurer, M. & Raulesfs, R. (2000a). Enhancement of multi-channel adc conversion by a code division multiplex approach, *IEEE 6th International Symposium on spread-spectrum technology and applications* .

Meurer, M. & Raulesfs, R. (2000b). Enhancement of multi-channel adc conversion by a code division multiplex approach, *IEEE 6th International Symposium on spread-spectrum technology and applications* pp. 1–6.

Mitchell, D. (1987). Generating antialiased images at low sampling densities, *Computer graphics, Imaging and visualization jouranl* 21(4): 65–72.

Morgado, A. & Domingues, J. (1991). Data acquisition and signal processing system based on tms320c50and on a imsa100 processing cascade, *Electro technical Conference* 1: 340–342.

Morgado, A., Domingues, J., Loureiro, C., Assuncaao, J. & Correia, C. (1991). Data acquisition and signal processing system based on tms320c50and on a imsa100 processing cascade, *Electro technical Conference* 1: 340–342, 22–24.

Nadeemm, S., Sodini, C. & Lee, H. (1994). 16 - channel oversampled analog-to-digital converter, *IEE journal of solid state circuits* 29(9).

Nallatech (n.d.). Virtex-4, dual 3 gsps adc, `http://www.nallatech.com/?node_id=1.2.2&id=63&request=2008update`.

Painter, J. & Sloan, K. (1989). Antialiased ray tracing by adaptive progressive refinement, *Computer graphics, Imaging and visualization jouranl* 23(3): 281–288.

Petrinovic, D. (1998a). High efficiency multiplexing scheme for multi-channel a/d conversion, *Midwest symposium on circuits and systems* 1: 534–537.

Petrinovic, D. (1998b). High efficiency multiplexing scheme for multi-channel adc conversion, *Midwest symposium on circuits and systems* pp. 534–537.

Pimentel, B., Filho, A., Campos, R., Fernandez, A. & Coelho, N. (2001). A fpga implementation of a dct-based digital electrocardiographic signal compression device, *IEEE,14th Symposium on Integrated Circuits and System Design* .

Posada, J. & Liou, J. (1991). Modeling the soil moisture sensor using an automated data acquisition system, *Industry Applications Society Annual Meeting* 2: 1678–1684.

Purgathofer, W. (1987). A statistical method for adaptive stochastic sampling, *Computer graphics, Imaging and visualization jouranl* 11(2): 157–162.

Rieger, R. & Taylor, J. (2009). An adaptive sampling system for sensor nodes in body area networks, *IEEE transactionson neural systems and rehabilitation engineering* 17(2).

Rigau, J., Feixas, M. & Sbert, M. (2002). New contrast measures for pixel supersampling, *Proceedings of CGI'02* pp. 439–451.

Rigau, J., Feixas, M. & Sbert, M. (2003a). Entropy-based adaptive sampling, *Proceedings of GI'03* .

Rigau, J., Feixas, M. & Sbert, M. (2003b). Refinement criteria based on f-divergences, *Proceedings of Eurographics Symposium on Rendering* .

Simmons, M. & Sequin, C. (2000). Tapestry: A dynamic mesh based display representation for interactive rendering, *Proceedings of the 11th Eurographics Workshop on Rendering* .

Sudars, K. & Ziemelis (2007). Expected performance of the sine-wave crossing data acquisition systems, *DASP Workshop)* .

Tamstorf, R. & Jensen, H. (1997). Adaptive sampling and bias estimation in path tracing, *Proc. of Eurographics Workshop on Rendering '97* pp. 285–295.

Technical series on data acquisition (n.d.). `http://www.kscorp.com/support/whitepapers`.

Theis, L. & Persyn, S. (2006). Development of a high-speed multi-channel analog data acquisitioning architecture, *IEEE aerospace conference* .

Whitted, T. (1980). An improved illumination model for shaded display, *ACM of Communications* 32(6): 343–349.

Widdershoven, F. & Hiasma, J. (2007). Signal processing device having frequency adaptive sampling, *US Patent Number 5299247* .

Xu, Q. & Sbert, M. (2007). A novel adaptive sampling by tsallis entropy, *Computer graphics, Imaging and visualization jouranl* .

Xv, W., Bing, H. & Wenbin, W. (2007). Design of logic control for micro-power a/d with a serial interface using fpga, *Electronic Measurement and Instruments* .

Part 2

Biomedical Intrumentations

8

Clinical Engineering

Pietro Derrico, Matteo Ritrovato,
Federico Nocchi, Francesco Faggiano,
Carlo Capussotto, Tiziana Franchin and Liliana De Vivo
IRCCS Ospedale Pediatrico Bambino Gesù, Rome,
Italy

1. Introduction

Clinical Engineering (CE) represents the part of *Biomedical Engineering* focused on the applications of theories and methodologies of the broad biomedical engineering field to improve the quality of health services. Its activities especially concern the appropriate management of biomedical technologies (from purchasing to risk controlling) and the development and the adjustment of hospital informative systems and telemedicine networks. CE combines with the medicine knowledge for conducing of healthcare activities by providing expertise in a wide spectrum of topics, from human physiology and biomechanics to electronics and computer science.

As biomedical technology developed towards ever more complex systems and spread in every clinical practice, so the field of CE grew. Such growth has been accompanied by an analogous expansion of biomedical and clinical engineering studies at the University and development of skills and tasks of CE professionals.

The main aim of CE is to support the use of biomedical technology by health professionals and hospital organizations with appropriate skills in order to reach the best compromise between clinical efficacy/efficiency, patient and operators safety, care quality and innovation, and management and equipment costs.

CE techniques and methodologies are mainly focused on safe, appropriate and economical management of technologies, as well as on governance and management (limited to specific responsibilities) of healthcare facility. Thus, CE covers all those knowledge and methods applied to the management of biomedical technologies, ranging from their early evaluation and assessment, to their technical conduct, to their dismissing. Thus the chapter will highlight different aspects of technology management by exploring technical and/or clinical, and/or economic issues related to the individuation and acquisition of appropriate equipment (i.e., Health Technology Assessment), acceptance testing, management of preventive and corrective maintenance, risk management, planning of quality testing, ICT management, management of maintenance contracts, equipments replacement planning, and so on.

2. Healthcare risk management

Because of the strong pressure on the health structures to optimize the services provided while lowering the associated costs and reducing the likelihood of adverse events, an organizational approach, in which a Healthcare Risk Management program plays a central role, becomes important.

Mistakes can be minimized, in fact, by creating organizational systems and using technologies to make it easier to do the right thing. It is clear that patient safety can be increased by means of appropriate procedures aimed at avoiding possible mistakes or correcting those that do happen.

In particular, the potential for biomedical equipment related adverse events needs to be analyzed in order to prevent their occurrence: healthcare structures have to use systematic analytical methods and instruments to manage technological risks to both patients and operators.

The aim of the health organizations is to take care of patients, by providing effective, appropriate and, in particular, safe treatments. The healthcare institutions (such as the clinicians themselves) have to ensure the care, as adequate as possible, of patients, avoiding or at least containing damage caused by human and system errors. Healthcare service activities connote, in fact, with the presence of several hazards that have the potential to harm patients and health operators.

Currently the best known approach is the Healthcare Risk Management program, with which it is possible to identify, assess, mitigate and control healthcare facilities risks, and thus realize the concept of "systemic safety".

Originally such approaches focused mainly, if not entirely, on the problem of reducing the "Clinical Risk" (Clinical Risk Management, CRM) with the aim of limiting enterprise liability-costs. In fact, over the course of the last several years healthcare institutions and practitioners have experienced a "malpractice crisis" that has led to the increase in jury verdicts, settlement amounts and insurance premiums, as well as dwindling insurance availability due to carrier withdrawals from the medical malpractice market (McCaffrey & Hagg-Rickert, 2010), and consequent increase of risk retention cost.

Gradually, the focus shifted to clinical problems and thus the term CRM now encompasses strategies to reduce the incidence and magnitude of harm and improve the quality of care (Taylor-Adams, et al., 1999) by focusing on patient safety and patient care related issues, including information gathering systems, loss control efforts, professional liability, risk financing and claims management activities.

2.1 Technological risk management

Dealing with clinical risk and patient safety means also dealing with biomedical technologies. In fact, as medical treatments have greatly progressed along with the analogous technological advances in medical equipment (ME), all medical procedures depend, to some extent, on technology to achieve their goals. Despite the (presupposed) inherent safety of MEs (also guaranteed by a plethora of laws and technical standards), device-related adverse events occur every day in hospitals around the world. Some can be very dangerous and occasionally even deadly.

An adverse event is (as defined by Medicines and Healthcare Products Regulatory Agency, MHRA) "an event that causes, or has the potential to cause, unexpected or unwanted effects involving the safety of device users (including patients) or other persons". ME related adverse events can occur for several reasons, ranging from incorrect choice and acquisition of the device, wrong installation, and poor maintenance, to use error and device obsolescence.

As stated before, a systemic approach is needed. Such an approach, identified as Medical Equipments Risk Management (MERM), is part of the global Technology Management

(Wilkins & Holley, 1998) as practised by the Clinical Engineering Department (CED) within the hospital. The specific activities of the MERM process are, as coded by several international standards (AS/NZS 4360:2004; ISO 14971:2007; ISO 31000:2009) regarding risk management applied to general production processes and specifically to the design and production of medical devices (but addressed to manufacturers, not the users, of medical equipment) as follows:

- risk identification
- risk analysis and assessment (including risk prioritization);
- planning of actions to mitigate the risk;
- tracking of information about the implemented actions;
- control and follow up.

All the standards stress that the task of risk assessment, along with risk identification,. is the most important element. This is mainly because all the measures the CED (as well as the healthcare organization as a whole) will take to reduce the level of risk will depend on the results of these two phases: an error in assessment would probably lead to several mistakes (and therefore waste of economical and human resources) in the subsequent phases.

Given below is a brief description of the methods available for addressing risk analysis and assessment. However, a thorough analysis of the remaining phases is left to the reader, since they require the active involvement of several lines of professionals, and thus are strongly dependent on the organizational and operational arrangements of the specific healthcare facility.

2.1.1 Methods and techniques

Risk identification and risk analysis are processes aimed at identifying the type of hazard and determining the potential severity associated with an identified risk and the probability that a harmful event will occur. Together, these factors establish the "seriousness of a risk" and guide the clinical engineer's choice of an appropriate "risk treatment" strategy (including preventive maintenance, user training, definition of a renewal plan, etc.).

Techniques for risk identification and assessment are various and dependent on the specific kind of hazard under assessment. In the healthcare sector, two techniques are widely and commonly used: Failure Mode and Effects Analysis and Root Cause Analysis.

Failure Mode and Effect Analysis (FMEA) is a systematic process for identifying potential process and technical failures, with the intent to eliminate them or minimize their likelihood, before they occur, that is in advance of the occurrence of the adverse event related to the analyzed risk (American Society for Healthcare Risk Management [ASHRM], 2002). Initiated in the 1940s by the U.S. Defense Department, FMEA was further developed by the aerospace and automobile industries, but it was only in the late 1960s that it was first applied to healthcare processes. Since then, in the healthcare sector, Failure Mode and Effects Analysis has been developed as a systematic, proactive method for evaluating clinical processes to identify where and how they might fail, and to assess the relative impact (in terms of damage to patients, workers and facilities) of different failures in order to identify the parts of the process that are most in need of change.

The rationale of FMEA is the acknowledgement that errors are inevitable and predictable, and thus can be anticipated and/or minimized by design.

As suggested by the name, the focus is on the *Failure Mode* (defined as the incorrect behavior of a subsystem or component due to a physical or human reason), on the *Effect* (defined as the consequences of a failure on operation, function or functionality, or status of some item) and, potentially (in which case the acronym becomes FMECA) on *Criticality* (defined as the combination of the probability that a failure will occur and the severity of its effect on the system or subsystem). In other words FMEA (or FMECA) analysis aims to identify and analyze

- All potential failure modes of a system and components of the system;
- The effects these failures may have on the system and parts of the system;
- How to avoid or reduce the probability of the failures, or mitigate the effects of the failures on the system.

Depicted below is a schematic, step-by-step description of how to conduct the FMEA process:

1. Define the FMEA topic.
    - Write a clear definition of the process to be studied.
    - Narrow the scope of the review so that it is manageable, and the actions are practical and able to be implemented.
2. Assemble the Team.
    - Guarantee the multidisciplinarity of the team by including expert representatives of all affected areas.
    - Identify the team leader/coordinator.
3. Prepare a graphic description of the process
    - Create and verify the flow chart.
    - Number each process step.
    - For complex processes, specify the area to focus on.
    - Identify and create a flow chart of the subprocesses.
4. Conduct a Hazard Analysis
    - List all possible/potential failure modes for each process/subprocess.
    - List all the possible causes of the *failure mode* (each failure mode may have multiple failure mode causes).
    - Determine the "severity (S)", "probability (P)" and "detectability (D)."
    - Determine the Risk Priority Number (RPN = S x P x D).
    - Determine if the failure mode warrants further action (e.g. RPN > 32).
5. Actions and Outcome Measures
    - identify actions or strategies to reduce the *Risk Priority Number* for each failure mode

The other widely adopted methodology is Root Cause Analysis (RCA) that aims to assess risks affecting healthcare activities by investigating the adverse events which have occurred. RCA is an analytic tool for performing a comprehensive, system-based review of critical incidents. It includes the identification of the root cause and contributory factors, determination of risk reduction strategies, and development of action plans along with measurement strategies to evaluate the effectiveness of the plans (Canadian Patient Safety Institute [CPSI], 2006). Unlike FMEA, which is a proactive and preventive process, RCA is carried out retrospectively in response to a specific, harmful event.

The main purpose of the RCA is to uncover the factor(s) that led to and caused the serious preventable adverse event. The preventable adverse event is very often the tip of the iceberg. Conducting and writing an RCA is an opportunity to examine how the systems for providing care function. The more areas investigated, the greater the possibility the system(s) will become better functioning and prevent the next event from occurring.

RCA focuses on the "how" and the "why", not on the "who". The goals of a root cause analysis are to determine:

- what happened;
- why it happened;
- what can be done to reduce the likelihood of recurrence.

A step by step description of the RCA may be depicted as follows:

1. Plan of action
   - strategies the organization intends to implement in order to reduce the risk of similar events occurring in the future.
   - responsibility for implementation, supervision, pilot testing as appropriate, time lines, and strategies for measuring the effectiveness of the actions.
2. What happened / Facts of the event
   - Information about the patient
   - Details of the event
   - Use of interviews, brain storming, or written description, etc.
3. Why it happened
   - Individuate the contributory factors
4. Identify root causes
   - Identification of the "Root Causes"
5. Minimize recurrence/monitoring
   - Implementation of each specific action that will be measured and communicated

The final goal of both methodologies is to address the commitment of healthcare organizations to reduce the likelihood or severity of adverse events. However, besides their technical, practical and philosophical differences, both present a major fault/drawback when applied to the specific case of medical equipment risk assessment. In fact, the methods themselves require some form of subjective assessment, mainly due to lack of quantitative data on which the assessment could be based. Moreover, to assess the risk related to the entire biomedical technological assets of healthcare facilities would certainly require a more systematic and structured method for collecting and processing data.

A possible solution to this problem could be an adapted implementation of the Risk Map or Risk Matrix (Ruge, 2004; Cox, 2008). A *risk matrix* (*risk map*) is a table (Cartesian diagram) that presents on its rows (y-axis), the category of *probability* (or *likelihood* or *frequency*) and on its columns (x-axis), the category of *severity* (or *impact* or *consequences*). Each cell of the table (or point in the Cartesian plane), which mathematically represents the product of the probability and severity values, is associated to a level of risk that eventually identifies the urgency or priority of the required mitigation actions.

The figure 1 shows an example of risk matrix, where probability and severity have been split into a range of five values, whereas risk level is categorized into three classes.

Thus, the risk assessment problem can be reduced to the estimate of probability and severity values. The estimate of severity does not present any particular concerns: by analyzing equipment design and features (such as, also, the FDA or CE risk classification), device user manual, clinical procedure and medical room in which the ME is used, it should be easy to determine the maximum possible damage the ME could do to the patient (or even to the operator). Moreover, such elements can be easily described by specifically defined numeric variables (for instance, all the considered aspects can be assigned values ranging from 1 to 5, in analogy with the main Risk Matrix axe values) and recorded in the equipment management system used by the CED. Lastly, by defining a computation method (whose complexity can vary from a very simple linear sum up to more complex fuzzy or neural network systems) the severity value can be associated to each ME owned by the healthcare facility.

However, the achievement of a robust, objective estimate of probability definitely presents more difficulties. In particular, it would be preferable to take into account only measurable characteristics, thus using easily quantifiable numeric variables.

			CONSEQUENCE				
			Minor	Moderate	Serious	Major	Catastrophic
			1	2	3	4	5
LIKELIHOOD	Rare	1					
	Unlikely	2					
	Likely	3					
	Expected	4					
	Certain	5					

<u>Harm occurrence Likelihood levels</u>

- -Certain: will occur on every occasion
- Expected: is expected to occur in most circumstances (e.g. more than 2 times a year)
- Likely: could occur in many circumstances (e.g. probable to happen up to 2 times a year)
- Unlikely: could occur occasionally (e.g. possibility of happening once a year)
- Rare: not expected to happen, but is possible (even if no occurrence registered)

<u>Harm severity levels</u>

- Catastrophic: multiple deaths
- Major: possibility of death or major permanent loss of function (motor, sensory, physiologic, or intellectual)
- Serious: major injury / adverse health outcome (e.g. possibility of permanent lessening of bodily functioning)
- Moderate : moderate injury / adverse health outcome (e.g. increased length of stay)
- Minor: no or minor injury/adverse health outcome;

<u>Estimated risk levels:</u>   –Red: unacceptable risk   –Yellow: tolerable risk   –Green: acceptable risk

Fig. 1. Example of Risk Matrix

The complexity of estimating probability stems from the fact that probability is dependent on three main different but inter-influenced issues: human factor, medical device functional reliability, medical device design and environmental characteristics (Brueley, 1989; Anderson, 1990; Dillon, 2000; FDA, 1997; FDA, 2000; Samore, et al., 2004). So, estimating the probability value must take into account the evaluation of these three elements. In estimating the human factor element, one must take into account not only those characteristics of the ME, of the process and/or of the environment that may facilitate a human error leading to an adverse event, but also the factors that may make the operator take corrective action for a ME or system failure. The ME functional reliability refers to the potential for device (material and/or functional) failure, potentially leading to an adverse event. Aspects to be considered are those related to the device reliability assessment such as the execution of safety checks, assessment of device obsolescence, and respect of a preventive maintenance plan. Medical device design and environmental characteristics are those related respectively to the possibility of the ME having specific features that could lead to an adverse event without the occurrence of material or functional failure or human error, and to the presence of environmental factors that could cause the ME to fail.

When defining the elements to be analyzed on each ME owned by the hospital, two considerations apply:

- Define measurable variables more quantitatively.
- Prefer elements (variables) already monitored by the organization and recorded in an information system (such as the ME management system used by the CED)

Table 1 shows an example of variables for probability estimation.

Human factor	Medical device functional reliability	Medical device design and environmental characteristics
Availability (at point of use) of complete written instructions (e.g., user manual) from the manufacturer	Device obsolescence	Appropriateness of wiring according to clinical activities and devices
Device ergonomics	Existence and respect of a preventive maintenance plan	Environmental conditions (noise, temperature, vibrations, electromagnetic interference, etc.)
Difficult working conditions (staff shortage, staff shifts, etc.)	Results of safety checks (cfr. IEC or ISO or EN safety standards)	The device is appropriate for the clinical needs for which it is intended
Environmental conditions (noise, temperature, lighting, space, etc.)		
Schedule and records of a training and education program on the use of specific ME and its related risks		

Table 1. List of possible variables for estimation of probability.

As is done for estimating severity, the last step consists of defining a computation method to elaborate the identified variables. Also, in this case the complexity of the method may vary from a very simple linear sum up to more complex fuzzy or neural network systems.

3. Health Technology Assessment

Nowadays many factors, ranging from the aging of population to the continuous fast-paced technology innovation, as well as the even more critical scarcity of economic resources, emphasize the importance of correct resource allocation at every level of a national health care system. This background adds to the criticality and complexity of decision-making, rendering essential a thorough evaluation which takes into consideration all the areas (health benefits, risks, costs, etc.) where health technology may have an impact..

A variety of specific methods and tools are available to support health care and medical decision making, for example Health Technology Assessment (HTA), a standardized methodology that can help decision makers select the most appropriate choice for their specific context.

HTA is a multidisciplinary process that systematically examines the technical performance, safety, clinical efficacy, effectiveness, cost, cost-effectiveness ratio, organizational implications, social consequences and legal and ethical considerations of the application of a health technology (EUNEHTA).

Advances in science and engineering
Intellectual property, especially patent protection
Aging population
"Cascade" effects of unnecessary tests, unexpected results, patient or physician anxiety
Emerging pathogens and other disease threats
Third-party payment
Inability of third-party payers to limit coverage
Financial incentives of technology companies, clinicians, and others
Clinician specialty training at academic medical centers
Malpractice avoidance
Provider competition to offer state-of-the-art technology
Public demand driven by consumer awareness, direct-to-consumer advertising, and mass media reports
Strong economies, high employment

Table 2. Factors that reinforce the market for health technology (Goodman 2004)

The term "health technology" is quite broad and includes the following categories: drugs, biologics, medical devices, equipment and supplies, medical and surgical procedures, support systems, organizational and managerial systems.

HTA may address the direct, intended consequences of technologies as well as their indirect, unintended consequences; its main purpose is to inform technology-related policy-making in health care.

HTA is increasingly used in American and European countries to inform decision- and policy-making in the health care sector and several countries have integrated HTA into policy, governance, reimbursement or regulatory processes.

3.1 Conducting an HTA process

An HTA process is conducted by interdisciplinary groups using explicit analytical frameworks drawing from a variety of methods: given the variety of impacts addressed and the range of methods that may be used in an assessment, several types of experts are needed in HTA.

Depending upon the topic and scope of assessment, these may include a selection of the following (Goodman, 2004):

- Physicians, nurses, dentists, and other clinicians
- Managers of hospitals, clinics, nursing homes, and other health care institutions
- Radiology technicians, laboratory technicians and other health professionals
- Clinical and biomedical engineers
- Pharmacologists
- Patients or patient representatives
- Epidemiologists
- Biostatisticians
- Economists
- Lawyers
- Social scientists
- Ethicists
- Decision scientists
- Computer scientists/programmers
- Librarians/information specialists

According to a recent study there are also significant differences in the practical application of HTA. Whereas in some countries HTA merely studies the clinical effectiveness and perhaps safety and cost-effectiveness of technologies, agencies in other countries apply a broader perspective and also consider other issues, such as ethics, and organizational, social or legal aspects of technology.

It is also known that the HTA activities can be carried out at different levels of health-care systems:

- macro level (international and national - i.e. decision-making within central government institutions)
- meso level (administrative level - i.e. regional or provincial health authorities, agencies, primary health-care units or hospitals);
- micro level (clinical practice)

At each of these levels, however, these activities should be carried out by a multidisciplinary staff, involving clinicians, clinical engineers, economists, epidemiologists, etc.) and, depending on the object of evaluation, also by specifically qualified professionals from the hospital departments.

Assessment reason	
New technology	Safety concerns
Changes in old technology	Ethical concerns
New indications for old technology	Economic concerns
New findings	Investment decisions
Structural/organizational changes	

Table 3. Reasons for performing an assessment (Velasco, et al., 2002)

3.2 The technical evaluation

As discussed in the previous paragraph, HTA now represents a multidimensional field of inquiry that increasingly responds to broad social forces such as citizen participation, accelerated technological innovation, and the allocation of scarce resources among competing priorities (Battista, 2006).

However,, this methodology was initially focused and applied on a small scale, concerning (clinical) engineering questions pertaining to a technology's safety and technical performances, and involving the investigation of one or more properties, impacts, or other features of health technologies or applications.

The *technical evaluation* represents, in fact, the core object of Clinical Engineering (CE) activity in HTA and is often conducted at a *meso* level. Many hospitals are increasingly developing HTA processes by means of *HTA Commissions* or structured *HTA Unit*, that include the CED.

In the *Health Technology*, CED are typically involved in the technical evaluation of the *medical electrical equipment* (as defined by the IEC 60601-1-1 normative) and sometimes of *medical devices*.

The main features characterizing these kinds of technologies can be summarized as follows:

- fast-changing technologies: their development is characterized by a constant flow of incremental product improvements;
- device impact on clinical and safety outcome depends on user training and experience that can vary and are hard to evaluate;

- the life cycle of a device is often as short as 18–24 months, which is considerably less than, for example, pharmaceuticals;
- the clinical application of the technology and potential utility for patients (accuracy or effectiveness) in comparison with the reference standard;
- improvement in the operating principle;
- state of development of technology (emerging, new, established);
- impact on organization (implementation phase, change in the treatment, users' qualification, IT requirements, etc.);
- impact on patient and user safety;
- economic aspects (acquisition, maintenance, spare parts, training, etc.);
- devices cannot be evaluated by RCTs – hard to blind and randomize. Early evaluation not possible

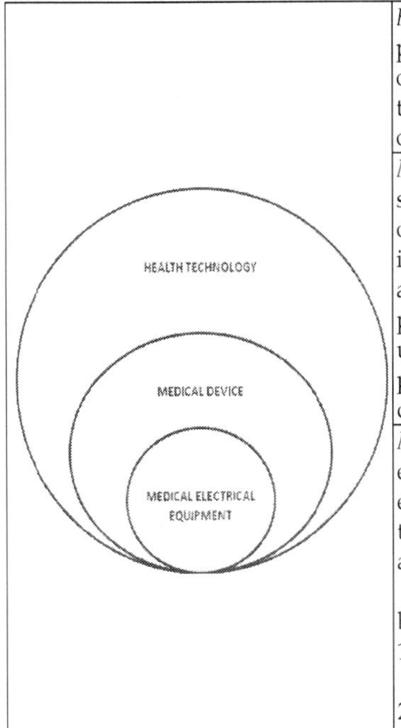

	Health technology: any intervention that may be used to promote health, to prevent, diagnose or treat disease or for rehabilitation or long-term care. This includes the pharmaceuticals, devices, procedures and organizational systems used in health care (INAHTA)
	Medical device: any instrument, apparatus, appliance, software, material or other article, whether used alone or in combination, including the software intended by its manufacturer to be used specifically for diagnostic and/or therapeutic purposes and necessary for its proper application, intended by the manufacturer to be used for human beings for the purpose of diagnosis, prevention, monitoring, treatment or alleviation of disease (European Directive 2007/47/EC)
	Medical electrical equipment (CEI EN 60601-1): electrical equipment having an applied part or transferring energy to or from the patient or detecting such energy transfer to or from the patient and which is: a. provided with not more than one connection to a particular mains supply; and b. intended by its manufacturer to be used: 1. in the diagnosis, treatment, or monitoring of a patient; or 2. for compensation or alleviation of disease, injury or disability

Fig. 2. Representation of Health Technology, Medical Device and Medical Electrical Equipment sets

A further classification of *medical electrical equipment* can be made according to their main characteristics or function. For instance, as can be found in the Italian CIVAB classification, *medical electrical equipment* can be grouped in three technological compartments:
- Functional explorations and therapeutic equipment;
- Medical laboratory or clinical chemistry equipment;
- Bio-imaging equipment.

The HTA process, while maintaining a uniform and systematic approach, may have to primarily focus on different characteristics because of the different weighting or different evaluation methodologies for the following aspects:

- Innovation
- Technology management
- Investment (big ticket technology; high volume purchase; service)
- Safety
- Efficacy
- Organization.

Functional explorations and therapeutic equipment often undergo relevant innovation, such as that involving the change of the physical or biological operating principle, which is difficult to evaluate empirically ("impossibility" of randomized controlled trial (RCT), short Time To Market vs short mean life). As regards safety, *electromedical equipment* are regulated by directives and technical norms that constitute not only a fair guarantee of their safety but also a valid guide to evaluate it for the specific context of its intended utilization. Moreover, patient safety strongly depends on user education and training in equipment use. Equipment's efficacy is often evaluated only by design data or in vitro or animal model tests. As such devices represent the greater part of an institute's biomedical equipment assets, organizational, economical and management issues become fairly important: uniformity of equipment can facilitate technological management (including risk issues), rationalize maintenance, take advantage of scale factors (equipment acquisition and renewal, consumables/spare parts).

Assessment of innovation for *Medical Laboratory equipment* has to accommodate the continuous introduction of new reagents and controls as well as the presence of homebrew technology, particularly in the most advanced fields such as Proteomics and Metabolomics. As concerns the management of these technologies, uniformity of equipment is also important for better and easier use by the operators, and ensures the availability of backup equipment. The most common mode of acquisition is by rental or service, where the cost of the equipment is included in the cost of the reagents.

Bio-Imaging equipment have been subject to innovations in virtually all aspects of their functioning, e.g. improvement of technical performances (e.g. spatial resolution), change in physical or biological operating principle (e.g. fMRI), safety for operators and patients (e.g. X-ray dose reduction). Their empirical evaluation is usually more practicable than for other kinds of equipment, particularly when testing no side-effects of technologies. Patient and operator safety relies on operational, technical and organizational issues (e.g. use of minimum dose setting for x-ray exams, implementing X-ray or magnetic shielding walls and ceilings, limiting access to exam room). As their complexity increases, so does the importance of user education and training to ensure a safe use of all the technological facilities. These kinds of technologies may have a very high cost both for their acquisition and for the necessary structural changes.

The aim of the HTA process, developed within a healthcare facility, is to guide decision-makers on the "correct" acquisition or implementation of a health technology, from different viewpoints:

- *clinical* : efficacy, risk/benefit rate, effect on current clinical procedures;
- *technological*: technical and technological efficacy, technical specifications (technological and structural interfaces), management and maintenance activities;
- *enterprise* : efficiency, productivity, impact on human (acceptability) and/or structural (e.g., need for building changes) and/or technological (e.g., need for HIS changes) resources.

3.1.1 Methods for technical evaluation

The evaluation of the technical characteristics of a device can be performed in different ways. A technique based on the European network for Health Technology Assessment (EUnetHTA) model is described below.

The EUnetHTA proposes an assessment scheme based on a basic unit, called assessment *element*. Each *element* defines a piece of information that describes the technology or the consequences or implications of its use, or the patients and the disease for which it is applied. An *assessment element* is composed of an *evaluation area, a macro key performance indicator* and *a micro key performance indicator* (see Figure 3a).

The *evaluation area* (*domain*) represents a wide framework within which the technology is considered. It provides an angle of viewing the use, consequences and implications of any technology. The following domains are considered:

The nature of the elements may vary across domains, since the consequences and implications are understood and studied differently in each domain. The following domains are considered:

1. Health problem and current use of technology
2. Technical specifications
3. Safety
4. Clinical effectiveness
5. Costs and economic evaluation
6. Ethical analysis
7. Organizational aspects
8. Social aspects
9. Legal aspects.

A *Macro Key Performance Indicator (Macro KPI or topic)* represents a more specific area of consideration within any of the *evaluation areas*. One *evaluation area* is divided into several *Macro KPIs*. Similar *Macro KPIs* may be assigned to more than one *evaluation area*. A *Micro Key Performance Indicator (Micro KPI or issue)* is a specific area of consideration within any of the *Macro KPI*. One *Macro KPI* typically consists of several *Micro KPIs*, but it may also contain only one *Micro KPI*.

The first task to accomplish in order to carry out the HTA process relates to the identification and definition of each KPI. To do this, the following steps are required:

Step 1. Literature search

A thorough literature analysis should be carried out by consulting the most important bibliographical sources such as clinical search engines (Pubmed, Medline, ISI Web of Knowledge, Cochrane Library, etc.), the national and international website of the HTA Agency (INAHTA, HTAi, EUnetHTA, Euroscan) or Institutes (ECRI, FDA, etc.), clinical practice guidelines, grey literature (technical reports from government agencies or scientific research groups, working papers from research groups or committees, white papers, or preprints). Other potential sources of data are manufacturers of the technology, clinicians, nurses, paramedics and patients.

The search can be performed by using main keywords for the technology in question (for example limiting the research in "abstract/title" OR "topic" fields). The most interesting results of these searches are selected and details investigated in order to intensify and develop the assessment.

Step 2. Identify the assessment elements

The analysis of the literature should therefore lead to the definition of the assessment elements, which are the core of the assessment. They are categorized into "evaluation area", "macro KPI" and "micro KPI". In order to make the assessment as objective as possible, the specific characteristics that support the assessment of a single area (and, subsequently, of the whole health technology) must be fully and measurably detailed, therefore objective and "instrumentally" measurable indicators are preferred. Moreover, those KPI that cannot be evaluated a priori should be excluded from the assessment.

Typically, the unit of measurement of KPIs may be:

- metric (e.g. spatial resolution, image uniformity, laser spot size, analytical specificity, etc.)
- expressed as a percentage of coverage of the clinical/production/technical needs (e.g. percentage of coverage of analytical test panel; percentage of coverage of nominal "productivity");
- ON/OFF (presence/absence of a specific feature or functionality)

Numerical Value	Verbal Scale	Explanation
1	Equal importance of both elements	Two elements contribute equally
3	Moderate importance of one element compared to another	Experience and judgment favor one element over another
5	Strong importance of one element compared to another	An element is strongly favored
7	Very strong importance of one element compared to another	An element is very strongly dominant
9	Extreme importance of one element compared to another	An element is favored by at least one order of magnitude
2, 4, 6, 8	Intermediate values	Used to reach a compromise between two judgments

Table 4. Saaty scale

Step 3. Weight of the indicators

After the assessment elements have been identified, it is necessary to define the decision-making framework and in particular to estimate the value of the weight of each element: such activity must involve the whole multidisciplinary evaluation team.

The definition of the weights, in fact, is a constituent part of the mathematical model of data processing, selected among those available in literature, such as the Analytic Hierarchy Process (AHP), expert systems based on Artificial Neural Network (ANN), and methodologies based on decision Fuzzy logic or Support Vector Machine (SVM).

With reference to AHP, for example, a structured questionnaire with a series of "pairwise comparisons" between the assessment elements can be used: each team member will be required, therefore, to compare on a qualitative scale e.g., Saaty scale, see table 4) the relative importance of the two compared elements. Finally, after the comparison of all pairs, the weight of each indicator will be calculated.

Step 4. Value of the indicators

The next step is to assess each technological alternative (the subject of the assessment) on the basis of the mathematical framework so far implemented. For this purpose, we assign values (quantitative or qualitative) to each lowest level KPI (usually a micro KPI, but also macro KPI and, rarely, even an evaluation area), on the basis of available literature data, and technical specifications or expert judgment. These values are then aggregated by the computational model to produce the value and rank of the single health technology.

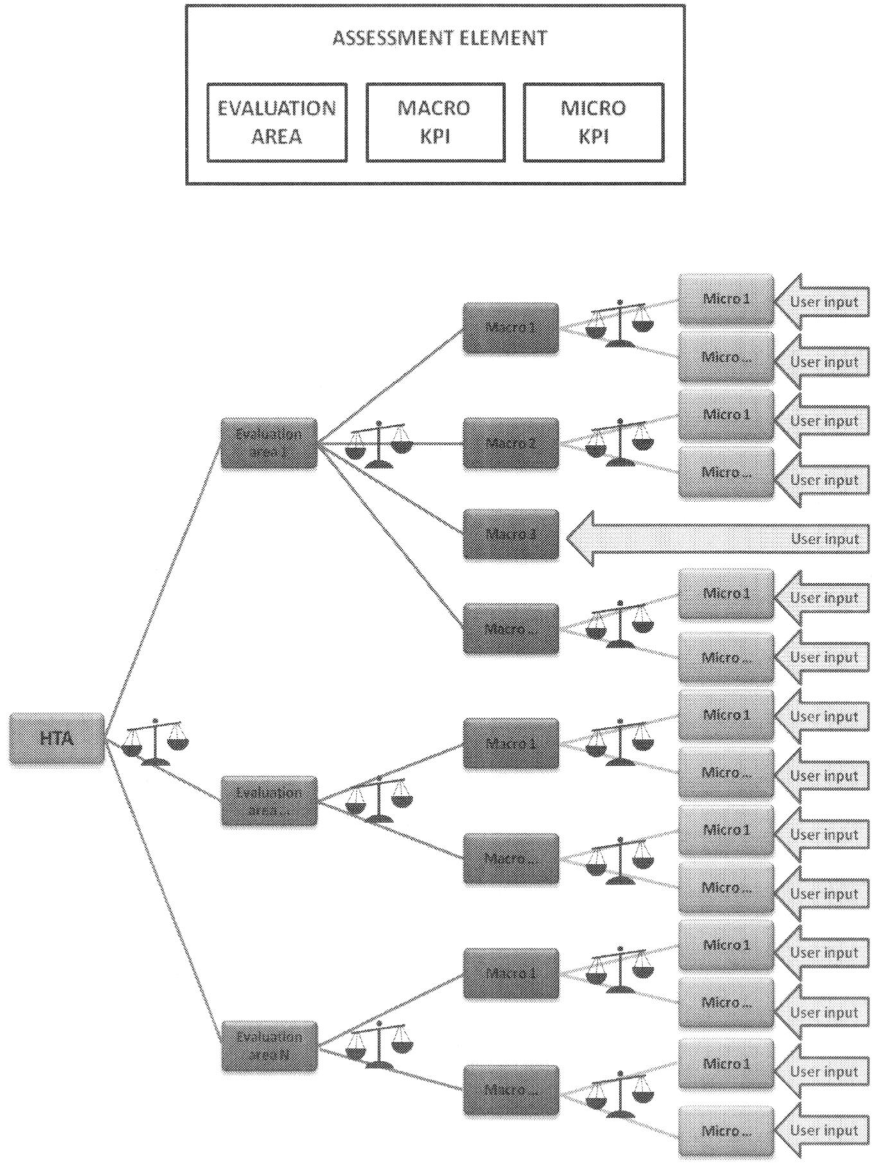

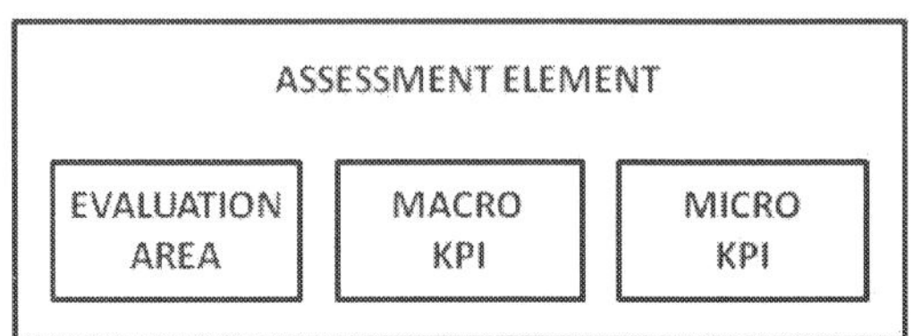

Fig. 3. a) The assessment element ; b) Combination of evaluation areas, macro KPI and micro KPI

Step 4. Results

The results obtained by aggregating the values can be represented graphically or through numerical reports. In particular, results can be processed to allow, for example:

- the comparison between the technological alternatives in order to show the performance on each evaluation area and/or macro KPI and/or Micro KPI;
- the comparison between weights of evaluation areas, macro and micro KPIs
- analysis of the evaluation tree with evidence of weighted values for each technological alternative
- etc.

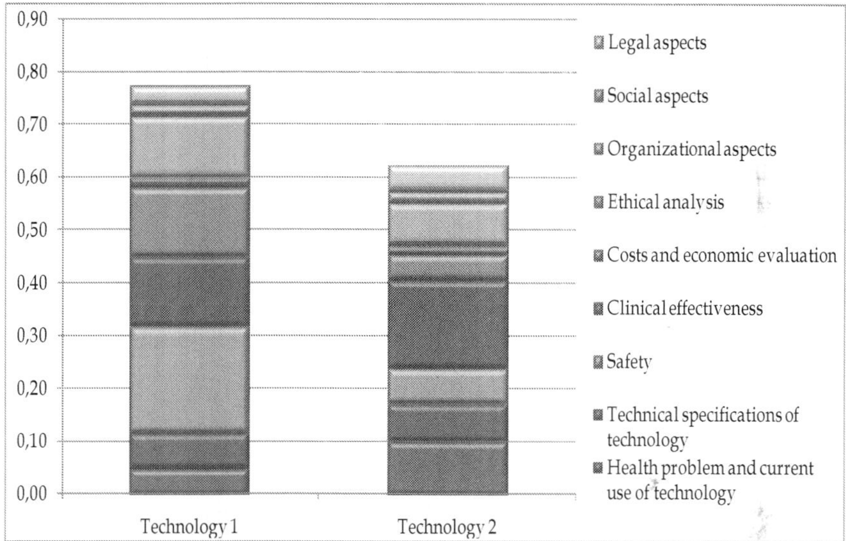

Fig. 4. Example of graphical representation of comparison of two health technologies

The *HTA* report

The final HTA report must provide the decision-makers with a clear, understandable summary of the information described above, in order to help them select the most appropriate technology. Moreover, it is essential to follow a standardized scheme, preferably one from a HTA agency or scientific community. However, it cannot be considered acceptable unless it contains the following sections:

- document summary;
- description of the technical characteristics and operating modalities of analyzed technologies;
- summary of findings of literature search;
- description of the criteria, indicators, macro and micro KPI;
- definition of weights;
- assigned values and mathematical processing method;
- results (e.g., ranking, charts, graphs, etc.)
- bibliography

4. Technology management

Hundreds to many thousands of medical devices may need to be managed in a healthcare facility, with several million Euros being invested each year for the acquisition of new health technologies and for planned technology replacement, while thousands of maintenance processes per year are required in order to maintain the efficiency of these devices. As evident from the analysis of adverse events occurring during the last few years, serious incidents can often be related to the malfunctioning of medical devices. In particular, a high degree of obsolescence of the technologies, as well as missed, inadequate or improper maintenance, are among the possible causes of failure not attributable to the manufacturer. Therefore, in every healthcare facility, responsibility for the safe management of medical devices should be identified. The CED can provide a relevant contribution to the prevention of adverse events resulting from medical device failures by the technical and clinical assessment of the technologies to be acquired and proper management of maintenance. Different organizational models can be used to manage the above mentioned activities (Italian Ministry of Health, 2009): an internal service with employees of the healthcare facility; a mixed service, with internal control by clinical engineers as well as by means of maintenance contracts with manufacturers and technicians who may either be employees of the healthcare facility or of specialized companies; finally, an external service, with technical assistance entirely outsourced to a "global service" provider. Each of these three models has advantages and disadvantages. The first approach allows timely intervention and a better control of maintenance activities; however it is only justified when there is a sufficiently large quantity of technological equipment in the healthcare facility, and also requires the continuous training of the technical staff: Furthermore, maintenance contracts with manufacturers are still necessary for high-technology equipment. The second model permits flexibility as regards the organizational structure of the healthcare facility, internal control of processes, and a better integration of skills. The last organizational model is often preferred by healthcare facilities that do not yet have a CED; it allows organizational flexibility, but requires a careful selection of a qualified external company and authoritative supervision by the healthcare facility staff, otherwise control of the processes will be progressively lost and the quality of service will deteriorate.

4.1 Preventive and corrective maintenance, safety and performance tests

Maintenance of medical devices has gradually evolved from the operational repair of out of order equipment to a management function aimed at preventing breakdown and failures, thus reducing risks associated with the use of medical devices, decreasing downtime and contributing to the improvement of diagnostic and therapeutic pathways, where technology is a key determinant. Healthcare facilities should identify responsibilities for maintenance and plan maintenance activities based on a detailed definition of methods, resources (i.e., operators, laboratories, measuring equipment, and maintenance contracts with external suppliers) and tools for supervision of the activities (e.g. dedicated software for the maintenance data management). To ensure adequate quality and safety standards and the rationalization of maintenance activities, a plan for maintenance and safety tests must be implemented, taking into account, for each device, the risks for patients and operators, degree of criticality and function of the device (e.g., therapeutic, diagnostic, or analytical). Within the European Community, preventive maintenance must be planned by the manufacturer prior to marketing the device. The 2007/47/EC Directive states that "the instructions for use must contain ... details of the nature and frequency of the maintenance and calibration needed to ensure that the devices operate properly and safely at all times". Preventive maintenance is of critical importance for ensuring the safe use of devices. Therefore, a preventive maintenance plan for each device must be defined, well documented and available at all operational levels to personnel responsible for maintenance tasks, including daily maintenance. Documentation should include informative documents and specific operating instructions which take into account both mandatory technical regulations and the service and user manuals provided by the manufacturer. Preventive maintenance is particularly relevant for life support devices, equipment for diagnosis and treatment, and devices identified as critical in relation to specific aspects such as the intended use of the device, class of risk, clinical features, type of location in which it is installed (e.g,. operating room, intensive care unit, ward), and presence of backup units. In carrying out the maintenance, the responsible technician must take into account all the maintenance instructions provided mandatorily by the manufacturer. Without affecting the liability of the manufacturer for any original product defects or faults, the person(s) performing maintenance will assume direct responsibility for all events deriving from this action. It is therefore essential that technicians, whether internal or external (see par. 5), have specific and proven experience. Training programs should be planned and preferably technicians should be trained by the manufacturers of the technologies which they maintain. Software for medical use deserves special consideration. Due to the complexity of systems and interactions, software behaviour may not be completely deterministic even when principles of good design practice are respected. Thus, software maintenance, which is usually performed by the manufacturer, should be supervised by the healthcare facility. Safety and performance tests must be periodically performed in order to ensure compliance with the essential safety requirements set by technical standards. The frequency of tests should be established taking into account criticality of device and according to reference guidelines. Particular attention is required in testing devices that can be used for critical applications (e.g., ventilators, anesthesia machines, infusion pumps, defibrillators, electrosurgical units) and for devices emitting or detecting ionizing radiations. Specific procedures and forms for different types of devices should be adopted to examine, measure, and verify the conformity of the device with the current mandatory technical standards and the instructions contained in the user manuals provided by the manufacturer. Dedicated equipment, for which calibration must be regularly performed and documented, should be used to measure parameters specific to each type of technology. Strategies for improving maintenance will only succeed if supervised effectively by external maintenance technicians in order to ensure their compliance with the agreed conditions (see par. 5). All relevant data relating to the life cycle of each device (from acceptance testing to disposal) must be recorded and made available at different operational levels. In order to ensure full traceability of the maintenance processes, preventive and corrective maintenance activities must be documented by detailed technical reports. In particular, preventive maintenance notice should be used to document the regularity of activities. Forms for maintenance requests to the CED must be defined and corrective maintenance notice should contain data useful for the identification of appropriate indicators (e.g. frequency of failures, time of first intervention, time to resolution, average downtime, distribution of failure types, maintenance costs, cost of spare parts), through which the condition of installed medical equipment can be analyzed.

4.2 Issues in inventory management

Establishing a complete and reliable inventory of medical equipment and ensuring the quality of the data is a complex task. Several different kinds of events, although rare, can lead to discrepancies between the inventory database and the technologies actually being used in a healthcare facility. These mismatches can be significantly reduced by establishing appropriate procedures and ensuring their strict observance. However, the large number of operators, devices and suppliers, the need to give priority to emergency care and the difficulty in directly and continuously monitoring the use of all devices in the healthcare facility, may inevitably produce such discrepancies. Failure to follow correct procedures for new equipment commissioning, for equipment transfer between departments, or for equipment disposal, are among the many possible events that could cause these mismatches. One possible solution is the use of Radio Frequency IDentification (RFID) tags and asset tracking systems. However, the use of this approach is limited because of ongoing debate about electromagnetic compatibility issues, and because the considerable cost of installation and management of these systems makes them still out of reach of most healthcare facilities. Until an advanced asset tracking solution is lacking in a healthcare facility, alternative strategies need to be implemented to keep the inventory data up-to-date. One way to monitor and update inventory data is through preventive and corrective maintenance or safety tests performed by CED technicians or by external service providers. Finally, it may be necessary to plan periodic inventory checks, which will be carried out independently or collaboratively by the CED and/or by the assets management office. Such controls may also provide an opportunity to remove devices that are no longer in use but are kept in stock and which may represent a source of risk.

4.3 Acquisitions and replacement plan

During the last decades, planning health technology acquisitions has become of strategic importance for healthcare organizations, both at the national and at facility level. Such planning is also essential task for the reduction of clinical risk associated with the use of medical devices. The importance of acquisition planning is also determined by the considerable increase in technology investments, which is due to the increase in number and rapid technological evolution of medical devices and systems.

Therefore, healthcare organizations should define specific methods for planning the acquisition of health technology. Such methods should take into account the obsolescence of devices, the evolution of technical standards, the possibility of improving safety for patients and healthcare operators, the possible availability of innovative technologies for improving clinical performance, as well as considerations about actual or expected clinical needs, economic or technical feasibility, organizational changes, and investment priorities (e.g., innovative technologies vs device renewal). Moreover, the availability of adequate infrastructure, staff and consumables for the equipment must be foreseen in order to ensure full use of the benefits provided by the new technology. The decision to proceed with the acquisition should be conditional on the presence of a detailed clinical, economic and technical assessment with well defined comparative criteria, carried out by qualified and multidisciplinary staff and inspired by the principles of HTA (see par. 2). An equipment replacement plan is aimed at better identification of investment priorities for device renewal and may be based on the definition of a replacement priority value (RPV). RPV is an index which represents synthetically the level of urgency for the replacement of each device, permitting determination of a replacement priority ranking and planning of a progressive replacement of technologies (Fennigkoh, 1992). Variables considered by the RPV computational algorithm may come from different sources, principally the CED database and clinical activities records. Variables must be carefully chosen, according to the organization of the healthcare facility and based on data availability. In fact, the effort needed for collecting new data and keeping it up-to-date must be considered in order to limit the amount of new data to be collected and to make the best use of the data already available. A typical model for computing the RPV is based on the use of component indexes, with each index highlighting the impact on a specific aspect of the device replacement. A coefficient must be assigned to each component index in order to weight its contribution to the RPV. Possible aspects that might be taken into account, by defining specific numeric variables, are obsolescence of the device, maintainability (e.g. cost and availability of spare parts), reliability (e.g. downtime or number of failures), criticality, strategic impact, clinical efficacy, efficiency, clinical risk, potential for performance improvement. For example, the cost of replaced spare parts, the number of technical activities performed by the technicians of the CED, the annual cost of contracts and the cost of technical assistance by external suppliers will be taken into account in the computation of the component index for maintenance costs.

5. Technical and economic issues in management of service contracts

A quality assurance requirement for clinical assistance is the implementation of related processes based on the principles of best/good practice standards. In the field of management of medical devices, this concept is fundamental for meeting the need of retaining costs and providing effectiveness in patient care.
CEDs are also evaluated as to their ability to implement a policy of Good Management Practice of biomedical technologies (Cheng & Dyro, 2004). Related economic aspects, such as medical equipment maintenance costs, are a critical issue of such management (Table 5).

Element	Financial	Internal processes	Customer satisfaction	Training and continuing education for CE staff
Measure	Staffing Beds per full-time equivalent employee Service/Acquisition ratio	Percent of IPM Complete IPM interval IPM time Repair time	Annual survey	Time spent on these activities Certifications obtained

Table 5. A balanced performance scorecard for Benchmarking CE departments (Gaev, 2010a)

Clinical engineers play a fundamental role in determining the proper strategy for medical equipment maintenance and in recognizing the best available option for supporting these activities. More specifically, the CED is in charge of setting the expected level of performance, monitoring the quality and integrity of the delivered services, dividing activities between internal and external BMETs, and pursuing the goal of an expense reduction policy. For this reason, before maintaining biomedical technologies, CEDs should plan rational acquisitions, allotting part of the organization budget for service contracts.

A service contract is an agreement between a company and a user for the maintenance, in this case, of medical equipment during a specific period of time, usually for a fixed price which may be subject to changes if maintenance activities are performed outside the user's location. The term "maintenance" typically includes inspection, preventive maintenance and repair. The terms and conditions of the contract usually stipulate the days and hours of service, the types of service, the response time, and which parts to be replaced are replaced free of charge" (Gaev, 2010b). This sort of contract can be extended to include the free loan of biomedical technologies. In this case, prices stated in the service contract are for consumables used for the equipment's functions, and are increased to include maintenance costs.

Reasons for having a service contract for a biomedical device are several. The first reason is the impossibility to provide a cost-effective service through in-house CED because of the lack of human and logistical resources. This is particularly common in hospitals where the problem of cost containment is approached with the sole objective of cost cutting and with no other financial or economic performance policy.

The second main cause is that healthcare governance is particularly reluctant to assume responsibility for equipment maintenance, and the belief that original equipment manufacturer (OEM) service contracts represent the "gold standard" is difficult to remove. On the other hand, for certain classes of medical devices (those characterized by high-technological complexity or high consumable costs, such as clinical chemistry analyzers), service contracts seem to be the only realistic solution for accommodating their management costs. The main issues which have to be discussed and negotiated in the drawing up of a service contract are: inspection and preventive maintenance, repair, spare parts, legal and financial aspects.

The term "Inspection and Preventive Maintenance (IPM)" covers all the activities involved in cleaning, lubricating, adjusting, checking for wear, and perhaps replacing components that could cause total breakdown or serious functional impairment of the equipment before the next scheduled inspection (Subhan, 2006).

These activities are well-described in the manufacturer's service manual and are aimed at avoiding the breakdown of a medical device in use, without any apparent warning of failure. Manufacturers are obliged to explicate preventive maintenance actions to healthcare operators or BMETs, and to suggest the minimum inspection frequency. The definition and respect of a timetable for IPM of all medical equipment is fundamental for reducing risk for patients and users, and preventing excessive repair costs by providing timely interventions; and it should be the CED's first priority, and should be decided before carrying out preventive maintenance activities.

Contracts should clearly explain the necessity of making known to all concerned the timetable for the maintenance by external technicians at the beginning of the year, in agreement with the CED and the healthcare personnel. This will allow the organization of clinical activities for healthcare operators and the possibility to enter the whole agenda into the biomedical technology maintenance management system. One other particular observation relates to the availability (at the charge of the contractor) of software update if required for the correct operation of the biomedical instrumentation. The last consideration relates to the possibility for CEDs (according to their competence) to evaluate the IPM requirements of medical equipment (Table 6) and to modify the service intervals recommended by the manufacturer, to obtain a more cost-effective maintenance without adversely affecting patient safety.

Repair (corrective maintenance) is a process to restore the physical integrity, safety and/or performance of a device after a failure. Aspects to be considered pertain to economic, safety and logistic concerns. Contracts should explain who can call for technical support: this aspect is fundamental for organizing the internal   maintenance process. One possible solution would be for the healthcare personnel to first of all attempt to resolve the problem by telephone (with proper manufacturer's customer support), and to define an internal procedure for advising the CED of the failure. In this way, the CED can monitor failure resolution time by the manufacturer's technicians by means of its maintenance management system.

Device	Shortest IPM Interval	Longest IPM Interval
Electrosurgical unit	6 months	12 months
Exam light	12 months	No IPM performer
Physiologic monitor	12 months	24 months
Pulse oximeter	12 months	No IPM performer

Table 6. Variations in IPM intervals for selected equipment, proposed by ECRI Inst. (2010)

Another significant aspect related to maintenance contracts is the definition of "bad-management" of biomedical technologies by healthcare personnel which may cause failure of the equipment. Some manufacturers are reluctant (or do not agree) to repair equipment under contract if abuse or improper use by hospital staff caused the failure. It is essential that the internal training of healthcare staff makes them aware of their responsibility for the correct use of biomedical equipment.

Moreover, in the contract, clinical engineers should define a way to evaluate the performance of OEM technicians, and stipulate the right to suspend the service contract in the event of low-quality maintenance work.

A common aspect of IPM and repair contracts is the possibility of a partnership for maintenance activities between the OEM technical support and the BMETs (internal or outsourced). Some manufacturers only permit maintenance activities by qualified (and certified by the OEM itself) technicians. Positive results of partnership contracts were showed just a few years ago. A first Italian joint project between OEMs and in-house service was started in 2002 (De Vivo et al., 2004): in-house personnel received adequate training, both generic (basic principles on which devices work) and specific (how to use, repair and maintain a particular model), for maintaining 90 medical devices (mostly monitoring equipment, ventilators and anesthesia units) in shared OEM/internal BMETs maintenance contracts.

Figure 5 summarizes the success of this program. One important effect was the increased awareness of the OEMs about the need for a rational selection of an effective preventive maintenance program in which service procedures and frequencies are based on real world feedback, efficacy of activities are measured and areas needing improvement are identified.

Clinical Engineers are also in charge of compiling technical reports related to maintenance activities (for instance, by means of an appropriate software system, see par. 6). These data are essential for monitoring the quality of OEM services, and claiming economic and legal penalties. Service contracts should also clearly explain the accuracy level of report writing, to avoid possible future disputes.

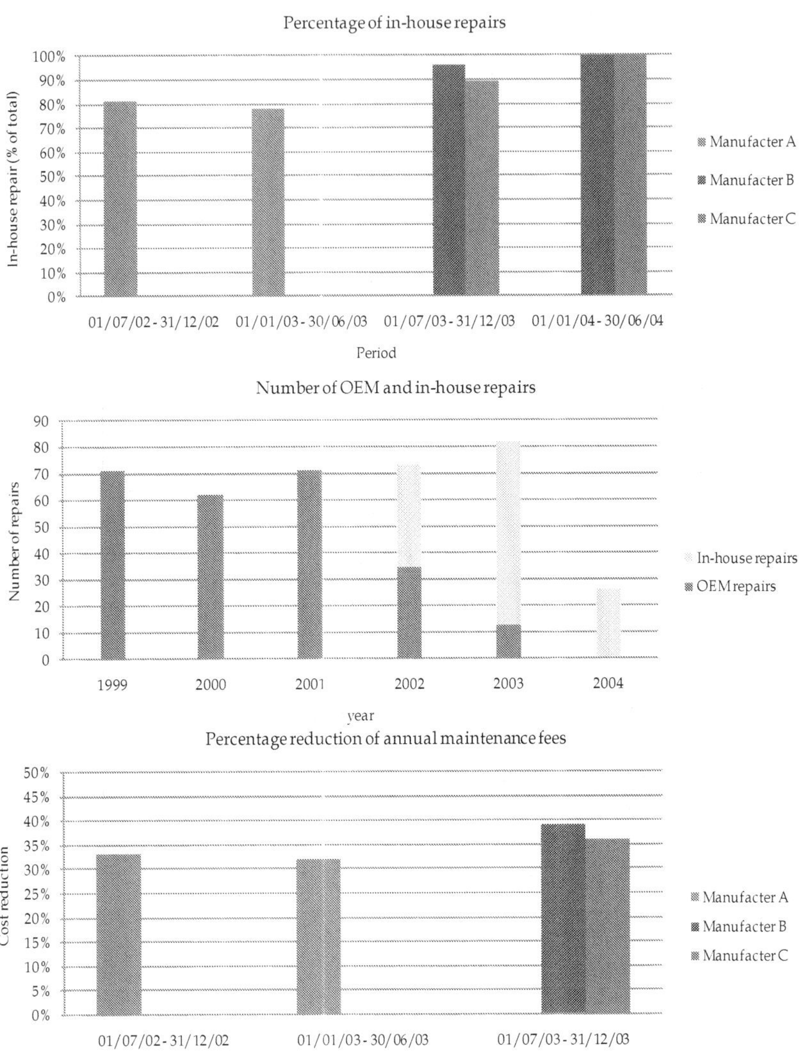

Fig. 5. a) Percentage of in-house repairs (July 2002-March 2004). The number of in-house repairs reached 90% and more after one year and continue to grow as in-house personnel sharpen their required basic skills. b) Number of OEM and in-house repairs (years 1999-2004). The decrease in OEM corrective maintenance was soon significant: as a consequence, OEMs were able to focus their attention on accurate preventive maintenance in order to prevent certain predictable failures. c) Percentage reduction of annual maintenance fees. Significant discounts were obtained based on the percentage of in-house corrective maintenance, justifying the cost related to internal technicians and the energies needed to set up the whole system.

Service contracts should include a specific paragraph on spare parts. OEM contracts usually lack the inclusion of them or any specification of the condition (e.g. new, refurbished) of parts used for maintenance and repair (Gaev, 2010b). It should be the duty of clinical engineers to assess the need for spare parts and include them in the contract, in dedicated annexes.

The economic assessment of service contracts is done using the definition of financial performance indexes. The most common index is the service cost/acquisition cost (S/A) ratio, i.e. the total cost to deliver a service, including parts and labor, divided by the acquisition cost of the equipment. Services delivered by OEMs (or third-party service suppliers) under a full-service contract usually include IPM and repair. The cost of same service delivered by an in-house CED is computed from the amount spent on parts and CED labor (labor hours) multiplied by the "loaded" rate including salary, benefits and other overhead expenses. In-house service is generally less expensive (50 percent less) than full-service OEM contract, even if this estimation varies significantly according to the equipment category. A recent ECRI review shows that imaging and high-tech laboratory equipment has a higher S/A ratio and is thus more costly to maintain than general biomedical equipment, even if this ratio may vary greatly due to institutional (e.g., teaching vs non teaching institution), logistics (e.g., urban vs rural hospital) as well as operational (e.g., low vs high negotiated acquisition price) differences (Gaev, 2010a).

Particular consideration should be given to the drawing-up of penalty clauses for the possibility of non-compliant service, the latter defined in terms of technical response time and equipment uptime/downtime. Moreover, competitive benchmarking for service contracts should also take into account fees for service outside of contract work hours, and any minimum charges required for travel time, service time, and work performed outside of the usual contract provisions. However, to make effective the use of penalty clauses, essential tools have to be set in place such as the computerized management of processes, implementation of a contact center (phone or online) for maintenance requests, systematic review of the quality of maintenance activities, failure analyses, and strict control of performance indicators and maintenance costs.

6. Issues in information technology and Clinical Engineering Department (CED) activities

Any action undertaken to improve the management/control of medical devices in a healthcare facility through an efficient and effective organization of maintenance and technology assessment activities, requires the implementation of operating procedures that enable the standardization of CED processes. However, the rapid evolution of health technologies during the last decades and the spread of heterogeneous technologies, besides bringing undeniable clinical improvements, have resulted in a considerable increase in technology investments, with the subsequent need for tools that can aid decision making in acquiring new technologies and managing the existing ones. To achieve the double goal of correctly applying and automating procedures and of implementing a model for the appropriate management of available resources and the proper definition of priorities, a comprehensive and reliable dataset for health technologies as well as an appropriate software tool to support data management will be required. Electronic archives are thus essential for storing all data and all events in the life of the medical devices managed by the CED, from the technology assessment that should always precede their acquisition until their disposal. Such a tool will permit safer documentation and reporting of the maintenance and management activities, sharing of information between the CED and other hospital staff, a dramatic improvement in data search, provision of summary statistics, and the definition of indicators that may contribute to the proper management of health technologies. The organization of this database may vary markedly depending on heterogeneous factors such as healthcare facility organization, technical and administrative management policies, number of devices, and resources dedicated to data management. The opportunity to support and significantly improve the management of medical equipment makes it advisable to implement a solution that can be configured and easily updated according to the evolution of specific needs. The configurable features of the system should include database design, user interfaces, queries, reports and statistics. The possibility to configure the database is useful not only for adding tables and fields, but also for the development of new features and adaptation of the software to the organizational structure of the healthcare facility. Configurable user interfaces should include at least the appropriate forms for inventory, acceptance testing, safety and performance tests, maintenance processes, preventive maintenance plan, maintenance contracts, disposal of devices, and administrative data management. Customizable configurations for different users should be guaranteed, in order to adapt the software according to the role and responsibilities of each user, with different data visualization and operating permissions. System users should be allowed to extract and export data in convenient formats (e.g., spreadsheets) for offline processing. Templates for standard documents (e.g. acceptance testing reports, maintenance reports) must be available and it should be easy to obtain automatically filled in and ready-to-print documents. It should be possible to analyze data with a configurable statistics dashboard. Such a system architecture would be suitable for developing methods for health technologies management and for defining indicators for the implementation of a technology replacement plan, the identification of maintenance priorities, and the optimization of resources allocation. Ultimately, being able to customize the software makes it possible to update the structure and configuration of the system according to the organization and evolution of operational requirements specific to a particular healthcare facility, and also makes it a suitable tool to support the development of processes. This feature is also particularly relevant for the purpose of satisfying the requirements for certification and the standards for national and international accreditation. The configuration should be performed or at least supervised by the CED staff, who best know the specific needs of the organizational context in which the software is to be used. Another advisable solution is to adopt systems that are accessible via the facility's intranet. Web-based systems that do not require any client-side software installation are useful for sharing information between the different actors involved and can improve the automation of processes for Health Technology Management (HTM). Moreover, with web-based systems it is possible for health operators to access many support features for the management of technologies. They can submit online requests for corrective maintenance, monitor the real-time evolution of submitted requests, search the database for devices, preventive maintenance plan or safety tests, and receive automatic e-mail notifications when certain events occur (e.g. , maintenance processes closed by biomed technicians, reminders for scheduled maintenance). This approach also has the advantage that only one data entry is needed (e.g., biomed technicians no longer have to re-enter data that have already been entered by the health operators on the maintenance request form). Obviously, all users should be trained in at least the basic principles of the system. The use of such a system for the management of medical devices can be extended to (or integrated with) the management of other technological facilities, ICT equipment, and other hospital assets.

6.1 Management of the acquisition process

A number of advantages for budget management can be gained by using computerized procedures for online submission of requests from heads of hospital units for the acquisition of new medical devices. Specification of medical device type according to a standard nomenclature system could be required, which would avoid the use of disparate terms for the same equipment. Also, the use of required fields in the electronic request form (e.g., reason for the acquisition, expected benefits, consumables needed) would ensure that all requests contain the essential information for their proper assessment. The medical board, with the support of the CED, would then have the right tools to manage the submitted requests in a uniform manner and make an objective analysis. assign a priority ranking to each request, and finally decide which ones to approve and which to reject. This approach could also be useful for the activation of hospital-based HTA (HB-HTA) processes (see par. 2). Furthermore, the authorization process (i.e., approval by department directors and medical board or medical devices committee) can be automated and differentiated according to the type of acquisition (e.g. property, loan, service, rental, clinical trial). Approval of the request will be automatically notified and immediately available online. The technology renewal plan managed by the CED may be integrated and partially automated in the software by implementing an algorithm for calculating the replacement priority value (see par. 4). Following the approval of requests for new acquisitions and replacement of medical devices, the automation of CED processes would provide valuable support for the management of data and documents relating to the assessment and acquisition of technologies. Information concerning single budget items (e.g., type of acquisition, number of requested devices, allocated budget) and on acquisition progress (i.e., end of the market survey, drafting and issuance of the technical assessment, date of order by the administration, supplier name) can be shared between the CED and the healthcare facility administration, with automatic update of acquisition progress and online availability of documents for each budget item. At all stages, starting from submission of the requests, only a single data entry is needed.

6.2 Acceptance testing and inventory management

In a computerized system for managing CED's processes, each medical device has its own inventory record containing the data relevant to its management (e.g., device model, accessories, system configuration, owner hospital unit, location, administrative data). Each device in the inventory must be uniquely identified, and the CED must place an identifying label on it. As stated above, the adoption of a standard medical device nomenclature for model identification is also strongly recommended. If a web-based system is used, health operators will be able to search for inventory records and obtain lists of devices that can be exported onto spreadsheets. For each device in the inventory, the acceptance testing must be registered in the system. The status of the device can be updated automatically and an e-mail notification sent upon completion of testing.. In order to keep the inventory data up-to-date, in addition to routine administrative tasks, periodic inventory checks must also be made. In this regard, mobile units (e.g., PDA) equipped with a tag (e.g. barcode, RFiD) reader, properly configured and synchronized with the CED software system, can be a useful tool. This approach allows easier tracking of devices and verification of equipment location and condition, as well as updating of system components. Another useful feature is the online availability of documents. These could include pre-acquisition documents (e.g., market survey, technical assessment, order form), user and service manuals, acceptance testing documents and training course forms, as well as pictures of system configurations and accessories.

6.3 Maintenance processes

Maintenance processes management could exploit the availability of an appropriate software tool. As stated above, a useful feature is the possibility for health operators, in case of failure of a medical device, to request corrective maintenance online. Maintenance activities should then be recorded in the system by CED biomed technicians. CED can enter and update the maintenance plan (i.e., the preventive maintenance activities for which both internal technicians and external maintenance personnel will be appointed) and share it, as well as related information (e.g. maintenance progress, e-mail notification of upcoming preventive maintenance), with all hospital units involved. Health operators should be allowed to retrieve and export lists of maintenance requests. Thousands of safety and performance tests are performed on medical devices each year by the CED. Thus the availability of test reports to health operators is only possible by implementing an automatic upload system. Radiology equipment deserves a particular mention in that it is usually managed by both CED and the Medical Physics Unit. This requires sharing of information on preventive and corrective maintenance and quality controls. Finally, the software tool can also be used to facilitate the management of spare parts. Online access to maintenance documents (i.e., preventive and corrective maintenance activities, safety and performance test reports, administrative documents) is another desirable feature. The availability of such electronic information enables the CED to analyze the history of maintenance processes for each device, to improve monitoring of maintenance activities performed both by CED technicians and by external maintenance personnel, to verify the compliance of suppliers with maintenance contracts, to gather downtime statistics, and to generate summaries of maintenance costs. Finally, algorithms can be defined and implemented to combine device replacement priority value (see par. 4) and maintenance priority rank for immediate identification of the most urgent corrective actions. Automated information sharing can also be helpful for the disposal of devices. The way this feature can be configured depends on the specific organization. For example, CED could be in charge of notifying the hospital unit of device disposal, while the physical removal of the device would be the responsibility of the facility handling service. An automatic e-mail notification of disposal confirmation to the CED would allow an easier tracking of out of order devices, thus reducing inconvenience and risk for patients and health operators.

7. References

American Society for Healthcare Risk Management. (2002). Strategies and tips for maximizing failure mode and effect analysis in an organization. *J Healthc Risk Manag* , 22(3), 9-12.

Anderson, F. A. (1990). Medical Device Risk Assessment. In *The Medical Device Industry: Science, Technology, and Regulation in a Competitive Environment* (p. 487-493). Marcel Dekker Ltd.

AS/NZS 4360:2004. *Risk Management Standard.*

Battista, R. (2006). Expanding the scientific basis of health technology assessment: a research agenda for the next decade. *Int J Technol Assess Health Care , 22(3)*, 275-80.

Brueley, M. (1989). Ergonomics and errors: who is responsible? *Proceedings of the first symposium on Human Factors in medical device,* (p. 6-10).

Canadian Patient Safety Institute. (2006). *CPSI, Canadian Root Cause Analysis framework: a tool for identifying and addressing the root causes of critical incidents in healthcare.*

CEI EN 60601-1 (n.d.). Medical electrical equipment, Part 1: General requirements for basic safety and essential performance.

Cheng, M.; Dyro, J.F. (2004). Good Management Practice for Medical Equipment, In: *Clinical Engineering Handbook,* J. F. Dyro, (Ed.), 108-110, Academic Press Inc., ISBN 978-0-12-226570-9, Burlington, Massachusetts, USA

Cox, L. J. (2008). What's Wrong with Risk Matrices? *Risk Analysis , 28 (2),* 497-512.

De Vivo, L.; Derrico, P.; Tomaiuolo, D.; Capussotto, C. ; Reali, A.   (2004). Evaluating alternative service contracts for medical equipment, *Proceedings of IEEE EMBS 2004 26th Annual International Conference,* pp. 3485-3488, IBSN 0-7803-8439-3, San Francisco, California, USA, September 1-5, 2004

Dillon, B. (2000). *Medical Device Reliability and associated areas.* CRC Press.

Draborg, E., Gyrd-Hansen, D., Poulsen, P. B., & Horder, M. (2005). International comparison of the definition and the practical application of health technology assessment. *Int J Technol Assess Health Care , 21(1),* 89-95.

EUNEHTA. (n.d.). *Work Package 4: HTA Core Model for Diagnostic Technologies.* Avaliable from www.eunethta.net.

European Directive 2007/47/EC.

FDA. (1997). *Design Control Guidance for Medical Device Manufacturers.*

FDA. (2000). *Guidance for Industry and FDA Premarket and Design Control Reviewers - Medical Device Use-Safety: Incorporating Human Factors Engineering into Risk Management.*

Fennigkoh - A Medical Equipment Replacement Model. *Journal of Clinical Engineering.* 17(1):43-47, January/February 1992

Gaev, J.A. (2010). Benchmarking Service Contracts, In: *TechNation,* June 2010, Available from https://www.ecri.org/

Gaev, J.A. (2010).Successful Measure: benchmarking clinical engineering performance, In: Health Facilities Management, February 2010, Available from https://www.ecri.org/

Garrido, V. M., Kristensen, F., Palmhøj Niel, C., & Busse, R. (2008). *Health technology assessment and health policy-making in Europe. Current status, challenges and potential.* Available from www.euro.who.int.

Goodman, C. (2004). *Introduction to Health Technology Assessment, HTA 101.*

INAHTA. (n.d.). *Glossary.* Available from www.inahta.org .

ISO 14971:2007. *Medical devices - Application of risk management to medical devices.*

ISO 31000:2009. *Risk management - Principles and guidelines.*

Italian Ministry of Health - Recommendation for the Prevention of Adverse Events Consequent to the Malfunctioning of Medical Devices/Electrical Equipment - Recommendation #9 April 2009

Mccaffrey, J., & Hagg-Rickert, S. (2010). Development of a Risk Management Program. In A. S. (ASHRM), *Risk Management Handbook for Health Care Organizations.*

Ruge, B. (2004). Risk Matrix as Tool for Risk Assessment in the Chemical Process Industries. *ESREL 2004*, (p. paper 0192).

Samore, M. H., Evans, R., Lassen, A., Gould, P., Lloyd, J., Gardner, R., et al. (2004). Journal of the American Medical Association. *Surveillance of medical device–related hazards and adverse events in hospitalized patients, JAMA. 2004;291(3):* , 325-334.

Subhan, A. (2006). Equipment Maintenance, Biomedical. In: *Encyclopedia of Medical Devices and Instrumentation,* J.G.Webster, 289-321, John Wiley & Sons, Inc., NJ USA

Taylor-Adams, S., Vincent, C., Stanhope, N. (1999). Applying human factors methods to the investigation and analysis of clinical adverse events. *Safety Science* , 31, 143-159.

Velasco, M., Perleth, M., Drummond, M., Gürtner, F., Jørgensen, T., Jovell, A. (2002). Best practice in undertaking and reporting health technology assessments. *Int J Technol Assess Health Care* , 18(2), 361-422.

Wilkins, R., & Holley, L. (1998). Risk management in medical equipment management. *Proceedings of the 20th Annual International Conference of the IEEE Engineering in Medicine and Biology Society. 6,* p. 3343-3345., Hong Kong Sar, China, October 1998

9

Integrated Power Management Circuit for Piezoelectronic Generator in Wireless Monitoring System of Orthopedic Implants

Chen Jia and Zhihua Wang
Tsinghua National Laboratory for Information Science and Technology
Institute of Microelectronics, Tsinghua University, Beijing,
China

1. Introduction

Wireless Monitoring System of Orthopedic Implants(WMSoOI), which is employed to detect the situations of implanted materials in patients as artificial joints, is one kind of Smart Biomedical MicroSystems(BMS). This kind of BMS is supplied by little mechanical energy. Due to the limit of input energy, there are a lot of challenges on power converter system, such as efficiency, volume, etc[1][2].

In this chapter, section 2 gives the application background of WMSoOI, and then according to the system requirements, a novel hybrid power management system is proposed in section 3. Section 4 illustrates the concrete circuit design of each block. In section 5, measurement results and simulation results are given. Finally, section 6 is a summary.

2. Application background of Wireless Monitoring System of Orthopedic Implants (WMSoOI)

Bone health is the precondition of a happy life. However, in China, 10% of the whole population suffers from osteoarthrosis, in whom many people don't have a normal life due to joint aging, joint diseases, etc. Artificial joint replacement surgery can help the patients to re-establish motor function, but there are many problems after surgery. When artificial materials have been implanted into human body, abrasion, loose and osteolysis not only affect the health and life quality of the patients, but also bother orthopedists.

In order to monitor the artificial material's situation, WMSoOI is proposed in figure 1[3]. As described, a piezoelectric(PZT) device is employed to generate electricity in an implanted bone prosthesis. When deformed by outside pressure, the PZT device can supply enough power to the whole information gathering system. In the above equipment, the PZT material not only plays a role as a sensor, but also plays a role as a generator.

In this work, a power management system is proposed to integrate several function modules into a chip to reach a small volume, which makes it possible to be implanted into human beings' body. The whole work process of the WMSoOI can be illustrated as the following. First, pressure information of artificial joint is gathered by PZT material and then these data can be stored in non-volatile memories. Second, all of these stored data can be read by other instruments with passive RFID technologies periodically, such as a couple of days. Finally, with the information data, medical information system can monitor the real situations of those artificial materials implanted in human beings. The gathered information will help doctors to get enough information in time, mitigate the patients' pain and also can help doctors to choose proper materials to be employed in implanted artificial joint instruments.

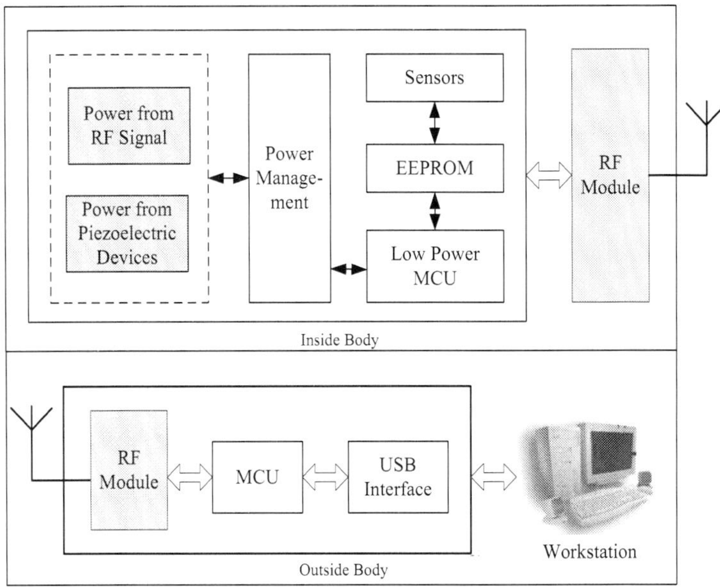

Fig. 1. Wireless monitoring system of the orthopedic implants

The difficulty to realize this integrated system lies on: PZT materials not only acts as sensors to detect the deformation of artificial joint, but also provides stable power for the functional circuits in the instrument. It is reported that the PZT device can only provide 4 mW power in a similar application background[4][5][6]. In addition, PZT materials have poor source characteristics, such as high output impedance, low output current, etc, which enhance the difficulty of designing power management circuit. In all, the power management system design of WMSoOI is a very challenging work.

3. Power management system of Wireless Monitoring System of Orthopedic Implants(WMSoOI)

In this section, in order to make full use of the energy generated by PZT materials in WMSoOI, the electrical characteristics of PZT materials and intermittent power supply mode will be illustrated first; then previous power management systems using PZT materials as power supply will be reviewed; finally, a power management system, which is suitable for intermittent power supply, is proposed to improve the convert efficiency.

3.1 Electrical characteristics of PZT material and intermittent power supply mode

Piezoelectric(PZT) materials are capable of converting the mechanical energy of compression into electrical energy. People have already used this characteristic to realize many kinds of sensors. But due to some intrinsic characteristics, such as high voltage, low current and high impedance, etc, the output power of PZT materials is very low and doesn't have the characteristics as an available power. But by now, with the advent of low power integrated circuits, it is possible to use ambient energy to provide power for an information system.

Electrical circuit model for PZT generators are typically represented by capacitors, resistors and inductance, as shown in figure 2[3][4]. F_{in} and V_{in} represent input force and input voltage respectively, and ϕ is the ratio of electrical output to mechanical input(V/N). R_e, L_e, C_e and C_p' are equivalent electrical circuit element parameters to reflect the mechanical element parameters. R at the right part of figure 2 is the load of the power generator.

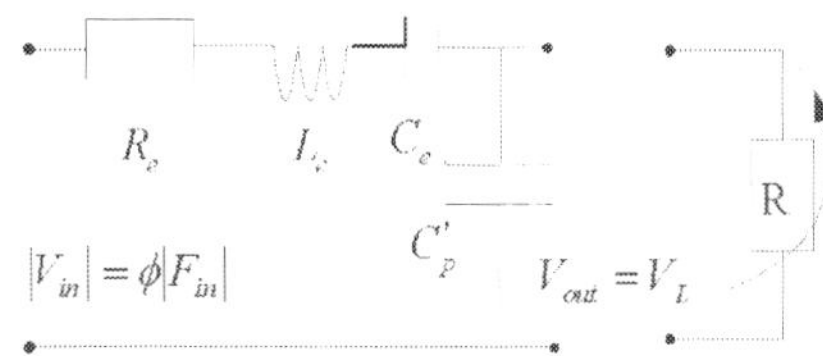

Fig. 2. Electrical Circuit Model of PZT

After being stored by power management system, the electrical energy generated by PZT materials, are converted into a stable power, which provides power for subsequent functional modules. The equivalent capacitor in the PZT generator is in parallel with the storage capacitor and the system load. There are two working situations. First, when the stored energy is not enough to provide power for the subsequent information system, the electrical energy generated by the PZT material is charged into the storage capacitor. At this time, the power consumption is just the leakage power, while the whole WMSoOI is in stand-by mode. Second, when the stored energy is enough for the whole system to finish functions, the storage capacitor is in a discharge situation, to provide power for the functional modules. The above whole process about energy convert and consumption is regarded as an intermittent work mode.

3.2 Current power management system in electrical system supplied by PZT materials

Figure 3 shows the system diagram to study the power converter of PZT materials[4]. This system is used to measure the electrical energy generated by three PZT devices in the artificial joint, where the situation is similar with the condition that human being is in a normal walking station. By diode rectifier and storage capacitor, about 4mW power is generated by these PZT devices. In [4][5][6], a big storage capacitor is employed to collect electrical energy and supply the subsequent functional circuits in each system. [4][5] use linear regulators to adjust the electrical energy in the storage capacitor to convert the energy into available power, whose converter efficiencies are 8.8% and 19%, respectively. [6] uses switcher to convert the energy stored in the capacitor, whose efficiency can reach 17.6%.

Furthermore, the systems in [4][5][6] employ commercial chips to fulfill power management functions. In rectifier circuit, because the output voltage of PZT material is very high, so the efficiency of the rectifier can reach 98%.

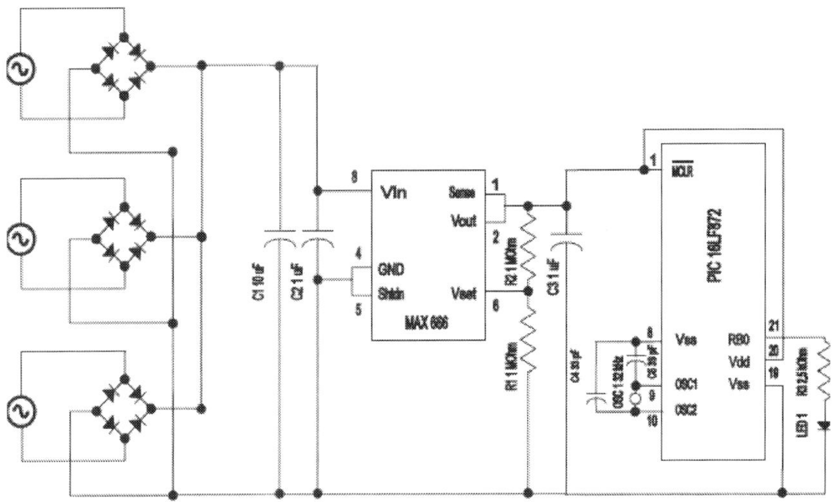

Fig. 3. Previous work of PZT generator [4]

These references prove that PZT materials have the ability to provide enough energy for microsystems and make sure that WMSoOI is feasible. But there are several problems[1]:

1. Previous works are principle experiments, without considering that the system volume when PZT materials implanted into the artificial joint.
2. The power system convert efficiency of storage capacitor is low that this little energy cannot provide enough power for the subsequent complicated function circuit, such as AD converter to sample PZT signals, MCU to process data and read-write EEPROM data circuits to interface data, etc.
3. The power system is lack of optimization. Monitoring circuit, control circuit, current limiting circuit, and other circuits are needed to improve power efficiency.

From above, a novel power management system is proposed to meet the requirements of WMSoOI in next section.

3.3 Power management system working in intermittent mode, using PZT materials as power supply

Regarding to the three problems illustrated in section 3.2, an integrated hybrid DC-DC converter is proposed to construct the main part of the power management system, which will be integrated with the rectifier, reduce the volume of the whole system and improve energy convert efficiency. In the same time, intermittent working mode is introduced to enhance the power management function to solve the technical problems in WMSoOI[1][2][7].

Due to human body's weight, PZT materials generate alternate current energy, which is rectified and then stored in the storage capacitor. Considering the output voltage ripple and convert efficiency, a 10μF capacitor is used as the storage capacitor to get a better trade-off in capacitor value. This power management system is in an intermittent working mode, the concrete working process is as following: 5V is set to be the threshold of this power converter system. When the voltage across C_{store} is lower than 5V, the power converter will stay in a standby mode until the PZT generator charges C_{store} above the threshold voltage. Otherwise, when the output voltage across C_{store} is higher than 5V, power converter begins to work. This is one measure to improve converter efficiency in system level.

In order to further improve the energy efficiency in a circuit level, a hybrid power management system is proposed, as shown in figure 4, including rectifier circuit, storage capacitor, input voltage monitoring circuit, variable step-down ratio SC(Switching Capacitor) converter, bandgap reference, output voltage monitoring circuit, start-up circuit and voltage limit circuit, etc .

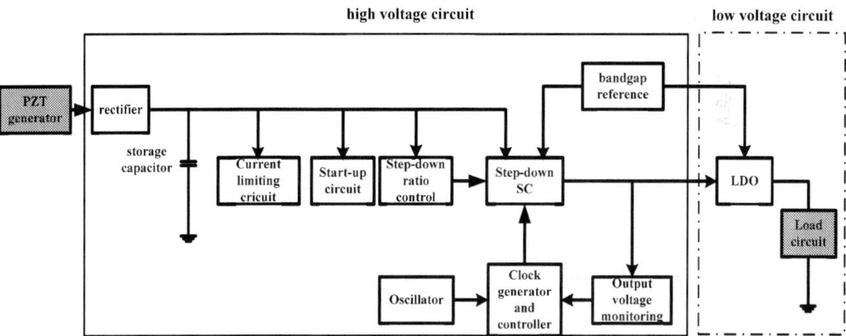

Fig. 4. Power converter system for PZT generator

The dominant blocks in the proposed power management system is serial connections of the variable step-down ratio SC converter and the low dropout linear regulator(LDO). Those circuits, surrounded by the dashed box, including bandgap reference, step-down SC, step-down ratio control circuit, oscillator, clock generator, clock control circuit and output voltage monitoring circuit, work in the high voltage supply region in this power management system, which is supplied by the storage capacitor. Oscillator, clock generator and clock controller are auxiliary parts for step-down SC circuit. Bandgap reference is employed to provide voltage reference and current reference for other modules. The LDO circuit and subsequent functional circuit, surrounded by dotted line, are supplied by the output of step-down SC circuit.

The function of variable step-down ratio SC circuit is to regulate the output voltage of storage capacitor, whose output voltage ranges from 5.5V to 15V, to 2V. The conversion ratio can be different, such as 2/3, 1/2 and 1/3. In order to realize variable step-down ratios, a SC converter with variable topology is employed. By choosing different switches, the concrete circuit topology can be set to implement different step-down ratios, which will be explained in detail in section 4.3. The function of LDO is to regulate the input voltage, which is about 2V, to 1V or even lower power supply with small ripples and high PSRR performance for analog circuits.

In the above power management circuits, those parts in high voltage region is designed in 0.35μm CMOS technology, while circuits in low voltage region is designed in 0.18μm CMOS technology, which is suitable for the integration of LDO circuit and the subsequent functional circuits.

This power management system operates according to the following rule. By monitoring the voltage on storage capacitor and the output voltage of step-down SC converter, the power management system can control the enable signal of variable step-down ratio of the SC circuit to improve the power convert efficiency of charges stored on storage capacitor.

4. Circuit design of the power management system in WMSoOI

In this section, several important circuit designs of the power management in WMSoOI are illustrated in detail.

4.1 Rectifier circuit

Rectifier is used to convert AC(alternative current) power into DC(direct current) power. Several papers have done a lot of work in fully integrated rectifier. [8] realizes half-wave rectifier of PZT material, which is used for low input voltage applications. [9] introduces fully integrated rectifiers working at high frequencies in commercial CMOS technology.

The rectifier in this system is a full wave rectifier composed of four diodes, as shown in figure 5. Its function is to change AC electrical energy into DC electrical energy. Diodes can be easily fabricated in commercial CMOS process, although they have larger threshold voltage comparing with CMOS devices.

When voltage on side A of the PZT material is higher than that of side B, D1 and D4 are shutoff while D2 and D3 are forward turned on. This ties the low voltage side of the PZT material to ground while passing the high voltage. Situation is reversed when the voltage of side B is higher than side A.

Due to low frequency, parasitic capacitance can be ignored. Diode area is set to be 30μmx30μm, to reduce the parasitic resistor when the diode is "ON" and so to improve convert efficiency. Storage capacitor also has the ability to filter output voltage ripple. Because the transistor gate breakdown voltage is 18V, which is enough for the storage capacitor to be charged into 15V. Higher voltage across the storage capacitor will provide more energy for subsequent circuits.

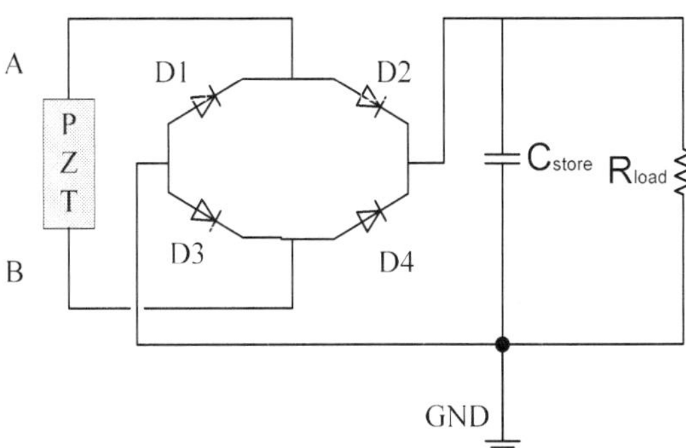

Fig. 5. Rectifier circuit

4.2 Bandgap reference

Bandgap reference circuit is a basic and important component in analog and mixed signal circuit. It not only provides precise voltage reference, but also provides precise bias currents. [10] summarizes bandgap reference circuits for low voltage operation, where current mode is often used to keep output voltage stable under conditions when supply changes. It is true that the variations of supply are small in low power supply. As far as large supply ranges are concerned, circuit topology including a voltage operational amplifier is a good solution. Figure 6 shows the system diagram of the proposed bandgap reference. In order to reduce the power dissipation of bandgap reference, transistors working in sub-threshold regions are used to reduce the supply current. At the same time, several high performance parameters of bandgap reference must be kept under different conditions such as supply voltage variations, temperature variations and different technology corners, etc. And a voltage buffer is integrated to increase the drive capacity of the bandgap reference.

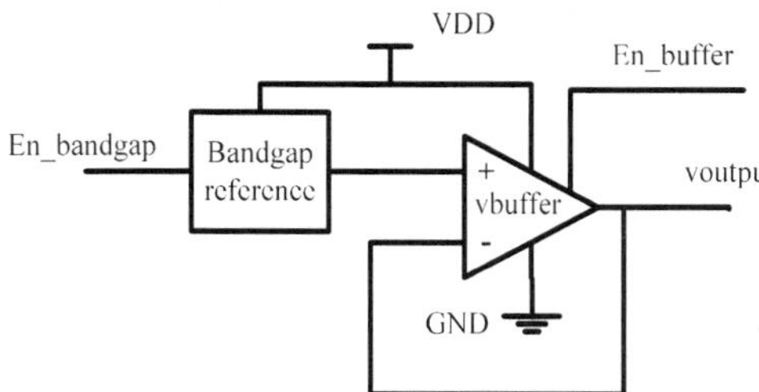

Fig. 6. System diagram of the proposed bandgap reference

Next is the principle of this bandgap reference working in subthreshold region. At the beginning, the Current performance of transistors working in subtreshold region is described. MOS transistors' drain-source current working in sub-threshold region can be expressed as

$$I_D = I_0 \frac{W}{L} e^{\frac{V_G - V_T}{n\phi_t}} \left(1 - e^{-\frac{V_{DS}}{\phi_t}} \right) \tag{1}$$

where I_0 is constant dependent on technology parameters, W and L are width and length of MOS transistors, respectively. V_T represents threshold voltage. n is a technology parameter dependent on process and ϕ_t is thermal voltage, which is about 26mV at room temperature 27°C. Equation (1) is suitable for general analysis when $V_G \ll V_T$. It is obvious that the drain source sub-threshold current is exponential to the minus of $(V_G - V_T)$. Therefore, sub-threshold current is sensitive to the variation of V_T.

And the transconductance of MOS transistors working in subthreshold region can be expressed as

$$g_m = \frac{I_D}{n\phi_t} \tag{2}$$

which discloses the relation between g_m and I_D in subthreshold region.

Selection of width and length of transisitor woking in sub-threshold region in the bandgap reference is explained in detail in this paragraph. Determining transistors' sizes is the key design in the process of circuit design. During this process, g_m / I_d is a very important design parameter and it represents the ratio of transconductance g_m to drain current I_D. In order to get high ratio of g_m / I_d to reduce power consumption[11][12], many people have already done a lot of work. In [13], Christian C. Enz and Eric A. Vittoz presented an EKV model for MOS transistors and this model can represent the MOS characteristics in different working regions using one equation, wherever the possible regions MOS transistors may work in. In [14], researchers proposed another MOSFET model, which has the common property that tries to use a unified model for MOS transistors in all regions, and the corresponding design methods. According to all of these papers, there are several equations available to design low power circuits.

$$I_D = 2\pi \cdot GBW \cdot C_L \cdot n \cdot \phi_t \left(\frac{1+\sqrt{1+if}}{2} \right) \tag{3}$$

$$\frac{W}{L} = \frac{2\pi \cdot GBW \cdot C_L}{\mu C_{ox}\phi_t} \left(\frac{1}{\sqrt{1+if}-1} \right) \tag{4}$$

$$V_{DS(sat)} \cong \left(\left(\sqrt{1+if}-1 \right) + 4 \right) \phi_t \tag{5}$$

$$f_t \cong \frac{\mu\phi_t}{\pi L^2} \left(\sqrt{1+if}-1 \right) \tag{6}$$

where I_D is the current of MOS transistor from the drain to the source, GBW is unity-gain bandwidth, C_L is load capacitance, n is the slope factor, ϕ_t is thermal voltage, i_f is inversion level, C_{ox} is oxide capacitance per area, f_t is the cut-off frequency of MOS transistor, W is the width of MOS transistor, L is the length of MOS transistor, μ is the mobility of electron or hole, V_{DS} is the drain to source voltage of MOS transistor.

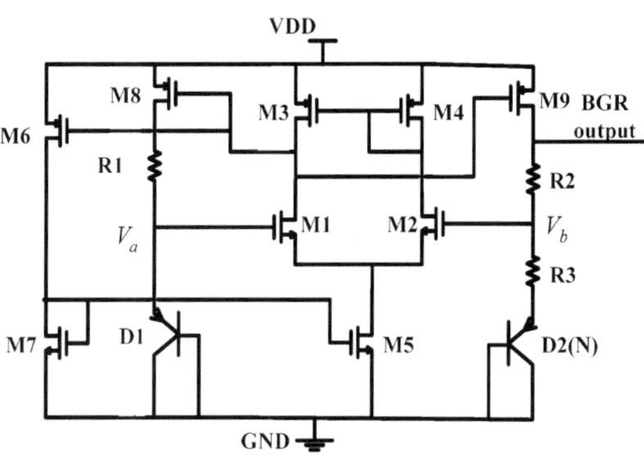

Fig. 7. Concrete circuit of the proposed bandgap reference

Figure 7 shows the concrete circuit of bandgap reference[15]. M1-M5 consist of an op-amp to keep the same voltage value of V_a and V_b. M6 and M7 provide the bias current for the op-amp. The output of op-amp is connected to the gate of M8 and M9. In order to reduce power consumption, all of these transistors are biased in sub-threshold regions or near the region to lower current consumption. Start-up circuit of bandgap reference is not drawn in figure 7.

Low current was assigned to every branch in figure 7. Every branch of the op-amp is less than 70nA and the bias current should be less than 140nA at 125°C, while the current through the resistors is less than 1.5µA. Because this system is not very stringent on circuit speed, its GBW is set to be 2.5KHz. By far the i_f parameter of transistor M1 and M2 can be obtained according to equation (3). Consequently, the W/Ls of transistors are obtained according to equation (4). At the same time, checking f_t parameters of transistors is necessary. If MOS transistors' parameters satisfy the requirement that unity gain frequency is greater than at least three times the GBW, the design space will avoid the parasitic diffusion and overlap capacitance to be of the same order of the load capacitance.

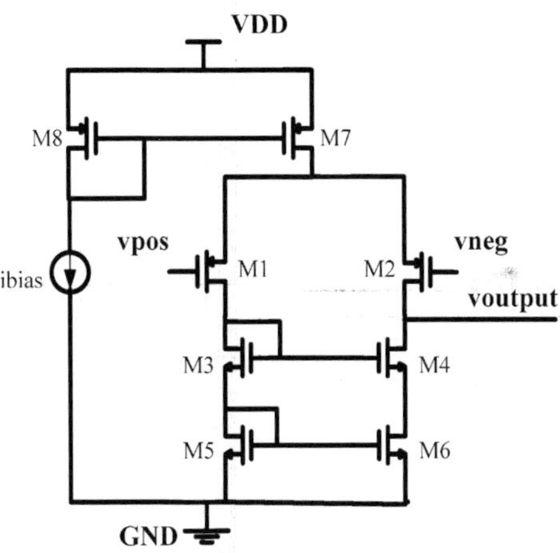

Fig. 8. Concrete circuit of the voltage buffer of bandgap reference

Voltage buffer of the bandgap reference is described in the next paragraph. Figure 8 shows the concrete circuit of the voltage buffer of the proposed bandgap reference. A traditional single stage amplifier is used as a voltage buffer to increase the drive capacity of the proposed bandgap reference. M1 and M2 are PMOS transistors as input transistors. M3, M4, M5 and M6 are used as current sources to form the active load of the input pair. ibias provides current reference for the amplifier. All the transistors in figure 8 are working in saturation region. The current through transistor M7 is about 3.2µA according to the simulation results.

4.3 Variable step-down ratio SC circuit

Circuit topology is shown in figure 9, which is illustrated in details in [16]. A and B are used to select different step-down conversion ratio. And P_1, P_2 and P_3 are logic combinations of A, B, clk1 and clk2, as illustrated in table 1.

VDD/Vout	1/3	1/2	2/3
A	0	1	1
B	1	1	0

Table 1. Relations between control signals and step-down conversion ratio

Equation (7) depicts the relationship between P_1, P_2, P_3 and other signals.

$$P_1 = (ck1)\bar{A} + (ck2)\bar{B}$$
$$P_2 = (ck1)A \eqno(7)$$
$$P_3 = (ck2)B$$

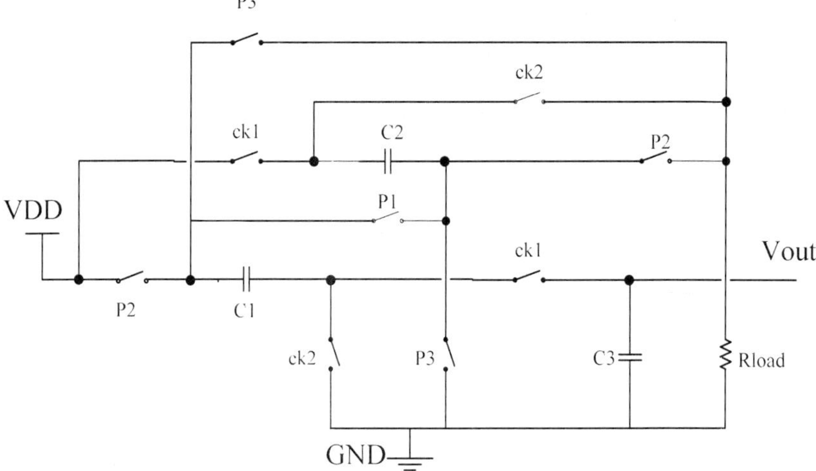

Fig. 9. SC converter circuit topology

Integrated capacitors are used to perform the DC-DC convert functions[17]. For integrated switched capacitor DC-DC circuits, there are three kinds of flying capacitors: MOS capacitors, PIP (poly-insulator-poly) capacitor and MIM (metal-insulator-poly) capacitor. Every capacitor has its own characteristics. MIM capacitors have good linear characteristic, but usually too much parasitic capacitance; PIP capacitors don't have good linear characteristic and they don't have too much parasitic capacitance; MOS capacitors have the biggest unit capacitance in CMOS technology because the distance between MOSFET gate and substrate is the smallest in the whole process. [18] compares parasitic capacitance among different kinds of integrated capacitance. After careful consideration and trade-off, MOS capacitance is preferred in this design.

One of the most important considerations of charge pump circuit design is to suppress the leakage current in the switching process. If PMOS's drain voltage or source voltage is 0.7V higher than supply voltage, the PN junction(drain or source of PMOS is regarded as p terminal, n well is regarded as n terminal) will be forward biased, which will lead to generation of leakage current.

There are two approaches to avoid leakage current generation. One is to properly set capacitors' values, second is to apply considerate clock sequence. When it comes to selection of capacitors' values, there are several considerations. The larger value the output capacitor has, the smaller output ripple the system has. At the same time, the ratio of output capacitor to flying capacitor determines the leakage current. If the ratio is large, then the voltage variation of flying capacitor will be large. This will add possibility of leakage current.

Another approach to suppress leakage current is to use proper clock sequences. 1/2 step-down conversion ratio is considered as a typical case, as shown in figure 10. After charge is delivered into C1 and C2, M1 and M3 are turned on, while M2 and M4 are turned off at this time. Then M1 is turned off to implement the redistribution between C1 and C2. If C1 is much smaller than C2, then the voltage across C1 is much larger than C2. If M2 and M4 are turned on simultaneously, the voltage at node2 is lower than ground. So during the selection of capacitor, C1 is not allowed to be much smaller than C2, although this will generate bigger output voltage ripple. In this case, C2 is set to be 10nF and C1 is set to be 1nF. In addition, if M4 is first turned on, and after several nano-seconds, M2 is then turned on. This method is named as stacked switches technique(those switches operate like stack), which will reduce the possibility of leakage current. But stacked switches technique needs complex clock sequence, figure 11 is an oscillator circuit to perform such a function.

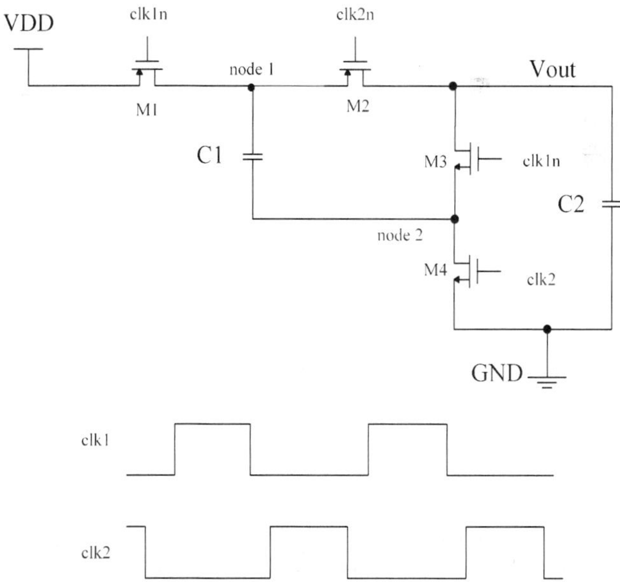

Fig. 10. 1/2 step-down conversion SC circuit

4.4 Clock generator and oscillator

Figure 11 shows the concrete circuit of the oscillator. Four comparators are used to implement the above mentioned clock scheme. Several logic operations of comparators' outputs are used to implement the clock scheme. TF, which is generated by clock output signals, is the signal to control turning on or off of M1 and M2, changing the charge stored in capacitor C and forming an oscillator. One of the advantages of this oscillator is that this scheme automatically realizes the controlled clock. When the output voltage of SC is lower than the settled value, through the control of TF signal, it will be convenient to achieve the enablement of clock, and then restart the SC converter. On the contrary, when the output of SC is higher than the settled value, clock will be disabled through the control of TF signal.

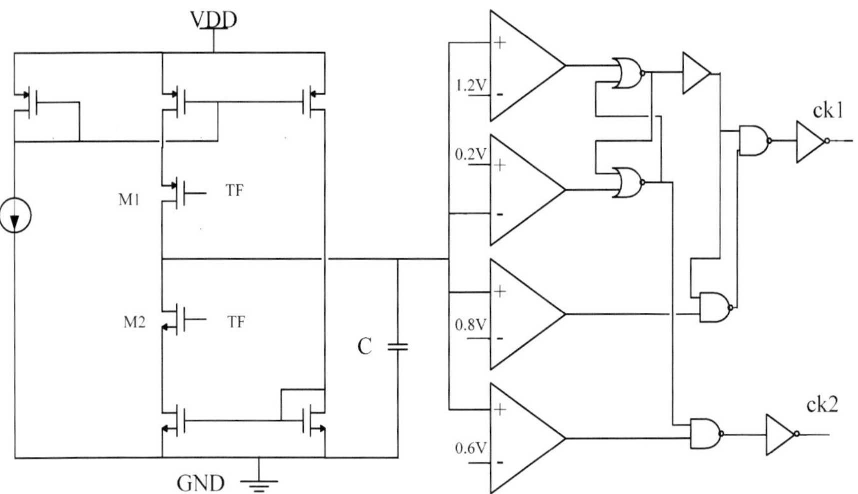

Fig. 11. Concrete circuit of oscillator

Comparators fabricated in CMOS technology have bigger DC offset. In addition, comparators working in switched capacitors are often affected by disturbance and noise. So hypothesis comparators are applied to reduce the above affects. Figure 12 shows the detailed circuit of hypothesis comparator.

The hypothesis comparator uses two-stage structure. In the first stage, M1-M7 consists of differential input stage, where M1 is the tail current, M2 and M3 are source coupled differential input pair, M4, M7 and M5, M6 are cross-coupled bi-stable current sources as load[19][20]. The ratios of width to length of M5, M6 are larger than M4, M7. M8-M11 consists of the second stage, which act as two inverters to increase drive capacity. The comparator consumes 1μA supply current when it is operating, which is a low power design, suitable for this system.

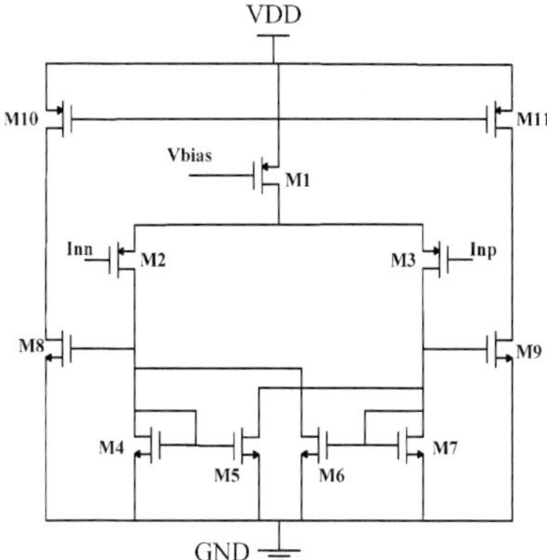

Fig. 12. Hypothesis Comparator Circuit

4.5 Step-down ratio decision circuit and output voltage monitoring circuit

The function of step-down ratio decision circuit is to monitor the voltage on storage capacitor. The output of this module is to dynamically set the step-down ratio of the SC circuit. The system block of this circuit is shown in figure 13. Vstore represents the voltage of storage capacitor.

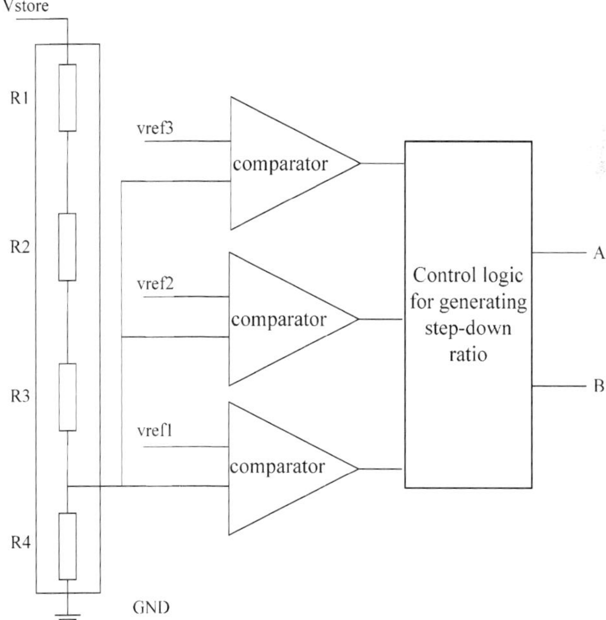

Fig. 13. Diagram of step-down ratio control circuit

The function of output voltage monitoring circuit is to detect the output voltage of variable step-down ratio SC circuit in real time. Its output determines whether enable the clock signal, in order to control the step-down SC circuit. The system diagram is shown in figure 14, where vout_sc is the output voltage of the variable step-down SC converter.

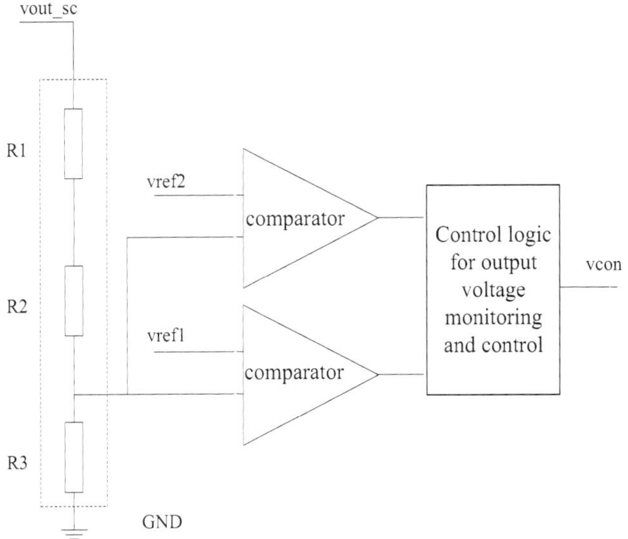

Fig. 14. Diagram of output voltage monitoring circuit

In figure 13 and figure 14, comparators are both realized by hypothesis comparator circuit, which is shown in detail in figure 12. In figure 13, 3 similar comparators are employed in the step-down ratio decision circuit while 2 similar comparators are employed in the output voltage monitoring circuit in figure 14.

4.6 LDO circuit

Traditional LDO circuit structure consists of three components: an error amplifier, a power transistor and a resistive voltage divider. The positive input of error amplifier is connected to the reference voltage and the negative one is connected to the resistive voltage divider of output voltage. The output voltage of error amplifier is to control the gate voltage of power transistor.

Because the subsequent functional circuits include analog components, such as AD converters and RF modules, PSRR(Power-Supply Rejection Ratio) of LDO is a very important characteristic, which is a measure of the ability of an output voltage to prevent noise from power supply noise. On one hand, high gain of error amplifier will lead to high PSRR; on the other hand, using PMOS transistor as power transistor will reduce power noise by offsetting power supply noise through power transistor and error amplifier [21].

In this case, error amplifier DC gain is more than 70dB and PMOS transistor is used as the power transistor. In order to suppress the supply noise from PMOS transistor, the error amplifier uses NMOS input differential pair and PMOS current-mirror load connected to the supply, as shown in figure 15.

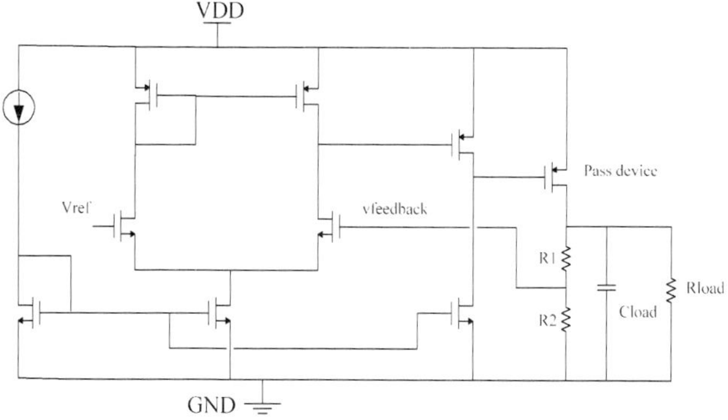

Fig. 15. Concrete LDO Circuit

5. Measurement results

Circuits of the power management circuit in high voltage region is taped out on 0.35µm CMOS EEPROM technology, while other circuits in low voltage region is to be taped out on 0.18µm CMOS technology. In this section, the measurement results of those parts in high voltage region and the simulation results of those parts in low voltage region are described.

5.1 Bandgap reference's measurement results

The proposed bandgap reference was fabricated on the above mentioned 0.35µm CMOS EEPROM technology[22]. Figure 16 shows the die photo of the proposed bandgap reference. The active area of the die is 370µm*454µm, including the voltage buffer.

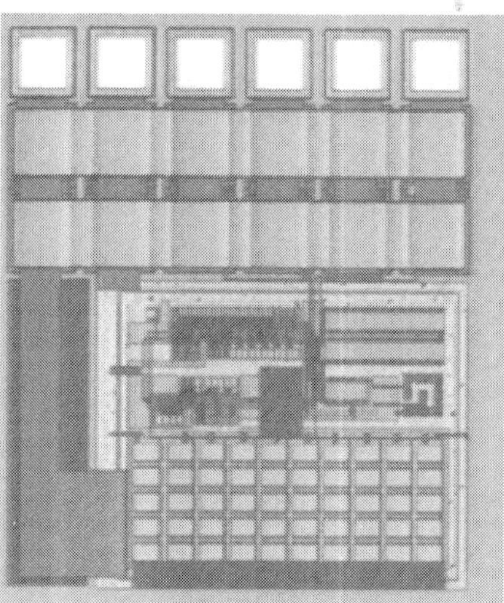

Fig. 16. Die photo of the proposed bandgap reference

Figure 17 shows the test image of the proposed bandgap reference when its supply voltage is 5V. On this typical working condition, the whole supply current is 6.87µA, including the voltage buffer, whose current is 3.6µA.

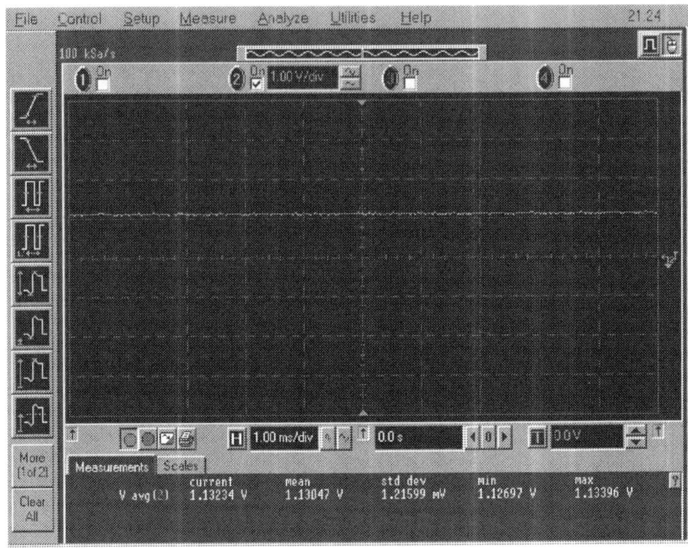

Fig. 17. Test image of the proposed bandgap reference

Figure 18 shows the output voltage characteristics of the proposed bandgap reference under different temperature. The measurement result shows the temperature coefficient is about 88.9ppm/°C at the range from 10°C to 100°C.

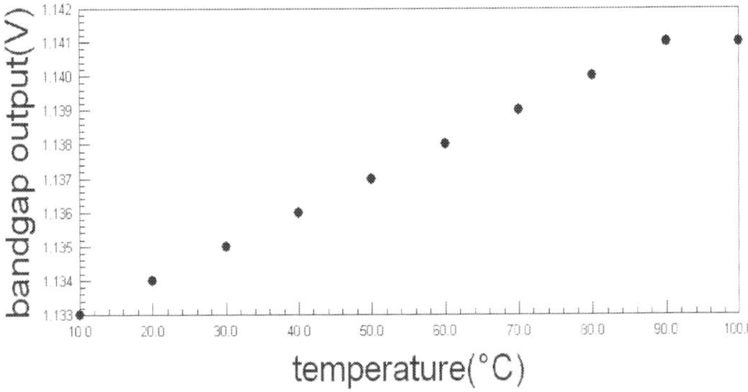

Fig. 18. Output voltage of the proposed bandgap versus temperature

Figure 19 shows the output voltage characteristics of the proposed bandgap reference under different power supply voltages. When the supply voltage changes from 3V to 11V, the output voltage of bandgap reference circuit varies about 0.875mV/V.

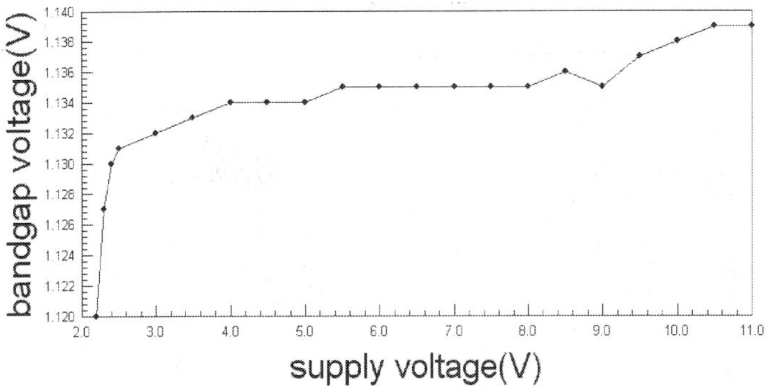

Fig. 19. Output voltage of the proposed bandgap versus supply voltage

In this system, one of the most important specifications is power consumption. All the power consumption listed below includes the power consumption of the voltage buffer. Table 2 shows the current consumption of the proposed bandgap reference at different temperature. With temperature increasing, the power supply consumption of the bandgap increases. Table 3 shows the current consumption of the proposed bandgap reference at different supply voltages. With increase of the supply voltage, the proposed circuit consumes more supply current. And the leaking current caused by PAD has been added to the total current consumption.

Temperature(°C)	10	20	30	40	50	60	70	80	90	100
supply current(μA)	6.81	6.87	6.95	7.12	7.37	7.62	7.96	8.33	8.71	9.12

Table 2. Current consumption of the proposed bandgap reference at different temperature

supply voltage(V)	3	4	5	6	7	8	9	10	11
supply current(μA)	6.54	6.71	6.87	7.04	7.26	7.62	8.14	8.79	10.56

Table 3. Current consumption of the proposed bandgap reference at different input supply voltage

This is a summary of the measurement results of the proposed bandgap reference. A bandgap working in sub-threshold region is proposed and measurement results have been shown in this paper. A voltage buffer working in saturation region has been added to increase the drive capacity of the proposed bandgap reference. When the supply voltage is 5V and at room temperature, the supply current is 6.87μA, including a voltage buffer whose current consumption is 3.6μA. The temperature co-efficiency can reach 88.9ppm at the range from 10°C to 100°C at the condition when supply voltage is 5V. And the line regulation can reach 0.875mV/V when supply voltage varies from 3V to 11V at room temperature. This design can be used widely in the power management unit in energy harvesting systems working in intermittent mode.

5.2 Variable step-down ratio SC converter's measurement results

The SC converter circuits have been taped out at the process of 0.35 μ m CMOS process with EEPROM technology, provided by Chartered Corporation. The micrograph of the proposed DC-DC converter is shown in figure 20. The size of core circuit is 600 μ m×800 μ m[23].

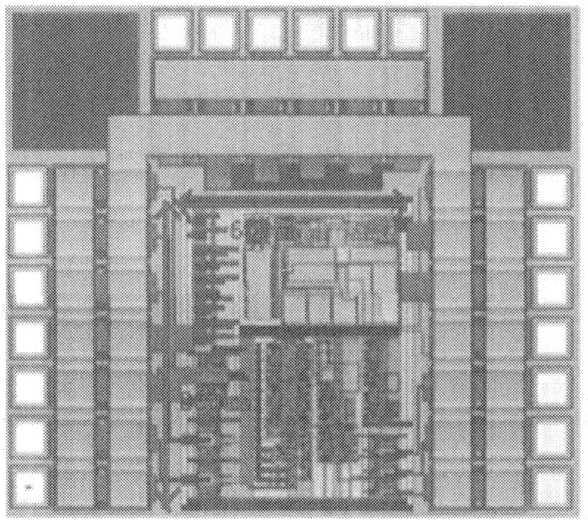

Fig. 20. The Micrograph of the proposed DC-DC converter

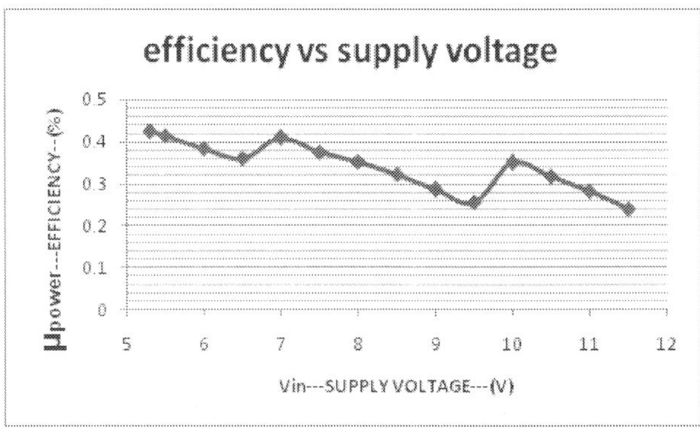

Fig. 21. The measured power converter efficiency varies with different input voltages.

It presents the measured power converter efficiency versus input voltage with the maximum load current in figure 21. The measured curve shows that the converter efficiency decreases with input voltage before changing the step-down conversion ratio. When the input voltage just exceeds the threshold voltage, the step-down conversion ratio is set to be maximum 2/3. With the input voltage increasing, the converter efficiency goes down, because system energy loss increases with supply voltage. When the input voltage reaches to the settled value, the ratio turns to 1/2 and efficiency bounces up because its no-load output voltage is closer to the load voltage desired. It also happens when the ratio changes from 1/2 to 1/3. The maximum efficiency occurs when the input voltage is 5V. It shows the waveform of output voltage and stacked clock in different step-down conversion ratios with the same load in figure 22. The higher input voltage is, the shorter converter works for in a period.

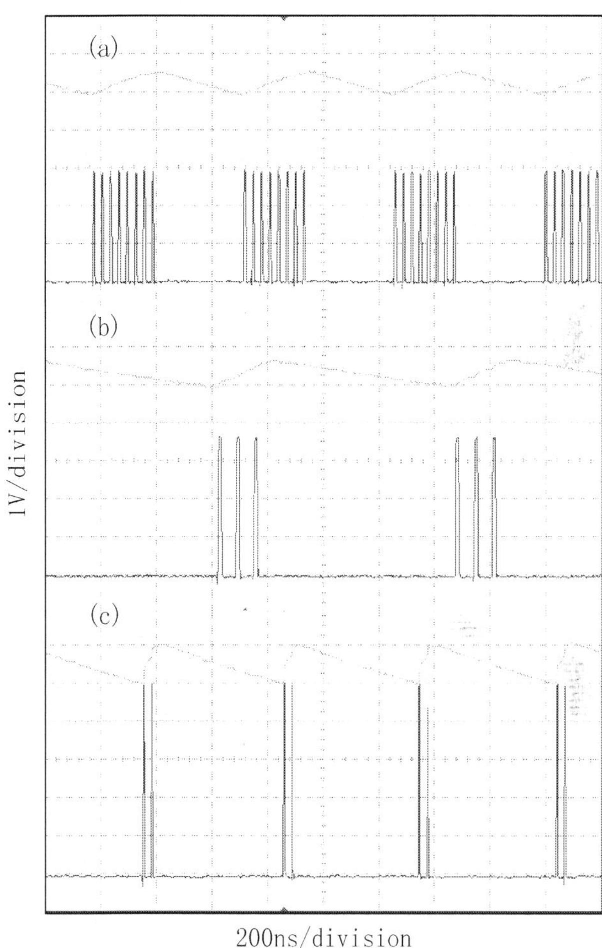

Fig. 22. The waveform of output voltage and stacked clock in different step-down conversion ratios (a) VDD=5.5V, ratio=2/3; (b) VDD=7V, ratio=1/2; (c) VDD=11V, ratio=1/3

Table 4 presents the whole circuit's performances. Measurement results show that the DC-DC converter can dynamically scale the charged capacitor supply from 5~15V to 2V and supply at least 560μA. The converter efficiency of SC converter can reach 61%, and the efficiency of the whole system is ranged from 28% to 42%, which is much higher than 17.6% in [6] and 19% in [5].

Symbol	Parameter	Testconditions	Min	Typ	Max	Units
Vin	Supply voltage	T=+27°C	5.3	9.5	14	V
Vout	Output voltage	RL=3.85KΩ	1.8		2.2	V
Iout	Supply current	5.5V<Vin<7.5V, RL=3.85KΩ		560		µA
		7.5V<Vin<11.5V, RL=3.85KΩ		580		
		11.5V<Vin<14V, RL=3.85KΩ		660		
Is	Quiescent Supply current	Iout=0mA	143		240	µA
fosc	Oscillator frequency			1	1.3	MHz
η1	SC Circuit efficiency	T=+27°C	49		61	%
η2	Total power efficiency	T=+27°C	28		42	%
Vpp	Output voltage ripple	RL=4KΩ	460		864	mV

Table 4. Measurement results of the variable step-down SC converter

This is a summary of the measurement results of the variable step-down ratio SC converter. A variable step-down conversion ratio switched capacitor DC-DC converter has been presented here to advance the converter efficiency of charge on the stored capacitor in a Wireless Monitoring System of Orthopedic Implants. The proposed converter works in intermittent mode to efficiently regulate from 15V down to approximately 2V. The SC topologies can be switched automatically to keep efficiency high over the entire supply voltage range. Stacked switches technique is also used to reduce leakage current in switching process of SC DC-DC converter. The whole converter efficiency can reach 42% including all auxiliary components' power consumption, which is far higher than previous work. This DC-DC converter could also be used in other similar intermittent energy harvesting systems.

5.3 LDO's simulation results

Table 5 shows LDO circuit's performances. Line regulation, load regulation and PSRR are important parameters for LDO design. LDO is expected to output a constant voltage even if input voltage changes a lot. Line regulation is such a measure of the ability of the power supply to maintain its output voltage given changes in the input line voltage. Usually it is simulated by changing input voltage at the range from low power supply to high power supply using DC analysis method. In the same way, LDO is expected to output a constant voltage even if load current changes a lot. Load regulation is a measure of the ability of an output voltage to remain constant given changes in the load. And it is simulated by sweeping load current from small load current to high load current using DC analysis method. PSRR shows the ability of an output voltage to prevent noise from power supply noise. It has become an important parameter because digital circuits and analog circuits have been integrated in a single chip. Switching noise from digital circuits will greatly affect the performance of analog circuits through power supply. For example, in this design, SC converter will bring much supply noise, so PSRR is a very important parameter.

	condition	*typical*	*ff*	*ss*
Line regulation	2V<input voltage<3V	122.99µV	144.99µV	99.16µV
Load regulation	1mA<load current<5mA	180.99µV	170.73µV	207.30µV
PSRR	input voltage =2V	41.96dB@1MHz 71dB@10kHz	43.05dB@1MHz 73dB@10kHz	43.06dB@1MHz 72dB@10kHz

Table 5. Simulation results of LDO circuit

Figure 23(a) shows the dynamic response of LDO when input voltage changes between 2V and 3V in 1µs. Figure 23(b) shows the dynamic response of LDO when load current changes between 1mA to 5mA in 1µs.

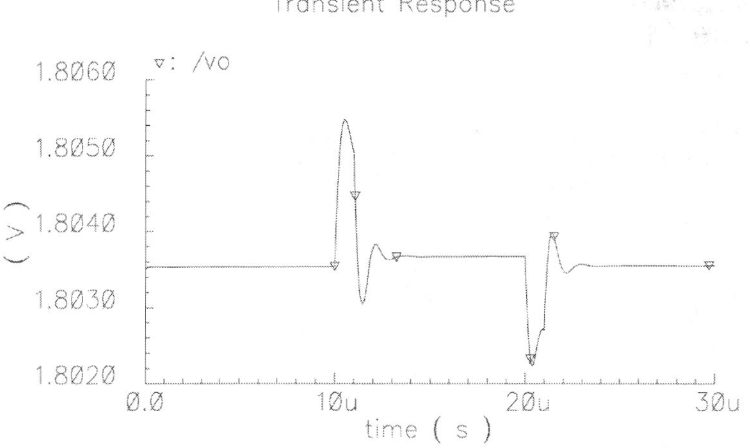

Fig. 23a. Dynamic response of input voltage

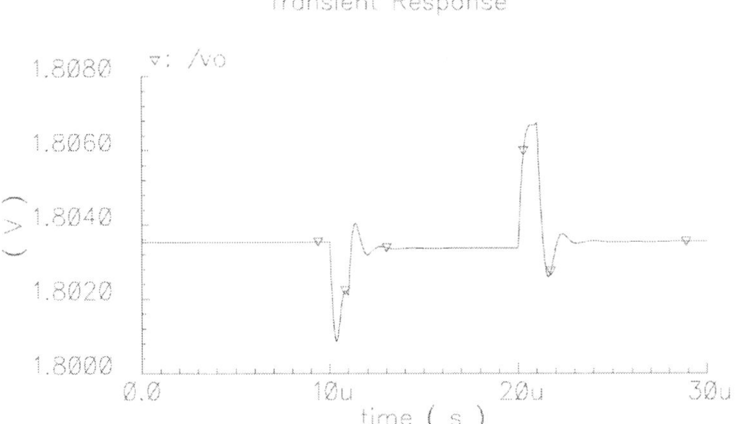

Fig. 23b. Dynamic response of load current

As is known, the efficiency of LDO is given by the product of output voltage and output current divided by the product of input voltage and input current. In this design, output voltage is 1.8V and input voltage ranges from 2V to 3V; output current is 1mA and input current is the summary of output current and the quiescent current of error amplifier, which is about 20μA. So, the efficiency of LDO ranges from 58.8% to 88.2%. If input voltage is settled less than 2.2V, then the efficiency can be larger than 80.2%.

In summary, the efficiency of whole system can be achieved by the product of the SC's efficiency and the LDO's efficiency. These components(including SC converter and auxiliary components) are working in high voltage region. According to the efficiency of the SC converter ranges from 49% to 61%, the efficiency of these parts working in high voltage region ranges from 28% to 42%. Assuming the efficiency of the LDO is 80%, the efficiency of the whole system is ranged from 22.4% to 33.6%, which is higher than 8.8%[5], 17.6%[6], 19%[4].

6. Conclusion

Based on the electrical circuit model, this paper chooses a proper storage capacitor for PZT generator. To improve converter efficiency of whole system, a hybrid DC-DC converter is proposed. A low power bandgap reference circuit working in sub-threshold region is also presented in order to reduce the power consumption of auxiliary circuits in this power system. When the supply voltage is 5V and at room temperature, the supply current is 6.87μA, including a voltage buffer whose current consumption is 3.6μA. The temperature co-efficiency can reach 88.9ppm at the range from 10°C to 100°C at the condition when supply voltage is 5V. The proposed variable step-down SC converter works in intermittent mode to efficiently regulate from 15V down to approximately 2V. The SC topologies can be switched automatically to keep efficiency high over the entire supply voltage range. Stacked switches technique is also used to reduce leakage current in switching process of SC DC-DC converter. The whole converter efficiency can reach 42% including all auxiliary components' power consumption. A LDO circuit is proposed and the efficiency of LDO ranges from 58.8% to 88.2% under different input voltage. Assuming the efficiency of the LDO is 80%, the efficiency of the whole hybrid converter is ranged from 22.4% to 33.6%, which is higher than previous work. And the proposed hybrid power management system working in intermittent mode could also be applied in other similar energy harvesting systems.

7. Acknowledgment

The author would like to thank Wenhan Hao, Hong Chen, Chun Zhang for their many contributions to this work.

8. References

[1] Chen Jia. 'Case study of kernel technologies for the power management circuits used in a smart medical micro-system'. Beijing :PhD thesis, Tsinghua University, 2009.(Chinese Version)

[2] Chen Jia, Hong Chen, Ming Liu, Chun Zhang, Zhihua Wang, 'Integrated power management circuit for piezoelectronic generator in wireless monitoring system of orthopaedic implants', IET circuit, device and system, Page(s): 485-494, Vol.2. Issue: 6, December 2008.

[3] Hong Chen, Ming Liu, Chen Jia, Chun Zhang, Zhihua Wang : 'Low Power IC Design of the Wireless Monitoring System of the Orthopedic Implants', Proceeding of 29th Annual International Conference of the IEEE Engineering in Medicine and Biology Society 2007, Lyon France, August 2007 pp.5766-5769.

[4] Stephen R. Platt, Shane Farritor, and Hani Haider: 'On Low-Frequency Electric Power Generation With PZT Ceramics', IEEE/ASME transactions on mechatronics, April 2005, Vol. 10, No. 2, pp.240-252.

[5] J. Kymissis, C. Kendall, J. J. Paradiso, and N. Gershenfeld: 'Parasitic power harvesting in shoes', Proc. 2nd IEEE Int. Conf.Wearable Computing, Los Alamitos, CA, Aug 1998, pp. 132–139.

[6] N. S. Shenck and J. A. Paradiso: 'Energy scavenging with shoe-mounted piezoelectrics', IEEE Micro, May-Jun. 2001, vol. 21, no. 3, pp. 30–42.

[7] Hong Chen, Chen Jia, Yi Chen, et al, 'A Low-Power IC Design for the Wireless Monitoring System of the Orthopedic Implants', IEEE Custom Intergrated Circuits Conference, 2008:363-366.

[8] Triet T. Le, Jifeng Han, Annette von Jouanne, Kartikeya Mayaram, and Terri S. Fiez: 'Piezoelectric Micro-Power Generation Interface Circuits', IEEE Journal of Solid State Circuits, , June 2006, Vol. 41, No. 6, pp.1411-1420.

[9] Maysam Ghovanloo and Khalil Najafi: 'Fully Integrated Wideband High-Current Rectifiers for Inductively Powered Devices', IEEE Journal of Solid State Circuits, November 2004, Vol. 39, No. 11, pp.1976-1984.

[10] Philip K.T. Mok and Ka Nang Leung: 'Design considerations of recent advanced low-voltage low-temperature-coefficient CMOS bandgap voltage reference', CICC, October 2004, Orlando, FL, USA, pp.635−642.

[11] F. Silveira, D. Flandre, and P. G. A. Jespers, A gm/Id based methodology for the design of CMOS analog circuits and its application to the synthesis of a silicon-on-insulator micropower OTA, IEEE J. Solid-State Circuits, vol. 31, pp. 1314–1319, Sept. 1996.

[12] D. Flandre, A. Viviani, et. Al: 'Improved Synthesis of Gain-Boosted Regulated-Cascode CMOS Stages Using Symbolic Analysis and gm/ID Methodology', J. Solid-State Circuits, July 1997, vol. 32, No. 7, pp 1006-1012.

[13] Enz, C.C. and Vittoz, E.A.: 'CMOS low-power analog circuit design', Designing Low Power Digital Systems, Emerging Technologies, 1996, pp.79-133.

[14] A. I. A Cunha, et al.: 'An MOS Transistor Model for Analog Circuit Design', IEEE Journal of Solid State Circuits, October 1998, Vol. 33, No.10, pp.1510-1519.

[15] Hironori Banba, Hitoshi Shiga, Akira Umezawa, Takeshi Miyaba, Toru Tanzawa, Shigeru Atsumi, and Koji Sakui: 'A CMOS bandgap reference circuit with sub-1-V operation', IEEE Journal of Solid State Circuits, May 1999, Vol. 34, No. 5, pp.670-674.

[16] Marek S. Makowski and Dragan Maksimovic,: 'performance limits of switched-capacitor DC-DC converters', PESC'95 Record, 26th Annual IEEE(2), 1995, Atlanta, Georgia, pp.1215-1221.

[17] Siamak Abedinpour, Bertan Bakkaloglu, and Sayfe Kiaei: 'A Multi-Stage Interleaved Synchronous Buck Converter with Integrated Output Filter in a 0.18μm SiGe Process, ISSCC 2006, San Francisco, CA, USA, pp.356-358.

[18] Pierre Favrat, Philippe Deval, and Michel J.Declercq: 'A high-efficiency CMOS voltage doubler', IEEE Journal of solid-state circuits, March 1998, Vol.33, No.3, pp.410-416.

[19] Gregorian Roubik. 'Introduction to CMOS Op-amps and Comparators'. New York: John Wiley &Sons，1999.

[20] D. J. Allstot. A Precision Variable-Supply CMOS Comparator. IEEE Journal of Solid-State Circuits, 1982, 17(6): pp1080~10

[21] Vishal Gupta, Gabriel A. Rincón-Mora: 'A 5mA 0.6μm CMOS Miller-Compensated LDO Regulator with -27dB Worst-Case Power-Supply Rejection Using 60pF of On-Chip Capacitance', ISSCC 2007, San Francisco, CA, USA, pp.520-521.

[22] Chen Jia, Wenhan Hao, Hong Chen, Chun Zhang, Zhihua Wang, 'A Low Power Bandgap Reference with buffer working in subthreshold region for Energy Harvesting Systems', Journal of Semiconducotors, pages:075014(1-5), Vol.30, No.7, July 2009.

[23] Wenhan Hao, Chen Jia, Hong Chen, Chun Zhang, Zhihua Wang, A variable step-down conversion ratio switched capacitor DC--DC converter for energy harvesting systems working in intermittent mode, Journal of Semiconducotors, pages: 125008(1-5), Vol.30, No.12, Dec 2009.

10

Design and Optimization of Inductive Power Link for Biomedical Applications

Kejie Huang[1,2], Yin Zhou[1,3], Xiaobo Wu[3], Wentai Liu[4] and Zhi Yang[1,4]
[1]Department of Electrical and Computer Engineering, National University of Singapore
[2]Data Storage Institute, Agency of Science, Technology and Research
[3]Institute of VLSI Design, Zhejiang University
[4]Department of Electrical Engineering, University of California at Santa Cruz
[1,2]Singapore,
[3]China,
[4]USA

1. Introduction

Powering biomedical devices is a major issue in the design of wearable and implantable electronics Chaimanonart et al. (2006); Chen et al. (2009); Kendir et al. (2004); Smith et al. (2002). Often, there is not space available for a battery that will last for the lifetime of the device, as batteries are limited both by total charge storage ability and number of recharge cycles Heller (2006). Replacement is often not an option, as the implant surgeries are both time consuming, require special expertise, and introduce the possibility of additional trauma to the patient. Percutaneous physical links Galbraith et al. (2007); Knutson et al. (2002) are prone to damage, because of the mismatch in material properties, scarring at the tissue interface Takura et al. (2006), and potential infections and skin irritation. In addition, these devices are difficult to keep sterile.

An alternative is inductive links, which are coupled coils forming an air core transformer Hamici et al. (1996); Li et al. (2005); Liu et al. (2000); Sauer et al. (2005); Sivaprakasam et al. (2005); Theogarajan & Wyatt (2006); Wang, Liu, Sivaprakasam, Weiland & Humayun (2005). As diagrammed in Fig. 1, an inductive link consists of two components of electronics. Those located externally or physically detached from the subjects are referred as primary side electronics, e.g., external battery, power transmitter, power control units, etc. Those located under the skin (implanted electronics) or along with the subjects (wearable electronics) are referred as secondary electronics, including resonant amplifier, rectifier, regulators, and power management units. Power-transmission efficiency and system miniaturization are major design specifications to evaluate a power link. Given application related constraints, these specifications are inherently correlated and a careful trade-off analysis is required to achieve an optimal performance.

This chapter is organized as follows. In Section 2, an introduction on power telemetry electronics is presented, followed by design analysis and simulation verifications. Section 3 focuses on inductor modeling, which correlates power efficiency with device size. Section 4 gives examples to quantify the achievable efficiency given design constraints.

2. Power telemetry electronics

2.1 Overview

The block diagram of an inductive power link is shown in Fig. 1 Kendir et al. (2005); Wang, Liu, Sivaprakasam & Kendir (2005). It consists of an external power supply, power amplifier, receiver resonant amplifier, inductive link and rectifier. The overall power load of secondary electronics are treated as a constant resistor for analysis.

Power efficiency of a telemetry link is defined as the ratio of the power consumed by load over the power derived from the battery. It is a most important parameter for performance evaluation. A second important parameter is the geometry size of the power receiver, where an inductor is the component of the largest footprint. In other words, a critical task in system miniaturization is to reduce the geometry size of the inductor used. In the rest of this section, modeling and analysis of individual circuit blocks are presented according to its relevance to power efficiency and device size.

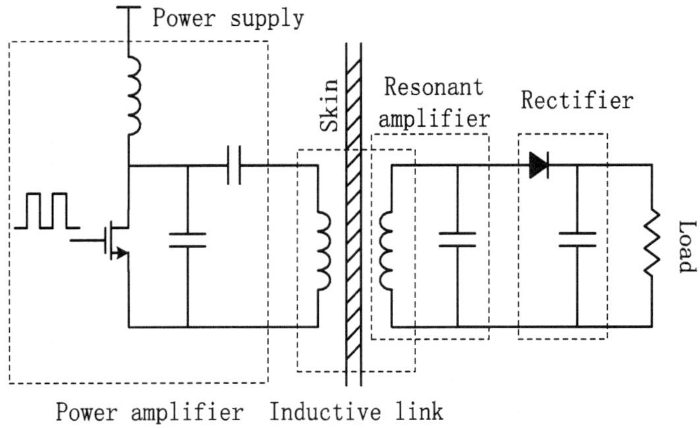

Fig. 1. Block diagrams of a generic inductive power telemetry link.

2.2 Power amplifier

There are different architectures available for building a power amplifier that converts a DC voltage to AC. Among the different designs, we choose Class-E power amplifier, because it achieves the highest power efficiency and suitable for implementation Kazimierczuk & Jozwik (2002); Sokal (2001). Compared with popular Class-D and Class-F amplifiers, it eliminates the power loss caused by shoot-through currents and achieves high impedance at harmonics Raab (2002).

As shown in Fig. 2, a class-E amplifier consists of two blocks: 1) a switching device and 2) an impedance network. The switch periodically turns on and off at the "zero-voltage" and "zero-current" point to avoid switching power losses. In practice this condition may not be 100% satisfied especially at a higher switching frequency, requiring careful tuning. The impedance network, on the other hand, is set up to attain resonance by minimizing the imaginary part of the impedance. The loading R_{load} consists of two part: equivalent series

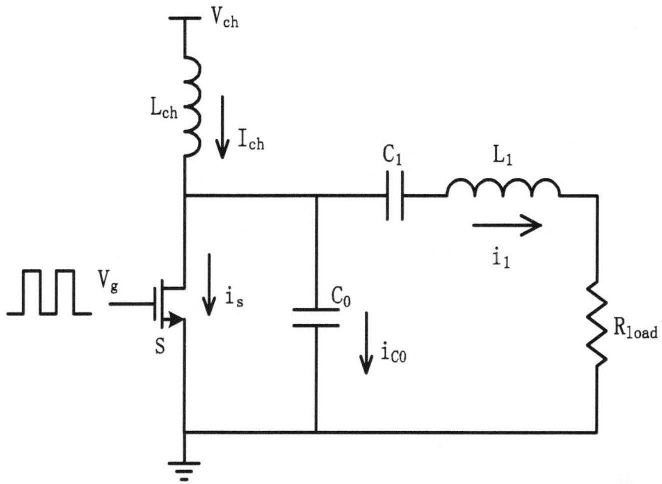

Fig. 2. Schematic of class E amplifier.

resistance(ESR) of inductor L_1 and the reflected resistance due to inductive link which will be discussed in detail in Section 2.3.

Several assumptions of Class-E power amplifier are made to facilitate further analysis Krauss et al. (1980); Rogers et al. (2010).

1. L_{ch} is large enough to ignore current ripples on I_{ch}.

2. Frequency harmonics are removed by the loop filter L_1 and C_1.

3. The variation in drain-to-source capacitor of the switch S is negligible compared with C_0.

4. "Zero voltage" turn on and "zero current" turn off conditions are precisely satisfied.

For illustration, we further assume switch S has a 50% duty cycle and is turned on at time $(2n + 1)\pi$. Under such conditions, closed-loop form expressions can be obtained.

The upper traces in Fig. 3 depict four crucial waveforms of Class E amplifier: the straight line I_{ch} is the DC current across L_{ch}. i_1 represents the current in the resonant tank and is expressed as $i_1 = I_1 sin(\omega t + \phi)$. The solid curve, i_s, and dotted curve, i_{C_0} are the currents flowing through the switch S and capacitor C_0, respectively. Note that i_s and i_{C_0} together make up a complete sinusoidal wave. The lower half of Fig. 3 gives the switch control signal V_g and drain to source voltage v_{C_0}. V_g forces the amplifier swapping between two alternative states: when S is on, i_s flows across the switch that shorts C_0; when S is off, i_{C_0} charges up the C_0. The current flowing through C_0 is

$$i_{C_0}(t) = \begin{cases} I_{ch} - I_1 \sin(\omega t + \phi), & 0 < \omega t < \pi \\ 0, & \pi < \omega t < 2\pi. \end{cases} \tag{1}$$

When the amplifier reaches its steady state, the voltage across C_0 is

$$v_{C_0}(t) = \frac{1}{C_0} \int i_{C_0}(t)dt = \begin{cases} \frac{1}{\omega C_0}(I_{ch} * \omega t + I_1 \cos(\omega t + \phi) - I_1 \cos\phi), & 0 < \omega t < \pi \\ 0, & \pi < \omega t < 2\pi \end{cases} \tag{2}$$

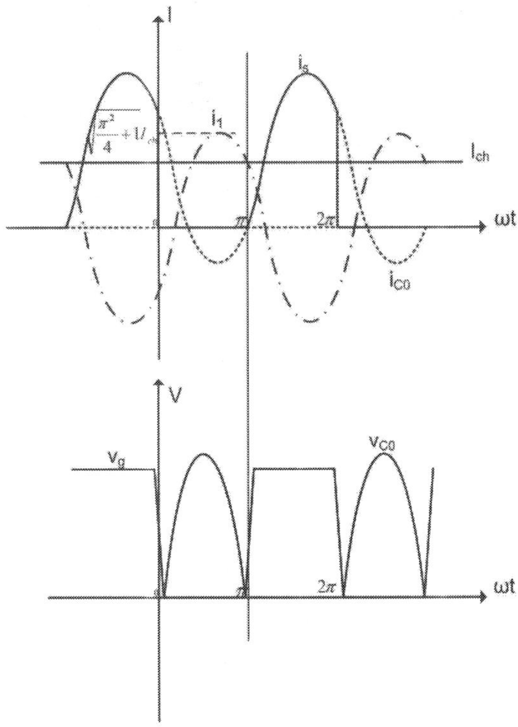

Fig. 3. Class E amplifier waveform when switch S has a 50% duty cycle and is turned on at time $(2n+1)\pi$

As reinforced conditions to further reduce switching power loss, Zero Differential Voltage Switching (ZDVS) and Zero Voltage Switching (ZVS) are added in designs Raab (1977).

$$\frac{dv_{C_0}(t)}{dt}\Big|_{t=\frac{T}{2}-} = 0, \quad v_{C_0}(t)\big|_{t=\frac{T}{2}-} = 0. \tag{3}$$

Equation 1 to 3 serve as key equations which prescribe a set of constraints for Class-E amplifier.

- Given the duty cycle, the relationship between the choke current (I_{ch}) and oscillation current across the inductor (i_1) is decided and can be numerically calculated by adding the turn on and turn off conditions. For example, when the duty cycle is 50%, $\phi \approx -32.5^0$, $I_1/I_{ch} = a = \sqrt{\frac{\pi^2}{4}+1}$, the equivalent input DC impedance is $R_{in,dc} = (\frac{\pi^2}{8}+\frac{1}{2})R_{load}$.

- The peak voltage across the switch (V_{peak}) appears when $dv_{C_0}(t)/dt = 0$ where $V_{peak} \approx -2\pi\phi V_{ch}$. The switch is required to be able to tolerate drain-to-source voltage drop several times higher than supply voltage;

- Once amplifier reaches a steady state, the averaged voltage across the switch is V_{ch}, making the choice of C_0 sensitive to the duty cycle and tank load. The larger the turn off duty cycle or tank load, the smaller C_0 should be and the more sensitive to parasitic capacitance. As a first order estimation, when duty cycle is 50%, $C_0 = 2/\omega R_{Load} a^2 \pi = 2 Q_{system}/\omega^2 a^2 \pi L$.

- The resonant thank is desired to have the peaked system Q at the operating frequency typically in sub-MHz or MHz range. If lower the frequency too much, the resonant tank becomes inefficient due to reduced inductor Q and large components values. If increase the frequency to GHz, the switching power loss and frequency related effects (detailed in Section 3), would significantly degenerate the power efficiency.

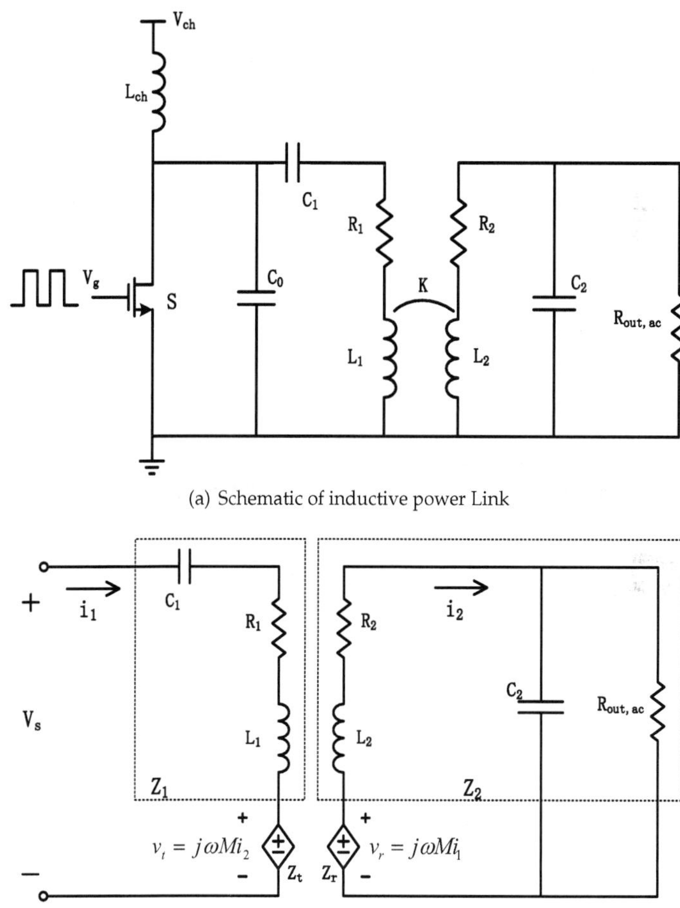

(a) Schematic of inductive power Link

(b) Equivalent model as an ideal transformer

Fig. 4. Inductive power link schematic and its equivalent circuit

2.3 Inductive link

Power efficiency is one of the major specifications for evaluating the performance of an inductive link Atluri & Ghovanloo (2005); Harrison (2007); Zierhofer & Hochmair (2002). In this section, emphasis is made to derive a set of analytic formulas to quantify a power telemetry efficiency, followed by discussions on performance optimization.

Fig. 4(a) illustrates a generic inductive power link, where R_1 and R_2 are *ESR* of inductor L_1 and L_2. $R_{out,ac}$ represents equivalent AC load resistance, which is half of its DC counterpart Ko et al. (1977). An equivalent model is shown in Fig. 4(b) Baker & Sarpeshkar (2007), where K is the coupling coefficient between L_1 and L_2, and $M = K\sqrt{L_1 L_2}$ is the mutual inductance. As the reflected impedance from the receiver and transmitter, Z_t and Z_r are

$$
\begin{cases}
Z_t = \dfrac{v_t}{i_1} = \dfrac{\omega^2 M^2}{Z_2} \\[2mm]
Z_r = \dfrac{v_r}{i_2} = j\omega M \dfrac{i_1}{i_2} \\[2mm]
Z_1 = R_1 + j\omega L_1 + \dfrac{1}{j\omega C_1} \\[2mm]
Z_2 = R_2 + j\omega L_2 + \dfrac{1}{j\omega C_2} \| R_{out,ac}
\end{cases}
\tag{4}
$$

where Z_1 and Z_2 are the impedance network shown in Fig. 4(a).

The transmitter efficiency (defined as the ratio of power consumed by the secondary electronics over the total power drained from a battery) and the receiver efficiency (defined as the ratio of power consumed by the load $R_{out,ac}$ over the total power consumed at the receiver side) are

$$
\begin{cases}
\eta_1 = \left| \dfrac{Z_t}{Z_1 + Z_t} \right| \leq \dfrac{K^2 Q_1 Q_2 R_{out,ac}}{K^2 Q_1 Q_2 R_{out,ac} + Q_2^2 R_2 + R_{out,ac}} \\[3mm]
\eta_2 = \left| 1 - \dfrac{R_2}{Z_2} \right| \leq \dfrac{Q_2^2 R_2}{Q_2^2 R_2 + R_{out,ac}} ,
\end{cases}
\tag{5}
$$

where $\eta_{1,2}$ reach its maximum if $Z_{1,2}$ has only real part left; Q_1 and Q_2 are quality factors of external and internal coils, respectively.

The total efficiency is product of η_1 and η_2

$$
\begin{aligned}
\eta_{link} &= \eta_1 * \eta_2 \\[2mm]
&\leq \frac{K^2 Q_1 Q_2^3 R_2 R_{out,ac}}{(K^2 Q_1 Q_2^3 R_2 R_{out,ac} + K^2 Q_1 Q_2 R_{out,ac}^2 + Q_2^4 R_2^2 + 2Q_2^2 R_2 R_{out,ac} + R_{out,ac}^2)} \\[2mm]
&= \frac{1}{1 + X}, \quad where \\[2mm]
X &= \frac{R_{out,ac}}{Q_2^3 Q_1 K^2 R_2} + \frac{R_{out,ac}}{Q_2^2 R_2} + \frac{2}{Q_2 Q_1 K^2} + \frac{R_2}{R_{out,ac} K^2 Q_1 / Q_2}
\end{aligned}
\tag{6}
$$

where η_{link} reaches its maximum if both η_1 and η_2 reach their maximums at the carrier frequency. In other words, the values of L_1, L_2, C_1 and C_2 must be carefully chosen to ensure that both Z_1 and Z_2 have only real part at the carrier frequency. In practice, load variation and mismatch of circuit parameters may degenerate the resonance, thus η_{link} in Eq. 6 is actually an efficiency upper bound.

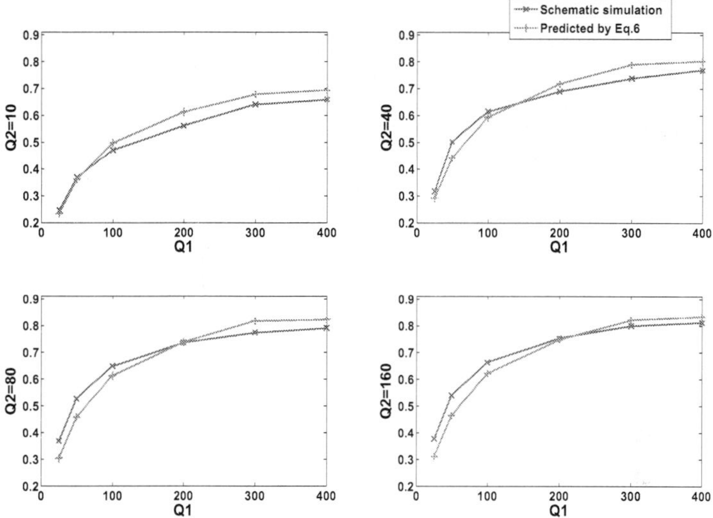

Fig. 5. Power efficiency with different coil quality factor

Note that the power efficiency is a monotonic function of X, lower X leads to higher efficiency. A conclusion we drawn from Eq. 6 is that the maximal achievable power efficiency is positively correlated with Q and coupling coefficient of the coils. It suggests that coils are the most important components for performance optimization. In section 2.4, both prediction based on Eq. 6 and circuit simulation results are given to sketch the function of power efficiency vs. different parameters, confirming above conclusion.

2.4 Simulation verifications

To quantitatively explore power efficiency and its sensitivity to different parameters, numeric simulations are performed and summarized in this section. A first set of simulations are designed to evaluate power efficiency as a function of Q. The external coil quality factor Q_1 is swept from 25 to 400 and internal coil quality factor Q_2 is swept from 10 to 160. The coupling coefficient K is set as 0.1 and both internal coil and external coil have 20uH inductance. Table 1 gives power efficiency under different combinations of Q_1 and Q_2, where a positive correlation between power efficiency and Q is observed. The simulation results are

Q_1	$Q_2 = 10$	$Q_2 = 20$	$Q_2 = 40$	$Q_2 = 80$	$Q_2 = 160$
25	0.24553	0.30505	0.31602	0.36770	0.37608
50	0.36763	0.44904	0.50174	0.52742	0.54013
100	0.46992	0.56561	0.61463	0.64740	0.66343
200	0.56127	0.63658	0.68944	0.73677	0.75357
300	0.64103	0.70081	0.73770	0.77357	0.79913
400	0.65824	0.72009	0.76860	0.79026	0.81193

Table 1. Power efficiency with different coil quality factor

K	$Q_1 = 25, Q_2 = 10$	$Q_1 = 25, Q_2 = 160$	$Q_1 = 400, Q_2 = 10$	$Q_1 = 400, Q_2 = 160$
0.01	0.0029	0.0074	0.0417	0.0721
0.04	0.0522	0.0794	0.3844	0.5110
0.07	0.1553	0.2102	0.5878	0.7463
0.10	0.2455	0.3261	0.6582	0.8119
0.13	0.3443	0.4394	0.6984	0.8440
0.16	0.3937	0.5131	0.7184	0.8644
0.20	0.4601	0.5932	0.7296	0.8901

Table 2. Power efficiency with different coupling coefficient

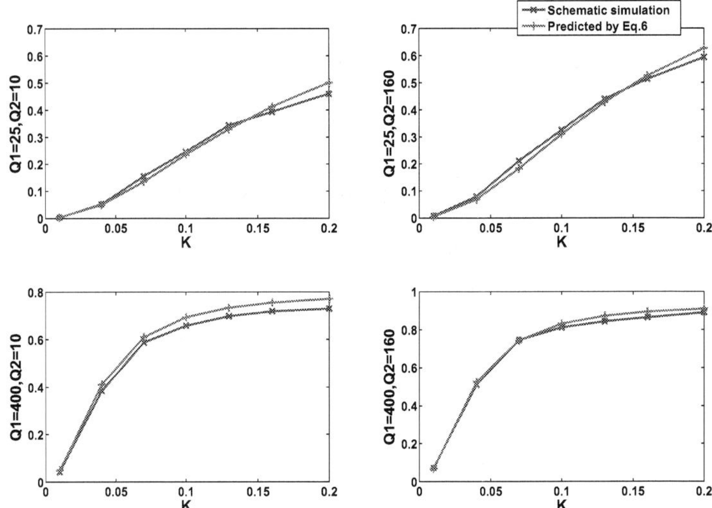

Fig. 6. Power efficiency with different coupling coefficient K

also plotted in Fig. 5 in comparison with analytical results predicted by Eq. 6. High Q coils can be used to improve power efficiency, however, the realization may violate the constraints on coil geometry size and weight. A critical optimization approach is to increase coil Q under given geometry and weight constraints, which is the focus of Section 3.

A second set of simulations is designed to evaluate power efficiency as a function of coupling coefficient K. K is swept from 0.01 to 0.2 under four combinations of Q_1, Q_2. The results in Table 2 show that higher coupling coefficient leads to higher power efficiency. In Fig. 6, schematic circuit simulation results are plotted in comparison with the analytical predicted results by Eq. 6, showing a close match. In practice, coupling coefficient is determined by coil separation and coil size, which are fixed parameters in many applications. Consequently, improving the Q factor of coils is a more practical approach to improve efficiency as shown in Section 3.

3. Inductor modeling

When coil operates at low frequency, its Q factor is defined as $Q = \frac{\omega L}{R}$, where ω is frequency, L is inductance, and R is series resistance. As frequency increases, frequency-related effects including skin effect, proximity effect Berleze & Robert (2003); Chen et al. (1993); Dwight (1945); Egiziano & Vitelli (2004); Lotfi et al. (1992); Murgatroyd (1989); Ravazzani et al. (2002) and self-resonance Massarini & Kazimierczuk (1997) modify both L and R, dramatically degenerating the Q factor. A formula predicting the Q factor is

$$Q(f) = \frac{2\pi f L}{R} \frac{1 - f^2/f_{self}^2}{1 + f^2/f_h^2},\tag{7}$$

where f_h is a parameter to quantify the impact from proximity effect(skin effect) and f_{self} is coil's self-resonant frequency. f_h and f_{self} are expressed by geometry and physical parameters, briefly

$$f_h \propto \frac{1}{r_s^2 \sigma \sqrt{N_t N_s}}, \quad f_{self} \propto \frac{1}{\sqrt{a \ln\frac{a}{r_t} \sum C_{p,k}(k-p)^2}}\tag{8}$$

where r_s, r_t, and a are the radius of a strand, a turn, and the coil loop (Usually litz winding is used, where one turn contains multiple strands; otherwise, $r_s = r_t$). N_s and N_t are the number of strands per turn and the number of turns of the coil winding. σ is the metal conductivity, $C_{p,k}$ is the parasitic capacitance between turn p and turn k.

For any given coil, there is an optimal frequency f_{peak} that has the maximal Q. To maximize the power efficiency, f_{peak}s of the coil pair should be designed in accordance with the power carrier frequency. Based on Eq. 7, an analytical form of f_{peak} is

$$\frac{1}{f_{peak}^2} \approx \frac{1}{f_h^2} + \frac{3}{f_{self}^2}.\tag{9}$$

Equation 9 represents a key design equation and a closed form analytical solution for f_{peak}. With this single equation of merit, the maximum Q, as well as the maximum efficiency of the telemetry system, can be determined. By changing the design parameters, one may tune f_{peak} close to the target frequency and maximize the power efficiency of the telemetry.

This section is a simplified introduction on inductor modeling basically according to the reference Yang et al. (2007) which has more detailed formula derivations.

3.1 Equivalent AC resistance

In the case that the radius of the cylindrical conductor is smaller or comparable to the skin depth, a first order approximation of Bessel functions allows the calculation of the AC resistance Ferreira (1992);Carter (1967)

$$R_{SK} = R_{DC}[1 + 0.021(r_s/\delta)^4],\tag{10}$$

where r_s is the radius of an individual strand, R_{DC} is the DC resistance, and δ is the skin depth $\delta = \sqrt{2/\mu_0 \sigma \omega}$. μ_0 and σ are the permeability and conductivity of the conductor, respectively. According to Ferreira (1994), the power dissipation from proximity effect in a single strand can be approximated as

$$P_{PRO} = \frac{\pi^3 r_s^4 \mu_0^2 \sigma f^2}{2} H_{peak}^2,\tag{11}$$

where H_{peak} is the peak H field through one strand.

By summarizing P_{PRO} over all strands, the power dissipation of the coil's winding from proximity effect is

$$P_{PRO.wind} = \frac{\pi^2 r_s^4 \mu_0^2 \sigma N_t^3 N_s I^2 f^2}{8 A_{winding}} \eta(b/t), \tag{12}$$

where $A_{winding}$ is the area of the cross section and η is a parameter defined to characterize a coil's geometry properties. Numeric values of η for different coils are shown in Figure 7.

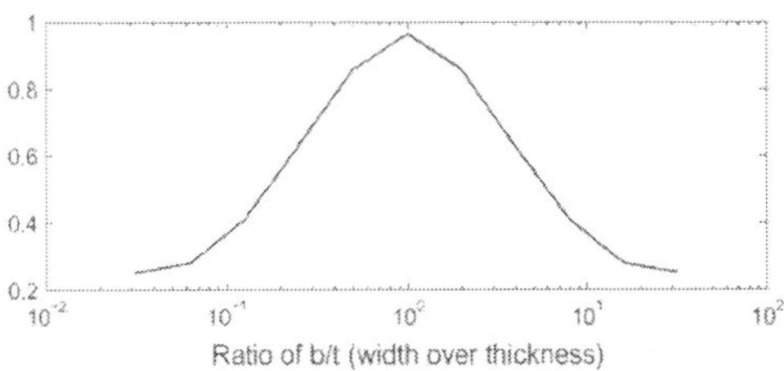

Fig. 7. Numeric values of η for coils with different cross sections. b and t are the coil's width and thickness.

Using Eq. 10 and Eq. 12, the AC resistance of a coil is derived as

$$R_{AC} = R_{DC} \frac{P_{SK.wind} + P_{PRO.wind}}{P_{DC.wind}} = R_{DC}\left(1 + \frac{f^2}{f_h^2}\right), \tag{13}$$

where f_h is the frequency at which the AC power dissipation is twice the DC power dissipation and expressed as

$$f_h = \frac{2\sqrt{2}}{\pi r_s^2 \mu_0 \sigma \sqrt{N_t N_s \eta \beta}}. \tag{14}$$

3.2 Coil self-resonant frequency

The equivalent distributive network of a coil at high frequency is shown in Figure 8.

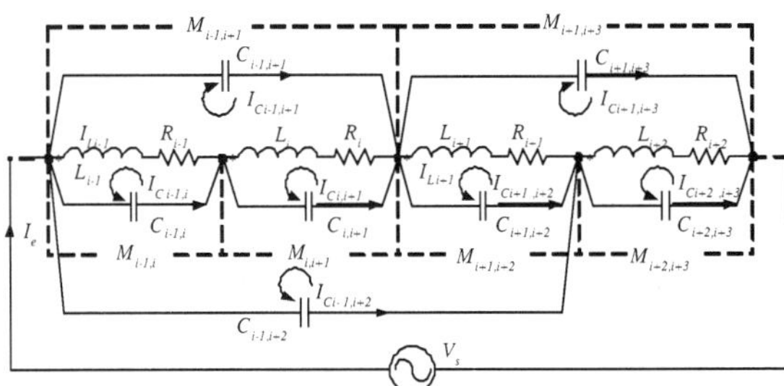

Fig. 8. Distributive equivalent model of a coil. I_{L_i} represents the current going through the inductive branch L_i, R_i is the equivalent ESR of the inductive branch L_i, $I_{C_{p,k}}$ denotes the mesh current through the parasitic capacitance $C_{p,k}$, I_e is the external driving current, and $M_{p,k}$ is the mutual inductance between turn p and turn k.

As illustrated in Figure 8, a coil is modeled as a distributive RCL network. Given that the voltage difference between two strands in the same turn is very small compared with the voltage difference between turns, the parasitic capacitance between strands in the same turn can be ignored. Each turn is then modeled as one node with unit inductance and AC resistance. Both inductive and capacitive couplings between turns (p and k) are modeled as mutual inductance $M_{p,k}$ and parasitic capacitance $C_{p,k}$. The analytical expression of the self-inductance of one turn is calculated as Sadiku (1994)

$$L_i = 0.5\mu_0 D_i \ln(D_i/OD), \tag{15}$$

where D_i is the diameter of the conductor loop and OD is the diameter of a single turn. Under the assumption that OD is negligible compared with the diameters of the conductor loops, mutual inductance $M_{p,k}$ can be calculated by Neumann formula

$$M_{p,k} = \mu_0 \int (\cos\theta/l) ds ds', \tag{16}$$

where θ is the angle of inclination between the two loop elements ds and ds', l is the radius vector between them, and the integration is to be taken over the contours of the two loops. R_i is used to model the series resistance of one turn and can be calculated using Eq. 13

$$R_i = \frac{R_{DC}}{N_t}\left(1 + \frac{f^2}{f_h^2}\right). \tag{17}$$

At a coil's self-resonance, the external driving current I_e reaches its minimum. The corresponding frequency (self-resonant frequency) can be found by solving the network as shown in Fig. 8. To obtain a convenient expression of the currents at different branches, the Mesh theorem is used Dorf (1993). Since the number of independent meshes is equal to the number of parasitic capacitors plus one, which comes from the external driving circuit, we construct the mesh currents based on individual parasitic capacitor.

Denoting the mesh current from node p to node k as $I_{C_{p,k}}$, and the external driving current as I_e, I_{L_i} is defined as the sum of mesh currents and external driving current

$$I_{L_i} = I_e - \sum_{p \le i, k \ge i+1} I_{C_{p,k}}. \tag{18}$$

Through the inductive branches, we obtain the voltage difference between node p and node k as

$$V_{p,k} = \sum_{p \le i < k} \omega L_i I_{L_i} + \sum_{p \le i < k}\sum_{j \ne i} \omega M_{j,i} I_{L_j} + \sum_{p \le i < k} I_{L_i} R_i, \tag{19}$$

where L_i is the unit inductance of turn i, $M_{j,i}$ the mutual inductance between turn j and turn i, and R_i the resistance of turn i, as shown in Fig. 8.

Given that a coil's cross section is much smaller than the area of the conductor loop ($b \ll D_{out}$, $t \ll D_{out}$), the coupling coefficient between two turns is close to 1. Therefore, Eq. 19 is simplified by assuming that the flux (Φ_{unit}) going through any individual turn is the same. Flux (Φ_{unit}) can be defined as

$$\begin{aligned}
\Phi_{unit} &= \sum_{i=1}^{N_t} L_i I_{L_i} = I_e \sum_{i=1}^{N_t} L_i - \sum_{i=1}^{N_t} L_i \sum_{p \le i, k \ge i+1} I_{C_{p,k}} \\
&\approx N_t L_i I_e - L_i \sum_{p < k} I_{C_{p,k}}(k - p),
\end{aligned} \tag{20}$$

where N_t is the number of turns. As a result, the voltage difference between node p and node k becomes

$$V_{p,k} = \omega(k-p)\Phi_{unit}\angle 90° + R_i \sum_{p \leq i < k} I_{L_i}. \tag{21}$$

Alternatively, the voltage difference can be computed through the capacitive branches as

$$V_{p,k} = \frac{I_{C_{p,k}}\angle - 90°}{\omega C_{p,k}}, \tag{22}$$

where $C_{p,k}$ is the parasitic capacitance between turn p and turn k. Equation 21 and 22 are combined to give the following expression for the mesh current $I_{C_{p,k}}$ as

$$I_{C_{p,k}} = -\omega^2 C_{p,k}(k-p)\Phi_{unit} + \omega R_i C_{p,k}\angle 90° \sum_{p \leq i < k} I_{L_i}. \tag{23}$$

To obtain a direct relationship between external driving current I_e and frequency, using the sum of $(k-p)I_{C_{p,k}}$, the resulting equation is

$$\sum_{p<k}(k-p)I_{C_{p,k}} = -\omega^2\Phi_{unit}\sum_{p<k}C_{p,k}(k-p)^2 + \omega R_i\angle 90°\sum_{p<k}C_{p,k}(k-p)\sum_{p \leq i < k}I_{L_i}. \tag{24}$$

Substituting 20 into 24 yields

$$\frac{1}{1-\alpha} = \omega^2 L_i \sum_{p<k}C_{p,k}(k-p)^2 - \omega R_i\angle 90°\sum_{p<k}C_{p,k}(k-p), \tag{25}$$

where

$$\alpha = \frac{N_t I_e}{\sum_{p<k} I_{C_{p,k}}(k-p)}. \tag{26}$$

The solution to Eq. 25 is

$$\omega_{self} = \frac{A \pm B}{G}, \tag{27}$$

where
$A = R_i\angle 90° \sum_{p<k}C_{p,k}(k-p)$
$B = \sqrt{\frac{1}{1-\alpha}4L_i\sum_{p<k}C_{p,k}(k-p)^2 - R_i^2[\sum_{p<k}C_{p,k}(k-p)]^2}$
$G = 2L_i\sum_{p<k}C_{p,k}(k-p)^2$.
To provide a simplified formula to predict the self-resonant frequency, additional approximations are made (a) $\alpha \approx 0$; (b) $4L_i\sum_{p<k}C_{p,k}(k-p)^2 \gg R_i^2[\sum_{p<k}C_{p,k}(k-p)]^2$. Consequently, the self-resonant frequency f_{self} can be calculated as Bartoli et al. (1996)

$$f_{self} = \frac{1}{2\pi\sqrt{LC_{self}}}, \tag{28}$$

where

$$L = N_t^2 L_i, C_{self} = \sum_{p<k}C_{p,k}(k-p)^2/N_t^2. \tag{29}$$

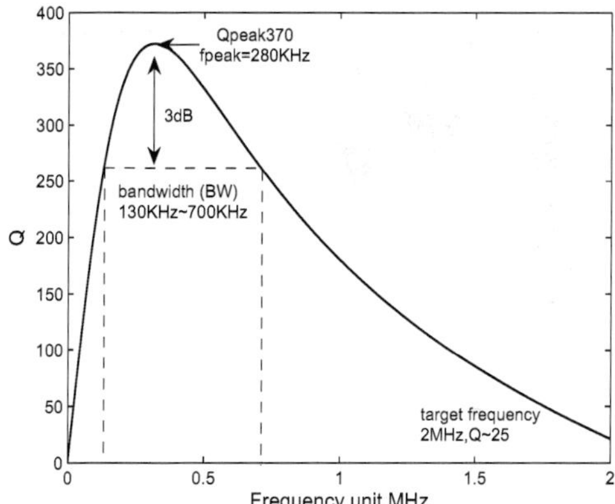

Fig. 9. Q vs Frequency curve. Coil specifications:
$N_t = 50, N_s = 30, D_{out} = 4.0cm, D_{in} = 2.8cm, r_s = 25um, L = 110uH, R_{DC} = 0.30ohm.$

3.3 Quality factor

Using lumped circuit model suggested by Eq. 28 and 29, the equivalent impedance of a coil
considering C_{self} is

$$Z_e = (j\omega L + R_{AC})\|\frac{1}{j\omega C_{self}} = \frac{R_{AC} + j\omega L}{(1 - \omega^2 L C_{self}) + j\omega R_{AC} C_{self}}. \tag{30}$$

The Q of a coil with impedance given in Eq. 30 is

$$Q(f) \approx 2\pi f L (1 - \frac{f^2}{f_{self}^2})/R_{DC}(1 + \frac{f^2}{f_h^2}), \tag{31}$$

where $f_h = 2\sqrt{2}/(\pi r_s^2 \mu_0 \sigma \sqrt{\eta \beta N_t N_s})$, $f_{self}^{-1} = 2\pi\sqrt{LC_{self}}$ and $R_{DC} = N_t(D_{out} + D_{in})/2\sigma\pi r_s^2 N_s$, as defined previously.

A typical curve to characterize the Q of a coil is shown in Figure 9. f_{peak} represents the
frequency at which a coil has the maximum Q, denoted as Q_{peak}. For telemetries, the power
transfer efficiency and the heat dissipation are the primary concerns, therefore it is desirable
to have the coil operating near f_{peak}.

Taking the derivative of the Q and setting it to zero allows the derivation of f_{peak}. f_{peak} is
approximately given as

$$f_{peak}^2 \approx f_h^2 \| \frac{f_{self}^2}{3} \tag{32}$$

Equation 32 represents a key design equation, and a closed form analytical solution for f_{peak}.
With this single equation of merit, the bandwidth(BW) and the maximum Q, and as well
as the maximum efficiency of the telemetry system, can be determined. By changing the
design parameters, one may tune f_{peak} close to the target frequency and maximize the power
efficiency of the telemetry.

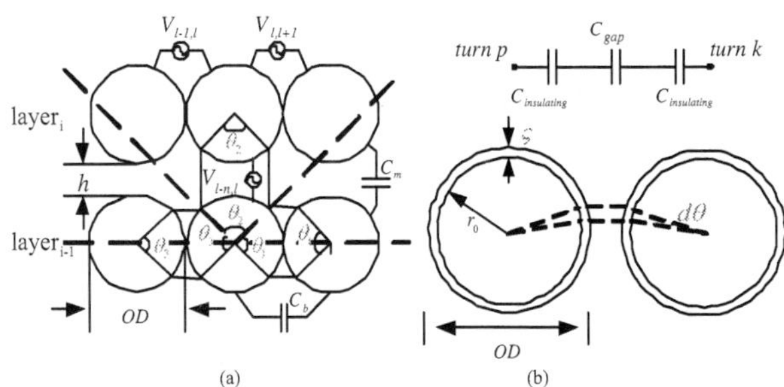

(a)   (b)

Fig. 10. Turn-to-turn parasitic capacitance. (a) Illustration of the parasitic capacitance in a coil winding. (b) Equivalent model to calculate the turn-to-turn parasitic capacitance.

3.4 Turn-to-turn parasitic capacitance

The cross section of a multiple-layer coil is shown in Figure 10, where C_m denotes the parasitic capacitance between turns in different layers, C_b the parasitic capacitance between turns in the same layer, and θ_i ($i = 1, 2, 3$) is the effective angle between two turns. As illustrated in Figure 10(b), the turn-to-turn parasitic capacitance is a combination of parasitic capacitances through the insulation layer and the nonconductive gap.

The parasitic capacitance contributed by the dielectric insulting layer per unit angle is Massarini et al. (1996)

$$C_{insulate} = \frac{\varepsilon_0 \varepsilon_r \pi D_i}{\ln \frac{r_0}{r_0 - \varsigma}}, \tag{33}$$

where ς is the thickness of the insulation layer, r_0 the radius of a single turn and D_i the average diameter of the conductor loop.

Assuming the dielectric constant of the gap is ε_0, the parasitic capacitance contributed by the gap per unit angle is approximately computed by

$$C_{gap} = \frac{\varepsilon_0 \pi D_i}{2(1 - \cos\theta) + \frac{h}{r_0}}, \tag{34}$$

where h is the separation between two turns.

As a result, the total parasitic capacitance per unit angle is approximated as

$$C_t = \frac{0.5 C_{gap} C_{insulate}}{C_{gap} + 0.5 C_{insulate}}. \tag{35}$$

Under the condition that $\varsigma \ll r_0$, the parasitic capacitance between two turns is

$$C_{p,k} = \varepsilon_0 \varepsilon_r \int_0^{\theta_e/2} \frac{\pi D_i r_0}{\varsigma + \varepsilon_r r_0(1 - \cos\theta) + 0.5 \varepsilon_r h} d\theta, \tag{36}$$

where θ_e is the effective angle between turn p and turn k.

As a first order approximation, assume that each turn except those on the perimeter of a coil is surrounded by four turns and $\theta_1 = \theta_2 = \theta_3 = 90°$.

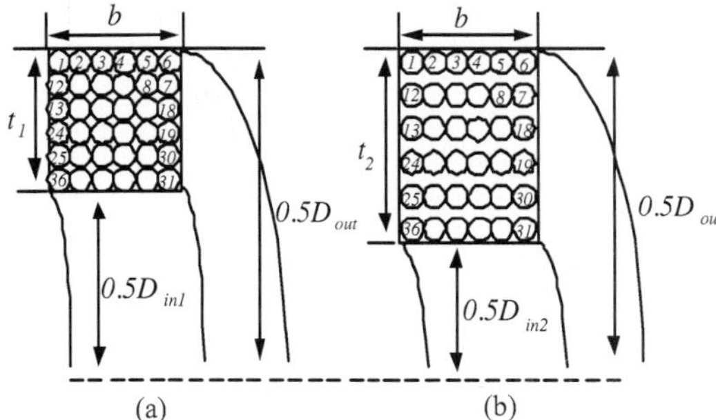

Fig. 11. Coils' cross sections. (a) Coil "I", tightly wound litz coil. (b) Coil "II", loosely wound litz coil with separation between layers.

4. Design examples

In this section, examples to illustrate the tradeoff between coil design parameters, f_{peak} and the Q are presented. Since the outer diameter, thickness, and inductance of a coil are typically specified for biomedical applications, design parameters available for optimization are the inner diameter, winding sequence, the number of strands per turn, and the diameter of an individual strand.

4.1 Inner diameter

When the target frequency is a few MHz or higher, a major design concern is the self-resonant frequency. To increase the self-resonant frequency of a coil and thus f_{peak}, an effective and practical method is to reduce a coil's inner diameter and increase the separation between layers, as shown in Fig. 11

According to Eq. 29, a general expression for the total parasitic capacitance for both coil I and "II", as illustrated in Fig. 11, is

$$C_{self} = \frac{1}{N_t^2}[C_b(l-1)m + C_m \sum_{i=1}^{l}(2i-1)^2(m-1)],$$ (37)

where C_b is the parasitic capacitance between two nearby turns in the same layer and C_m the parasitic capacitance between different layers, as shown in Figure 10.

For a tightly wound coil, e.g., coil "I", the parasitic capacitance between two nearby turns other is

$$C_b = C_m = \varepsilon_0\varepsilon_r \int_0^{\frac{\pi}{4}} \frac{\pi D_i r_0}{\varsigma + \varepsilon_r r_0(1-\cos\theta)} d\theta$$ (38)

For coils with spacing between layers, e.g., coil "II", the parasitic capacitance is

$$\begin{cases} C_b = \varepsilon_0\varepsilon_r \int_0^{\frac{\pi}{4}} \frac{\pi D_i r_0}{\varsigma + \varepsilon_r r_0(1-\cos\theta)} d\theta \\ C_m = \varepsilon_0\varepsilon_r \int_0^{\frac{\pi}{4}} \frac{\pi D_i r_0}{\varsigma + \varepsilon_r r_0(1-\cos\theta)+0.5\varepsilon_r h} d\theta, \end{cases}$$ (39)

where h is the separation between two layers.

Coil	D_{in}	C_b	C_m	L	C_{self}	f_{self}
$I, h = 0$	$2.76cm$	$15pF$	$15pF$	$85uH$	$17pF$	$4.1MHz$
$II, h = r_0$	$2.66cm$	$15pF$	$1.0pF$	$77uH$	$1.5pF$	$15MHz$

Table 3. Parasitic capacitance, self-resonant frequency of coil "I" and "II". Coil Specification $D_{out} = 3cm, OD = 200um, h = 100u, \varsigma = 3um, \varepsilon_r = 3.$

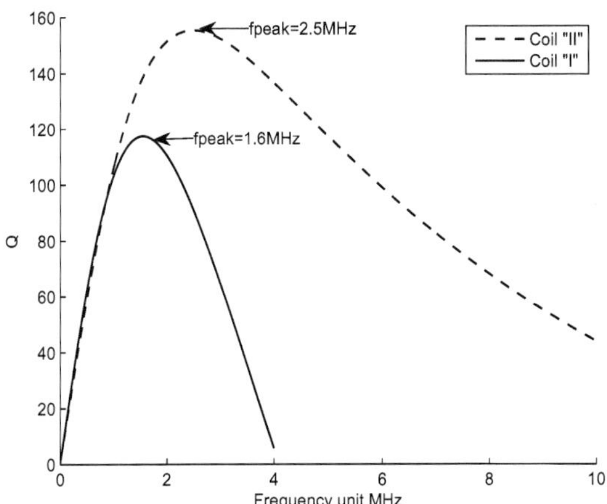

Fig. 12. Q vs Frequency curves of coil "I" and "II".

Using proposed formulae, the total parasitic capacitance and the self-resonant frequency can be calculated directly. An example of the result is shown in Table 3.

As shown in Table 3, Coil "I" and "II" have similar geometry parameters, inductances, and DC resistances. The only difference between them is that coil "II" has an additional air gap between two layers. In practical coil design, such a gap can be achieved by increasing the bundle level insulation coating. The values in the last column of Table II demonstrate that coils with spacing between layers (e.g., Coil "II") have a much higher self-resonant frequency than tightly wound coils (e.g., Coil "I"). As a result of layer to layer spacing, the inner diameter of coil "II" is reduced to $2.66cm$, while the inner diameter of coil "I" is $2.76cm$. The Q vs Frequency curves for both coil "I" and "II" are shown in Fig. 12, assuming AWG44, 7 strand litz wire ($OD = 200\ um$) is used to wind the coils.

As Fig. 12 illustrates, at low frequencies, the Q for both coil "I" and "II" are similar. This is because the frequency of operation is well below the self-resonant frequency and the AC power dissipation is close to the DC power dissipation. At higher frequencies, coil "II" has a higher Q than coil "I", mainly due to lower parasitic capacitance.

4.2 Winding sequence

The winding sequence of the turns of a coil also affects the total parasitic capacitance and the self-resonant frequency. Two coils with the same geometry parameters but different winding sequences are shown in Fig. 13.

In Fig. 13, the numbers in the wire cross section indicate the winding sequence. The total parasitic capacitance for coil "III", due to the altered winding sequence is expressed as

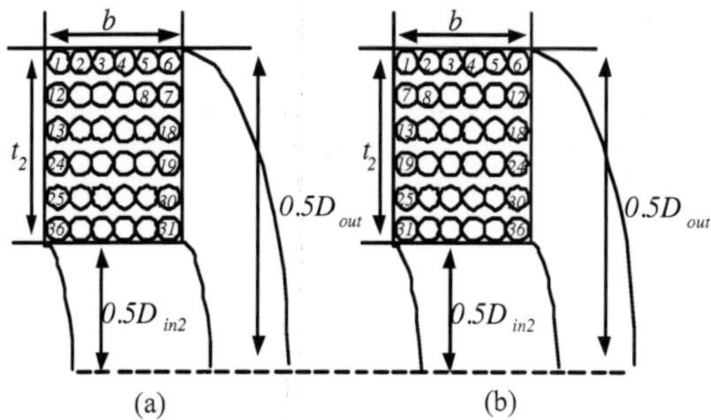

Fig. 13. Coils' cross sections. (a) Coil "II", loosely wound litz coil with normal winding sequence and separation between layers. (b) Coil "III", loosely wound litz coil with different winding sequence and separation between layers.

$$C_{self} = \frac{1}{N_t^2}[C_b(l-1)m + C_m l^3(m-1)] \tag{40}$$

Coil	C_b	C_m	L	C_{self}	f_{self}
$II, h = OD/2$	$15pF$	$1.0pF$	$77uH$	$1.5pF$	$15MHz$
$III, h = OD/2$	$15pF$	$1.0pF$	$77uH$	$1.2pF$	$17MHz$

Table 4. Parasitic capacitance, self-resonant frequency of coil "II" and "III". Coil Specifications $D_{out} = 3cm, D_{in} = 2.66cm, OD = 200um, h = 100u, \varsigma = 3um, \varepsilon_r = 3$.

4.3 The number of strands

If the cross section of the winding is fixed, reducing the number of strands is an effective way to increase f_{peak} and the Q at higher frequencies for two reasons. First, f_{self} increases, due to the increased separation between nearby turns, as shown in Fig. 14. Second, f_h increases, since the total number of strands in the winding decreases. Therefore, both f_{peak} and the Q are larger at higher frequencies. For the purpose of demonstration, numeric comparisons of several coils with different geometry parameters are given in Table 5.

Coil	N_s	R_{DC}	f_{self}	f_{peak}	Q_{peak}	$BW(bandwidth)$
IV	3	$9.5 ohm$	$26MHz$	$8.5MHz$	198	$2.5 - 15.5MHz$
V	7	$4.1 ohm$	$19MHz$	$4.2MHz$	215	$1.8 - 8.5MHz$
VI	15	$1.9 ohm$	$14MHz$	$2.1MHz$	222	$0.9 - 4.5MHz$
VII	30	$0.95 ohm$	$5.6Mhz$	$1.1MHz$	219	$0.4 - 2.2MHz$

Table 5. Self-resonant frequency, quality factor, bandwidth of coil "IV"-"VII". Coil Specifications $D_{out} = 3.2cm, D_{in} = 2.7cm, b = 2.5cm, t = 2.5mm, d_s = 50um, N_t = 36, \varsigma = 3um, \varepsilon_r = 3, AWG44$.

The Q vs Frequency curves of coils in Table 5 are plotted in Fig. 15. Even though the DC resistance of a coil is much higher when fewer strands are used per winding, the f_{peak} and f_{self} increase significantly. Since telemetry efficiency is a function of the operating frequency, the coil with fewer strands represents a significant improvement compared with conventional implant telemetry design.

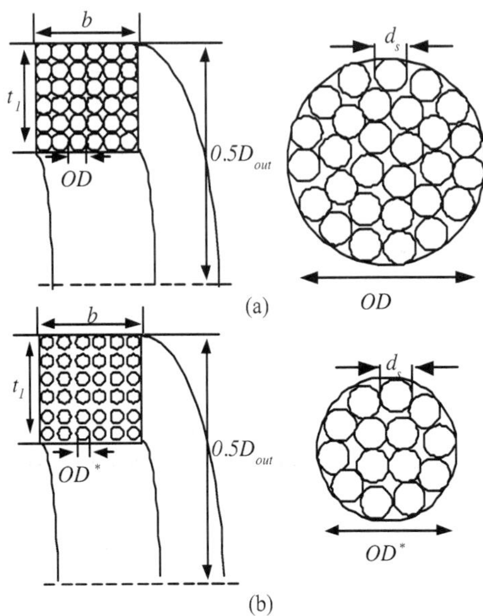

(a)

(b)

Fig. 14. Coils' cross sections. (a) Tightly wound litz coil with the maximum number of strands. (b) Loosely wound litz coil with less strands.

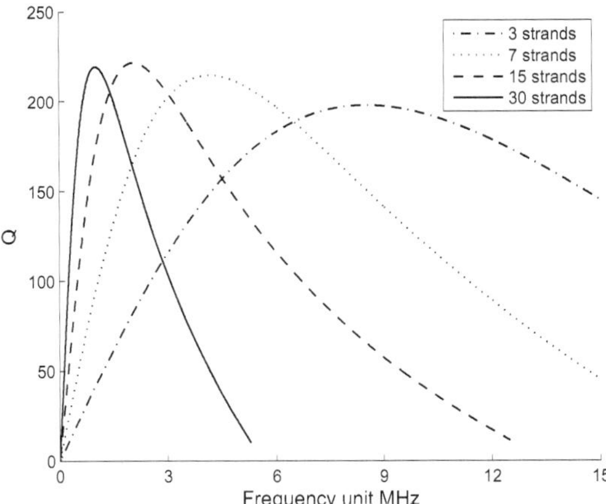

Fig. 15. Q vs Frequency curves for coils with the same cross sections but different numbers of strands.

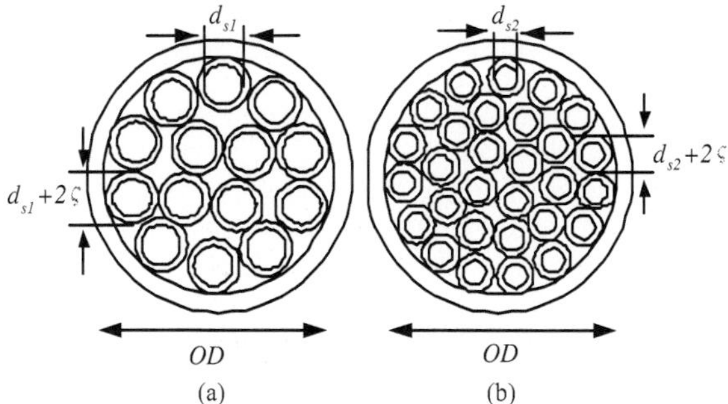

Fig. 16. Cross sections of individual turns. (a) Bigger wire is used. (b) Smaller wire is used.

4.4 Diameter of single strand

Under the assumption that a coil's cross section, inductance, and area efficiency are fixed, the only method to reduce the power consumption from proximity effect is to decrease the size of a single strand and keep the OD unchanged, as shown in Fig. 16.

If the displaced current is not a concern, a reduction of wire size helps to reduce the power dissipation from proximity effect. Reduction of the wire size is limited in practical coil design for several reasons.

First, once the target frequency is lower than f_h, the power dissipation from proximity effect is less than the DC power dissipation, thus a further decrease of r_s only slightly reduces the AC power dissipation.

Second, given the thickness of coating, cross section and inductance, reducing the size of a single strand inevitably decreases area efficiency of an individual strand, thus increasing the DC power dissipation.

Third, experimental results show that an increase of the number of strands increases strand-level displaced currents hence reduces the self-resonant frequency of a coil [Bartoli et al. (1996)].

Fourth, small wire is more expensive.

When f_h is equal to or greater than the target frequency, power dissipation from proximity effect should not be a major concern.

For coils used in an inductive link, the Q and f_{self} are critical. Using the assumption that coils are restricted to a particular geometry set, an analytical closed form solution is derived to determine the Q and f_{self}. Not only providing a close form solution, our derivation also allows the designer to set criticality on parameters and find an optimal solution.

5. References

Atluri, S. & Ghovanloo, M. (2005). Design of a wideband power-efficient inductive wireless link for implantable biomedical devices using multiple carriers, *Proceedings of the 2nd International IEEE EMBS Conference on Neural Engineering*, pp. 533–537.

Baker, M. & Sarpeshkar, R. (2007). Feedback analysis and design of RF power links for low-power bionic systems, *IEEE Transactions on Biomedical Circuits and Systems* 1(1): 28–38.

Bartoli, M., Noferi, N., Reatti, A. & Kazimierczuk, M. (1996). Modeling litz-wire winding losses in high-frequency power inductors, *IEEE Power Electronics Specialists Conference (PESC)*, pp. II: 1690–1696.

Berleze, S. & Robert, R. (2003). Skin and proximity effects in nonmagnetic conductors, *IEEE Transactions on Education* 46(3): 368–372.

Carter, G. (1967). *The electromagnetic field in its engineering aspects*, Longman.

Chaimanonart, N., Olszens, K., Zimmerman, M., Ko, W. & Young, D. (2006). Implantable RF power converter for small animal in vivo biological monitoring, *International Conference of the Engineering in Medicine and Biology Society(EMBS)*, IEEE, pp. 5194–5197.

Chen, Q., Konrad, A. & Biringer, P. (1993). A hybrid approach to the solution of open boundary eddy current problems under tm field excitation, *IEEE Transactions on Magnetics* 29(6): 2485–2487.

Chen, Q., Wong, S., Tse, C. & Ruan, X. (2009). Analysis, design, and control of a transcutaneous power regulator for artificial hearts, *IEEE Transactions on Biomedical Circuits and Systems* 3(1): 23–31.

Dorf, R. (1993). *The Electrical Engineering Handbook*, CRC Press, Boca Raton.

Dwight, H. (1945). *Electrical Coils and Conductors*, New York: McGraw-Hill.

Egiziano, L. & Vitelli, M. (2004). Time-domain analysis of proximity effect current driven problems, *IEEE Transactions on Magnetics* 40(2): I: 379–383.

Ferreira, J. (1992). Analytical computation of ac resistance of round and rectangular litz wire windings, *IEEE Proceedings of Electric Power Applications, Part B* 139(1): 21–25.

Ferreira, J. (1994). Improved analytical modeling of conductive losses in magnetic components, *IEEE Transactions on Power Electronics* 9(1): 127–131.

Galbraith, D., Soma, M. & White, R. (2007). A Wide-band efficient inductive transdennal power and data link with coupling insensitive gain, *IEEE Transactions on Biomedical Engineering* 34(4): 265–275.

Hamici, Z., Itti, R. & Champier, J. (1996). A high-efficiency power and data transmission system for biomedical implanted electronic devices, *Measurement Science and Technology* 7(2): 192–201.

Harrison, R. (2007). Designing efficient inductive power links for implantable devices, *IEEE International Symposium on Circuits and Systems(ISCAS)*, IEEE, pp. 2080–2083.

Heller, A. (2006). Potentially implantable miniature batteries, *Analytical and Bioanalytical Chemistry* 385(3): 469–473.

Kazimierczuk, M. & Jozwik, J. (2002). Resonant dc/dc converter with class-E inverter and class-E rectifier, *Industrial Electronics, IEEE Transactions on* 36(4): 468–478.

Kendir, G., Liu, W., Bashirullah, R., Wang, G., Humayun, M. & Weiland, J. (2004). An efficient inductive power link design for retinal prosthesis, *Proceedings of the 2004 International Symposium on Circuits and Systems(ISCAS)*, Vol. 4, IEEE.

Kendir, G., Liu, W., Wang, G., Sivaprakasam, M., Bashirullah, R., Humayun, M. & Weiland, J. (2005). An optimal design methodology for inductive power link with class-E amplifier, *IEEE Transactions on Circuits and Systems I: Regular Papers* 52(5): 857–866.

Knutson, J., Naples, G., Peckham, P. & Keith, M. (2002). Electrode fracture rates and occurrences of infection and granuloma associated with percutaneous intramuscular electrodes in upper-limb functional electrical stimulation applications, *Journal of Rehabilitation Research and Development* 39(6): 671–684.

Ko, W., Liang, S. & Fung, C. (1977). Design of radio-frequency powered coils for implant instruments, *Medical and Biological Engineering and Computing* 15(6): 634–640.

Krauss, H., Bostian, C. & Raab, F. (1980). *Solid state radio engineering*, Wiley New York.

Li, W., Rodger, D., Weiland, J., Humayun, M. & Tai, Y. (2005). Integrated flexible ocular coil for power and data transfer in retinal prostheses, *International Conference of the Engineering in Medicine and Biology Society (EMBS)*, pp. 1028–1031.

Liu, W., Vichienchom, K., Clements, M., DeMarco, S., Hughes, C., McGucken, E., Humayun, M., De Juan, E., Weiland, J. & Greenberg, R. (2000). A neuro-stimulus chip with telemetry unit for retinal prosthetic device, *IEEE Journal of Solid-State Circuits* 35(10): 1487–1497.

Lotfi, A., Gradzki, P. & Lee, F. (1992). Proximity effects in coils for high frequency power applications, *IEEE Transactions on Magnetics* 28(5): II: 2169–2171.

Massarini, A. & Kazimierczuk, M. (1997). Self-capacitance of inductors, *IEEE Transactions on Power Electronics* 12(4): 671–676.

Massarini, A., Kazimierczuk, M. & Grandi, G. (1996). Lumped parameter models for single- and multiple-layer inductors, *IEEE Power Electronics Specialists Conference (PESC)*, pp. I: 295–301.

Murgatroyd, P. (1989). Calculation of proximity losses in multistranded conductor bunches, *IEE Proceedings, Part A, Science, Measurement and Technology* 136(3): 115–120.

Raab, F. (1977). Idealized operation of the class E tuned power amplifier, *IEEE Transactions on Circuits and Systems* 24(12): 725–735.

Raab, F. (2002). Class-E, class-C, and class-F power amplifiers based upon a finite number of harmonics, *IEEE Transactions on Microwave Theory and Techniques* 49(8): 1462–1468.

Ravazzani, P., Ruohonen J., Tognola, G., Anfonsso, F., Ollikainen, M., Ilmoniemi, R. & Grandori, F. (2002). Frequency-related effects in the optimization of coil for magnetic stimulation of nervous system, *IEEE Transactions on Biomedical Engineering* 49(5): 463–471.

Rogers, J. & Plett, C. (2010). *Radio frequency integrated circuit design*, Artech House Publishers.

Sadiku, N. (1994). *Elements of Electromagnetics*, Orlando, FL: Sounders College Press.

Sauer, C., Stanacevic, M., Cauwenberghs, G. & Thakor, N. (2005). Power harvesting and telemetry in cmos for implanted devices, *IEEE Transactions on Circuits and Systems I* 52(12): 2605–2613.

Sivaprakasam, M., Liu, W., Humayun, M. & Weiland, J. (2005). A variable range bi-phasic current stimulus driver circuitry for an implantable retinal prosthetic device, *IEEE Journal of Solid-State Circuits* 40(3): 763–771.

Smith, B., Tang, Z., Johnson, M., Pourmehdi, S., Gazdik, M., Buckett, J. & Peckham, P. (2002). An externally powered, multichannel, implantable stimulator-telemeter for control of paralyzed muscle, *Biomedical Engineering, IEEE Transactions on* 45(4): 463–475.

Sokal, N. (2001). Class-E RF power amplifiers, *QEX [published by American Radio Relay League, 225 Main St., Newington, CT 06111-1494, USA], Issue* 204: 9–20.

Takura, T., Somekawa, T., Sato, F., Matsuki, H. & Sato, T. (2006). Improvement of communication area for implantable signal transmission system with ferrite chip core, *Journal of Applied Physics* 99.

Theogarajan, L. & Wyatt, J. (2006). Minimally invasive retinal prosthesis, *IEEE International Solid-State Circuits Conference (ISSCC)*, pp. 54–55.

Wang, G., Liu, W., Sivaprakasam, M. & Kendir, G. (2005). Design and analysis of an adaptive transcutaneous power telemetry for biomedical implants, *IEEE Transactions on Circuits and Systems I: Regular Papers* 52(10): 2109–2117.

Wang, G., Liu, W., Sivaprakasam, M., Weiland, J. & Humayun, M. (2005). High efficiency wireless power transmission with digitally configurable stimulation voltage for retinal prosthesis, *International Conference of the Engineering in Medicine and Biology Society (EMBS)*, pp. 543–546.

Yang, Z., Liu, W. & Basham, E. (2007). Inductor modeling in wireless links for implantable electronics, *IEEE Transactions on Magnetics* 43(10): 3851–3860.

Zierhofer, C. & Hochmair, E. (2002). High-efficiency coupling-insensitive transcutaneous power and data transmission via an inductive link, *IEEE Transactions on Biomedical Engineering* 37(7): 716–722.

11

Pressure Measurement at Biomedical Interfaces

Vincent Casey[1], Pierce Grace[2] and Mary Clarke-Moloney[2]
[1]Physics Department, University of Limerick
[2]Vascular Research Unit, Mid Western Area Regional Hospital, Limerick
Ireland

1. Introduction

The science of pressure measurement is mature with many available pressure measurement technologies some of which have their origins dating back to steam power and the industrial revolution. Along with temperature, the use of pressure as a general physiological parameter is well established and it may be accurately and reliably determined for a wide range of medical applications and environments involving liquids and gases (Mootanah & Bader, 2006). However, pressure is also commonly used in biomedical engineering and medicine to quantify the mechanical interaction between biomedical interfaces such as those arising between tissue and support surfaces (Tissue Viability Society, 2010; Shelton et al, 1998), e.g. beds, seats, prosthesis, and between tissue and pressure applying devices such as tourniquets (Doyle & Taillac, 2008), bandages (Partsch et al, 2006), and surgical instruments. The term interface pressure may be used in such contexts. The materials constituting such interfaces are, in general, not fluidic but connective and so they may support shear and torsional forces in addition to the normal hydrostatic force quantified as pressure/interface-pressure (average normal force per unit area).

The non-fluid nature of many biomedical interfaces means that current mature quantitative pressure measurement technologies are not well matched to the biomedical interface environment, i.e. they are not media compatible. Pressure measurement devices may also contribute to erroneous and anomalous data since they need to be deployed at the interface site and so are necessarily intrusive (Casey et al, 2001; O'Brien & Casey, 2002). These problems have acted as a barrier to the more general use of pressure measurement to characterise mechanical interactions at biomedical interfaces. In cases where such measurements have been used, the resulting data is often degraded due to interface and sensor contact artifacts ultimately leading to difficulties with reproducibility and reliability (Buis & Convery, 1997; Fay & Brienza, 2000).

Significant benefits would arise if a reliable low cost interface pressure measurement technology were available for emergency, acute and home medical care environments as well as areas such as Intravenous Regional Anaesthesis (Casey et al, 2004), compression therapy and pre-hospital emergency care. Such a technology would allow improved diagnostics and treatments, early hazard warning and could save lives (Kragh et al, 2009; Noordin et al, 2009). In this chapter, modifications to readily available MEMS devices are described which render the devices suitable for general purpose non-invasive pressure and pressure gradient measurement at biomedical interfaces. Sample data is presented for a range of biomedical application environments including pneumatic and non-pneumatic tourniquets, bandages and support stockings. It is hoped that this will stimulate more extensive on-body testing and verification of the technology resulting in pressure measurement solutions which will contribute to a better understanding of the biomedical interface environment ultimately leading to improved efficacy of treatments and procedures and simple standardised measurement protocols.

2. Background

The forces that occur in many biomedical contexts are distributed over areas rather than being discrete, i.e. applied at a point with a well defined (arbitrary) direction. Consequently, pressure (defined as the average force per unit area acting normal to the surface) is the parameter of choice in quantifying many biomechanical interactions. In the case of static fluids acting on surfaces, pressure reliably quantifies the forces involved since we may neglect shear forces and the only forces acting will be perpendicular to the surface (i.e., hydrostatic). Common pressure measurement sensors and transducers will provide high integrity data for such applications, e.g. arterial blood pressure, urethral pressure and intra compartmental pressure.

In this work we are concerned with interfaces between two continuum phases one of which is living tissue and the other a biomedical device or support surface. Specifically we are interested in the non-invasive measurement of pressures at such biomedical interfaces. These arise, for instance, in compression therapy using bandages (Ferguson-Pell et al, 2000; Ghosh et al, 2008), which is the mainstay of venous leg ulcer treatment (Grace, 2003). In these situations specific pressures are required to achieve the desired clinical outcome. If the pressure is too low no clinical benefit will accrue while if the pressure is too high an adverse outcome may result. Pneumatic tourniquets are routinely used in intravenous regional anaesthesia to occlude arteries and to control anaesthetic and provide a bloodless operating field (McEwen, 1994). Tourniquets are also deployed in combat (Kragh et al, 2009; Noordin et al, 2009; Tien et al, 2008), in civilian emergency settings (Lee et al, 2007) and for remote emergency care (Fludger & Bell, 2009). Patient tissue is also compressed by support surfaces, e.g. beds, wheelchairs and prosthetics (Ferguson-Pell et al, 1993). With most of these applications one may expect shear (Wertheim et al, 1998) and torsional forces to coexist with normal forces, giving rise to resultant compound forces. Standard pressure measurement solutions that assume fluidic transmission of pressure will not yield reliable quantitative data in such applications.

Ideally, the physician would like to know the actual forces acting (e.g. normal and shear forces at a limb/organ surface; radial force near an arterial wall; tensile force on nerve tissue) at specific locations in order to inform decisions in relation to patient well-being and diagnosis. However, such detailed information is not routinely available (Shear Force Initiative, 2010) unless through expensive MRI (Oomens et al, 2010) and other imaging techniques. Standard pressure sensors and transducers are often used at biomedical interfaces because of their ready availability. However, the conditions under which verifiable data may be obtained for such use are rather restrictive. For instance, in the case where tissue of Poisson's ratio 0.5 is being perfectly hydrostatically compressed, i.e. the entire volume of the tissue is subject to a uniform normal force per unit area, then, the pressure within the tissue or at interfaces, will correlate exactly with the hydrostatically applied pressure. However, this is rarely the case in practice. Poisson's ratio for real tissue may vary over a range from about 0.2 to 0.4 (Cristalli et al, 1993). With departures of Poisson's ratio from 0.5 (incompressible), deformation of the tissue will occur and with connective tissue, shear forces, as well as compressive forces, will arise

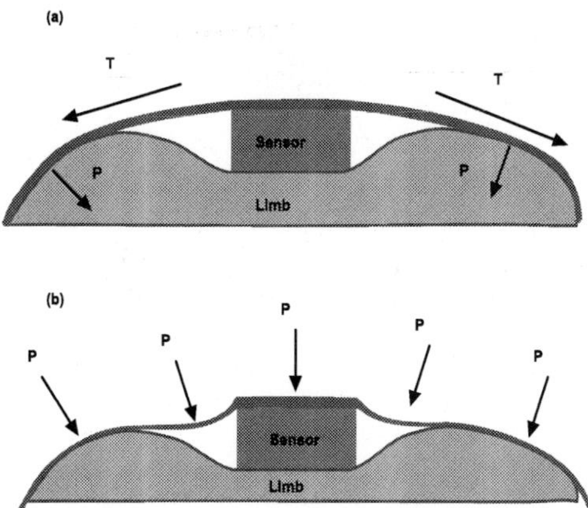

Fig. 1. Deformation of interface region due to intrusive rigid sensor. The 'Hammocking' effect for (a) Tension devices such as bandages and combat application tourniquets (CATs), (b) Pneumatic tourniquet type devices.

at the surface of the tissue and within its bulk. Additionally the pressure applicator rarely encompasses the entire body but is more usually applied to a localised section or sections of tissue. Time variant deformation of the compressed tissue is likely in such instances due to migration of tissue fluids from the compressed region. Inclusions such as bones and other hard tissue further complicate the situation. This makes it very difficult to compare values of interface pressure obtained by different research groups and has lead some groups to seek an alternative metric (e.g. statistical (Shelton et al, 1998), Limb Occlusion Pressure, LOP (Aziz, 2009; McEwen et al, 2002), deformation (Oomens et al, 2010), etc.) to reliably quantify the effects of compression on real tissue. Others question whether pressure or interface pressure should be used at all (Fay & Brienza, 2000; Oomens et al, 2010).

Further complications (Allen et al, 1993; Buis & Convery, 1997) arise with the measurement of pressure at biomedical interfaces using pressure sensors deployed at the interface since such sensors are in the main intrusive and may introduce measurement artifacts and errors. For instance, rigid sensors will prise the interface materials away from each other, Fig. 1 and give rise to the so called hammocking effect (O'Brien & Casey, 2002) which is pressure dependent and leads to anomalously high readings and difficulties with calibration. Low profile(van Hout et al, 2003), minimally intrusive, conformal sensors (Polliack et al, 2000) are available which allow localized (Picopress, 2009; van den Kerckhovea et al, 2010) and full body interface pressure mapping (distributed pressure) (Lai & Li-Tsang, 2009; Pliance, 2011). The latter systems can involve sophisticated signal processing and special calibration procedures tailored to the application environment. For such applications the most important technical performance parameters are repeatability, resolution, drift, creep and accuracy in that order (Skelton & Lott, 2007). Low cost, universal biomedical pressure and pressure gradient measurement systems with high spatial resolution which provide continuous, accurate, dynamic data flow for important biomedical applications are currently not readily available.

Our objective is to develop an inexpensive biomedical interface pressure transducer (BIPT) with minimum cross sensitivity to shear forces. We believe that such a sensor would provide reproducible and reliable data for a wide range of application environments without overly complicated measurement procedures and protocols. This would increase the confidence of practitioners in the use of biomedical interface pressure data. The realisation of such a technology would represent a significant milestone in a much larger project seeking to develop an integrated sensor solution with capability to discriminate between, and quantify, both shear and pressure at biomedical interfaces.

3. Functional specification for an optimal biomedical interface pressure transducer

An optimal pressure transducer (Paris-Seeley et al, 1995) for non invasive pressure measurement at biomedical interfaces should combine the following features (Partsch et al, 2006):

- be capable of measuring the pressure applied by any one of a specified number of medical devices to a portion of a human body surface or tissue, in the pressure range 0-750 mmHg (0-100 kPa);
- permit fast, convenient and intuitive calibration checking in the target application environment;
- typical measurement errors should be less than 1% of full scale;
- hysteresis/creep over a one-hour time period should be less than $\pm$ 1% of full scale;
- allow easy compensation for ambient pressure and temperature variations;
- be digitally compatible, i.e. easily interfaced to modern microcontrollers;
- have similar compliance to that of the target tissue;
- conform to curved, compliant tissue surfaces with radii of curvature as low as 2 cm (pediatric cuffs);
- be low profile (<2 mm high) with very small footprint (<1 cm^2)
- must not significantly alter the tissue device interface;
- be made from biocompatible materials;

In addition to the above the transducer should be immune to electromagnetic interference, conform to relevant electrical standards, must not present electrosurgical or thermal hazards, must fail safe and, for reusable devices, must be sterilizable using at least one of the various conventional sterilization techniques. The performance to cost ratio must be high to allow deployment in disposable devices.

4. MEMS as a candidate technology for pressure measurement at biomedical interfaces

The specification for an optimal BIPT is very demanding. However, the combination of electrically excited solid state sensors/transducers with modern microcontroller/digital processors provides an excellent platform for the development of high performance, versatile, application specific measurement system solutions (Barker, 2000). Miniature general purpose pressure sensor devices are typically piezoresistive, i.e. transform a mechanical stress into a resistance signal. Of the various electrical device properties, electrical resistance is the easiest one to measure precisely over a wide range at moderate cost. The piezoresistive

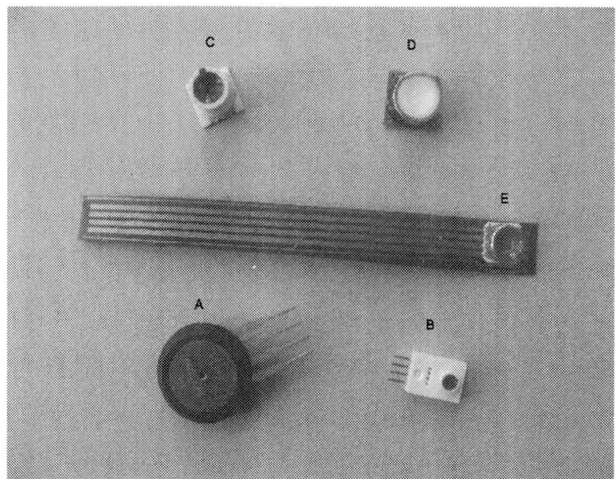

Fig. 2. Some MEMS pressure sensors: A, MPX2000 and B, MPX2300DTI, Freescale Semiconductor Inc.; C, MS Series, Merit Sensor Systems; D, HRPF0100, Hope RF (Rhopoint Components); E, MS5201, Measurement Specialties (Intersema) as mounted on flex-circuit.

silicon pressure transducer is a solid state, microelectromechanical system (MEMS) (Wise, 2007) sensor fabricated using silicon integrated circuit processing technology. Therefore, it benefits from the economies of scale and enhanced performance associated with silicon technology yielding devices with high performance to cost ratios. Devices may be voltage or current excited. They may be simple transducers, i.e. convert pressure/pressure changes to resistance or may be complete pressure transmitters converting the pressure signal to a standard electrical signal (analogue or digital) via integrated processing electronics. Consequently, MEMS technology deserves serious consideration as a candidate technology for the development of transducers for the measurement of pressure at biomedical interfaces. High performance, low cost MEMS pressure sensors, Fig. 2 are used extensively in fluidic pressure measurement for medical and biomedical applications (Wise, 2007). Their use in consumer goods such as wrist-watch altimeters and depth gauges is providing a technology push to lower profile, compact, devices (Epcos, 2009). Similarly, biomedical applications are providing an incentive to develop so called 'media compatible' devices (Lucas Novasensor, 2010). Recently, progress has been reported with the development of prototype MEMS devices having tissue compatibility, i.e. capable of measuring tissue contact pressures directly without gas/liquid lines/interfaces (Casey et al, 2010).

The delicate silicon micromachined membrane in MEMS pressure sensors must be mounted on a rigid chip carrier and it, plus any integrated circuitry and bond wires, must be protected from the ambient and target measurement environments to avoid drift in specifications and/or failure. Consequently, MEMS pressure sensors necessarily involve rigid packaging which may be many times the volume of the enclosed microchip, in order to confer the desired mechanical and chemical immunity. Typical package heights, without coupling nozzles, range from 3 to 5 mm for off-the-shelf devices. This, combined with package footprints of $1cm^2$ or more, and cumbersome electrical interconnects (Fig. 2) has made this attractive technology overly intrusive for general medical interface pressure measurement applications. Furthermore, these devices are optimized for measurement of pressure in fluid environments where shear coupled forces either do not exist or are negligible compared to the normal hydrostatic forces which are easily coupled to the sensing diaphragm either directly or via a soft gel barrier layer. Therefore, the many benefits of MEMS pressure sensing technology could be exploited in pressure measurement at biomedical interfaces if the devices could be rendered media/tissue compatible while simultaneously making them minimally intrusive so as to reduce sensor related artifacts. Modifications to off-the-shelf MEMS pressure sensors are therefore necessary in order to address these coupled challenges.

5. MEMS sensor selection

Pressure sensors including MEMS pressure sensors, are generally categorised according to the reference pressure used with them. Three categories are common: absolute pressure sensors measure pressure relative to vacuum; differential pressure sensors measure pressure relative to a reference pressure line; gauge pressure sensors measure pressure relative to ambient atmospheric pressure. Differential devices tend to be formed with a fluid line connector to the reference port thereby adding to the overall size/profile of the device. Gauge devices, on the other hand, need only an in-plane hole to port to the atmosphere and so can have minimal overall size and profile. Absolute devices have a sealed reference chamber typically enclosing a high vacuum. MEMS biomedical pressure transducers normally operate at ambient atmospheric pressure and so either gauge or absolute devices may be used.

The sensor pressure range is dictated largely by the end application and the sensitivity required. Bandage and support surface environments, for instance, require relatively low range sensors, e.g. 0-100 mmHg or lower, while IVRA and general tourniquet measurements require a dynamic range stretching to in excess of 500 mmHg while prosthetic interface measurement devices require higher ranges again. Another important range related sensor parameter is the overpressure rating. Because of the necessary direct tissue-MEMS contact, devices must be able to withstand and recover from burst pressures and directly applied forces that are multiples of the maximum rated pressure. Overpressure ratings of two to three times the maximum rated pressure should be considered in order to ensure a reasonable engineering safety margin.

In addition to the normal electrical performance characteristics of high accuracy, high sensitivity, low drift, linearity, fast response time and low hysteresis desirable in all sensors, a full bridge configuration, energized by a unipolar supply is an additional desirable characteristic for biomedical pressure logging applications and digital product development. Small size is critically important in order to reduce the intrusiveness of the device and thereby minimize artifacts due to hammocking (Casey et al, 2001) and shear and to increase spatial resolution. The device must also be mechanically robust and so a packaging technology which provides good mechanical and chemical protection combined with low profile package interconnects is essential. Surface mount (SM) packaging is a low cost assembly and interconnect technology which meets these needs and at the same time offers a route to low cost automated product assembly.

The size of the sensor port exposed to the target media is also critically important in selecting a MEMS sensor for the measurement of pressure at biomedical interfaces. This port must be filled with a tissue compatible layer (interface layer) which couples the media/tissue pressure to the MEMS sensing element. The interface layer must be soft but durable and must not adhere to the target media. If the port opening is narrow, surface tension forces between the barrier medium/gel and the port walls can detrimentally affect sensor performance, particularly response time. It can also introduce hysteresis and significantly reduce device

Manufacturer	Merit	Measurement Specialties Inc.			Hope RF
Type	MS Series	MS5401	MS1451	MS5201	HRP0100
Range (mmHg)	0-774	0-750	0-258	0-750	0-750
(kPa)	0-103	0-100	0-34	0-100	0-100
Type	Diff.	Abs.	Gauge	Gauge	Gauge
Package	Cer.	Cer.+Met.	Cer.+Plas.	Cer.+Met.	HR4+Met.
Length (mm)	6.4	6.4	7.6	7.6	9.2
Width (mm)	6.4	6.2	7.6	7.6	9.2
Height (mm)	2.94	2.8	3.68 (3.2mm)	2.8	4.5
Port Dia. ϕ (mm)	4.4	4.4	4.0	6.0	7.4
AAR	0.31	0.38	0.22	0.34	0.51
Contacts	8 DIL	8 DIL	8 DIL	8 DIL	4 Pads

Table 1. Sample sensors used in modified MEMS Biomedical Interface Pressure Transducers (AAR - Active Area ratio).

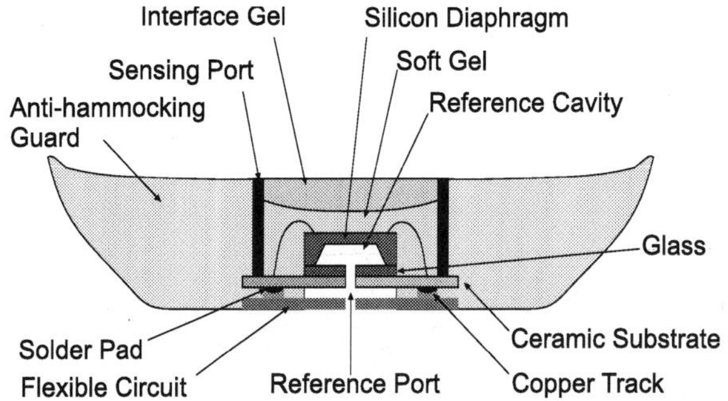

Fig. 3. Schematic representation of a gel modified MEMS pressure sensor with conformable anti-hammocking guard.

sensitivity (see Sec. 7 below). A useful index in selecting a suitable MEMS device for interface pressure measurement is the Active Area Ratio (AAR), i.e. device port size to footprint ratio. Ideally this should be as close to unity as possible but values of 0.3-0.5 are common with current technologies, see Table 1. Of course the overall footprint size will determine the spatial resolution in array configurations designed for gradient measurement and so should be as small as possible, e.g. less than one square centimetre. The package should preferably be made from biomedically compatible materials. Fortunately, many MEMS pressure sensor vendors provide SM package options designed for medical/biomedical applications. Many devices have on-chip processors which provide digital output. While this is desirable in many instances, it can add to package size, device cost, and impose constraints on follow on circuitry in the signal path.

The data in Table 1 summarises key specifications for a sample range of commercially available MEMS pressure sensors meeting the above design criteria or which may be easily modified to meet the criteria. The table is not a comprehensive survey of all vendors and their matching products but rather is a sample of devices that were tested by this group.

6. MEMS sensor modifications

Many MEMS devices come with barbed or plain molded plastic front port connection tubes (Meas. Specialties Inc., MS5201) but otherwise match the selection criterion outlined for biomedical interface sensors. For such devices the package tube and chamber top cap were removed using a cutting jig specially made for the purpose. The jig holds the sensor firmly in place while providing a reference surface along which a sharp blade is moved in order to slice off the cap and tube in a single clean movement, i.e. without sprinkling debris onto the isolation gel and sensitive chip/diaphragm.

Sensors were reflow soldered onto flexible circuit, see Fig. 3, to facilitate electrical interconnection while deployed on body. Polimide flexible circuit with copper cladding was patterned with pad landing areas matched to the sensor surface mount device to be used. Copper tracks extended from the bridge excitation and bridge output pads along a flying lead section where the track pitch was matched to that of standard zero insertion force (ZIF) connectors, i.e. pitch of 1.27 mm. Solder paste was spread onto the pads using a stencil cut from polimide tape. The sensor device was placed onto the substrate and manually aligned with the solder coated pads. The combination was placed in a solder reflow oven with a plateau temperature of 185° C.

Once the sensor was mounted on the flexible circuit, and in cases where a protective gel die coating was not already present, a soft ion free silicone gel (Dow Corning Sylgard 527) with viscosity less than 1000 cps and low hardness (Intersema, 2004), was added, after vacuum degassing, to protect the sensor die and bond wires and to provide a humidity barrier while leaving head room for the interface layer. The protective gel was allowed set for at least two hours before adding interface gel. The interface gel fills the cavity completely and provides a durable non-stick surface which may be brought directly into contact with body tissue or pressure applying materials/parts. Room temperature vulcanising silicon rubber with hardness in the range, Shore A, 23-30, was found to work reasonable well for this purpose. The two gel combination resulted in robust, durable, zero volume displacement devices.

A polydimethylsiloxane (PDMS) anti-hammock guard was moulded around the sensor assembly in order to provide a constant well defined sensing area/volume at the target interface. The rear end of the guard was flush with the rear surface of the flexible circuit and the guard front surface was flush with the top surface of the port interface gel surface. The objective of the symmetrical design is to ensure that all top and bottom guard-contact-forces, apart from those coming to bear on the sensing area, are mutually canceled. The overall geometry of the guard was diamond shaped with contoured side walls and a slight lip on the front surface perimeter which gives an air-tight cupping effect against tissue. The PDMS/flexible circuit in the region of the rear port of the MEMS sensor (gauge devices) was drilled to provide an opening to the rear port of the sensor thereby allowing equilibration of the device with ambient atmospheric air pressure. A composite teflon/PDMS anti-hammock guard was also tested but did not offer any benefits over a pdms guard on its own. A photograph of various biomedical interface pressure transducer (BIPT) configurations is shown in Fig. 4.

7. Results

Preliminary device testing and characterisation was carried out using an isolated nominal 6V supply. A teflon nozzle was machined to fit over the MEMS sensor front port to allow device testing and calibration under air. The other end of the nozzle was connected to an

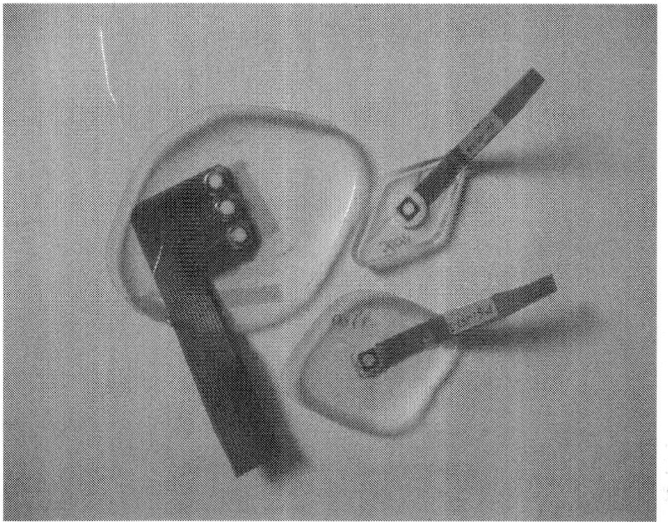

Fig. 4. Discrete and array Biomedical Interface Pressure Transducers (BIPT) incorporating modified MEMS pressure sensors.

inflation bulb via a mercury manometer. A soft silicone washer provided an airtight seal between the nozzle and the sensor port. This allowed easy, reliable testing of the transducers in the 0-300 mmHg pressure range. The stiffness of the interface gel is critical to device performance. PDMS (Shore A, 50) was found to be too stiff introducing large zero offsets and drift plus hysteresis. Q-gel which is a very soft silicone gel strongly adhered to tissue and other media and divided when separated from the support tissue. Room temperature vulcanising silicones on the lower end of the hardness scale (Shore A 23-30) such as that supplied by Rubson for general domestic sealing applications were found to be very durable and non-stick while still being soft enough to allow in-specification MEMS performance. Mould makers' silicone rubber (T20 and T30, Alec Tiranti Ltd, www.tiranti.co.uk) was also used successfully as MEMS media interface gel as was room temperature vulcanising silastic rubber from Dow Corning. The hardness of both the mold makers' rubber and the silastic rubber could be lowered by dilution with silicone fluid. In addition, it was possible to vacuum degas these rubbers to reduce air bubble entrapment which can lead to dimensional instability, over time, in the cured rubber. Device specifications (zero offset, sensitivity and response time), after gel modifications, remained within the manufacturer's specifications for all devices tested, see calibration curve, Fig. 5.

7.1 Pressure measurement under a surgical pneumatic tourniquet

On body data logging was carried out using a National Instruments USB data acquisition card (USB-6008) to interface the transducers to a laptop computer running NI Labview 8.5. This device can accommodate 4 differential analogue input channels and also has an analogue output voltage channel which may be programmatically controlled within the range 0-5V. This was used to provide a reference voltage (3V) to a unity gain operational amplifier powered by the USB-6008 5V supply. The output of the buffer amplifier was used to

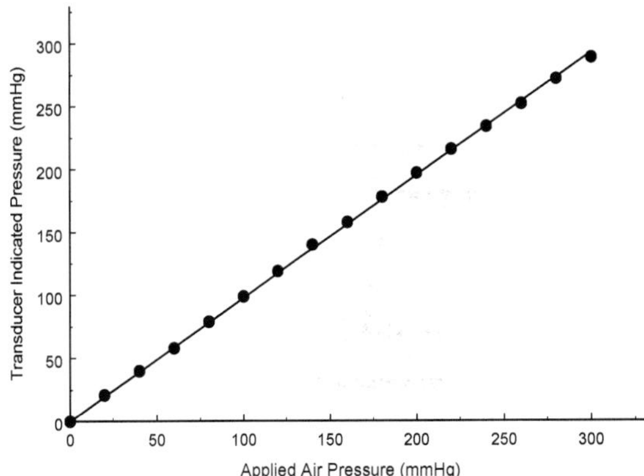

Fig. 5. BIPT calibration curve using air applied pressure (inflate-deflate cycle).

energise the MEMS sensor(s). An interconnect card with 4 Berg, 4-way sockets allowed easy make-break connections between the transducers and the USB-6008. A Labview program (Virtual Instrument) was developed to facilitate transducer calibration, data display and data storage. This configuration allowed data logging of up to four transducers simultaneously. One channel was generally reserved as a reference channel to monitor tourniquet inflation pressure or ambient atmospheric pressure.

The following protocol was adopted for on-body measurements using a 100 mm wide Zimmer pneumatic tourniquet cuff. Subjects were seated with their arm (normally left arm) resting on the bench and extended. Measurements were made at two locations on each subject's arm: the inner lower arm and the inner upper arm (biceps). The BIPT was zeroed and calibrated at 150 mmHg set-point (air applied pressure using the same bulb/manometer as used for cuff inflation). The BIPT was placed directly onto the tissue with the sensing volume facing the tissue and the interconnect lead taped in place. One round of cotton wool was loosely wrapped around the arm and sensor to cushion the tourniquet. The tourniquet was centered over the sensor and fitted so that it gave a snug fit to the arm. The measurement sequence comprised initial zeroing of the transducer on the bench; application of the sensor and tourniquet; inflate/deflate cycle (0, 20, 50, 100, 150....300, 250,...100, 50, 20, 0); zeroing of the BIPT in situ under cuff if required; repeat inflate/deflate cycle.

The results for two complete log sequences are shown in Fig. 6. The BIPT indicated pressures track the tourniquet applied pressure but at slightly elevated values particularly at the higher inflation pressures. A slight negative BIPT pressure is indicated after completion of the first inflate-deflate cycle. This is largely due to the temperature sensitivity of the device's zero pressure offset voltage which drops as the sensor temperature rises to body temperature. Re-zeroing the transducer at zero tourniquet pressure while still under the cuff (see second 'Lower Arm' cycle) after body-temperature equilibration increases the degree of elevation in indicated pressures, i.e. + 25 mmHg at 300 mmHg tourniquet inflation pressure. The

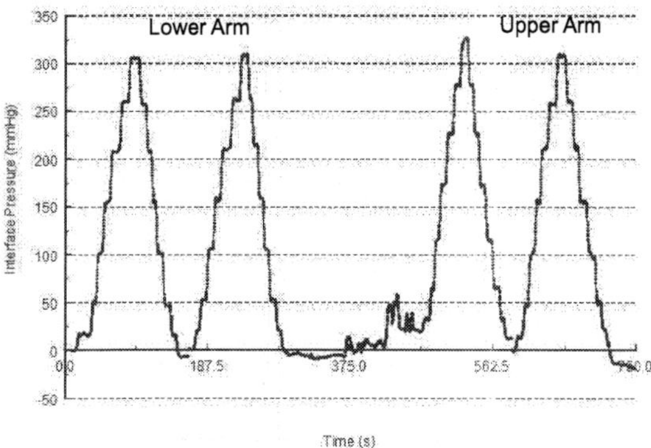

Fig. 6. Interface pressure measured under 10 cm Zimmer Cuff on Lower and Upper Arm

sharp pressure transitions after 375 s in Fig. 6 occur as the tourniquet cuff is tightly re-fitted onto the arm over the transducer prior to inflation. The BIPT therefore allows one judge the tightness of fit of the cuff (not detectable using the cuff inflation pressure gauge). This initial cuff applied pressure provides a further elevation in the indicated pressures which may be compensated/nulled by re-zeroing the transducer once it has settled onto the arm, i.e. after a complete inflate-deflate cycle. The elevated BIPT indicated pressures are probably due to residual sensitivity of the transducer to shear forces and tissue contact artifacts.

Data-log sequences were carried out on 11 healthy volunteers in order to gauge the spread in BIPT indicated pressures for a sample of limb sizes and tissues. Subjects comprised 4 females (age range 22-52) and 7 males (age range 18-54). The mean and standard deviation of the sub-tourniquet pressure readings obtained for all 11 subjects at the inflate/deflate set-points (second cycle) for both lower and upper arm locations is presented in Table 2. The error is the ratio of the standard deviation to set-point value at each set-point expressed as a percentage, i.e. relative set-point error. The relative errors are highest at low pressures where offset is most pronounced. In the critical range for intravenous regional anaesthesia (100-300 mmHg) errors can be as large as 8%. The composite data for all 11 subjects plotted in Fig. 7, also displays a positive skew in the error particularly at higher pressures, as noted earlier with the single inflate-deflate plots and attributed to residual shear sensitivity.

In tests where large positive offset errors were indicated, (upper arm Fig. 8) flexing of the arm muscle, i.e. tensioning and relaxing it a number of times, while the cuff was inflated to pressures greater than 200 mmHg reduced the offset error. This supports the view that errors in BIPT indicated pressures, where they arise, are largely due to the coupling of shear forces to the BIPT sensing area.

7.2 Emergency and Military Tourniquet (EMT) and Combat Application Tourniquet (CAT®)

Body extremities - arms and legs - bear the brunt of traumatic injury in both civilian and military settings. Quickly addressing life-threatening hemorrhage from an extremity with the

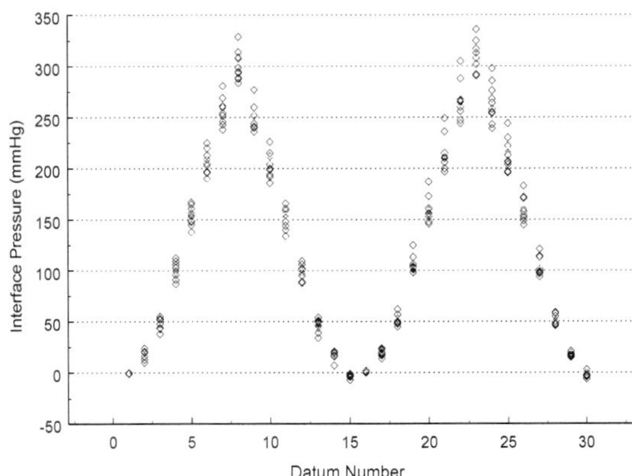

Fig. 7. Measured interface pressure data from the upper and lower arms (second inflate/deflate cycle) of 11 subjects. Inflate-deflate sequence, 0, 20, 50, 100 ..300, 250, ..50, 20,0 mmHg.

	Lower Arm			Upper Arm		
P (mmHg)	Mean (mmHg)	SD	Error	Mean (mmHg)	SD	Error
0	0	0		1	1	
20	18	4	22%	20	3	14%
50	48	5	11%	51	4	9%
100	101	8	8%	104	8	8%
150	153	8	5%	159	11	7%
200	206	10	5%	214	14	7%
250	255	12	5%	265	17	7%
300	301	13	4%	314	18	6%
250	252	12	5%	264	17	7%
200	205	11	6%	214	14	7%
150	151	9	6%	160	11	7%
100	98	6	6%	104	8	8%
50	47	6	11%	51	4	9%
20	15	4	22%	19	3	15%
0	-4	1		-2	3	

Table 2. Mean and standard deviation of readings for all 11 subjects at the inflate/deflate set points for both lower and upper arm locations.

use of a relatively simple maneuver such as applying a tourniquet can reduce morbidity since limb-injury exsanguination is a leading cause of preventable trauma deaths on the modern

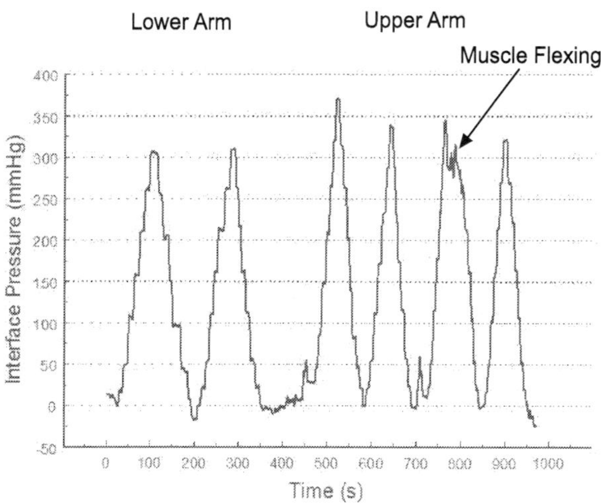

Fig. 8. Interface pressure on arm of subject with large shear artifacts relieved by muscle flexing.

battlefield (Rush et al, 2009). The primary function of the tourniquet is to occlude major arteries in order to save life (Walters et al, 2005). However, in cases where the limb may be salvageable, it is important that the tourniquet pressure should not be excessive and should be evenly and uniformly applied around the limb (Glinz & Jameson, 2010). In these and many other biomedical settings, interface pressure gradients are as important as peak or local pressure values (Oomens et al, 2010). It is a relatively simple matter to arrange the BIPT described here into multisensor arrays, see Fig. 4. The planar three sensor array configuration is useful for determining the local pressure and pressure gradients under cuffs, bandages and other extensive biomedical pressure applying devices. Clearly the spacing may be varied to suit the particular pressure applicator, and more sensors may be added as desired since the flexible carrier circuit is easily customised. Gradient data for a pneumatic emergency and military tourniquet (EMT, Delfi Medical Innovations Inc.) (Lee et al, 2007), is presented in Fig. 9. In this case the gradient transducer comprised three gel modified Measurement Specialties Inc., MS5201-AD MEMS sensors mounted linearly onto a single flexible circuit substrate on 1 cm centres. A PDMS anti-hammock guard was moulded around the combination with similar profile to that described earlier for individual devices. First inflate-deflate cycle data indicate anomalously high readings for set-points in excess of 100 mmHg. However, second cycle data shows much better correlation between set-point data and sub-EMT pressure measurements. This is attributed to cuff settling and consequent reduction in shear forces acting on the overall transducer structure. The second cycle pressure data indicates a drop in pressure of about 20 mmHg/cm either side of the centre of the cuff at pressures greater than 200 mmHg, i.e. a relatively low pressure gradient.

Corresponding data obtained for different transducer positions under a combat application tourniquet (CAT, Composite Resources, USA) applied to the upper leg is shown in Fig.

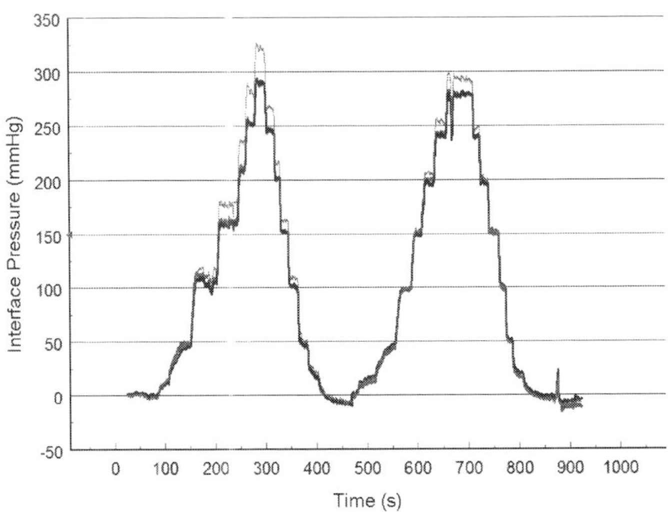

Fig. 9. Concurrent interface pressure from a BIPT three sensor array placed transversely under an EMT (Delfi Medical Innovations Inc.) on the upper leg for two inflate deflate cycles. Sensor positions: central, black; distal, red; proximal, blue.

10. The transducer was placed transversely under the CAT and tightened by turning the windlass handle through four full revolutions before reversing the procedure to release the applied pressure. The first cycle shows data for the transducer placed centrally under the CAT. The subsequent two cycles correspond to transducer positions progressively closer to the CAT distal edge. The last two cycles correspond to CAT positions off-centre and progressively closer to the proximal edge of the CAT. The CAT position was not changed during these measurements. The first spike plus plateau with pressures in the range 20-40 mmHg is due to tightening of the CAT velcro strap. The subsequent spikes followed by plateaus in pressure correspond to full turns of the windlass handle. The spikes are largely due to the requirement to twist the windlass rod/handle past the securing structure before allowing it to untwist slightly back into the securing hook (Casey & Little, 2010). The pressure gradients indicated for the CAT (250-300 mmHg/cm for peak applied pressures of 300-400 mmHg) are considerably greater than those for the EMT consistent with previously published results (Noordin et al, 2009) with particularly high gradients close to the CAT edges. Data for the gradient transducer placed longitudinally under the CAT is presented in Fig.11 indicating relatively small pressure variations circumferentially under the CAT. While shear forces are also likely to contribute to indicated BIPT pressure values for the CAT, a fully independent pressure measurement is needed in order to access the degree of shear contribution. One possibility is to incorporate a dynamometer into the tensioning strap of the CAT (Casey & Little, 2010) from which pressure might be inferred using the LaPlace rule and the limb dimensions.

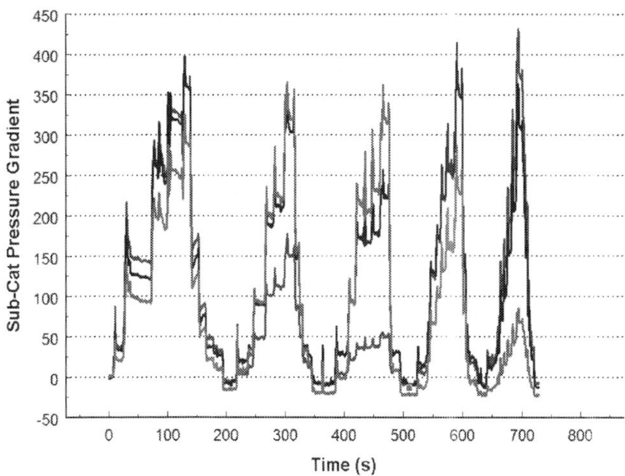

Fig. 10. Concurrent interface pressure for a Combat Application Tourniquet (CAT) on the upper leg with BIPT three sensor array placed centrally (A) and at two positions distal to (B) and proximal to (C) the central position. (Array sensor positions: central, black; distal, red; proximal, blue)

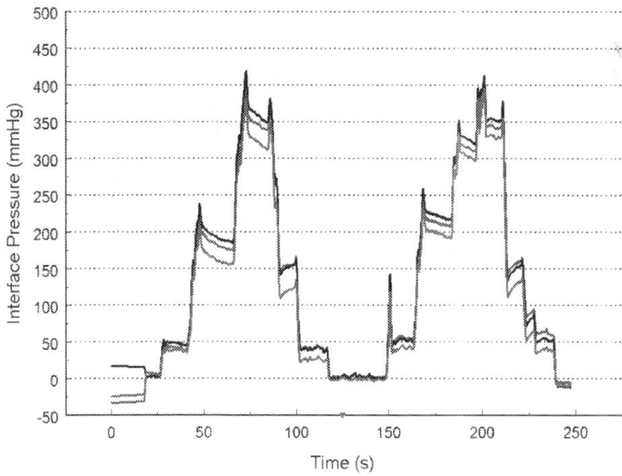

Fig. 11. Concurrent interface pressure for a CAT on the upper leg with the BIPT three sensor array placed longitudinally under the CAT. First cycle - outer leg position; second cycle - inner leg position.

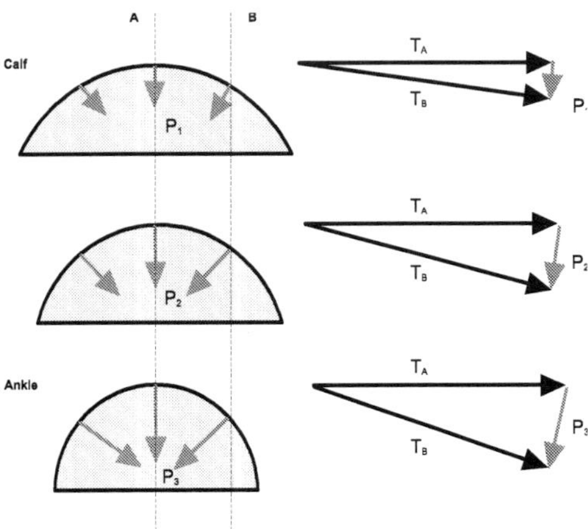

Fig. 12. According to the law of LaPlace, a constant tension membrane produces a pressure which is proportional to the local curvature.

7.3 Bandages and support stockings

In compression therapy, bandages or support stockings are used to aid venous return and reduce venous hypertension which results from chronic venous insufficiency. The pressures involved are much lower than those encountered in tourniquet applications (artery occlusion) and are typically in the 20-50 mmHg range. The tension in the bandage or stocking membrane produces a compression or normal pressure on the supporting limb according to the so called 'Law of LaPlace'. The pressure is proportional to the membrane tension, the number of turns (membrane layers) and the curvature of the limb, $P \propto TN\kappa$ where the curvature $\kappa = 1/R$ for a cylindrical geometry of radius R. For a bandage applied with constant tension and extending from foot/ankle up to and including the calf, regions of high curvature such as the region around the ankle, see Fig. 12, will be subject to high interface pressure compared to a region of low curvature such as the calf. A properly applied bandage should, therefore, produce a pressure profile which decreases from ankle to calf. Such a pressure profile is believed to aid venous return of blood from the ankle region and produce a favourable effect on subcutaneous interstitial pressures (Giswold & Moneta, 2005)

Bandages are designed to generate a pressure in the ankle region of about 40 mmHg dropping to about 20 mmHg just distal to the knee. A sub-bandage interface pressure transducer based on micromoulded (soft-lithography) elastomer springs and flexible circuit technology has been used to measure sub-bandage pressures (Casey et al, 2010). The modified MEMS devices described here were also tested under bandages and support stockings. The interface pressure transducer was placed 5 cm above the medial malleolus facing the limb and held in place using adhesive tape. The bandages were applied to the leg by a trained practitioner and the interface pressure data was logged. The results obtained for a Smith & Nephew *ProGuide* bandage are shown in Fig. 13. The bandage generates a steady pressure of around 40 mmHg in the subject while seated. The fast dynamic response of the sensor also shows the effect of muscle flexing, i.e. the muscle pump action. Previous studies have shown that muscle contraction in the presence of a compression bandage or stocking results in a significant increase in venous blood flow (Lyons et al, 2002). Standing and elevation produce

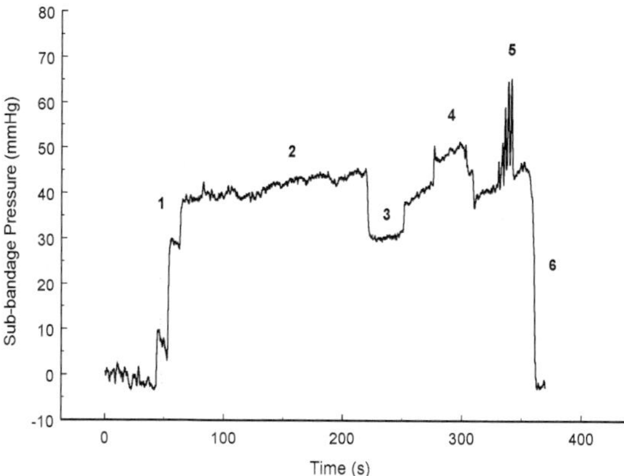

Fig. 13. Interface pressure measured with BIPT located above the medial malleolus under a Smith & Nephew ProGuide bandage: 1 Bandage Application, 2 Sitting with foot on floor, 3 Foot elevated, 4 Standing, 5 Flexing calf muscle, 6 Bandage removal.

pressure fluctuations above and below the value for a seated subject respectively, as expected. Similar results were obtained using Smith & Nephew, *Profore* bandages. The interface pressure measured above the medial malleolus under a Medivan CCL1 support bandage is shown in Fig. 14. According to the manufacturers, the CCL1 should generate pressures in the region of 30-40 mmHg at the malleolus.

8. Discussion and conclusions

The measurement of pressure at biomedical interfaces is complicated on the one hand by the continuum nature of the interface media and on the other by the intrusiveness of the pressure transducer. The latter problem may be ameliorated to some extent using low profile, small foot print transducers with flexible contoured packaging designed to conform to the biomedical interface shape. Biomedical media compatibility is a more difficult problem to solve. However, the results obtained with modified MEMS BIPT devices presented here for a range of biomedical interface environments are encouraging. These transducers have been rendered bio-media compatible by filling the sensor port with two gels, a MEMS protection gel and an interface gel. The first gel protects the delicate silicon diaphragm, chip and bond wires while the second interface gel couples the biomedical tissue or pressure applying element to the sensor. A contoured anti-hammocking guard ensures there is no void or lift-off zone created by the sensor at the interface. Since MEMS pressure sensors are manufactured to operate across a wide range of pressures, devices may be matched to specific applications, i.e. 0-100 mmHg for sub-bandage pressure measurement; 0-500 mmHg for sub-tourniquet measurements and 0-750 mmHg or higher for prosthetics.

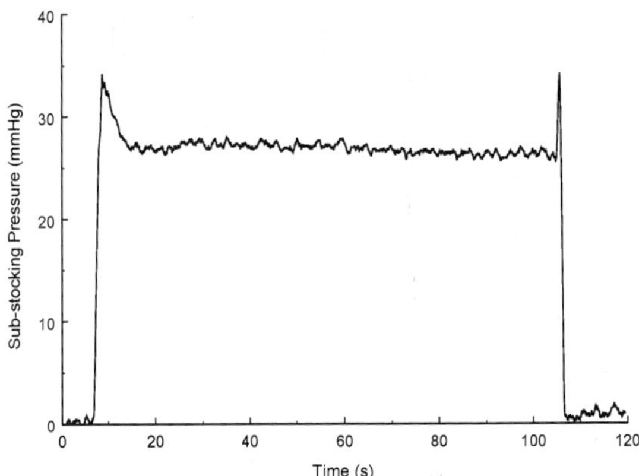

Fig. 14. Interface pressure measured under a Medivan CCL1 support stocking with the sensor located above the MM.

While the primary operating mechanism of the BIPT is the deflection of an elastic diaphragm, the actual deflections involved are microscopic and therefore negligible on the scale of the overall BIPT size. The transducer is effectively a constant volume device. In particular, the sensing volume comprising the two-gel filled sensor port does not change under typical biomedical pressures and so pressure dependent hammocking artifacts are avoided. Transducers may be reliably calibrated using inflated bladders, set-point loads or, as done routinely in this work, by using a pressure air-line coupled to a suitable sensor shroud, i.e. plastic chamber which provides an air-tight seal around the sensing area. The latter approach has the advantage of being independent of the actual interface/application environment. The sensor performance characteristics, such as calibration stability, sensitivity, response time and hysteresis of these devices stays within or very close to the MEMS pressure sensor manufacturer's specification.

MEMS modified BIPTs may also be configured as multisensor arrays. With footprints less than 0.25 cm^2 linear arrays with sensor density of 2/cm are feasible. Two sided flexible circuit interconnect with vias/through-holes would allow two dimensional arrays with sensor density of 4/cm^2. Lower density two dimensional arrays could be implemented using single sided flexible circuit provided there is space to route the interconnect tracks between the devices. While it is useful to know absolute or peak pressures in many medical and biomedical settings, there are many instances when knowledge of the local pressure gradients is equally important. For example, in the management of venous leg ulcer disease, establishing a pressure gradient from ankle to knee using compression is an essential part of the treatment. A wide-spacing extensive linear array of BIPTs would facilitate the application of the correct pressure gradient and provide objective evidence of good bandaging technique which is 'operator dependent' thereby improving safety and aiding training. Equally, the simple close-spaced three sensor configuration described here can provide useful information on pressure gradients under pneumatic and non pneumatic tourniquets indicating hazard conditions and cuff tightness.

In close-spaced array form, the PDMS guard/flexible-circuit combination acts as a carrier for the individual sensors. The overall structure can conform to limb curvature while maintaining a stable interface contact zone. For instance a linear BIPT paediatric array could accommodate in excess of 20 pressure sensors on a limb with radius of curvature of 2 cm using currently available devices (array thickness less than 3 mm). However, while PDMS is compliant, it is significantly stiffer than the target soft tissue for some biomedical applications. In the measurement of biomedical interface pressures there is, in general, a trade off between compliancy and accuracy. Compliant, totally conformable sensors present very significant calibration and stability challenges in real applications. Rigid structures provide the highest performance specifications but are intrusive and may be subject to significant measurement artifacts. The design used here minimizes the compromise on performance while addressing the compliance/conformability need to a useful extent for applications involving sub-bandage and sub-tourniquet settings.

The temperature change from room to body temperature produces changes in the span and zero offset voltage in simple voltage driven piezoresistive MEMS devices. There are many standard temperature compensation techniques available for full-bridge piezoresistive elements ranging in sophistication from simple passive component circuits to microcontroller implemented correction algorithms using integrated temperature measurement. As the offset voltage temperature-sensitivity is significantly larger than that of the span sensitivity, it is possible to compensate for offset, in many instances, by simply re-zeroing the sensor when on-body after allowing sufficient time for the device to reach body temperature. Gauge and differential sensor configurations should not require ambient pressure compensation provided the reference port is vented to the ambient atmosphere. However, this may not always be possible or advisable in biomedical interface pressure measurement since the open port can present a contamination risk and compromise the integrity of the sensor as well as presenting sterilisation problems for reusable devices. If the reference port is sealed or if absolute devices are used, then ambient pressure variations may be monitored using a reference sensor, and appropriate corrections applied to measured interface pressures.

The BIPT devices show residual sensitivity to shear and frictional forces. These can vary with body tissue properties as seen in the sample population data presented. Such shear forces can be reduced using protocols specific to the particular application. For instance, shear contributions with pneumatic tourniquet cuffs may be reduced by using an initial inflate-deflate cycle to 'settle' the cuff onto the limb. However, even with such protocols, standardised procedures and controls, there is still significant scope for variability in results, since 'no two humans, even of the same weight and stature, are anatomically identical' (Shelton et al, 1998). This situation is likely to continue unless a completely shear independent biomedical interface pressure transducer emerges. Clearly, a lubrication gel may be added to the sensor-tissue interface to decouple such shear forces. However, the use of such gels could pose a contamination problem in surgical applications and has therefore been avoided in this work which targets a fully solid state biomedical interface pressure measurement solution.

On-going developments in the MEMS pressure sensor industry in the area of miniature altimeters and depth gauges as well as navigation technology is resulting in ever smaller devices. The availability of such small MEMS devices will allow for further reduction in the intrusiveness of BIPTs, and, increases in the spatial resolution of BIPT arrays. Clearly, for volume market applications, custom MEMS package designs optimised for the measurement of pressures at biomedical interfaces could be justified using bare chip MEMS available from many foundries. Bond wire strain-relief-loops to the top-side of MEMS silicon die adds to overall device. Custom devices with under-side bonding of the MEMS die to the substrate carrier would significantly reduce overall transducer height. Combined with flexible surface mount technology, integrated 16 bit analogue to digital converters and digital interfaces, it should be possible to develop biomedical interface pressure measurement products and applications which are minimally intrusive, compliant, temperature and ambient pressure compensated, and which can be reliably calibrated, all at relatively low cost. Further reduction or complete elimination of the residual shear sensitivity of these devices will be the focus of future work aimed at developing a general purpose biomedical interface pressure transducer which does not call for any special 'standardised' procedures or application specific protocols, in order to yield reliable biomedical interface pressure data.

9. Acknowledgements

The authors would like to acknowledge the provision of copper clad polimide flexible circuit by PPI Ltd., Waterford, a range of Profore and Proguide bandages from Smith & Nephew Ltd., an Emergency and Military Tourniquet (EMT) from Delfi Medical Innovations Inc., Vancouver and sample MS1451 devices from Measurement Specialties Ltd, Shannon.

10. References

Allen, V., Ryan, D. W., Lomax, N. & Murray, A., (1993) Accuracy of interface pressure measurement systems, *J. Biomed. Eng.*, Vol. 15:344-348

Aziz, E. S., (2009) Tourniquet use in orthopaedic anaesthesia, *Current Anaesthesia & Critical Care*, Vol. 20:55-59

Tissue Viability Society (2010) Laboratory measurement of the interface pressures applied by active therapy support surfaces: A consensus document, *J. Tissue Viability* Vol. 19:2-6

Barker, B., (2000) Interfacing Pressure Sensors to Microchip's Analog Peripherals, Microchip Technology Inc., Data Sheet AN695.

Buis, A. W. P. & Convery, P., (1997) Calibration problems encountered while monitoring stump/socket interface pressure with force sensing resistors: Techniques adopted to minimise inaccuracies, *Prosthetics and Orthotics International*, Vol. 21:179-182

Casey V., Griffin, S. & O'Brien, S. (2001) An investigation of the hammocking effect associated with interface pressure measurements using pneumatic tourniquet cuffs. *Medical Engineering and Physics*, Vol. 23:511-517

Casey, V., O'Sullivan, S. & McEwen, J. (2004) Interface pressure sensor for IVRA and other biomedical applications, *Medical Engineering & Physics* Vol. 26(No.2):177-182

Casey, V. & Little, E., (2010) Novel Interface Pressure Transducers for Tourniquets and Other Medical Devices, *CMBEC 33*, Vancouver, Canada.

Casey, V., McAree, B., Moloney & M.C., Grace, P. (2010) Wearable sub-bandage pressure measurement system, *IEEE Sensors Applications Symposium (SAS)*, Limerick, pp.41-45.

Cristalli, C. Ursino, M. Palagi, F. & Bedini, R., (1993) FEM simulation and experimental evaluation of the 'squeezing' phenomenon in Riva-Rocci blood pressure measurement, *Computers in Cardiology*, 655-658

Doyle, G. & Taillac, P. (2007) Tourniquets: A review of current use with proposals for expanded prehospital Use, *Prehospital Emergency Care*, Vol. 12(No.2):241-256

See 'World's smallest barometric sensor'; URL:*http://www.epcos.com* Also ABS1200E data sheet.

Fay, B. & Brienza, D., (2000) What is Interface Pressure?, *Proc. 22nd Annual EMBS Conf.*, Chicago, pp.2254-2255

Ferguson-Pell, M. & Cardi, M. D., (1993) Prototype development and comparative evaluation of wheelchair pressure mapping system, *Assist. Technol.*, 78-91

Ferguson-Pell, M., Hagisawa, S. & Bain, D.(2000) Evaluation of a sensor for low interface pressure applications, *Medical Engineering & Physics*, Vol.22:657-663

Fludger, S. & Bell, A., (2009) Tourniquet Application in a Rural Queensland HEMS Environment, *Air Medical Journal* Vol.28:291-293

Giswold, M.E. & Moneta, G.L., (2005). Non operative treatment of chronic venous insufficiency, *in* Rutherford R.B. (ed.), *Vascular Surgery* 6th Ed., Vol.2, Philadelphia, pp.2241-2250

Glinz, K.L. & Jameson, M., (2010) Development and technical evaluation of military tourniquets and emergency tourniquets for pre-hospital settings, *CMBEC 33*, Vancouver, Canada.

Ghosh, S., Mukhopadhyay, A., Sikka, M. & Nagla, K.S., (2008) Pressure mapping and performance of the compression bandage/garment for venous leg ulcer treatment, *J Tissue Viability*, Vol.17:82-94

Grace, P. A. (2003) The Management of Leg Ulcers, Editorial, *Irish Medical Journal*, Vol. 96:37

Intersema Application Note, AN508, "Mounting of Pressure Sensor Dice", Intersema Sensoric SA, URL:www.intersema.ch

Kragh Jr., J.F., Walters, T.J., Baer, D.G., Fox, C.J., Wade, C.E., Salinas, J. & Holcomb, J.B. (2009) Survival with emergency tourniquet use to stop bleeding in major limb trauma, *Ann Surg*, Vol.249:1Ű7

Lai, C. H. Y. & Li-Tsang, C. W. P., (2009) Validation of the Pliance X System in measuring interface pressure generated by pressure garment, *Burns*, Vol. 35:845-851

Lee, C., Porter, K. M, & Hodgetts, T. J., (2007) Tourniquet use in the civilian prehospital setting, *Emerg Med J*. Vol.24:584-587

See 'NPI-12 Stainless Steel Media Isolated Sensor' Lucas NovaSensor, URL:http://www.ge-mcs.com/en/pressure-mems/mems-sensors/npi-12-series-novasensor.html

Lyons, G.M., Leane G.E. & Grace P.A., (2002) The effect of electrical stimulation of the calf muscle and compression stocking on venous blood flow velocity *Eur J Vasc Endovasc Surg* Vol.23:564-566

McEwen, J. A. (1994) Apparatus for Intravenous Regional Anesthesia, *US Patent Number 5352195*

McEwen, J.A., Inkpen K. B. & Younger A., (2002) Thigh tourniquet safety. Limb occlusion pressure measurement and a wide contoured cuff allow lower cuff pressure. *Surgical Technologist*, Vol.21:55-62)

Mootanah, R. & Bader, D. (2006) *Pressure Sensors*, Wiley Encyclopedia of Biomedical Engineering, Online Publication, Wiley

Noordin, S., McEwen, J., Kragh, J., Eisen, A. & Masri, B., (2009) Surgical Tourniquets in Orthopaedics, *J Bone Joint Surg Am* Vol.91:2958-2967

O'Brien, S. & Casey, V., (2002) Numerical and asymptotic solutions for hammocking. *Quart J Mech App Math* Vol.55:409-420

Oomens, C., Loerakker, S. & Bader, D., (2010) The importance of internal strain as opposed to interface pressure in the prevention of pressure related deep tissue injury, *Journal of Tissue Viability*, Vol.19:35-42

Paris-Seeley N.L., Romilly D.P. & McEwen J.A. (1995) A compliance-independent pressure transducer for biomedical device/tissue interfaces. Proceedings of RESNA (Rehabilitation Engineering Society of North America Conference), Montreal

Partsch, H., Clark, M., Bassez, S., Benigni, J.P., Becker, F, Blazek, V., et al. (2006) Measurement of lower leg compression in vivo: recommendations for the performance of measurements of interface pressure and stiffness: consensus statement. *Dermatol Surg*, Vol.32(No.2):224-232

PicoPress Compression Measurement System, Microlab Elettronica, Italy, URL:*www.microlabitalia.it*

Pliance System, novel Germany, URL:*http://novel.de/novelcontent/pliance*

Polliack, A. A., Sieh, R. C., Craig, D. D., Landsberger, S., McNeil, D. R. & Ayyappa, E, (2000) Scientific validation of two commercial pressure sensor systems for prosthetic socket fit, Prosthetics and Orthotics International, Vol.24:63-73

Rush, R.M., Beekley, A.C., Puttler, E.G. and Kjorstad, R.J., (2009) The mangled extremity, *Curr Probl Surg*, Vol.46:851-926

Shelton, F., Barnett, R & Meyer, E. (1998) Full-body interface pressure testing as a method for performance evaluation of clinical support surfaces, *Applied Ergonomics*, Vol.29(No.6):491-497

Shelton, F. & Lott, J. W., (2007) Conducting and interpreting interface pressure evaluations of clinical support surfaces, *Geriatric Nursing*, Vol.24:222-227

Shear Force Initiative, National Pressure Ulcer Advisory Panel (US).

Tien, H.C., Jung, V., Rizoli, S.B., Acharya, S.V. & MacDonald, J.C. (2008) An evaluation of tactical combat casualty care interventions in a combat environment, *J Am Coll Surg*, Vol.207:174-178

Van den Kerckhovea, E., Fieuwsc, S., Massagéd, P., Hierneri, R., Boeckxe, W., Deleuzef, J.P., Laperreg, J & Anthonissenh, M., (2010) Reproducibility of repeated measurements with the Kikuhime pressure sensor under pressure garments in burn scar treatment, *Burns*, Vol.33:572-578

van Hout, J., Scheurer, J. & Casey, V. (2003) Elastomer microspring arrays for biomedical sensors fabricated using micromachined silicon molds, *J. Micromech. Microeng.*, Vol.13:885-891

Walters, T.J., Wenke, J.C., Kauvar, D.S., McManus, J.G., Holcomb, J.B. & Baer, D.G., (2005) Effectiveness of self-applied tourniquets in human volunteers *Prehosp Emerg Care* Vol.9(No.4):416-422

Wertheim, D., Melhuish, J., Llewellyn, M., Hoppe, A., Williams, R. & Harding, K., (1998) An integrated instrumentation approach to the study of wound healing, Proceedings 20th Annual International Conference of the IEEE Engineering in Medicine and Biology Society, Vol. 20:1760-1761

Wise, K. D., (2007) Integrated sensors, MEMS, and microsystems: Reflections on a fantastic voyage, *Sensors and Actuators A: Physical*, Vol.136:39-60

12

Sensor Developments for Electrophysiological Monitoring in Healthcare

Helen Prance
University of Sussex
United Kingdom

1. Introduction

Recent years have seen a renewal of interest in the development of sensor systems which can be used to monitor electrophysiological signals in a number of different settings. These include clinical, outside of the clinical setting with the subject ambulatory and going about their daily lives, and over long periods. The primary impetus for this is the challenge of providing healthcare for the ageing population based on home health monitoring, telehealth and telemedicine. Another stimulus is the demand for life sign monitoring of critical personnel such as fire fighters and military combatants. A related area of interest which, whilst not in the category of healthcare, utilises many of the same approaches, is that of sports physiology for both professional athletes and for recreation. Clinical diagnosis of conditions in, for example, cardiology and neurology remain based on conventional sensors, using established electrodes and well understood electrode placements. However, the demands of long term health monitoring, rehabilitation support and assistive technology for the disabled and elderly are leading research groups such as ours towards novel sensors, wearable and wireless enabled systems and flexible sensor arrays.

All of these areas could, in principle, benefit from advances in telehealth and telerehabilitation (Winters, 2002). In the case of neurological disorders there is, for example, a recognized need for in-home and unsupervised rehabilitation (Johnson et al., 2007). The problems of taking data from individuals and interfacing with remote data networking systems are being solved by many workers and organizations, using a wide range of wireless communication technologies (see, for example, Dabiri et al., 2009; Ruffini et al. 2007). In addition, some of the interactive gaming technology is beginning to find a place in rehabilitation and as assistive technology for the physically disabled. However, there is still a need for the acquisition of high quality signals at the front-end, using sensors which are easy to attach, comfortable to wear for extended periods, and which provide reliable data under a wide range of operating conditions.

This chapter begins by considering the range of electrophysiological signals and the challenges of acquisition; introduces the application of electrophysiology to healthcare; briefly reviews the standard electrodes and sensors used and their limitations; and then considers in detail two specific areas of development which have particular relevance for the healthcare applications of interest.

2. Classes of electrophysiology signals

The human body generates a wide range of electrical potentials. Most of these arise through the firing of neurons, and associated electrical signal pathways, which respond to stimuli and control the body's physiological responses. These electrical potentials can be detected at the surface of the body and the measurements are classed according to the functional source of the potential. Thus, the electrocardiogram (ECG, or EKG) is a measure of the heart's electrical activity; the electroencephalogram (EEG) arises from the firing of neurons in the brain; the electromyogram (EMG) results from muscular activity; and the electroretinogram (ERG) records the electrical response of cells in the retina. The electrooculogram (EOG) has a rather different source, due to changes in the direction of the standing potential across the eye, and is a useful indicator of eyeball movement. Most of these measurements can be performed subcutaneously and, for clinical diagnosis, such invasive measurements give the most accurate and complete information. For example, in the clinical setting, needle EMG measurements provide the most accurate, spatially resolved measurements. However, their invasive character means that they are unsuitable for extended monitoring, particularly in non-clinical and unsupervised settings such as the home (Hogrel, 2005; Stegeman et al., 2000). In the context of long term monitoring of state of health, it is necessary for measurement techniques to be non-invasive and straightforward for non-specialist personnel to undertake. This dictates, among other things, that the signals be acquired from the surface of the body, or off-body, and this chapter is concerned solely with these types of measurement.

The ease with which surface potentials can be measured depends primarily on their amplitude and the spatial resolution with which they must be acquired. For a typical surface ECG measurement the peak deviation of the QRS complex is around 1-2 mV on the chest (V1–V5 lead positions) and 0.3-0.8 mV on the periphery (I-lead position) (Hampton, 1992). More challenging is the detection of the foetal ECG which is typically an order of magnitude smaller, of order 100 µV at the surface of the mother's abdomen, and is difficult to deconvolute from the maternal ECG (Martens et al., 2007). The surface EEG also represents a weak signal, typically of order 10-100 µV (Ruch & Fulton, 1960). The spatial resolution with which an electrophysiology measurement must be made also varies widely. For cardiac function, and with the most sensitive electrodes (see section 5.1.2), a good ECG can be acquired anywhere across the heart, from a pair of electrodes spaced across the chest to a pair located on opposite wrists. On the other hand, meaningful information about muscular activity must be obtained with closely spaced EMG electrodes. In the most advanced high density arrays, there may be multiple electrodes each of diameter, or length, 1-10 mm and spaced by 2-10 mm (Merletti et al., 2001). For neuroelectrophysiology, using arrays of EEG electrodes, the spacing is typically a few cm. However, a high density array may have 256 electrodes located over the surface of the scalp, in which case the accuracy of placement is similar to that for EMG.

All electrophysiology signals are at relatively low frequency, a bandwidth of up to a few hundred Hertz will usually suffice, so high frequency response is not a problem. If clinical quality information is to be obtained from surface electrodes, then the signal bandwidth must be sufficient to capture all of the notable features. Clinical standards have been set such as those prescribed by the American Heart Association for the ECG (Kligfield et al. 2007). In this case, a bandwidth of 50 mHz to 150 Hz is required for high quality adult ECG measurements and this may need to be extended to 250 Hz for infant ECGs. Interference from other low frequency sources, including mains (line) noise, movement artefacts, and even competing surface potentials, does have to be addressed. This can determine the choice of electrode, as discussed in following sections, and will also dictate the signal conditioning and processing required in a given application.

All of the signals described above have been discussed in the context of measurements made on the surface of the body. However, with a sensor capable of detecting electrical potential or electric field, it is possible to detect a signal caused by body movements if the electrode is spaced off from the surface of the body. Although not in the same class of electrophysiology measurement as those discussed previously, this can provide valuable information. For example, the correlation of respiration, detected via chest wall movement, with heart rate variability is of interest for both the care of the elderly and in sports physiology. The detection of restricted limb movements could have application for assistive technology and human-machine interfacing. Finally, the straightforward detection of whole body movement may be of interest for monitoring single occupants of rooms in both a care home (Scanaill et al., 2006) and a custody setting (Ebling & Thomas, 2008). The source of such a signal is the change in ambient electric field caused by the movement of a dielectric and conducting object, the human body, (Beardsmore-Rust et al., 2010) and the significance of such a signal as both a problem and an opportunity is discussed further in section 5.1.2.

3. Applications of electrophysiology to healthcare

The areas of healthcare which can benefit from electrophysiological measurements include; the monitoring of long term, chronic conditions; the rehabilitation of patients following trauma; and the facilitation of assistive technology for the disabled. Amongst the most familiar applications of electrophysiology is the monitoring of heart conditions through measurement of the surface ECG. Less familiar, perhaps, is the use of the surface EMG for the assessment of muscle function. However, it provides a suitable set of illustrations of these applications to healthcare and will be used here as an exemplar.

3.1 Monitoring chronic conditions

The role of electrophysiological measurement in this area is well illustrated by considering the assessment of muscle function. There is a significant amount of published research which shows that the measurement of the surface EMG provides useful clinical information for the assessment and evaluation of neuromuscular conditions. It is considered particularly useful for the assessment of motion (gait), multiple muscle groups, response times, tremors, chewing and breathing (Pullman et al., 2000). The type of useful data which may be obtained includes the firing rate and shape of muscle activation signals, changes in muscle fibre conduction velocity (MFCV), muscle responses to electrical or magnetic stimulation, and evidence of reinnervation zones in motor neurone disease. The timing and activation of contraction between different muscles is considered particularly useful for neurological studies (DeLuca, 2008). All of the above parameters can be used to track changes in the progress of disease due to pathology, intervention or ageing (Maathuis et al., 2008), provided a system is available which allows for long term monitoring of the surface EMG. In order to compete with the quality of measurements provided by the needle EMG, it has been necessary to demonstrate that surface EMG systems can provide high spatial resolution, overcome cross-talk from adjacent muscles and include techniques to deconvolute spatial filtering due to volume conduction (Pullman et al., 2000).

3.2 Rehabilitation

In the area of rehabilitation, for example, of neuromuscular conditions such as stroke, there is a great deal of interest in designing techniques which motivate patients to develop and strengthen the correct voluntary muscle movements. The surface EMG is capable of detecting isometric muscle signals, that is, ones which are too weak to result in muscle movement (Reaz et al., 2006; Saponas et al, 2008). In principle, it can be used to provide early indication of voluntary muscle activation and, with visual feedback, promote the correct patterns of activity. However, it is significant that, while surface EMG may be used in a clinical setting to evaluate protocols and assess the use of equipment, many rehabilitation exercises currently use other technologies for data collection, such as position sensors and video (Johnson et al., 2007). This is usually because surface EMG electrodes are considered to be too complicated and awkward to place correctly, attach securely and wear for extended periods of time. In summary, there is a clear need for surface EMG systems to be made more robust, reliable and user-friendly if their capabilities are to be realized for rehabilitation and these requirements apply equally to other applications of electrophysiology to rehabilitation.

3.3 Assistive technology

Assistive technology for the promotion of access for people with severe disabilities aims to utilize whatever limited control an individual possesses. Much effort has been put into exploiting any residual muscle signals for the control of assistive systems. In addition, this area of research crosses over into the two fields of electronically controlled prostheses and of human-computer interaction (HCI) for the gaming and virtual reality industries (Reddy & Gupta, 2007; Saponas, et al., 2008). Often the only muscles under the patient's control are in awkward locations (face, eyes, shoulders, single finger, wrist). Some workers are exploring the use of the EOG signal as an eye tracker for human-computer interaction (Bulling et al., 2009) whilst others are exploring the use of muscle signals for the control of prostheses (Garcia et al., 2007). The same limitations of surface EMG for rehabilitation apply here; the difficulty of attaching existing electrodes securely, of wearing them for extended periods and the limited spatial resolution of most systems. As a result, simpler technologies are often employed, such as active capacitive sensors for the eye and brow (Rantanen et al., 2010), piezoelectric sensors for the brow (Felzer & Nordmann, 2008) and force sensitive resistors for the forearm (Amft et al., 2006). However, new developments in electrode technology for surface EMG, which are beginning to address these issues, are described in section 5.

4. Electrophysiology sensors

The techniques used to detect electrophysiological signals from the surface of the body are well reviewed in the literature (see, for example, Prutchi & Norris, 2005; Searle and Kirkup, 2000). The following brief overview of standard approaches illustrates some of the challenges being addressed by the more recent developments discussed in section 5.

The detection of electrophysiological signals has, for many years, relied on the use of 'wet' silver-silver chloride (Ag/AgCl) transducing electrodes which convert ionic current on the skin surface to electronic currents for amplification and signal conditioning. Such electrodes are cheap and disposable (thus avoiding potential cross-contamination) but require the use of a conducting gel between the electrode and the skin. Changes in the electrochemistry between the skin and the electrode do cause problems with baseline drift (DeLuca, 2008). Both this, and interference from the larger ECG signal, are a particular problem for surface EMG measurements (Allison et al., 2003). In addition, the use of the conducting gel is associated with problems of drying out, potential skin irritation, discomfort and shorting between adjacent electrodes in an array if not carefully placed. These problems make wet electrode systems unsuitable for use outside of the clinical environment and particularly unsuitable in terms of wearability for long term use.

A further complication is introduced by the development of high density electrode arrays, the most recent examples being for surface EMG mapping. A recent review editorial describes the difficulty of distributing gel to all of the electrodes such that it provides a high conductivity contact, whilst at the same time not shorting adjacent electrodes, and providing good contact stability during movement. It concludes that alternative, non-conducting electrodes could provide a better solution (Merletti, 2010).

A more user-friendly approach to surface measurements is to use 'dry' conducting electrodes, which make a resistive contact to the skin without the need for gel or paste (Chi et al., 2010; Searle & Kirkup, 2000). The electrode surface metal must be non-irritant, e.g. stainless steel. However, these electrodes still require careful skin preparation such as abrasion, suffer from changes in contact resistance due to sweating or skin creams, tend to be noisier than wet electrodes and can suffer from movement signal artefacts and charge sensitivity (Searle & Kirkup, 2000) if not very securely attached.

A different approach is to dispense with a DC, resistive coupling to the skin and instead couple to the surface potential capacitively, through a thin insulating layer (Clippingdale et al., 1991; Spinelli & Haberman, 2010). Because the signal fidelity does not rely on a good resistive contact, these electrodes do not necessitate skin preparation, or suffer from changes in contact resistance. As with dry electrodes, they can suffer from movement artefact and charge sensitivity (Searle & Kirkup, 2000). However, insulated electrode sensors are considered among the most promising for healthcare applications and their development is discussed in detail in section 5.1.

Much of the problem with noise is due to the impedance mismatch between the high source impedance and the following electronics. This is overcome by the use of active electrodes, commonly used for the detection of very low level EEG signals. These usually comprise an impedance buffer integrated into the wet or dry electrode structure. The disadvantage of active electrodes is that they can be bulky, require power to be supplied and, in most implementations, are not highly miniaturized for good spatial resolution. However, the use of high impedance, active electrodes is recommended for surface EMG (Clancy et al., 2002).

There has been considerable interest, driven by the demands of the applications described in section 3, in developing electrodes which can be deployed through, or embedded in, clothing. A number of workers have attempted to achieve this, using dry or insulating electrodes. For example, Kang et al. have designed both wet and dry, active electrodes fabricated using a nonwoven conductive fabric and flexible thick film circuitry which can be integrated into clothing (Kang et al. 2008). Measurements of the ECG from the torso, at rest and during exercise, indicate that the mounting is secure enough to minimize the movement artefact. However, the system will suffer from the same limitations as other wet and dry electrode structures and its durability remains to be proven. There have been attempts to realize non-contact electrodes by using dry electrodes to acquire electrophysiological signals through clothing; in all cases cotton-based to avoid electrostatic charging effects from man-made fabrics. The problem with this approach is that cotton is not a good, low-leakage insulator (Chi et al., 2010), so the noise performance of the sensor is compromised. A better solution is to use active, insulated electrodes to couple through clothing and the performance of these types of sensor is reviewed in section 5.1.3.

Whichever type of electrode is chosen, they are usually employed as either bipolar pairs or in linear arrays. For example, in the case of surface EMG systems for neurological disorders, it is recommended that some form of array is used (Merletti et al., 2001, 2003). This allows for; the acquisition of signals from multiple sites over a muscle to aid placement decisions; improved spatial resolution; improved noise elimination, through the comparison of signals from different electrodes; and the deconvolution of cross-talk between interfering muscle fibres. Linear arrays are available commercially but developments of high density two-dimensional arrays are also underway and described in section 5.2.

5. Electrophysiology sensor developments

Recent developments in sensor technology have seen progress in a number of areas, all of which have the potential to allow the healthcare challenges described in the Introduction to be addressed. Two aspects in particular are discussed below; advances in non-invasive electrophysiology measurement offered by a particular type of active, insulated sensor; and advances in the development of high-density and flexible electrode arrays.

5.1 The Electric Potential Sensor

There has long been a recognition that the reliance on wet electrodes does not allow for ease of use and long-term monitoring. As a result, steady progress has been made in the development of dry and insulating electrodes. In particular, the performance of active, insulated electrode sensors depends on the high input impedance at the front end. This performance was given a boost over a decade ago by the introduction of the Electric Potential Sensor (EPS) (Clippingdale et al., 1991, 1994a, 1994b; R.J. Prance et al., 1998). This is a generic electric field measurement technology which has a wide range of applications beyond electrophysiology, including materials testing and characterisation (Gebrial et al., 2006a), imaging of static charge distributions for forensic applications (Watson et al., 2010c), detection of pressure induced voltages in rocks (Aydin et al., 2009) and electric field detection of nuclear magnetic resonance signals (R.J. Prance & Aydin, 2007). As an insulated, active electrode sensor, it requires no resistive contact with the source and relies on the displacement current through a capacitively coupled, thin, dielectric electrode coating.

The EPS is a good example of the cross-fertilisation of ideas from different branches of research. It was originally developed as part of the Sussex group's fundamental physics investigations into superconducting devices for quantum technologies (R.J. Prance et al., 1981; Skinner et al., 2010). There was a need to monitor the charging of a quantum regime weak link capacitor non-perturbatively, that is, without drawing real charge. The extreme experimental requirements precluded the use of a standard laboratory electrometer. The sensor needed to be located in a cryogenic chamber, at a considerable distance from room temperature. This, along with the necessity of non-perturbative monitoring, dictated an active, ultra-high input impedance sensor. In the event, the cryogenic version was not realized at that stage. However, the suitability of the design for room temperature electric potential measurements was quickly recognised and further development undertaken, leading to the first published implementation as a sensor of ECG signals both on-body and up to 5 cm off-body (Clippingdale et al., 1991).

5.1.1 Design of the Electric Potential Sensor

In order to produce a sensor with ultra-high input impedance, the design of the active front-end should be based on a high impedance amplifier configuration. In addition, a technique must be found to provide the DC bias required by the device, without compromising this input impedance. There are a number of methods used to achieve this, including the use of a low-leakage diode as the biasing component (R.J. Prance et al., 1998) or careful circuit board design which, through on-chip guarding and control of parasitics, precludes the need for a specified DC bias path (R.J. Prance et al., 2000). The resistance of the DC bias component has a significant effect on the output noise performance of the sensor, as illustrated in figure 1 which shows a continuous reduction in noise voltage measured up to resistances of order 10^{12} Ω. Well understood bootstrap and guarding circuit techniques (Graeme, 1973; Yeager & Hrusch-Tupta, n.d.) are used to maintain the effective input impedance as close as possible to the intrinsic device specifications. Whilst these techniques do not enhance the signal to noise, neither do they degrade it and they are crucial to retaining good low frequency operation, particularly in weakly coupled applications, as explained in due course.

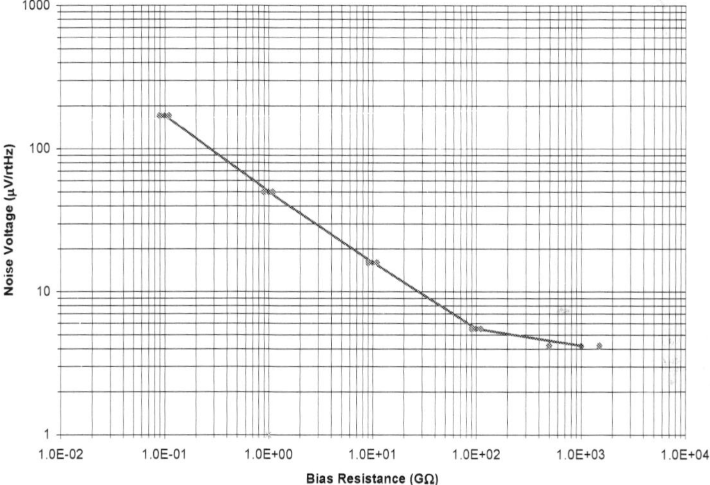

Fig. 1. Plot of input noise voltage at 1 Hz as a function of bias resistance value. Resistor tolerances, shown in red, are +/-10% up to 100 GΩ and +/-50% for 1 TΩ.

A generic block diagram of the EPS is shown in figure 2. It has been configured with a range of implementations and the details of the techniques used are covered by a suite of University of Sussex patents.

The combination of such a high input impedance, active front-end with an insulating electrode means that the EPS draws no real current from the source and can be thought of as approaching an 'ideal voltmeter'. Its performance as a non-perturbative detector of local electric fields has recently been verified by comparing measurements of the electric field between two large capacitor plates with finite-element simulations of the field (Aydin et al., 2010). This work demonstrates that the sensor causes no significant perturbation of the field and is capable of measuring fields as low as 2.6 µV/m with 2% accuracy.

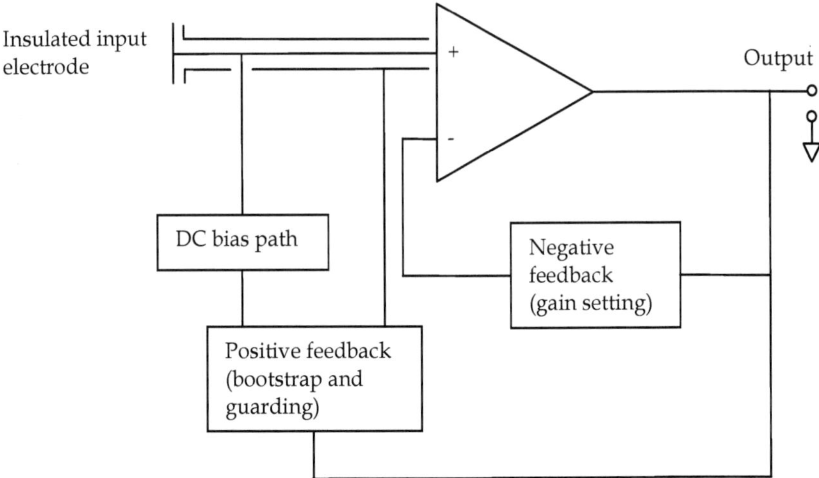

Fig. 2. Generic block diagram of the Electric Potential Sensor (EPS).

The standard limitation of high input impedance laboratory electrometers is that, with a true DC response, any charge present causes the input to drift to the power supply rail. Such electrometers therefore have to be reset repeatedly and are unsuitable for use in open, noisy environments. In addition, with an ambient atmospheric electric field of the order of 100 V/m present over the surface of the earth (Feynman et al., 1964), any movement of a sensor with a DC response will generate an associated AC movement artefact. The EPS is designed for both stability and usability. It overcomes the limitation of standard electrometers by dispensing with a true DC response and, in so doing, achieves excellent stability in standard working environments. Some commentators have perceived the lack of a true DC response as a limitation of insulated electrode sensors (Chi et al., 2010). However, it is worth noting that, in practice, almost every measurement made of voltage (potential) does not require knowledge of the true DC level. What is usually of interest at very low frequency is the variation, i.e. trend, in the signal. The EPS can be designed to provide any frequency response necessary for a given application, from the order of 30 mHz (R.J. Prance et al., 2000) to over 100 MHz (Gebrial et al., 2002), with either a broadband (R.J. Prance et al., 1998, Watson et al., 2010b) or tuned response (Clippingdale et al., 1994b), as required. The ability to set both upper and lower corner frequencies by design has a number of advantages. As would be expected, sensitivity to out of band noise is reduced by restricting the upper cut-off frequency. Restriction of the lower cut-off frequency minimises the DC drift problems as described above. In addition, the ability to choose the lower cut-off, by careful design of the bootstrap and guarding circuitry, is a benefit which has not been widely recognized. In particular, for weak coupled applications such as through clothing, it is essential to ensure that the appropriate standard operating bandwidth for a given electrophysiology application is retained. The design of the EPS manages to achieve this with no offset adjustments required at construction, set-up or in use. For example, for clinical quality adult ECGs, the operating bandwidth is typically 50 mHz to 150 Hz.

The physical embodiment of the EPS has developed over the years and been optimized for different applications. Figure 3 shows a typical pair of sensors and differential amplifier electronics used for on-body or through clothing electrophysiology measurements. The electrodes range from 1-5 cm in diameter and contain the active front-end electronics. The output is buffered to drive a long length of screened cable without sensitivity to mains (line) interference or cable movement. The metal electrode surface is coated with a thin, very low leakage dielectric and is guarded by a conducting ring. As an active sensor, the EPS electrode is not disposable by design. However, the electrodes can be completely potted in an inert compound which is inherently electrically safe and allows for sterilisation. They benefit from all of the advantages of insulated electrodes, requiring no skin preparation and being immune to changes in skin conductivity caused by sweating. For many electrophysiology applications, a differential measurement from a single pair of sensors is sufficient. The differential amplifier on the output is configured with minimal filtering, just a notch filter at the line frequency and a switchable low pass filter, as well as switchable gain. In practice the notch filter is not usually required due to the high quality differential measurement.

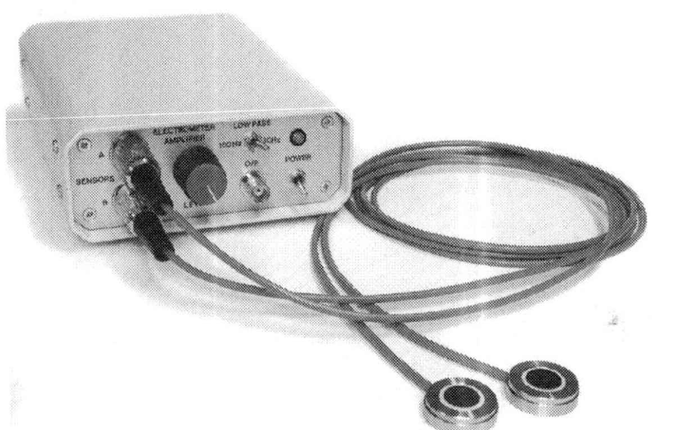

Fig. 3. Photograph of one embodiment of the EPS electrophysiology system, comprising a pair of insulating electrodes and a differential amplifier with analogue output.

5.1.2 Performance of the Electric Potential Sensor

Typical raw data, with no averaging or additional post-processing is shown in figure 4, which shows the electrocardiogram acquired from the wrists in an open, noisy environment. The performance of the sensor is such that comparable quality ECG signals can also be acquired through clothing, provided the material does not introduce electrostatic charge interference. Other workers have followed the EPS developments and implemented their own versions of active, insulated electrodes for through clothing electrophysiology. Sullivan et al., for example, use a circuit which incorporates bipolar transistor reset switches to combat the effect of the preamplifier input bias current drift (Sullivan et al., 2007) . However, the insulation and reset circuitry are not low leakage and both the signal to noise and bandwidth of the measurement are compromised in this implementation. The performance of this, and other, competing electrode technologies are compared in section

5.1.3. Spinelli & Haberman followed the EPS developments very closely and recently independently verified that ECG signals comparable to those from contact wet electrodes could be acquired through clothing using high input impedance active, insulating electrodes (Spinelli & Haberman, 2010).

For insulated electrodes in contact with the skin, the EPS technology has been proven to acquire clinical quality signals and even the His bundle feature, usually only observed with catheter ECG electrodes (Harland et al., 2002b). For example, the ECG signal measured in a 10 mHz to 100 Hz bandwidth with a small, 4-element array of EP sensors placed on the chest has been shown to provide equivalent information to the conventional 7-lead ECG (Harland et al., 2005).

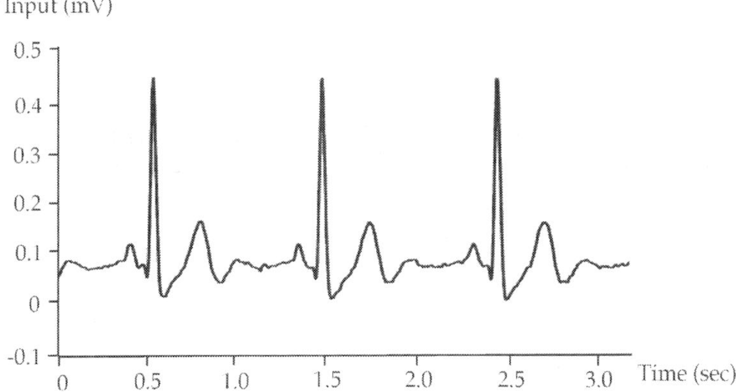

Fig. 4. I-lead ECG acquired from a differential pair of EPS electrodes positioned on the wrists. Signal acquired in real time, with no averaging, in a 0.5 - 30 Hz bandwidth.

The front-end electronics is low power and has been implemented with a wireless link, to monitor the ambulatory ECG, as a proof-of-principle (Harland et al., 2003a). The same demonstration shows that, provided the sensors are securely attached to the body, in this case by mounting each of the pair of electrodes in a wristwatch type fixture, the signal is not disrupted by strenuous movement.

The EPS has also been shown to have the sensitivity required for the weaker electrophysiology signals described in section 2. The alpha-blocking phenomenon in the EEG has been acquired through hair, and up to 3 mm off-body in a screened environment (Harland et al., 2002a). In addition EMG signals acquired from miniature sensors placed on the forearm show early indications of single motor unit action potential activity (H. Prance et al., 2009). In this case, three EPS electrodes; a closely spaced differential pair plus one mounted on the wrist; were used. By contrast, the EOG due to eyeball movement and blinking is of larger amplitude and can be acquired straightforwardly using a single pair of electrodes, with no reference, placed on the forehead (Harland et al., 2003b).

In the applications described above, the active electrodes are screened by physical contact with, or close proximity to, the surface of the body. They are therefore relatively immune to interference from external noise, including from the mains (line) supply, and what interference is picked up can be easily removed by the differential output amplifier.

However, if the electrodes are spaced off from the body in an unscreened environment, then the problems of interference must be addressed. It is not sufficient to limit the output bandwidth with a low pass filter, even if the application allows this. This is because large interference fluctuations at the input of the sensor may cause saturation. As a result, the signal of interest cannot be extracted satisfactorily by post-processing in either hardware or software. The EPS design has addressed this problem by enhancing the dynamic range of the sensor. One approach is to use an analogue comb filter to suppress the mains (line) frequency and its harmonics (H. Prance et al., 2007). An alternative solution uses high selectivity notch filters, digitally tuned in a smart sensor configuration to reject unwanted frequencies by up to 95 dB, thereby taking the level to below the intrinsic noise floor of the sensor (Beardsmore-Rust et al., 2009a; R.J. Prance et al., 2007, 2008). In both cases, the filters are incorporated into the feedback loop of the sensor, to reduce the front-end sensitivity at the unwanted frequencies and so enhance its dynamic range.

Whereas a previous design of EPS allowed the remote detection of electrophysiology signals in a screened room (Harland et al., 2002a, 2008); as a result of the developments described above, it has been possible to demonstrate the acquisition of both cardiac and respiration signals as a distance of up to 40 cm off-body, in an open, noisy laboratory environment (Beardsmore-Rust et al., 2009a; R.J. Prance et al., 2008). It is important to recognize that the ECG represents a body potential signal and, as such, cannot be measured by electrodes spaced by an air-gap from the body. This is demonstrated by comparing the phase of a cardiac electrical signal measured at the surface of the body, and at increasing distances off-body, with the phase of the arterial pulse, as measured by a pulse oximeter (Harland et al. 2002b). The signal at the surface of the body is, as expected, out of phase with the arterial pulse but it gradually moves into phase as the separation from the body increases. The cardiac signal acquired off-body will comprise a combination of electrical potential variation due to the electric field of the heart and a movement signal caused by the arterial pulse moving the chest wall. The movement signal will predominate at separations of over a few centimeters. The effects of body movement, and the phase dependence of the cardiac signals, are also observed, although the latter is not commented on, by Luna-Lozano & Pallas-Areny (Luna-Lozano & Pallas-Areny, 2010).

At significant sensor to body separations, relative movement between the two will result in an additional signal, as noted in section 2 and above, which is typically much larger than bioelectric signals. This can be a problem and secure attachment of electrodes is required to eliminate this source of interference. However, as explained in section 2, the ability to detect, and potentially track, the movement of persons does have application in home healthcare as well as security. An EPS sensor has been used to detect the movement of an individual through a wall (Beardsmore-Rust et al., 2009b; Harland et al., 2008) and a 4-element array of sensors was also used to track the movement of an individual within a 6 m x 6 m area (Beardsmore-Rust et al., 2011). The advantage of this, over competing techniques based on video or infra-red cameras or radar surveillance, is that the method is low bandwidth, low power and inherently passive, using the ambient electric field of the earth as the signal source.

5.1.3 Characterisation of the Electric Potential Sensor

We have termed the two extreme modes of application, one in physical, but not resistive, contact with the source and the other spaced off from the source; contact and remote modes respectively. The challenge for characterising sensor performance is that of accurately defining a coupling capacitance which reflects that expected for each mode of operation. In the case of contact mode, coupling capacitances are typically from 1 nF down to around 1 pF, and these can be replicated using good quality lumped components. However, for remote mode, the coupling is significantly weaker because the self capacitance of the electrode structure, which couples to the local electric field, is typically of the order of 100 fF. Here, suitable lumped components are not available and instead custom-made, well characterized, guarded capacitors have been used to couple to the EPS in order to characterize its performance for remote and weakly coupled operation, including for microscopic imaging applications (Watson et al., 2010b). Figure 5 shows typical frequency responses and noise spectra for two extreme coupling scenarios (Harland et al., 2002b).

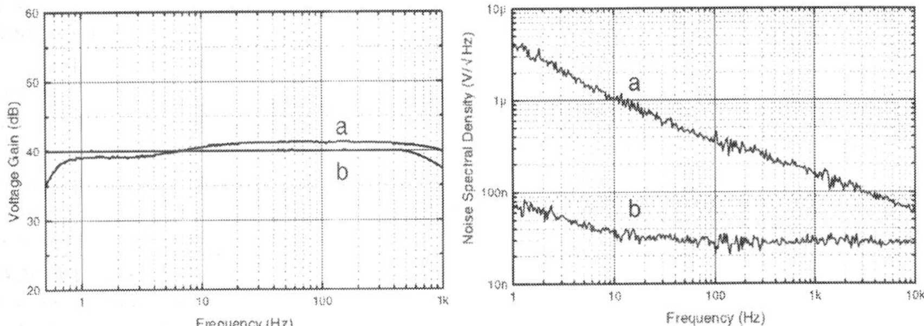

Fig. 5. (Reproduced with permission of IOP Publishing, from Harland et al., 2002b, figs 2 and 3). Frequency response (left) and noise spectra of an EPS sensor (right) for a) remote coupling through less than 1 pF and b) contact coupling through of order of 1 nF.

In the case of coupling through very small air-gaps, or through hair or clothing, the situation is much less well-defined. However, the sensor performance in these cases will lie between the two extremes depicted in Figure 5. Table 1 shows typical specifications for an EPS sensor for the three cases of; contact mode, for on-body electrophysiology measurements in contact with the skin; the weaker, through clothing, mode; and remote mode, for off-body applications such as the remote detection of life signs. These specifications are compared, where possible, to those presented by a number of authors who have reported active electrode systems similar to, or in competition with, the EPS.

5.2 High density and flexible electrode arrays

The use of arrays of electrophysiology sensors, for example for cardiac imaging, accurate EMG detection and EEG investigations, allows for the real time mapping of surface potentials. The increasing emphasis on non-invasive techniques for diagnosis and health monitoring has extended to this area and the use of large numbers of electrodes has also been aided by advances in data acquisition and processing. The advantages of body surface mapping in electrocardiography, for example, are that high spatial resolution images of surface potentials improve the early detection of abnormal activity (Lefebvre & Hoekstra, 2007). Similarly, high density arrays for surface EMG offer the capability of identifying and tracking single motor unit action potentials.

	EPS	Chi et al. 2010 dry	Chi et al. 2010 wet	Spinelli 2010	Sullivan et al. 2007	Oehler et al. 2008
Contact mode						
Input impedance	10^{15} Ω, 1 pF	1.3 MΩ, 12 nF	350 kΩ, 25 nF			
Coupling capacitance	1 nF			100 pF	(0.1 mm spacing)	
Frequency response	10 mHz – 200 MHz			< 10 mHz – 500 kHz	3 – 70 Hz	200 mHz – 80 Hz
Input noise per root Hz at 1 Hz	70 nV	1.5 µV	2.5 µV	1 µV	0.3 µV (at 3 Hz)	20 µV
Weaker mode, e.g. through clothing						
Input impedance	10^{15} Ω, 10^{-13} F	305 MΩ, 34 pF				
Coupling capacitance	Between extremes of contact and remote modes	1 pF		10 pF	(3.2 mm spacing)	
Frequency response				~ 10 mHz – 200 kHz	4 – 60 Hz	200 mHz – 70 Hz
Input noise per root Hz at 1 Hz		2.7 µV		10 µV	2 µV (at 3 Hz)	
Remote mode						
Input impedance	10^{18} Ω, 10^{-16} F					
Coupling capacitance	0.4 pF					
Frequency response	10 mHz – 200 MHz					
Input noise per root Hz at 1 Hz	4 µV					

Table 1. Comparison of selected electrophysiology sensor specifications under three different source-electrode coupling schemes. All electrodes, including the EPS, are active and insulating, except where stated.

The EPS has been used in array format since its earliest implementations. A 25-element array of spring coupled electrodes; mounted in a bench and designed to conform to the surface of the chest when laid upon; was used to image the electrical activity of the heart across the chest in real time (Clippingdale et al., 1994a). In a further development, a 7 cm diameter, 4-element array of EPS electrodes placed on the chest was used to recreate the conventional 7-lead ECG vectors (Harland et al., 2005). A similar approach was taken later by Oehler et al., who used a 15-element array of flexibly mounted, active, insulated electrodes with integral tablet PC to image chest cardiac activity in real time (Oehler et al., 2008). In this case, the diameter of the array was 185 mm and, with an input noise performance of 20 μV/rtHz at 1 Hz, the patient had to be grounded to improve signal to noise. However, the detection of 15 ECG channels through cotton clothing was also demonstrated.

The potential of the EPS for use in high density arrays, for example for EMG detection, is illustrated by work done for materials and semiconductor sensing applications. This demonstrates that the sensors are highly scaleable, with spatial resolutions demonstrated down to 6 μm (Watson et al., 2010a, 2010c). In addition, the high input impedance and lack of a conducting interface to the source ensures that adjacent sensors in an array do not cross-couple to each other and can therefore be closely packed. Finally, the requirement to match sensor elements in an array, for straightforward data processing, is simply a matter of incorporating a small numerical correction factor in software to normalize the outputs of the array. In this way seamless data acquisition has been achieved without hardware adjustment or component selection (Gebrial et al., 2006b).

Large element arrays for electrocardiographic imaging, for example over 200 electrodes, have been developed (Ramanathan et al., 2004; Rosik et al., 2007). These are based on dry electrodes, for ease of use. Similarly, dry electrodes have been used in an attempt to make the imaging of brain activity, in this case for human-computer interfacing, simpler and more convenient than with the traditional, wet electrode, EEG cap array (Popescu et al., 2007).

Whilst cardiac imaging arrays can be relatively easily incorporated into a vest for chest mounting, the need to detect muscle activity in locations such as the jaw, for the assessment of swallowing (McKeown et al., 2002), or on curved limb surfaces is more challenging. A high density two-dimensional surface EMG array has been implemented using dry electrodes but in a very bulky system with uncomfortable, and somewhat painful, pointed electrodes (Blok et al., 2002, 2006; Huppertz et al., 1997; Rau & Disselhorst-Klug, 1997). Ideally, the array should be flexible and easily positioned and recent work has shown great progress in this direction. A flexible, high density two-dimensional array format based on wet electrodes has been developed for use on the face (Lapatki et al., 2003, 2004, 2010; Maathuis et al., 2008). In other work, the performance of flexible, washable dry electrodes for surface EMG was compared with conventional electrodes (Laferriere et al., 2010). This work concluded that, while the wet electrodes were lower noise, the dry electrodes used had sufficient sensitivity for mobility monitoring applications.

As yet, no-one has implemented an insulating electrode array for EMG. However, a pair of contactless electrodes, based on active, insulated sensors, has been used to acquire an EMG signal from the biceps through cotton (Gourmelon & Langereis, 2006). The noise performance is not optimum, at 10 μV/rtHz at 1 Hz, and the subject had to be grounded for through clothing measurements. The high spatial resolution acquisition of an EMG signal using three EPS electrodes, referred to in section 5.1, shows more promise and work is underway to implement a multi-element high density array for surface EMG investigations.

6. Conclusion

The development of novel electrophysiological sensors, based on active, insulated or dry electrodes, and of high density sensor arrays are both highly active research areas. This is driven by the needs of healthcare monitoring, including the demands of home health monitoring, telehealth and sports physiology, as well as the related fields of human-computer interfacing and security. The acquisition of surface EMG signals, for the assessment of muscle activity, has been offered here as an exemplar to illustrate how electrophysiology measurements can be used to monitor chronic conditions, to support rehabilitation and to provide assistive technology for the elderly and disabled.

For these types of application, it has been noted that active, insulated electrode systems out-perform both wet and dry electrode systems in terms of signal to noise, immunity to interference and ease of use. They are able to offer all of the advantages of competing dry electrodes, active electrodes and electrode arrays but without the problems of skin preparation, skin irritation, motion artefact and cross-coupling between adjacent electrodes.

Having reviewed developments in active, insulated electrode sensor technology, it is clear that, by careful design, it is possible to retain the low noise performance and stable operation even in the weakly coupled limit of signal acquisition through clothing or an air gap. In addition, even in this coupling limit, it is possible to achieve the correct low, as well as high, frequency performance required for high quality electrophysiology measurements, as demonstrated by both the Prance group, with their EPS, and later by Spinelli et al.

Significant progress has been made in the development of high density, two-dimensional electrode arrays, particularly in the relatively new field of surface EMG imaging. However, whilst they are able to provide for a flexible array, wet electrodes are far from ideal for this application due to their inferior noise performance and susceptibility to cross-talk. Dry electrode high density arrays also have limitations in terms of the measures that are required to ensure good contact with the skin and it is likely that insulated electrodes will offer the best performance with the highest isolation between array elements and hence the highest spatial resolution. The ultimate goal is to develop flexible arrays of miniaturized, active, insulated electrodes, capable of high spatial resolution surface potential measurements. Such an array would find application in all of the areas of healthcare reviewed here, and particularly for both electrocardiographic and electromyographic imaging.

7. Acknowledgment

Support for research into the applications of the Electric Potential Sensor has been provided by the Engineering and Physical Sciences Research Council, UK (grant numbers GR/R87550/01 and EP/E042864/1). I am grateful for useful discussions with my colleagues Professor Robert Prance, Dr Christopher Harland and Philip Watson.

8. References

Allison, G.T (2003). Trunk muscle onset detection technique for EMG signals with ECG artefact. *Journal of Electromyography and Kinesiology*, Vol.13, pp. 209-216 ISSN 1050-6411

Amft, O.; Junker, H.; Lukowicz, P.; Troster, G. & Schuster, C. (2006). Sensing Muscle Activities with Body-Worn Sensors, *Proceedings of the International Workshop on Wearable and Implantable Body Sensor Networks BSN 2006.*, pp. 138–141, IEEE press, April 2006.

Aydin, A.; Prance, R.J.; Prance, H. & Harland, C.J. (2009). Observation of pressure stimulated voltages in rocks using an electric potential sensor, *Applied Physics Letters*, vol. 95, p. 124102 (3 pages), ISSN 0003-6951

Aydin, A.; Stiffell, P.B.; Prance, R.J. and Prance, H. (2010). A high sensitivity calibrated electric field meter based on the electric potential sensor, *Measurement Science and Technology*, Vol. 21, p. 125901 (5 Pages), ISSN 0957-0233

Beardsmore-Rust, S.T.; Prance, R.J.; Aydin, A.; Prance, H.; Harland, C.J. & Stiffell, P.B. (2009a). Signal specific electric potential sensors for operation in noisy environments, *Journal of Physics Conference Series*, Vol. 178, p. 012011 (6 pages), ISSN 1742-6956

Beardsmore-Rust, S.T.; Watson, P.; Stiffell, P.B.; Prance, R.J.; Harland, C.J. & Prance, H. (2009b). Detecting electric field disturbances for passive through wall movement and proximity sensing, in *Smart Biomedical and Physiological Sensor Technology VI*, Cullum, B.M. & Porterfield, D. Marshall (Eds.), Proceedings of SPIE Vol. 7313, pp. 73130P-1-8, ISSN 1605-7422

Beardsmore-Rust, S.T.; Stiffell, P.B.; Prance, H.; Prance, R.J. & Watson, P. (2010). Passive tracking of targets using electric field sensors, *Proceedings of SPIE Defense Security + Sensing 2010*, 6-8 April, 2010, Orlando, Florida, USA, Vol. 7666, pp. 766622-1-8

Beardsmore-Rust, S.T.; Prance, H.; Stiffell, P.B. & Prance, R.J. (2011). Sensing presence, movement and position with passive electric field measurements, in preparation

Blok, J.H.; van Dijk, J.P.; Drost, G.; Zwarts, M.J. & Stegeman, D.F. (2002). A high-density multichannel surface electromyography system for the characterization of single motor units, *Review of Scientific Instruments*, Vol. 73, No. 4, pp.1887-1897, ISSN 0034-6748

Blok, J.H. (2006). New perspectives for surface EMG in clinical neurophysiology: From biophysics to applications. PhD thesis, Radboud Universiteit Nijmegen, ISBN 90-8559-125-2

Bulling, A.; Roggen, D. & Troster, G. (2009). Wearable EOG goggles: Eye-based interaction in everyday environments, *Proceedings of CHI – Interactivity – Look, Hear, Wear*, pp. 3259-3264, Boston, MA, April 4-9, 2009

Chi, Y.M.; Jung, T-P & Cauwenberghs, G. (2010). Dry-Contact and Noncontact Biopotential Electrodes: Methodological Review, *IEEE Reviews in Biomedical Engineering*, Vol. 3, pp. 106-119, ISSN 1937-3333

Clancy, E.A.; Morin, E.L. & Merletti, R. (2002). Sampling, noise-reduction and amplitude estimation issues in surface electromyography, *Journal of Electromyography and Kinesiology*, Vol.12, pp. 1-16, ISSN 1050-6411

Clippingdale, A.J.; Prance, R.J.; Clark, T.D.; Prance, H. & Spiller, T. (1991). Ultra-high impedance voltage probes and non-contact electrocardiography, In: Sensors: Technology, systems and applications, K.T.V. Grattan (Ed.), pp.469-472, ISBN 0-7503-0157-0

Clippingdale, A.J.; Prance, R.J.; Clark, T.D. & Watkins, C. (1994a). Ultra-high impedance capacitively coupled heart imaging array, *Review of Scientific Instruments*, Vol. 65, No. 1, pp.269-270, ISSN 0034-6748

Clippingdale, A.J.; Prance, R.J.; Clark, T.D. & Brouers, F. (1994b). Non-invasive dielectric measurements with the scanning potential microscope, *Journal of Physics D: Applied Physics*, Vol. 27, pp. 2426-2430, ISSN 0022-3727

Dabiri, F.; Massey, T.; Noshadi, H.; Hagopian, H.; Lin, C.K.; Tan, R.; Schmidt, J. & Sarrafzadeh, M. (2009). A Telehealth Architecture for Networked Embedded Systems: A Case Study in In Vivo Health Monitoring, *IEEE Transactions on Information Technology in Biomedicine*, Vol. 13, No. 3, pp. 351-359, ISSN 1089-7771

De Luca, C.J. (2008). A Practicum on the Use of sEMG Signals in Movement Sciences, Delsys Inc. ISBN: 978-0-9798644-0-7

Ebling, D. & Thomas, G. (2008). Review of life signs monitoring in custody cells: The cell occupancy monitoring system produced by COSATT, Home Office Scientific Development Branch, Horsham, UK (2008)

Felzer, T. & Nordmann, R. (2008). Using Intentional Muscle Contractions as Input Signals for Various Hands-free Control Applications, In: *Proceedings of the 3rd International Convention on Rehabilitation Engineering & Assistive Technology*, pp. 87–91, Bangkok, Thailand, 13-18 May 2008

Feynman, R.P.; Leighton, R.B. & Sands, M. (1964). *The Feynman Lectures on Physics Volume II*, p. 9-1, Addison-Wesley, ISBN 0-201-02117

Garcia, G.A.; Zaccone, F.; Ruff, R.; Micera, S.; Hoffmann, K.-P. & Dario, P. (2007). Characterization of a new type of dry electrodes for long-term recordings of surface-electromyogram, *Proceedings of the 2007 IEEE 10th International Conference on Rehabilitation Robotics*, pp. 849-853, Noordwijk, Netherlands, June 12-15, 2007, ISBN 1-4244-1320-6

Gebrial, W.; Prance, R.J.; Clark, T.D.; Harland, C.J.; Prance, H. & Everitt, M. (2002). Noninvasive imaging of signals in digital circuits, *Review of Scientific Instruments*, Vol. 73, No. 3, pp.1293-1298, ISSN 0034-6748

Gebrial, W.; Prance, R.J.; Harland, C.J.; Stiffell, P.B.; Prance, H. & Clark, T.D. (2006a). Non-contact imaging of carbon composite structures using electric potential (displacement current) sensors, *Measurement Science and Technology*, Vol. 17, pp. 1470-1476, ISSN 0957-0233

Gebrial, W.; Prance, R.J.; Harland, C.J. & Clark, T.D. (2006b). Noninvasive imaging using an array of electric potential sensors, *Review of Scientific Instruments*, Vol. 77, pp. 063708 (6 pages), ISSN 0034-6748

Graeme, J.G. (1973). *Applications of operational amplifiers: Third generation techniques*, McGraw-Hill, ISBN 0-07-123890-1

Gourmelon, L. & Langereis, G. (2006). Contactless sensors for surface electromyography, *Proceedings of the 28th IEEE EMBS Annual International Conference*, Section FrB05.4, pp. 2514-2517, New York, USA, Aug 30-Sept 2, 2006, ISBN 1-4244-0033-3

Hampton, J.R. (1992). *The ECG in Practice*, Churchill Livingstone, London 1992

Harland, C.J.; Clark, T.D. & Prance, R.J. (2002a). Remote detection of human electroencephalograms using ultrahigh input impedance electric potential sensors, *Applied Physics Letters*, Vol. 81, No. 17, pp. 3284-3286, ISSN 0003-6951

Harland, C.J.; Clark, T.D. & Prance, R.J. (2002b). Electric potential probes – new directions in the remote sensing of the human body, *Measurement Science and Technology*, Vol. 13, pp. 163-169, Institute of Physics Publishing, ISSN 0957-0233, DOI 10.1088/0957-0233/13/2/304

Harland, C.J.; Clark, T.D. & Prance, R.J. (2003a). High resolution ambulatory electrocardiographic monitoring using wrist-mounted electric potential sensors, *Measurement Science and Technology*, Vol. 14, pp. 923-928, ISSN 0957-0233

Harland, C.J.; Clark, T.D. & Prance, R.J. (2003b). Applications of Electric Potential (Displacement Current) Sensors in Human Body Electrophysiology, *Proceedings of the 3rd World Congress on Industrial Process Tomography*, pp. 485-490, Banff, Canada.

Harland, C.J.; Clark, T.D.; Peters, N.S.; Everitt, M.J. & Stiffell, P.B. (2005). A compact electric potential sensor array for the acquisition and reconstruction of the 7-lead electrocardiogram without electrical charge contact with the skin, *Physiological Measurement*, Vol. 26, pp. 939-950, ISSN 0967-3334

Harland, C.J.; Prance, R.J. & Prance, H. (2008). Remote monitoring of biodynamic activity using electric potential sensors, *Journal of Physics Conference Series*, Vol. 142, p. 012042 (4 pages), ISSN 1742-6956

Hogrel, J.-Y. (2005). Clinical applications of surface electromyography in neuromuscular disorders, *Neurophysiologie Clinique*, Vol. 35, pp. 59–71, ISSN 0987-7053

Huppertz, H.J.; Disselhorst-Klug, C.; Silny, J. & Heimann, G. (1997). Diagnostic yield on non-invasive high spatial resolution electromyography in neuromuscular diseases, *Muscle and Nerve*, November 1997, pp. 1360-1370

Johnson, M.J.; Feng, X.; Johnson, L.M. & Winters, J.M. (2007). Potential of a suite of robot/computer-assisted motivating systems for personalized, home-based, stroke rehabilitation, *Journal of NeuroEngineering and Rehabilitation*, Vol. 4, No. 6, 1743-0003

Kang, T.-H.; Merrit, C.R.; Grant, E.; Pourdeyhimi, B. & Nagle, H.T. (2008). Nonwoven Fabric Active Electrodes for Biopotential Measurement During Normal Daily Activity, *IEEE Transactions on Biomedical Engineering*, Vol. 55, No. 1, pp. 188-195, ISSN 0018-9294

Kligfield, P.; Gettes, L.S.; Bailey, J.J.; Childers, R.; Deal, B.J.; Hancock, W.; van Herpen, G.; Kors, J.A.; MacFarlane, P.; Mirvis, D.M.; Pahlm, O.; Rautaharju, P. & Wagner, G.S. (2007). Recommendations for the Standardization and Interpretation of the Electrocardiogram Part I: The Electrocardiogram and Its Technology, *Journal of the American College of Cardiology*, Vol. 49, No. 10, pp. 1109-1127, ISSN 0735-1097

Laferriere, P.; Chan, A.D.C. & Lemaire, E.D. (2010). Surface Electromyographic Signals using a Dry Electrode, *Proceedings of the IEEE International Workshop on Medical Measurements and Applications*, pp. 77-80, April 30 – May 1, 2010

Lapatki, P.G.; Stegeman, D.F. & Jonas, I.E. (2003). A surface EMG electrode for the simultaneous observation of multiple facial muscles, *Journal of Neuroscience Methods*, Vol. 123, pp. 117-128, ISSN 0165-0270

Lapatki, P.G.; van Dijk, J.P.; Zwarts, M.J.; Jonas, I.E. & Stegeman, D.F. (2004). A thin, flexible multielectrode grid for high-density surface EMG, *Journal of Applied Physiology*, Vol. 96, pp. 327-336, ISSN 8750-7587

Lapatki, P.G.; Oostenveld, R.; van Dijk, J.P.; Jonas, I.E.; Zwarts, M.J. & Stegeman, D.F. (2010). Optimal placement of bipolar surface EMG electrodes in the face based on single motor unit analysis, *Psychophysiology*, Vol. 47, pp. 299-314

Levebvre, C. & Hoekstra, J. (2007). Early detection and diagnosis of acute myocardial infarction: the potential for improved care with next-generation, user-friendly electrocardiographic body surface mapping, *American Journal of Emergency Medicine*, Vol. 25, pp. 1063-1072, ISSN 0735-6757

Luna-Luzano, P.S. & Pallas-Areny, R. (2010). Microphonics in biopotential measurements with capacitive electrodes, Proceedings of the 32nd Annual International Conference of the IEEE EMBS, pp. 3487-3490, Buenos Aires, Argentina, Aug 31-Sep 4, 2010, ISBN 978-1-4244-4124-2

Maathuis, E.M.; Drenthen, J.; van Dijk, J.P.; Visser, G.H. & Blok, J.H. (2008). Motor unit tracking with high-density surface EMG, *Journal of Electromyography and Kinesiology*, Vol.18, pp. 920-930 ISSN 1050-6411

Martens, S.M.M.; Rabotti, C.; Mischi, M. & Sluijter, R.J. (2007). A robust fetal ECG detection method for abdominal recordings, *Physiological Measurement*, Vol. 28, pp. 373-388, ISSN 0967-3334

McKeown, M.J.; Torpey, D.C. & Gehm, W.C. (2002). Non-invasive monitoring of functionally distinct muscle activations during swallowing, *Clinical Neurophysiology*, Vol. 113, pp. 354-366, ISSN 1388-2457

Merletti, R.; Rainoldi, A. & Farina, D. (2001). Surface electromyography for noninvasive characterisation of muscle, *Exercises and Sports Sciences Reviews*, Vol. 29, No. 1, pp. 20-25, ISSN 0091-6631

Merletti, R.; Farina, D. & Gazzoni, M. (2003). The linear electrode array: a useful tool with many applications, *Journal of Electromyography and Kinesiology*, Vol.13, pp. 37-47 ISSN 1050-6411

Merletti, R. (2010). The electrode–skin interface and optimal detection of bioelectric signals: Editorial, *Physiological Measurement*, Vol. 31, p. E01, ISSN 0967-3334

Oehler, M., Ling, V., Melhorn, K. & Schilling, M. (2008). A multichannel portable ECG system with capacitive sensors, *Physiological Measurement*, Vol. 29, pp. 783-793, ISSN 0967-3334

Popescu, F., Fazli, S., Badower, Y., Blankertz, B. & Muller, K.-R. (2007). Single Trial Classification of Motor Imagination Using 6 Dry EEG Electrodes, *PLoS ONE*, Vol. 2, No. 7: e637. doi:10.1371/journal.pone.0000637

Prance, H.; Prance, R.J. & Stiffell, P.B. (2007). Hardware comb filter enhances dynamic range and noise performance of sensors in noisy environments, *Review of Scientific Instruments*, Vol. 78, pp. 074701 (6 pages), ISSN 0034-6748

Prance, H.; Watson, P.; Prance, R.J.; Harland, C.J.; Beardsmore-Rust, S.T. & Aydin, A. (2009). High spatial resolution dry-electrode surface EMG acquisition system, *Assistive technology from adapted equipment to inclusive environments - Proceedings of AAATE 2009*, P.L. Emiliani (Ed.), pp 109-113, IOS Press, ISBN 978-1-60750-042-1

Prance, R.J; Long, A.P.; Clark, T.D.; Widom, A.; Mutton, J.E.; Sacco, J.; Potts, M.W.; Megaloudis, G. & Goodall, F. (1981). Macroscopic quantum electrodynamic effects in a superconducting ring containing a Josephson weak link, *Nature*, Vol. 289, pp. 543-549

Prance, R.J.; Clark, T.D.; Prance, H. & Clippingdale, A. (1998). Non-contact VLSI imaging using a scanning electric potential microscope, *Measurement Science and Technology*, Vol. 9, pp. 1229-1235, ISSN 0957-0233

Prance, R.J.; Debray, A.; Clark, T.D.; Prance, H.; Nock, M.; Harland, C.J. & Clippingdale, A. (2000). An ultra-low-noise electrical-potential probe for human-body scanning, *Measurement Science and Technology*, Vol.11, pp. 291-297, ISSN 0957-0233

Prance, R.J. & Aydin, A. (2007). Acquisition of a nuclear magnetic resonance signal using an electric field detection technique, *Applied Physics Letters*, vol. 91, p. 044103 (3 pages), ISSN 0003-6951

Prance, R.J.; Beardsmore-Rust, S.T.; Prance, H.; Harland, C.J. & Stiffell, P.B. (2007). Adaptive electric potential sensors for smart signal acquisition and processing, ultra-low-noise electrical-potential probe for human-body scanning, *Journal of Physics Conference Series*, Vol. 76, p. 012025 (5 pages), ISSN 1742-6956

Prance, R.J.; Beardsmore-Rust, S.T.; Watson, P.; Prance, Harland, C.J. & Prance, H. (2008). Remote detection of human electrophysiological signals using electric potential sensors, *Applied Physics Letters*, vol. 93, p. 033906 (3 pages), ISSN 0003-6951

Pullman, S.L.; Goodin, D.S.; Marquinez, A.I.; Tabbal, S. & Rubin, M. (2000). Clinical utility of surface EMG: Report of the therapeutics and technology sub-committee of the American Academy of Neurology, *Neurology*, Vol. 55, pp. 121-177, ISSN 0028-3878

Prutchi, D. & Norris, M. (2005). Design and Development of Medical Electronic Instrumentation, John Wiley and Sons New Jersey, ISBN 0-471-67623-3

Ramanathan, C.; Ghanem, R.N.; Jia, P.; Ryu, K. & Rudy, Y. (2004). Noninvasive electrocardiographic imaging for cardiac electrophysiology and arrhythmia, Nature Medicine, Vol. 10, No. 4, pp. 422-428

Rantanen, V.; Niemenlehto, P.-H.; Verho, J. & Lekkala, J. (2010). Capacitive facial movement detection for human–computer interaction to click by frowning and lifting eyebrows, *Medical and Biological Engineering and Computing*, Vol. 48, pp. 39-47

Rau, C. & Disselhorst-Klug, C. (1997). Principles of high-spatial-resolution surface EMG (HSR-EMG): Single Motor Unit Detection and Application in the Diagnosis of Neuromuscular Disorders, *Journal of Electromyography and Kinesiology*, Vol.7, No. 4, pp. 233-239, ISSN 1050-6411

Reaz, M.B.I.; Hussain, M.S.; Mohd-Yasin, F. (2006). Techniques of EMG signal analysis: detection, processing, classification and applications, *Biological Procedures Online*, Vol. 8, No. 1, pp.11-35

Reddy N.P. & Gupta, V. (2007). Toward direct biocontrol using surface EMG signals: Control of finger and wrist joint models, *Medical Engineering & Physics*, Vol. 29, pp. 398-403, ISSN 1350-4533

Rosik, V.; Karas, S.; Heblakova, E.; Tysler, M. & Filipova, S. (2007). Portable Device for High Resolution ECG Mapping, *Measurement Science Review*, Vol. 7, Section 2, No. 6, pp. 57-61

Ruch, T.C. & Fulton, J.F. (1960). *Medical Physiology and Biophysics*, Chapter 21, W.B. Saunders Company, Philadelphia and London

Ruffini, G.; Dunne, S.; Farres, E.; Cester, I.; Watts, P.C.P.; Silva, S.R.P.; Grau, C.; Fuentemilla, L.; Marco-Pallares, J. & Vandecasteele, B. (2007). ENOBIO dry electrophysiology electrode; first human trial plus wireless electrode system, Proceedings of the 29th Annual International Conference of the IEEE EMBS, pp. 6689-6693, Lyon, France, 23-26 August, 2007, ISBN 104244-0788-5

Saponas, T.S.; Tan, D.S.; Morris, D. & Balakrishnan, R. (2008). Demonstrating the Feasibility of Using Forearm Electromyography for Muscle-Computer Interfaces, *Proceedings of CHI 2008*, pp. 515-524, April 5-10, 2008, Florence, Italy, ISBN 978-1-60558-011-1

Scanaill, C.N., Carew, S., Barralon, P., Noury, N., Lyons, D. & Lyons, G.M. (2006). A Review of approaches to mobility telemonitoring of the elderly in their living environment, *Annals of Biomedical Engineering*, Vol. 34, No. 4, pp. 547-563

Searle, A. & Kirkup, L. (2000). A direct comparison of wet, dry and insulating bioelectric recording electrodes, *Physiological Measurement*, Vol. 21, pp. 271-283, ISSN 0967-3334

Skinner, J.C.; Prance, H.; Stiffell, P.B. & Prance, R.J. (2010). Sisyphus Effects in a Microwave-Excited Flux-Qubit Resonator System, *Physical Review Letters*, Vol. 105, p. 257002 (4 pages), ISSN 0031-9007

Spinelli, E. & Haberman, M. (2010). Insulating electrodes: a review on biopotential front ends for dielectric skin-electrode interfaces, *Physiological Measurement*, Vol. 31, pp. S183-S198, ISSN 0967-3334

Stegeman, D.F.; Blok, J.H.; Hermens, H.J. & Roeleveld, K. (2000). Surface EMG models: properties and applications, *Journal of Electromyography and Kinesiology*, Vol.10, pp. 313-326, ISSN 1050-6411

Sullivan, T.J., Deiss, S.R. & Cauwenberghs, G. (2007). A low-noise, non-contact EEG/ECG sensor, *Proceedings of the IEEE Biomedical Circuits and Systems Conference, BIOCAS 2007*, pp. 154_157, 27-30 Nov. 2007, Montreal Canada, ISBN 978-1-4244-1524-3

Watson, P.; Prance, R.J.; Prance, H. & Beardsmore-Rust, S.T. (2010a). Imaging the time sequence of latent electrostatic fingerprints, *Proceedings of SPIE: Optics and Photonics for Counterterrorism and Crime Fighting VI and Optical Materials in Defence Systems Technology VII*, Vol. 7838, p. 783803-1-6, Toulouse, France, September 2010

Watson, P.; Prance, R.J.; Beardsmore-Rust, S.T.; Aydin, A. & Prance, H. (2010b). Imaging the microscopic properties of dielectrics via potential and charge, *Proceedings of the ESA Annual Meeting on Electrostatics 2010*, Paper K1, Charlotte NC, June 2010

Watson, P.; Prance, R.J.; Beardsmore-Rust, S.T. & Prance, H. (2010c). Imaging electrostatic fingerprints with implications for a forensic timeline, accepted for publication in *Forensic Science International*, DOI: 10.1016/j.forsciint.2011.02.024, ISSN 0379-0738

Winters, J.M. (2002). Telerehabilitation Research: Emerging Opportunities, *Annual Review of Biomedical Engineering*, Vol. 4, pp. 287-320, ISSN 1523-9829

Yaeger, J. & Hrusch-Tupta, M.A. Eds. (n.d.). *Low Level Measurements*, 5th edition, Keithley Instruments Inc., USA

Part 3

Biomedical Signal Processing

13

Time-Frequency Based Feature Extraction for Non-Stationary Signal Classification

Luis David Avendaño-Valencia, Carlos Daniel Acosta-Medina
and Germán Castellanos-Domínguez
Universidad Nacional de Colombia, Sede Manizales
Colombia

1. Introduction

Biosignal recordings are useful for extracting information about the functional state of an organism. For this reason, such recordings are widely used as tools for supporting medical decision. Nevertheless, reaching a diagnostic decision based on biosignal recordings normally requires analysis of long data records by specialized medical personnel. In several cases, specialized medical attention is unavailable, due to the high quantity of patients and data to analyze. Besides, the access to this kind of service may be difficult in remote places. As a result, the quality of medical service is deteriorated. In this sense, automated decision support systems are an important aid for improving pathology diagnosis and treatment, specially when long data records are involved. The successful performance of automatic decision systems strongly depends on the adequate choice of features. Therefore, non-stationarity is one of the most important problems to take into account. Non-stationarity is an inherent property of biosignals, as the underlying biological system has a time dependant response to environmental excitations. Specially, changes in physiological conditions and pathologies may produce significant variations.

It has been found that non-stationary conditions give rise to changes in the spectral content of the biosignal (Hassanpour et al., 2004; Quiceno-Manrique et al., 2010; Sepúlveda-Cano et al., 2011; Subasi, 2007; Tarvainen et al., 2009; Tzallas et al., 2008). Therefore, time-frequency (t–f) features have been previously proposed for examining the dynamic properties of the spectral parameters during transient physiological or pathological episodes. It is expected that t–f features reveal the correlation between the t–f characteristics of abnormal non-stationary behavior (Debbal & Bereksi-Reguig, 2007). For this reason, t–f methods should outperform conventional methods of frequency analysis (Tzallas et al., 2008). Besides, t–f features are expected to behave slowly enough along the time axis, so the usual stationary restrictions imposed on short-term intervals should work out better than when straightforwardly analyzing over the raw input biosignal.

Among t–f features, *time-frequency representations* (TFR) are one of the most common and widely used features. TFRs are the most complete characterization method for non-stationary biosignals, as they display the energy distribution of a signal in time and frequency domains. Several TFR estimators have been proposed, which can be classified as non-parametric (linear and quadratic) and parametric (Marchant, 2003; Poulimenos & Fassois, 2006). The selection of a particular TFR estimator should be led by its estimation properties, the expected precision and the computational resources. *Time–frequency dynamic features* (TFDF) based on spectral sub-band methods, summarize t–f information in a compact fashion. TFDF set has also demonstrated its capability for discriminating between normal and pathological patterns (Quiceno-Manrique et al., 2010; Sepúlveda-Cano et al., 2011). In this sense, the TFDF set can be suitably estimated by filter bank methods, such as sub-band spectral centroid, sub-band spectral centroid energy, linear cepstral coefficients, or discrete wavelet transform. These features have a lower dimensionality than the original TFR, but they still contain a stochastic dependance along time axis that has to be considered in the analysis.

In order to make pattern recognition problems solvable, it is necessary to convert t–f patterns into feature vectors, which become condensed representations, ideally containing only relevant information. From the viewpoint of managing large quantities of data, it is even more useful if irrelevant or redundant attributes could be segregated from relevant and important ones (Cvetkovic et al., 2008). A direct approach is to use linear transform methods, such as principal component analysis (PCA) or partial least squares (PLS), to reduce the feature space dimensionality resulting from the t–f plane. A reduced feature set obtained by PCA can be effectively accommodated to loosely structured TFR planes, when quantitative and decision based analysis is required (Bernat et al., 2007; Englehart et al., 1999). However, for classification purposes, the obtained components are not always related to the most discriminative information, as their transformation is based only on feature variability while class labels are neglected. Supervised methods, like PLS, can be used to improve performance of linear transform methods taking into account label variability as well as feature variability (Avendano-Valencia et al., 2010).

Nonetheless, computing transformation matrices of linear transform methods becomes more expensive as the dataset dimension increases. This is the case of t–f patterns, which may contain thousands of data points. Thus, it might be necessary to select *a priori* a confined portion of relevant data from the t–f feature to achieve computational stability during the feature extraction process. Classification based on local regions of the t–f plane has achieved higher success rates than those based on the entire t–f plane (Tzallas et al., 2008), but there is a significant unsolved issue associated with local-based analysis, which is the selection of the size and location of relevant regions. As a result, the choice of the feature extractor in the t–f domain is highly dependent on the final application (Sejdic et al., 2009). Relevance analysis is a tool that may serve to select the most informative t–f features from a discriminative viewpoint. In relevance analysis, a relevance measure is defined to determine the dependence of the features with regard to the each class label. The application of relevance measures has demonstrated a significant improvement compared to when no relevance measure is used, as proven in the case of TFR based classification (Avendaño-Valencia et al., 2010), and in frequency sub-band feature based classification (Sepúlveda-Cano et al., 2011).

Despite the large efforts in designing appropriate t–f based feature extraction for biosignal classification, there are still some issues to be solved. Particularly, as time-frequency data has a natural order, feature extraction methods can benefit if the data is treated as stochastically dependent, thus capturing the evolving information of the structure. A former approach was to use multidimensional linear transform methods, separately taking into account time and frequency dependence. When PCA transformations are used, these methods are known as two dimensional PCA (2D-PCA) (Yang et al., 2004). Two dimensional methods can be extended for different kinds of linear transforms, as in the case of PLS

(Avendano-Valencia et al., 2010), with improved classification performance. Nonetheless, these methods do not impose a priori a dynamic structure for the t–f feature ordering.

In summary, both TFR and TFDF are features that describe the non–stationary behavior of a biosignal and allow the analysis of different kinds of dynamic behavior. These features should contain all the available information for discriminating among different classes. Nevertheless, from the pattern recognition point of view, this class of features is troublesome to use, due to two important aspects: *multiple dimensions* and *high dimensionality*. In contrast to conventional characterization methods, TFR and TFDF are multidimensional features. Thus, while a conventional feature vector lies on $\mathbb{R}^{N}$ vector space, TFR and TFDF lie on $\mathbb{R}^{N \times T}$ matrix space. A multidimensional nature is important for describing temporal dynamics and relationships between spectral bands and should be exploited by the pattern recognition framework. Moreover, the intrinsic dimensionality of TFR and TFDF features is very high, and can normally lead to thousands of feature points. In that case, the performance of the classifier is compromised, as stated by *the curse of dimensionality*. So, in order to decrease the computing and storage requirements, as well as improving the generalization capabilities of the classifier, it is mandatory to reduce the dimensionality of TFR and TFDF features. Therefore, the dimensionality reduction approach should encompass with the following properties:

– Should be able to exploit the multidimensional nature of the data, taking into account both temporal dynamics and relationships between spectral bands.

– Should be able to extract the most informative data and fully describe the multidimensional features into a small set of features, as well as avoiding all irrelevant information.

This chapter is devoted to the review and comparison different time-frequency based feature extraction methods for classifying non-stationary biosignals. Subsequently, based on previous work in (Avendano-Valencia et al., 2010), a new methodology is proposed, oriented to reducing the dimensionality of t–f based features. The proposed methodology consecutively performs both the selection of the most relevant features as well as a linear transform of the t–f planes. Initially, the most relevant features extracted from the TFR are selected using a relevance measure that selects the most discriminative t–f features. Therefore, both the irrelevant information and the computational burden are significantly decreased. Then, the data is projected into a lower dimensional subspace using linear transform methods. Special attention will be drawn to different forms of improving linear transform methods for the case of dynamic t-f features. For the sake of comparison, conventional state of the art approaches for t–f based classification, and proposed linear transform and relevance analysis methods are included in this study.

Comparison is made with reference to the problem of identifying normal, inter-ictal and ictal records from publicly available non-stationary electroencephalographic biosignal database for detection of epilepsy (Andrzejak et al., 2001). Most representative non-parametric and parametric TFR estimators are under comparison: short time Fourier transform (STFT), smoothed pseudo Wigner-Ville distribution (SPWVD), and parametric TFR based on smoothness priors time varying autoregressive moving average models (SP–TAR). Spectral sub-band and discrete wavelet transform are also considered in the analysis. The accuracy, computational effort and ease of use are analyzed to check the advantages and drawbacks of conventional and proposed t–f based classification approaches.

2. Materials and methods

2.1 Time-Frequency Representations and Time-Frequency Dynamic Features

Time-Frequency Representation is a joint representation of the energy distribution of a signal in both time and frequency domains. The TFR of a signal $x_i(t) \in L_2(\mathbb{R})$ is mathematically represented as a function of time and frequency $X_i(t, \omega) \in L_2(\mathbb{R}^2)$. TFR should be used when there is evidence of time-varying or non-stationary conditions on the signal. In such cases, the time or the frequency domain descriptions of the signal alone cannot provide comprehensive information for analysis and classification, thus t–f methods should outperform conventional analysis methods (Sejdic et al., 2009; Tzallas et al., 2008).

In the past, different forms of estimating TFR have been proposed. These estimation methodologies can be grouped into the following main approaches (Marchant, 2003; Poulimenos & Fassois, 2006): (*i*) non–parametric TFR (*linear TFR* and *quadratic -Cohen class-TFR*); and (*ii*) *parametric TFR*.

Linear TFR makes use of t–f functions derived from translating, modulating and scaling a basis function with a definite time and frequency localization (Sejdic et al., 2009). Thus, for a signal $x_i(t)$, the TFR is given by,

$$X_i(t, \omega) = \int_{-\infty}^{\infty} x_i(\tau)\phi_{t,\omega}^*(\tau)d\tau = \langle x_i(t), \phi_{t,\omega} \rangle \tag{1}$$

where $\phi_{t,\omega}$ represents the basis function which defines the specific transform method, and * represents the complex conjugate. The basis functions are assumed to be square integrable, this is $\langle \phi_{t,\omega}, \phi_{t,\omega} \rangle^{1/2} < \infty$. Short time Fourier transform – STFT, wavelets, and matching pursuit approaches are typical examples of this class of transforms.

Quadratic TFR are defined as the Fourier transform of the local autocovariance function, given by the product $x_i(t + 1/2\tau)x_i^*(t - 1/2\tau)$. Also, different t–f kernels might be used in order to attain the desired properties on the transform. Thus, a quadratic TFR is defined by,

$$X_i(t, \omega) = \frac{1}{4\pi^2} \int_{-\infty}^{\infty} \int_{-\infty}^{\infty} \int_{-\infty}^{\infty} x_i\left(u + \frac{1}{2}\tau\right) x_i^*\left(u - \frac{1}{2}\tau\right) \phi(\theta, \tau)e^{-j\theta t - j\tau\omega + j\tau u}dud\tau d\theta \tag{2}$$

where $\phi(\theta, \tau)$ is a two-dimensional kernel function, defining the specific representation and its properties. Wigner-Ville, Choi-Williams, and spectrogram, are some exemplary methods belonging to this category.

Parametric TFR are based on a parametric signal model, like a TARMA model. The model should be fitted to the analyzed signal, and then, the TFR can be derived from the time-varying parameters and residual variance (Poulimenos & Fassois, 2006). A TARMA(n_a, n_c) model is defined as,

$$x_i(t) = -\sum_{n=1}^{n_a} a_{i,n}(t)x_i(t - n) + \sum_{n=1}^{n_c} c_{i,n}(t)e_i(t - n) + e_i(t), \quad e_i(t) \sim \mathbf{N}(0, \sigma_{e_i}^2(t)) \tag{3}$$

where $a_{i,n}(t), n = 1, \ldots, n_a$ and $c_{i,n}(t), n = 1, \ldots, n_c$ are the time-varying AR/MA parameters, and $e_i(t)$ is the residual sequence assumed as zero mean white gaussian noise with time-dependant variance $\sigma_{e_i}^2(t)$, noted as $\mathbf{N}(0, \sigma_{e_i}^2(t))$. The parametric TFR derived from

TARMA model is defined as,

$$X_i(t,\omega) = \left| \frac{1 + \sum\limits_{n=1}^{n_c} c_{i,n}(t)e^{-j\omega n}}{1 + \sum\limits_{n=1}^{n_a} a_{i,n}(t)e^{-j\omega n}} \right|^2 \sigma_e^2(t) \tag{4}$$

which would be the power spectral density of the signal if the system were made stationary at time instant t. The effectiveness of this method mainly lies in the accurate selection of model orders n_a and n_c as well as the temporal change assumed form of the parameters $a_{i,n}(t)$ and $c_{i,n}(t)$, and residual variance $\sigma_{e_i}^2(t)$. If these conditions are met, the parametric TFR can improve in accuracy, resolution and tracking of time-varying dynamics compared with linear and quadratic TFR.

Further discussion on the properties and advantages/disadvantages of each TFR estimation approach is out of the scope of this study. For more information on this subject, the reader can refer to the following papers: linear, quadratic and parametric TFR (Marchant, 2003); parametric t–f analysis (M Tarvainen & Karjalainen, 2004; Poulimenos & Fassois, 2006); comparison of different TFR on EEG classification (Tzallas et al., 2008); parametric TFR based classification (Avendano-Valencia et al., 2010).

Time-frequency Dynamic Features – TFDF are a set of variables describing the temporal dependency of some spectral–related quantity. The TFDF set of the signal $x_i(t)$ can be mathematically represented as a set of ... N functions $\boldsymbol{x}_i(t) = [x_{i,1}(t), \ldots, x_{i,N}(t)]^\top$ describing the dynamics on a particular frequency band. When sampled, these features can be arranged as a matrix $\boldsymbol{X}_i \in \mathbb{R}^{N \times T}$. The following dynamic variables are under consideration: *linear frequency cepstral coefficients – LFCC, subband spectral centroids – SSC, subband spectral centroid energy – SSCE*, and *discrete wavelet transform – DWT*. The TFDF set describes the quantity of energy that the analyzed signal has on each of the n–frequency bands defined by the specific approach. In the case of LFCC, the TFDF are extracted using the following expression:

$$LFCC_{i,n}(t) = \sum_{m=1}^{n_M} \cos\left(n\frac{\pi(m-1)}{2N}\right) \log s_m(t) \tag{5}$$

$$s_m(t) = \int_{-\infty}^{\infty} F_m(\omega) X_i(t,\omega) d\omega$$

where N is the number of desired LFCCs to be considered, $F_m(\omega), m = 1, \ldots n_M$ is a set of n_M triangular log–filter banks, and $s_m(t), m = 1, \ldots, n_M$ is the weighted sum of each frequency filter response set. On the other hand, SSCs are computed following the equation:

$$SSC_{i,n}(t) = \frac{\int\limits_{-\infty}^{\infty} \omega F_n(\omega) X_i(t,\omega) d\omega}{\int\limits_{-\infty}^{\infty} F_n(\omega) X_i(t,\omega) d\omega} \tag{6}$$

where the set of filters $F_n(\omega)$, $n = 1, \ldots, N$ are linearly distributed along the spectrum. Additionally, the energy for each SSC (SSCE) can also be considered as a time–variant feature, which for a fixed bandwidth $\Delta\omega$ is computed by means of:

$$SCCE_{i,n}(t) = \int\limits_{SSC_{i,n}(t)-\Delta\omega}^{SSC_{i,n}(t)+\Delta\omega} X_i(t,\omega)d\omega \qquad (7)$$

where $SSC_{i,n}(t)$ is the value of the SSC estimated using (6). Both LFCCs from Equation (5) and SSCE from Equation (7) measure the average energy on the frequency band defined by each filter bank $F_m(\omega)$, whereas SSCs from Equation (6) measure the average frequency for each one of the defined spectral subbands. On the estimation of the TFDF any of the TFRs defined in equations (1), (2) and (4) can be used.

The *discrete wavelet transform* is also a means for analyzing the signal at different frequency bands, with different resolutions by decomposing the signal into approximation and detail coefficients. The DWT describes the signal $x_i(t)$ using the wavelet orthogonal basis $\{\psi_{j,k}\}_{(j,k)\in\mathbb{Z}}$ as:

$$x_i(t) = \sum_{j=-\infty}^{\infty} \sum_{k=-\infty}^{\infty} \langle x_i(t), \psi_{j,k}\rangle \psi_{j,k}(t) \qquad (8)$$

$$\psi_{j,k} = \frac{1}{\sqrt{2^j}} \psi\left(\frac{t - 2^j k}{2^j}\right)$$

So, each partial sum

$$d_{i,j} = \sum_{k=-\infty}^{\infty} \langle x_i(t), \psi_{j,k}(t)\rangle \psi_{j,k}(t)$$

can be interpreted as the detail variations at the scale 2^j. As a result, the signal is defined in terms of the coefficients, representing their energy content in a specified time-frequency region, determined by the mother wavelet $\psi_{j,k}$ at scale j and time shift k (Mallat, 2008).

Both TFR and TFDF can be arranged into matrices. In the case of the estimated TFR, any of the methods from equations (1), (2) or (4) when evaluated on specific discrete time and frequency points will yield a TFR matrix $X_i \in \mathbb{R}^{N\times T}$, as

$$X_i = \begin{bmatrix} X_i(t_1,\omega_1) & X_i(t_2,\omega_1) & \dots & X_i(t_T,\omega_1) \\ X_i(t_1,\omega_2) & X_i(t_2,\omega_2) & \dots & X_i(t_T,\omega_2) \\ \vdots & \vdots & \ddots & \vdots \\ X_i(t_1,\omega_N) & X_i(t_2,\omega_N) & \dots & X_i(t_T,\omega_N) \end{bmatrix}$$

where N and T are the number of time and frequency sampling points, respectively. Similarly, for the estimated TFDF obtained from (5), (6), (7) or (8), evaluation on different time points yields a TFDF matrix $X_i \in \mathbb{R}^{N\times T}$, as

$$X_i = \begin{bmatrix} x_i(t_1) & x_i(t_2) & \dots & x_i(t_T) \end{bmatrix}$$

2.2 State of the art approaches for TFR based classification

Within the context of feature extraction in TFR and dynamic features, two main approaches are to be considered:

- **Distance based approaches:** (Aviyente, 2004; Sejdic et al., 2009; Sejdic & Jiang, 2007) For this approach, a geometrical or statistical distance function is computed between the analyzed TFR and a template TFR. Furthermore, considering the resemblance between TFR and probability density functions, distance measures between probability density functions can be extended to the t-f plane (Michel et al., 64-67). The most common distance measure used for probability functions is the Kullback-Leibler divergence measure, that can be adapted to TFR as follows:

$$d_{KL}(X_1, X_2) = \int \int X_1(t, \omega) \log \frac{X_1(t, \omega)}{X_2(t, \omega)} dt d\omega \qquad (9)$$

  where $d_{KL}(X_1, X_2)$ is the Kullback-Leibler divergence. The measure $d_{KL}(X_1, X_2)$ is non-symmetrical and therefore, non-metric. By applying $d_{KLS}(X_1, X_2) = d_{KL}(X_1, X_2) + d_{KL}(X_2, X_1)$ the Kullback-Leibler divergence is converted into a symmetric measure.

  Once a distance measure is selected, the classifier decision is based on the shortest distance to any of the template TFRs. Choosing an effective template often requires familiarity with the problem, otherwise, the template can be obtained as a group average or by cluster analysis. Another solution is to compare the analyzed TFR with a properly labeled TFR set and use the nearest neighbor rule. As in every distance-based nearest neighbor approach, this approach suffers when the data dimensionality is very high, and as a result, poor performance can be obtained. For this reason, the choice of a feature extractor can have a strong influence on the obtained results.

- **Regional analysis approaches** (Bernat et al., 2007; Cvetkovic et al., 2008; Hassanpour et al., 2004; Subasi, 2007; Tzallas et al., 2008) In this approach, the TFR is decomposed in regions of interest and further analysis is carried out with respect to the behavior on each of such regions defined on the t-f plane (Tzallas et al., 2008). For example, a partition of the t-f plane can be regarded, defining a grid depending on some *a priori* information known about the information distribution over the plane. As it is recommended in Tzallas et al. (2008) for the case of EEG classification, a partition of the time domain into 8 s equal sized windows is defined, while the frequency domain is divided into five sub-bands corresponding to the EEG frequency bands defined by medical experts (0-2.5 Hz, 2.5-5.5 Hz, 5.5-10.5 Hz, 10.5-21.5 Hz, and 21.5-43.5 Hz). Then, the feature vector z_i is built as,

$$z_i = \begin{bmatrix} \bar{X}_{11} \dots \bar{X}_{1K} & \bar{X}_{21} \dots \bar{X}_{2K} & \dots & \bar{X}_{L1} \dots \bar{X}_{LK} & \bar{X} \end{bmatrix} \qquad (10)$$

$$\bar{X}_{lk} = \int_{t_l} \int_{\omega_k} X_i(t, \omega) d\omega dt, \qquad\qquad \bar{X} = \int \int X_i(t, \omega) d\omega dt$$

  where $t_l, l = 1, \dots, L$ is the l-th time window, $\omega_j, k = 1, \dots, K$ is the k-th frequency band, and L, K are the number of time windows and frequency bands respectively. Each feature represents the fractional energy of the signal in a specific frequency band and time window. Besides the total energy of the signal is included as an additional feature. Then, the feature vector z_i depicts the energy distribution of the signal. This method is less computationally expensive compared to distance based approaches, but an adequate selection of the regions of interest should be attained in order to achieve accurate results. Other regional decomposition can be accomplished by transform methods as proposed in (Bernat et al., 2007; Hassanpour et al., 2004) or wavelet sub–band decompositions (Cvetkovic et al., 2008; Subasi, 2007).

2.3 Dimensionality reduction on TFR and TFDF using orthogonal transforms

The TFR or TFDF–based pattern recognition approach can be described within the following framework. Let ξ_i be an object from object space ξ. The object ξ_i is associated with a class label $c_i = 1, \ldots, N_c$ from the class label space $\mathcal{C} \subset \mathbb{N}$. A set of N features are estimated on different times T from the object ξ_i, yielding the TFR/TFDF matrices $\boldsymbol{X}_i$ lying on a subspace $\mathcal{X}$ of $\mathbb{R}^{N \times T}$. A dimensionality reduction mapping is used to convert such matrices into a set of lower dimensionality features $\boldsymbol{z}_i$ in a reduced feature subspace $\mathcal{Z}$ of $\mathbb{R}^p$. Then, features $\boldsymbol{z}_i$ are used as inputs for training and classification. It is assumed that both subspaces $\mathcal{X}$ and $\mathcal{Z}$ contain the discriminant information of space ξ and thus the relationship between ξ and $\mathcal{C}$ can be recovered. A set of M objects are sampled from object space ξ, yielding the subset $\{\xi_i, i = 1, \ldots, M\}$. The estimated features from this subset are written as $\{\boldsymbol{X}_i, i = 1, \ldots, M\}$, and the features in reduced feature space are written as $\{\boldsymbol{z}_i, i = 1, \ldots, M\}$. Figure 1 depicts the space definitions within the relationships between them.

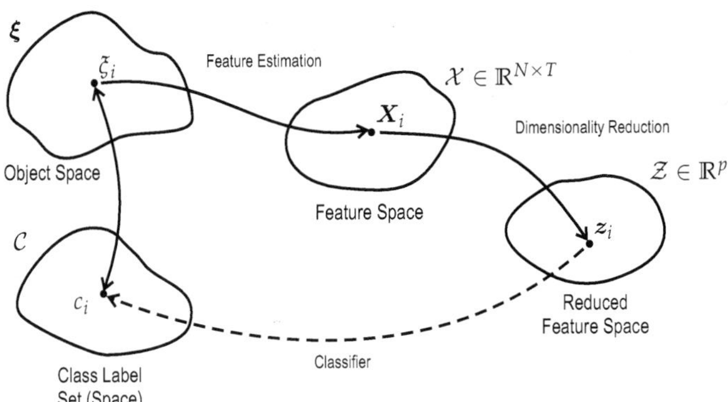

Fig. 1. Definition of object, class label, feature and reduced feature spaces, as well as mappings between spaces.

Within the explained framework, both TFR and TFDF are regarded as the *feature estimation* step, mapping from the object space (raw signals) to the feature space (space of feature matrices). Then, each one of the feature matrices, $\boldsymbol{X}_k \in \mathbb{R}^{N \times T}$ is described as follows:

$$\boldsymbol{X}_i = \left[\boldsymbol{x}_{c1}^{(i)}, \boldsymbol{x}_{c2}^{(i)}, \ldots, \boldsymbol{x}_{cT}^{(i)} \right] = \begin{bmatrix} \boldsymbol{x}_{r1}^{(i)} \\ \boldsymbol{x}_{r2}^{(i)} \\ \vdots \\ \boldsymbol{x}_{rN}^{(i)} \end{bmatrix} = \begin{bmatrix} x_{11}^{(i)} & x_{12}^{(i)} & \ldots & x_{1T}^{(i)} \\ x_{21}^{(i)} & x_{22}^{(i)} & \ldots & x_{2T}^{(i)} \\ \vdots & \vdots & \ddots & \vdots \\ x_{N1}^{(i)} & x_{N2}^{(i)} & \ldots & x_{NT}^{(i)} \end{bmatrix},$$

where $\boldsymbol{x}_{ck}^{(i)}$ is the k–th column vector and $\boldsymbol{x}_{rl}^{(i)}$ is the l–th row vector of the feature matrix $\boldsymbol{X}_i$. Besides, $x_{lk}^{(i)}$ is the element in the l–th row and k–th column of the feature matrix $\boldsymbol{X}_i$.

Straightforward *dimensionality reduction* on matrix data by means of orthogonal transforms can be carried out, just by stacking matrix columns into a single vector, as follows:

$$x_i = \left[(x_{c1}^{(i)})^\top \ (x_{c2}^{(i)})^\top \ \cdots \ (x_{cT}^{(i)})^\top \right] \tag{11}$$

where $x_i \in \mathbb{R}^{NT}$ is the vectorized feature. Then, in order to reduce data dimensionality, a transform matrix $V \in \mathbb{R}^{NT \times p}$, with $p \leq NT$ ($p \ll NT$) is defined to transform original feature space $\mathbb{R}^{NT}$ into a reduced feature space $\mathbb{R}^{p}$, by the linear operation $z_i = x_i V$. The transformation matrix V can be obtained using a non–supervised approach, such as *principal component analysis – PCA*, or a supervised approach, such as *partial least squares – PLS* using data set matrix X and the class label matrix c, defined as (Barker & Rayens, 2003),

$$X = \begin{bmatrix} x_1 \\ x_2 \\ \vdots \\ x_M \end{bmatrix}; \qquad c = \begin{bmatrix} 1_{M_1 \times 1} & 0_{M_2 \times 1} & \cdots & 0_{M_{N_c} \times 1} \\ 0_{M_1 \times 1} & 1_{M_2 \times 1} & \cdots & 0_{M_{N_c} \times 1} \\ \vdots & \vdots & \ddots & \vdots \\ 0_{M_1 \times 1} & 0_{M_2 \times 1} & \cdots & 1_{M_{N_c} \times 1} \end{bmatrix}$$

where N_c is the number of class labels and $M_n, n = 1, \ldots, N_c$ is the number of samples for each class in the training set. The vectorization approach in Equation (11) will be referred to as *vectorized PCA/PLS*, depending on the specific transform used. Vectorized PCA transform has been previously used in image recognition applications with the name of eigenfaces (Turk & Pentland, 1991). The vectorization approach was also used in (Bernat et al., 2007) to decompose and analyze TFR from P300 data, and in (Avendano-Valencia et al., 2010) for TFR–based classification. Nonetheless, this approach has several drawbacks, as the multidimensional structure of the data is not exploited nor analyzed; besides computational cost and memory requirements are increased.

When the feature matrix X_i is considered, a transform matrix $U \in \mathbb{R}^{q \times N}$ can be used to reduce the number of rows in data matrix, as $z_i^{(L)} = U X_i$, where $z_i^{(L)} \in \mathbb{R}^{q \times T}$. Also, a transform matrix $V \in \mathbb{R}^{T \times p}$ can be used to reduce the number of columns of data matrix, as $z_i^{(R)} = X_i V$, where $z_i^{(R)} \in \mathbb{R}^{N \times p}$. If both transforms are combined, further dimensionality reduction can be achieved, as

$$z_i = U X_i V \tag{12}$$

where U and V are the same as defined above, and $z_i \in \mathbb{R}^{q \times p}$ is the reduced dimensionality feature. Estimation of the transformation matrices U and V is carried out on the data matrices $X^{(L)}$ and $X^{(R)}$ respectively, which are defined as,

$$X^{(L)} = \begin{bmatrix} X_1^\top \\ X_2^\top \\ \vdots \\ X_M^\top \end{bmatrix}; \qquad X^{(R)} = \begin{bmatrix} X_1 \\ X_2 \\ \vdots \\ X_M \end{bmatrix}$$

In image recognition literature this approach is known as 2D–PCA (Yang et al., 2004; Zhang & Zhou, 2005) when the transformation matrices U and V in (12) are obtained with PCA. 2D–PCA and 2D–PLS have also been used for TFR–based classification in (Avendano-Valencia et al., 2010).

Increased insight can be achieved if the functional structure of the data is taken into account. Let each column of the feature matrix $x_{ck}^{(i)}$ be modeled as the weighted sum of basis functions ϕ_{jk},

$$x_{ck}^{(i)} = \sum_{j=1}^{p} \alpha_j^{(i)} \phi_{j,k} = \alpha_1^{(i)} \phi_{1,k} + \alpha_2^{(i)} \phi_{2,k} + \ldots + \alpha_p^{(i)} \phi_{p,k} \tag{13}$$

where $\phi_{j,k}, j = 1, \ldots, p$ is a set of p basis functions evaluated in column k, and $\alpha_j^{(i)} \in \mathbb{R}^N, j = 1, \ldots, p$ is the parameter vector of the model for the i-th object and the j-th base function. Then, the dynamic information is coded into the basis functions $\phi_{j,k}$ while the object information is coded in the set of parameter vectors $\alpha_j^{(i)}$. Equation (13) can be rewritten as,

$$x_{ck}^{(i)} = \begin{bmatrix} \alpha_{11}^{(i)} \\ \alpha_{21}^{(i)} \\ \vdots \\ \alpha_{N1}^{(i)} \end{bmatrix} \phi_{1,k} + \begin{bmatrix} \alpha_{12}^{(i)} \\ \alpha_{22}^{(i)} \\ \vdots \\ \alpha_{N2}^{(i)} \end{bmatrix} \phi_{2,k} + \ldots + \begin{bmatrix} \alpha_{1p}^{(i)} \\ \alpha_{2p}^{(i)} \\ \vdots \\ \alpha_{Np}^{(i)} \end{bmatrix} \phi_{p,k} = \begin{bmatrix} \alpha_{11}^{(i)} & \alpha_{12}^{(i)} & \ldots & \alpha_{1p}^{(i)} \\ \alpha_{21}^{(i)} & \alpha_{22}^{(i)} & \ldots & \alpha_{2p}^{(i)} \\ \vdots & \vdots & \ddots & \vdots \\ \alpha_{N1}^{(i)} & \alpha_{N2}^{(i)} & \ldots & \alpha_{Np}^{(i)} \end{bmatrix} \begin{bmatrix} \phi_{1,k} \\ \phi_{2,k} \\ \vdots \\ \phi_{p,k} \end{bmatrix}$$

$$x_{ck}^{(i)} = A_i \phi_{ck} \tag{14}$$

then, the complete matrix can be written as,

$$X_i = \begin{bmatrix} x_{c1}^{(i)} & x_{c2}^{(i)} & \ldots & x_{cT}^{(i)} \end{bmatrix} = A_i \begin{bmatrix} \phi_{c1} & \phi_{c2} & \ldots & \phi_{cT} \end{bmatrix} = A_i \Phi \tag{15}$$

where the matrix $A_i \in \mathbb{R}^{N \times p}$ accounts for the information in the object ξ_i, while the matrix $\Phi \in \mathbb{R}^{p \times T}$ accounts for the temporal information. The complete set of measurements from M objects X can be represented in the following form,

$$X = \begin{bmatrix} X_1 \\ X_2 \\ \vdots \\ X_m \end{bmatrix} = \begin{bmatrix} A_1 \Phi \\ A_2 \Phi \\ \vdots \\ A_m \Phi \end{bmatrix} = \begin{bmatrix} A_1 \\ A_2 \\ \vdots \\ A_m \end{bmatrix} \Phi = A\Phi \tag{16}$$

where $A \in \mathbb{R}^{NM \times p}$ is a matrix containing the model parameters of the complete set of measurements from M objects. For the representation given in Equation (15), a procedure similar to 2D–PCA/PLS can be applied, using a transform matrix U to reduce the number of rows (measured variables) in data X_i by the linear operation,

$$z_i^{(L)} = UX_i = UA_i\Phi \tag{17}$$

where $U \subset \mathbb{R}^{q \times N}, q \leq N$ and $z_i^{(L)} \in \mathbb{R}^{q \times T}$. Likewise, a transform matrix V can be used to reduce the number of columns (time points) in data X_i by the linear operation,

$$z_i^{(R)} = X_i V = A_i \Phi V = A_i W \tag{18}$$

with $V \in \mathbb{R}^{T \times \tau}, \tau \leq T, W = \Phi V \in \mathbb{R}^{p \times \tau} z_i^{(R)} \in \mathbb{R}^{N \times \tau}$. Combining both operations, temporal information and measurements can be compressed into a smaller representation, as follows

$$z_i = U X_i V = U A_i \Phi V = U A_i W \tag{19}$$

where U, V and W are as explained above, and $z_i \in \mathbb{R}^{q \times \tau}$. Notice also that if the matrix Φ has orthogonal rows and also $V = \Phi^\top$, then $W = \Phi \Phi^\top = I_{p \times p}$, thus,

$$z_i = U A_i \Phi \Phi^\top = U A_i \tag{20}$$

subsequently, the dimensionality reduction can only be carried out in the parameter matrix A_i. Transform matrix U can be computed in the same way as in 2D–PCA/PLS approach, whereas Φ can be any truncated orthogonal basis, for example, trigonometric basis, polynomial basis, etc. This approach will be referred to as *functional PCA/PLS (fPCA/fPLS)* in accordance with the specific transform method.

2.4 The concept of relevance in dynamic variables

Relevance analysis distinguishes variables that effectively represent the subjacent physiological phenomena according to an evaluation measure. Such representative variables are named *relevant features*, whereas the evaluation measure is known as *relevance measure*. Variable selection tries to reject those variables whose contribution to the representation target is none or negligible (*irrelevant features*), as well as those variables that have repeated information (*redundant features*). Therefore, the first issue concerning variable selection is selecting an appropriate relevance definition. Previous efforts have been made in this area by (Yu & Liu, 2004) and (Sepúlveda-Cano et al., 2011) for the case of static variables under non-supervised framework.

The notion of relevance can be cast into the supervised framework by considering the object set $\mathcal{X}_s = \{X_i, i = 1, \ldots, M\} \subset \mathcal{X}$ including M observation samples from the feature subset $\mathcal{X}$. Each observation sample is associated with a class label $c_i \in \mathbb{N}$ constituting the sampled class label (sub)set $\mathcal{C}_s$ from class label set $\mathcal{C}$. Then, given $\mathcal{X}_s$ and $\mathcal{C}_s$, for each one of the x_{lk} features, the relevance function ρ is defined as follows:

$$\rho : \mathbb{R}^{N \times T} \times \mathbb{N} \times \mathbb{R} \to \mathbb{R}$$
$$(\mathcal{X}_s, \mathcal{C}_s, x_{lk}) \mapsto \rho(\mathcal{X}_s, \mathcal{C}_s, x_{lk}) \in \mathbb{R} \tag{21}$$

where the feature relevance function ρ satisfies the following properties (Sepúlveda-Cano et al., 2011):

- *Non–negativity,* i.e. $\rho(\mathcal{X}_s, \mathcal{C}_s, x_{lk}) \geq 0, \forall l, k$.

- *Nullity,* the function $\rho(\mathcal{X}_s, \mathcal{C}_s, x_{lk})$ is null if and only if the feature x_{lk} has not relevance at all.

- *Non–redundancy,* if a feature $\boldsymbol{x}' = \alpha\boldsymbol{x} + \eta$, where the real–valued $\alpha \neq 0$ and η is some noise with mean zero and ε variance, then, the difference $|\rho(\mathcal{X}_s, \mathcal{C}_s, \boldsymbol{x}') - \rho(\mathcal{X}_s, \mathcal{C}_s, \boldsymbol{x})| \to 0$ as $\varepsilon \to 0$.

The value of the function $\rho_{lk} = \rho(\mathcal{X}_s, \mathcal{C}_s, \boldsymbol{x}_{lk})$ for the feature $\boldsymbol{x}_{lk}$ is called *relevance weight*. When all the features are considered, a relevance matrix can be built as $\boldsymbol{R} = [\rho_{lk}]$ for $l = 1,\ldots,N$ and $k = 1,\ldots,T$. Also, when relevance is concerned over any of the axes (rows or columns of the feature matrix), a relevance estimate can be obtained by averaging on rows or columns, thus obtaining

$$\rho_r = \frac{1}{T}\sum_{k=1}^{T}\rho_{ck} \qquad\qquad \rho_c = \frac{1}{N}\sum_{l=1}^{N}\rho_{rl} \tag{22}$$

where, within the specific TFR and TFDF framework, ρ_r accounts for the relevance of each time-varying feature, while ρ_c describes how relevance change through time. Then, the variable selection process is carried out by selecting those x_{lk} features whose relevance value ρ_{lk} is over a certain threshold δ. It is likely that most relevant time-varying features can be selected, extracting those time-varying features $\boldsymbol{x}_{rl}$ whose relevance value ρ_{rl} is over certain threshold ρ_{min}.

Within the literature several relevance measures have been considered, such as linear correlation, conditional entropy, symmetrical uncertainty and transformation–based measures (Avendano-Valencia et al., 2010; Yu & Liu, 2004). Among them, *symmetrical uncertainty* is capable of measuring both linear and complex non-linear relationships between variables. The symmetrical uncertainty is defined as follows

$$\rho_{su}(x_i, c) = 2\frac{H(x_i) - H(x_i|c)}{H(x_i) + H(c)}, \quad \rho_{su}(x_i, c) \in [0,1], \forall i = 1,\ldots,m \tag{23}$$

where $H(x_i)$ is the entropy of the features and $H(x_i|c)$ is the conditional entropy of the features given the classes, both defined as

$$H(x_i) = -\int_{x_i} P(x_i)\log P(x_i)dx_i, \quad \forall i = 1,\ldots,m \tag{24}$$

$$H(x_i|c) = -\int_c P(c)\int_{x_i} P(x_i|c)\log P(x_i|c)dx_i dc, \quad \forall i = 1,\ldots,m \tag{25}$$

A value of $\rho_{su}(x_i, c) = 1$ indicates that the feature x_i completely predicts the values of the class labels c. Since the computation of Equation (23) requires the estimation of both $P(x_i)$ and $P(x_i|c)$, histogram–driven estimates might be used. Therefore, the integrals in Equations (24) and (25) become sums that are carried out along the histogram bins.

2.5 Selection of most informative areas from dynamic t–f variables

Once the relevance measure is properly determined, the selection of the feature vectors is carried out by choosing those variables with a relevance that exceeds a given threshold. Nonetheless, managing dynamic variables requires special handling since the considered features are no longer organized as vectors. Within this framework two approaches are proposed: a) *1D-Relevance:* Evaluate the relevance measure for each point of the TFR, and then select the most relevant time–frequency points to appraise a reduced feature vector that will be later processed by conventional linear transform methods (PCA or PLS); this approach is described in Algorithm 1. b) *2D-Relevance:* Evaluate the relevance measure on rows or columns of the dynamic feature set as in Equation (22) and then select the most relevant time instants or frequency bands to appraise a TFR–based feature matrix, which will be further reduced using either the matricial approach: 2D–PCA, 2D–PLS; this approach is described in Algorithm 2. c) *Functional Relevance:* The relevance measure is evaluated as in b) to select the most relevant time instants of frequency bands and later, the most relevant data is further reduced using ĚƒPCA or ƒPLS. The approach is described in Algorithm 3. The approach is described in Algorithm 3..

Algorithm 1 1D-Relevance: Selection of TFR–based features using relevance measures and dimensionality reduction

---

Input: TFR dataset $\{X_1, X_2, \ldots, X_M\}$, relevance threshold ρ_{min}.
Output: Reduced feature vector set $\{z_1, z_2, \ldots, z_M\}$.

1. Convert TFR matrices into vectors
   for $i = 1$ to M **do**
   $$x_i = \text{vec}(X_k) = \left[(x_{c1}^{(i)})^\top, (x_{c2}^{(i)})^\top, \ldots, (x_{cT}^{(i)})^\top \right]$$
   end for

2. Compute the relevance measure vector $\rho(x)$ of the feature vectors $\{x_1, x_2, \ldots, x_M\}$, using the relevance measure defined in Equation (23).

3. Select the most relevant variables from vectorized TFRs
   for $i = 1$ to M **do**
   $$\hat{z}_i = \left\{ x_{lk}^{(i)} \ \forall k, l : \rho(x_{kl}) \geq \rho_{min} \right\}$$
   end for

4. Compute the transformation matrix V of PCA or PLS using the relevant feature vector set $\{\hat{z}_1, \hat{z}_2, \ldots, \hat{z}_M\}$.

5. Transform the feature vectors $\hat{z}_i$ into the reduced feature vector z_i, as
   for $i = 1$ to M **do**
   $$z_i = \hat{z}_i V$$
   end for

---

3. Experimental set–up

3.1 EEG database

The EEG signals correspond to 29 patients with medically intractable focal epilepsies. They were recorded by the Department of Epileptology of the University of Bonn as explained in (Andrzejak et al., 2001). The database comprises five sets (denoted as A-E) composed of 100 single channel EEG segments, which were selected and extracted after visual inspection from continuous multichannel EEG to avoid artifacts (e.g. muscular activity or eye movements). Datasets A and B consist of segments taken from scalp EEG records of five healthy subjects using the standard $10 - 20$ electrode placements. Volunteers were woken up, and relaxed with their eyes open (A) and eyes closed (B), respectively. Datasets C, D and E were selected

---

Algorithm 2 2D-Relevance: Frequency band selection from TFR using relevance measures and dimensionality reduction by matricial approach

---

Input: TFR matrix dataset $\{X_1, X_2, \ldots, X_M\}$, relevance threshold $\rho_{\min}$.
Output: Reduced feature vector set $\{z_1, z_2, \ldots, z_M\}$.

1. Follow steps 1. and 2. of Algorithm 1

2. Compute the average relevance value of row axis ρ_r as defined by Equation (22).

3. Select the most relevant frequency bands from TFR

    for $i = 1$ to M **do**
$$\hat{X}_i = \left\{ x_{rl}^{(i)} \quad \forall l : \rho_{rl} \geq \rho_{\min} \right\}$$
    end for

4. Compute the transformation matrices U and V of 2D–PCA (or 2D–PLS), using the reduced TFR matrices set $\{\hat{X}_1, \hat{X}_2, \ldots, \hat{X}_M\}$.

5. Transform the reduced TFR matrices $\hat{X}_i$ into the reduced feature vector z_i, as

    for $i = 1$ to M **do**
$$Z_i = U \hat{X}_i V^\top$$
$$z_i = vec(Z_i)$$
    end for

---

from presurgical diagnosed EEG recordings. The signals were selected from five patients who achieved a complete control of the epileptic episodes after the dissection of one of the hippocampal formations, which was correctly diagnosed as the epileptogenic zone. Segments of set D were recorded in the epileptogenic zone, and segments of C in the hippocampal zone of the opposite side of the brain. While sets C and D only contain activity measured on inter–ictal intervals, set E only contains records with ictal activity. In this set, all segments were selected from every recording place exhibiting ictal activity. All EEG signals were recorded with an acquisition system of 128 channels, using average common reference. Data was digitized at 173.61 Hz with 12 bits of resolution.

In this study, the database described above is organized to create one classification task, where all the EEG segments are sorted into three different classes: A and B types of EEG segments were combined in a single class (Normal); C and D types were also combined in a single class (Interictal); and type E completes the third class (Ictal). This set is the one closest to real medical applications which include three categories: normal (i.e., types A and B) with 200 recordings, seizure free (i.e., types C and D) with 200 recordings, and seizure (i.e., type E) with 100 recordings. Validation of the classifier is carried out by 10 fold cross-validation, where the database is divided into 10 folds containing different records from each class. Nine of these folds are used for training and the remaining one for validation purposes. Training and validation folds are changed until the ten folds are used for validation.

3.2 Feature estimation

Time-Frequency Representations: Time-frequency analysis of EEG signals is carried out using STFT, SPWVD and parametric TFR based on SP-TARMA modeling. Analysis is performed in the frequency range from 0 to 43.4 Hz as recommended for EEG signals (Subasi, 2007). STFT is computed using a 512 point gaussian window with a 504 sample overlap. SPWV parameters

---

Algorithm 3 Functional Relevance: Frequency band selection from TFR using relevance measures and dimensionality reduction by functional approach

---

Input: TFR matrix dataset $\{X_1, X_2, \ldots, X_M\}$, relevance threshold $\rho_{\min}$.
Output: Reduced feature vector set $\{z_1, z_2, \ldots, z_M\}$.

1. Follow steps 1. and 2. of Algorithm 1

2. Compute the average relevance value of row axis ρ_r as defined by Equation (22).

3. Select the most relevant frequency bands from TFR

   for $i = 1$ to M do
   $$\hat{X}_i = \left\{ x_{rl}^{(i)} \quad \forall l : \rho_{rl} \geq \rho_{\min} \right\}$$
   end for

4. Compute the representation coefficients A_i of the basis Φ

   for $i = 1$ to M do
   $$\hat{A}_i = \hat{X}_i \Phi^{-1}$$
   end for

5. Compute the transformation matrices U and of fPCA (or fPLS), using the representation coefficient matrix set $\{\hat{A}_1, \hat{A}_2, \ldots, \hat{A}_M\}$.

6. Transform the reduced TFR matrices $\hat{A}_i$ into the reduced feature vector z_i, as

   for $i = 1$ to M do
   $$Z_i = U \hat{A}_i$$
   $$z_i = vec(Z_i)$$
   end for

---

are adjusted as suggested in (Tzallas et al., 2008), using 64-point Hamming window for time and frequency smoothing window. For parametric SP-TAR, estimation, model order selection and validation is implemented following the recommendations in (Poulimenos & Fassois, 2006). The model order selection approach consists in finding the elbow of the *log likelihood function* computed for each record in the database using SP-TAR(n_a) models, with $n_a = 2, \ldots, 20$. The achieved selected orders n_a are between 10 to 14 for the SP–TAR model. The estimation parameters of each estimation methodology are summarized in Table 1. For all the methods considered, a set of TFRs with size $T = 512$ and $N = 256$ was obtained.

Time-Frequency Dynamic Features: Analysis by TFDF is carried out with SSC, SSCE, LFCC and DWT coefficients. Spectral centroids and cepstral coefficients are computed from STFT, using 8 frequency sub-bands. Filters banks are designed using gaussian functions with a 10% overlap between bands. DWT is computed using Daubechies 4 mother wavelet up to the fifth decomposition level as suggested in (Subasi, 2007). For each EEG recording, both wavelet coefficients and reconstructed time series for each decomposition level are considered in the analysis. The information regarding to estimation of each dynamic feature is summarized in Table 1.

Figure 2 shows exemplary TFRs obtained with the three different estimation approaches. Each column refers to a different estimation approach: STFT - short time Fourier transform, SPWVD - smoothed pseudo Wigner-Ville distribution, and SP-TAR - parametric TFR based

Estimation Method	Parameters
STFT	Window parameters: Gaussian window, length 512 samples, overlap 504 samples.
SPWV	Time and frequency smoothing window: Hamming 64 point window. Number of points in frequency axis 256.
SP-TARMA	Model order selection criteria: elbow of *log likelihood function*. Variance tradeoff parameter of Kalman filter/smoother $v = 0.01$. Smoothness priors order $\kappa = 2$. Number of points in frequency axis 256.
TFDF	Parameters
SSC & SSCE	Filter bank function: Gaussian function. Band overlap: 10%. Number of sub-bands: 10. Energy estimation bandwidth: $\Delta\omega$ 10.85 Hz.
LFCC	Number of sub-bands: 10. Number of LFCC: 8.
DWT	Mother wavelet: Daubechies 4. Decomposition level 5.

Table 1. Implementation details of TFR and TFDF estimation methods.

on SP-TAR model. Likewise, each row shows TFRs associated with some typical recordings from a database class (A to E).

3.3 Dimensionality reduction

The dimensionality reduction scheme considers a linear transform approach to the set of most relevant features extracted from the t–f feature set. Most relevant features are selected according to the symmetrical uncertainty relevance measure, described in Equation (23). The symmetrical uncertainty is evaluated on the TFR dataset yielding the relevance matrices and vectors shown in Figure 3. Plots in the left column show the average relevance measure over the frequency axis; plots in the central column show the TFR relevance average for each training fold set; plots in the right column show the sorted relevance measures vs. the percentage of features. In the case of the TFDF set, the relevance measure is evaluated and the relevance of each TFDF is obtained by averaging all of the relevance outcomes along time. The relevance measure obtained for each one of the analyzed TFDF sets is shown in Figure 4. After evaluating the relevance measure on each dataset, the most relevant features are further reduced using vectorized, 2D and functional linear transform approaches. The representation coefficients in functional linear transform method are computed by means of discrete cosine transform. The basis is truncated up to the first coefficient with 0.5% of the power of the largest coefficient. The number of features in the reduced feature space is selected as the minimum number that explains 95% of the complete dataset variance.

3.4 Results

The classification performance is measured the accuracy, sensitivity and specificity, defined by,

$$\text{Acc }(\%) = \frac{N_C}{N_T} \times 100; \quad \text{Sens }(\%) = \frac{N_{TP}}{N_{TP} + N_{FN}} \times 100; \quad \text{Spec }(\%) = \frac{N_{TN}}{N_{TN} + N_{FP}} \times 100$$

where N_C is the number of correctly classified patterns, N_T is the total number of patterns used to feed the classifier, N_{TP} is the number of true positives (objective class accurately classified), N_{FN} is the number of false negatives (objective class classified as reference class), N_{TN} is the

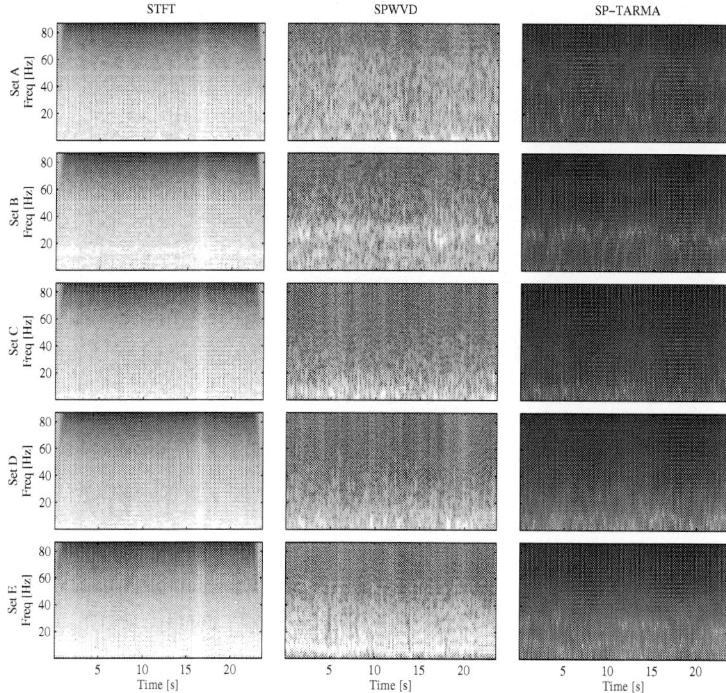

Fig. 2. Estimated TFR using the three different estimation approaches considered for exemplary signals from each class (A to E). STFT - short time Fourier transform, SPWVD - smoothed pseudo Wigner-Ville distribution, and SP-TARMA - parametric TFR based on SP-TARMA model.

number of true negatives (reference class accurately classified), and N_{FP} is the number of false positives (reference class classified as objective class). Mean and standard deviations of the accuracy, sensitivity and specificity are calculated for all the validation folds. The following approaches are analyzed:

- Conventional approaches: *t–f* grid energy approach (TF-grid), TFR Kullback-Leibler distance based nearest neighbors approach (TFR-KNN) and statistical measures extracted from DWT coefficients (DWT-averages).

- Relevance analysis and linear transform based approaches: symmetrical uncertainty based vectorized PCA/PLS on TFR matrices and on TFDF (1D- PCA TFR, 1D- PLS TFR, 1D- PCA TFDF, and 1D-PLS TFDF); symmetrical uncertainty based 2D–PCA/PLS on TFR matrices and on TFDF (2D-PCA TFR, 2D-PLS TFR, 2D-PCA TFDF, and 2D- PLS TFDF); and symmetrical uncertainty based functional PCA/PLS on TFR matrices and on TFDF (*f*PCA TFR, *f*PLS TFR, *f*PCA TFDF, and *f*PLS TFDF).

Table 2 shows the performance outcomes of the conventional approaches. The feature vectors obtained with TF-grid and DWT-averages are further reduced by PCA, using a

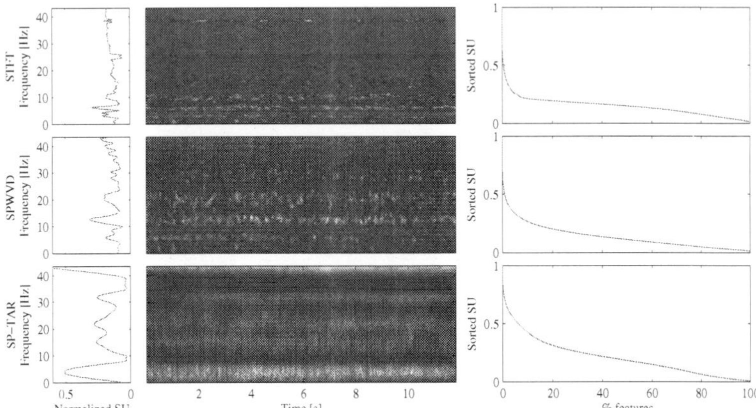

Fig. 3. Average symmetrical uncertainty values for TFR sets of EEG database. Left plots, relevance average on the frequency axis; center plots: fold average of the TFR relevance matrix; right plots: sorted relevance measure. Top–bottom: TFR estimator, STFT, SPWVD and parametric SP–TAR.

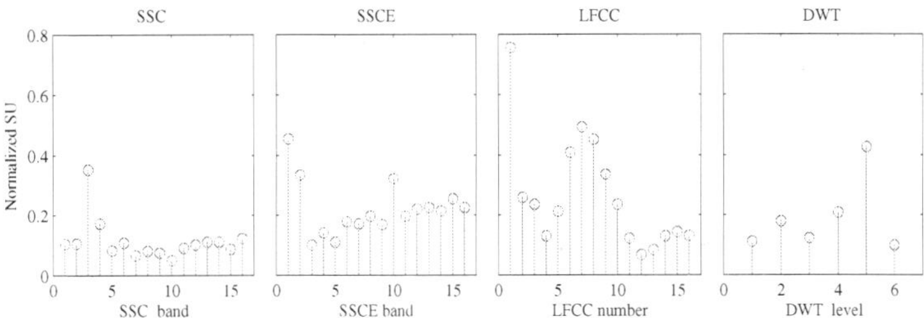

Fig. 4. Average symmetrical uncertainty values for TFDF sets of EEG database. Each plot shows the relevance value for each TFDF set, SSC, SSCE, LFCC and DWT level coefficients.

number of features accounting for 95% of the variability of the original data. All TFR–based approaches are tested with STFT, SPWVD and SP-TAR based TFR estimates. Table 3 shows the performance outcomes of the 1D-Relevance, 2D–Relevance and Functional Relevance methods described by Algorithms 1, 2, and 3, respectively. A comparison is made between linear transforms on the complete data and on the 50% of the most relevant variables. All TFR–based approaches are tested with STFT, SPWVD and SP-TAR based TFR estimates, whereas all TFDF–based approaches are tested with SSC, SSCE, LFCC and DWT subband coefficients. For all approaches, a 3 nearest neighbor classifier is used. In addition to classifier performance, the computing times and size of the reduced feature set are taken into account in the analysis. The average computing times during training for each method are shown in the Figure 5(a). Size of the reduced feature set for each method is shown in the Figure 5(b). Values for TFR–based approaches are shown on the left plot, and those for TFDF–based approaches in the plot on the right.

	Method	Accuracy	Sensitivity	Specificity
	STFT	91.20 ± 3.16	92.00 ± 2.58	94.33 ± 4.98
TF-grid	SPWVD	92.20 ± 3.94	94.50 ± 4.97	96.33 ± 3.67
	SP-TAR	91.40 ± 1.65	96.50 ± 2.42	93.67 ± 2.46
	STFT	88.60 ± 4.12	97.00 ± 3.50	97.33 ± 3.06
TFR-KNN	SPWVD	88.00 ± 4.90	96.00 ± 4.59	97.67 ± 2.74
	SP-TAR	85.20 ± 3.43	98.50 ± 2.42	92.00 ± 5.26
DWT-averages		88.40 ± 3.86	93.00 ± 5.37	92.67 ± 4.39

Table 2. Performance outcomes of conventional t–f based classification approaches for epilepsy diagnosis on EEG database.

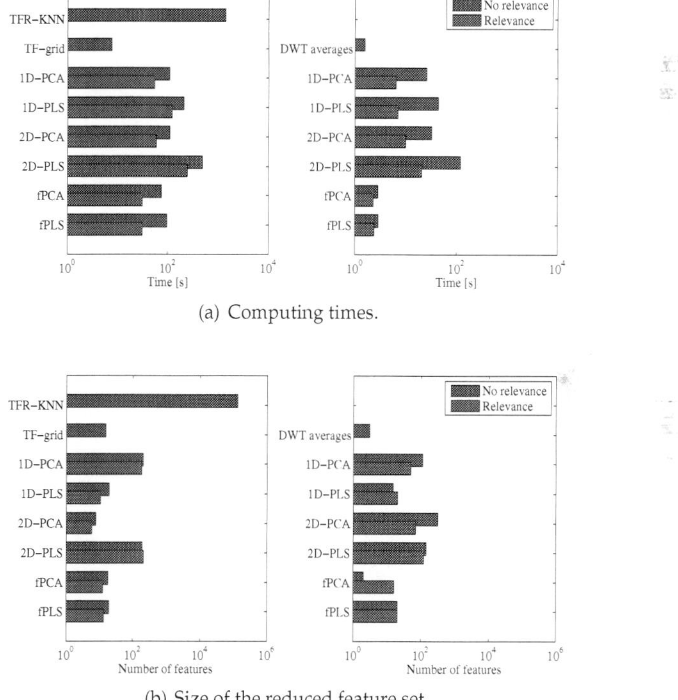

(a) Computing times.

(b) Size of the reduced feature set.

Fig. 5. Computing times and size of the reduced feature set of each one of the analyzed t–f based classification approaches. The left plot show the values for TFR–based approaches, the right plot show the values for TFDF–based approaches.

			Complete feature set			50% most relevant variables		
	Method		Accuracy	Sensitivity	Specificity	Accuracy	Sensitivity	Specificity
1D–Relevance	1D-PCA TFR	STFT	92.20 ± 3.58	94.00 ± 5.16	98.00 ± 2.33	92.20 ± 4.26	93.50 ± 5.80	97.33 ± 3.44
		SPWVD	90.60 ± 4.99	91.50 ± 4.74	99.33 ± 1.41	92.60 ± 4.22	90.00 ± 4.08	98.33 ± 2.36
		SP–TAR	85.80 ± 3.94	93.00 ± 5.87	91.67 ± 4.23	91.00 ± 3.02	97.00 ± 3.50	93.67 ± 4.83
	1D-PLS TFR	STFT	96.60 ± 3.13	98.50 ± 2.42	97.67 ± 2.25	96.00 ± 3.27	97.00 ± 3.50	97.33 ± 2.63
		SPWVD	97.40 ± 2.50	99.50 ± 1.58	98.00 ± 2.33	95.40 ± 3.13	97.50 ± 2.64	98.00 ± 3.22
		SP–TAR	96.60 ± 2.99	100.00 ± 0.00	96.67 ± 3.51	96.80 ± 2.70	99.00 ± 2.11	97.33 ± 3.06
	1D-PCA TFDF	SSC	76.00 ± 7.72	74.50 ± 11.65	92.00 ± 5.92	78.40 ± 6.10	74.50 ± 8.96	91.33 ± 6.89
		SSCE	63.20 ± 10.38	63.50 ± 13.95	79.00 ± 12.18	60.40 ± 6.59	64.00 ± 14.49	73.67 ± 7.45
		LFCC	62.00 ± 7.42	57.00 ± 9.78	72.67 ± 6.44	64.00 ± 6.99	58.00 ± 8.56	76.67 ± 5.88
		DWT	85.20 ± 5.90	82.00 ± 11.35	90.00 ± 4.44	78.20 ± 5.20	71.50 ± 11.32	90.67 ± 3.06
	1D-PLS TFDF	SSC	86.20 ± 4.37	85.00 ± 7.45	96.00 ± 4.66	87.20 ± 3.91	85.50 ± 6.85	94.33 ± 3.53
		SSCE	93.40 ± 2.50	93.00 ± 4.83	98.33 ± 2.36	89.80 ± 3.58	88.00 ± 6.32	97.33 ± 2.63
		LFCC	91.00 ± 3.80	94.00 ± 7.38	93.33 ± 3.51	89.00 ± 4.55	91.50 ± 5.80	92.33 ± 4.17
		DWT	93.40 ± 3.53	97.00 ± 3.50	94.00 ± 3.44	91.20 ± 3.16	94.00 ± 3.16	93.67 ± 5.54
2D–Relevance	2D-PCA TFR	STFT	86.20 ± 3.94	69.00 ± 10.75	99.33 ± 2.11	85.40 ± 3.78	67.50 ± 10.87	99.33 ± 2.11
		SPWVD	90.60 ± 2.67	79.00 ± 9.66	99.33 ± 2.11	89.80 ± 3.82	76.50 ± 11.32	99.67 ± 1.05
		SP–TAR	90.00 ± 3.53	95.00 ± 2.36	94.33 ± 3.87	96.40 ± 2.80	98.50 ± 2.42	97.00 ± 3.31
	2D-PLS TFR	STFT	92.80 ± 3.16	88.50 ± 7.09	99.00 ± 2.25	92.00 ± 3.27	88.00 ± 7.15	98.67 ± 2.33
		SPWVD	94.20 ± 2.39	94.00 ± 5.16	98.00 ± 2.33	95.20 ± 2.53	95.00 ± 6.24	98.00 ± 2.81
		SP–TAR	92.80 ± 4.44	98.50 ± 2.42	94.33 ± 5.68	96.60 ± 2.50	98.50 ± 3.37	97.67 ± 2.74
	2D-PCA TFDF	SSC	78.00 ± 8.16	60.00 ± 15.09	99.33 ± 1.41	78.00 ± 8.27	61.50 ± 14.35	99.00 ± 1.61
		SSCE	93.00 ± 5.10	95.00 ± 6.24	96.67 ± 3.14	82.60 ± 4.62	87.00 ± 7.89	89.33 ± 5.40
		LFCC	79.40 ± 9.24	81.50 ± 16.84	87.00 ± 3.99	80.00 ± 10.02	83.00 ± 16.36	87.33 ± 4.66
		DWT	92.20 ± 3.71	96.50 ± 4.12	90.33 ± 4.57	94.60 ± 2.32	99.50 ± 1.58	92.67 ± 4.10
	2D-PLS TFDF	SSC	85.60 ± 3.63	81.50 ± 7.47	94.00 ± 3.44	87.00 ± 3.56	82.50 ± 7.91	94.33 ± 3.16
		SSCE	82.60 ± 6.11	75.00 ± 8.16	95.00 ± 2.36	83.60 ± 5.23	79.50 ± 7.98	92.67 ± 5.16
		LFCC	88.80 ± 4.02	91.50 ± 7.84	93.33 ± 3.51	89.80 ± 4.16	92.00 ± 8.23	94.33 ± 3.16
		DWT	92.80 ± 2.70	97.50 ± 3.54	92.33 ± 4.17	92.80 ± 4.13	97.50 ± 3.54	92.67 ± 6.05
Functional Relevance	_f_PCA TFR	STFT	95.20 ± 2.86	96.00 ± 3.16	98.00 ± 3.22	90.00 ± 5.16	92.50 ± 4.86	93.00 ± 4.83
		SPWVD	92.40 ± 2.95	95.00 ± 4.08	94.67 ± 3.58	91.00 ± 3.68	92.50 ± 4.86	94.67 ± 3.58
		SP–TAR	96.60 ± 3.41	99.50 ± 1.58	98.00 ± 2.81	92.80 ± 6.48	98.50 ± 3.37	94.67 ± 4.77
	_f_PLS TFR	STFT	94.80 ± 3.29	96.00 ± 3.16	97.67 ± 3.16	93.00 ± 2.87	95.50 ± 4.38	95.00 ± 4.23
		SPWVD	94.80 ± 2.35	97.00 ± 3.50	97.00 ± 2.92	91.80 ± 2.90	94.00 ± 6.15	95.33 ± 3.58
		SP–TAR	97.00 ± 2.87	99.50 ± 1.58	97.67 ± 2.74	97.40 ± 2.50	99.50 ± 1.58	98.00 ± 2.33
	_f_PCA TFDF	SSC	84.60 ± 4.53	86.50 ± 5.80	90.67 ± 4.66	85.80 ± 5.29	80.50 ± 8.32	92.00 ± 4.22
		SSCE	93.80 ± 2.20	94.00 ± 3.16	98.67 ± 1.72	85.20 ± 3.91	83.50 ± 5.30	93.00 ± 2.92
		LFCC	87.40 ± 4.72	89.00 ± 7.38	91.33 ± 3.22	79.20 ± 6.75	79.00 ± 15.06	87.33 ± 4.39
		DWT	86.80 ± 4.54	90.50 ± 5.50	89.67 ± 7.61	88.00 ± 3.89	94.50 ± 3.69	90.67 ± 6.99
	_f_PLS TFDF	SSC	78.40 ± 5.48	72.00 ± 10.06	90.67 ± 4.66	84.80 ± 5.18	82.00 ± 7.53	94.00 ± 4.66
		SSCE	72.60 ± 5.58	45.00 ± 13.94	95.67 ± 3.16	90.20 ± 6.00	92.50 ± 6.35	95.33 ± 4.50
		LFCC	55.60 ± 3.24	39.50 ± 8.64	73.00 ± 5.32	88.20 ± 4.05	90.50 ± 6.85	93.00 ± 2.46
		DWT	73.20 ± 4.34	55.50 ± 9.26	89.00 ± 4.73	89.20 ± 3.29	94.50 ± 3.69	92.00 ± 5.02

Table 3. Performance outcomes of t–f classification approaches based on linear transforms for epilepsy diagnosis on EEG database.

4. Discussion

4.1 Time–Frequency Representations and Time–Frequency Dynamic Features

Three different TFR estimators have been studied in the experimental framework, STFT, SPWVD and parametric TFR based on SP-TAR modeling. Accurate estimation of the TFR is very important to achieve adequate performance of the classifier. Nonetheless, after proper adjustment of TFR estimators, it is possible to obtain good results. The results in tables 2 and 3 show that the performance outcomes attained by STFT, SPWVD and parametric TFR are very similar. According to the dimensionality reduction approach, each TFR estimator shows either better or worse results. The best results are found with parametric TFR and SPWVD, but, in general, there is no tendency of the best performance. Both STFT and SPWVD are easy to adjust and compute, whereas parametric TFR requires an increased set up time and user expertise to achieve proper performance. So, in terms of the problem addressed in this study, it may be enough to use simple TFR estimators. Nevertheless, more specialized approaches may be needed for other applications under different non–stationary conditions.

On the other hand, four TFDF sets have been considered in this study, SSC, SSCE, LFCC and DWT coefficients. Those features are shown to be easier to manage than TFR features and require less computing time, as they are more compact representations (see Figure 5). The performance of the TFDF based approach is lower than the performance of its TFR counterpart. The performance obtained using different dimensionality reduction approaches is random and the dispersion values are high. Only the SSCE and DWT coefficients show proper performance. The best performance is achieved using DWT coefficients.

4.2 Classification based on $t\text{--}f$ features

Several approaches for TFR and TFDF have been analyzed. Such approaches can be grouped into conventional approaches, vectorization transform methods, bidimensional (2D) transform methods and functional transform methods. Distance based and local averaging techniques are grouped within the conventional approaches. Nearest neighbor classifier based on computation of Kullback-Leibler distance between TFR matrices is shown to be the most computationally expensive approach with the worst performance. Also, distance computation is carried out using the entire dataset, so the generalization capabilities of the classifier are poor, explaining the low performance on the EEG database. Local averaging techniques like the $t\text{--}f$ grid approach and DWT averages are very easy to implement, fast to compute and yield acceptable results. These properties make them an appealing choice for making former tests on a database and for fixing TFR and wavelet parameters. Nevertheless. Nevertheless, as dynamical properties of the $t\text{--}f$ features are lost, local averaging techniques cannot reach highest performance.

Vectorization transform methods are a straightforward application of the conventional linear transform methods to functional and matricial data. Advantages of this method are ease of use and accurate results. In fact, the best performance of the TFDF set is obtained using a vectorization approach, which can be explained by the unidimesional structure of these features that fits better the representation as vector. Difficulties lie in the management of huge data matrices which require large memory resources, for example, when covariance matrices should be computed in the 1D–PCA approach. Moreover, the performance outcomes are very different when supervised and non–supervised methods are used, specially when the TFDF set is used. Bidimensional transform reduces the memory requirements of data matrices, but increases the computational cost, as transform matrices should be computed for each dimension. These methods demonstrate stable performances for supervised and non–supervised methods, but seem to work inappropriately with TFDF features. Functional transform methods exhibit the best performance among the studied approaches. Computational requirements are low, the classification performance is high and stable, and lowest reduced representation space is achieved amongst all the considered dimensionality reduction methods. This approach is well suited to TFR–based classification, for both supervised and non–supervised linear transform methods. In general, all the linear transform methods can extract maximum information from the $t\text{--}f$ feature set, thus achieving adequate performance rates, but may require more attention the selection of an adequate reduced feature set size.

Relevance analysis is shown to be a highly beneficial tool for analyzing high dimensional data, as shown by the results on t–f feature sets from EEG biosignals. By means of the symmetrical uncertainty measure, it is possible to reduce the feature set by 50%, before linear transform methods are applied. Thus computational requirements and time are significantly reduced and numerical stability is improved. Besides, in most of the cases, the performance rates remain stable, and performance even improves in some cases. More stable behavior might be achieved, for example, if the relevance threshold were selected according to the accuracy rate of the classifier.

5. Conclusion

Throughout this chapter, several t–f based dimensionality reduction methods for classification of non–stationary biosignals were presented and discussed. A novel approach, based on feature selection by relevance analysis and linear transform of the most relevant features, was presented. Vectorized and bidimensional linear transform approaches were defined and reviewed, and the functional linear transform approach, specially designed to manage matricial and functional data, was proposed. The recommended *functional relevance* approach was tested on the detection of epileptic events on a public non–stationary electroencephalographic database. Comparison was made with other conventional state of the art approaches. Results show the benefits of the proposed functional linear transform approach and relevance analysis. Thus, it is demonstrated that the proposed *functional relevance* approach is able to exploit the multidimensional nature of data, while the relevance analysis facilitates the extraction of the most informative data.

Several questions are still open for further research. To begin with, the influence of the selected number of variables on the final classification performance is still to be analyzed. In this study, the explained variability of each eigenvector was used to select the size of the reduced feature set, but an automatic discriminative criterion could improve the classifier performance. On the other hand, the automatic selection of the relevance threshold is more difficult. A criterion, based on the classification rates could be used, but this increases the computational effort in the training stage. If the redundance of the feature set is also regarded, the most informative variables would be chosen as those that have the highest relevance value among similar redundant variables. In regard to the proposed functional linear transform, it is also important to compare different basis functions, as the final performance is compromised when coupling the basis function to the analyzed data. Finally, the importance of the relevance measure and the large influence that it has on the proposed methodology should be highlighted. For this reason, other approaches can also benefit if a relevance measure is considered in the design. Moreover, it is still to be analyzed the influence of different relevance measures on the performance of the methodology.

6. Acknowledgements

This research is carried out under grant *"Servicio de monitoreo remoto de actividad cardiaca para el tamizaje clinico en la red de telemedicina del departamento de Caldas"*, funded by Universidad Nacional de Colombia and Universidad de Caldas.

7. References

Andrzejak, R., Lehnertz, K., Rieke, C., Mormann, F., David, P. & Elger, C. (2001). Indications of nonlinear deterministic and finite dimensional structures in time series of brain electrical activity: Dependence on recording region and brain state, *Phys. Rev. E* 64: 71–86.

Avendano-Valencia, L. D., Godino-Llorente, J., Blanco-Velasco, M. & Castellanos-Dominguez, G. (2010). Feature extraction from parametric timeŰfrequency representations for heart murmur detection, *Annals of Biomedical Engineering* .

Avendaño-Valencia, L., Martínez-Vargas, J., Giraldo, E. & Castellanos-Domínguez, G. (2010). Reduction of irrelevant and redundant data from tfrs for eeg signal classification, *Engineering in Medicine and Biology Society (EMBC), 2010 Annual International Conference of the IEEE*.

Aviyente, S. (2004). Information processing on the time-frequency plane, *Acoustics, Speech, and Signal Processing, 2004. Proceedings. (ICASSP '04). IEEE International Conference on*, pp. 617–620.

Barker, M. & Rayens, W. (2003). Partial least squares for discrimination, *Journal of chemometrics* 17(3): 166–173.

Bernat, E. M., Malone, S. M., Williams, W. J., Patrick, C. J. & Iacono, W. G. (2007). Decomposing delta, theta, and alpha time-frequency ERP activity from a visual oddball task using PCA., *International journal of psychophysiology : official journal of the International Organization of Psychophysiology* 64(1): 62–74.

Cvetkovic, D., Ubeyli, E. & Cosic, I. (2008). Wavelet transform feature extraction from human ppg, ecg, and eeg signal responses to elf pemf exposures: A pilot study, *Digital Signal Processing* 18(5): 861–874.

Debbal, S. & Bereksi-Reguig, F. (2007). Time-frequency analysis of the first and the second heartbeat sounds, *Applied Mathematics and Computation* 184(2): 1041 – 1052.

Englehart, K., Hudgins, B., Parker, P. A. & Stevenson, M. (1999). Classification of the myoelectric signal using time-frequency based representations, *Medical Engineering and Physics* 21(6-7): 431 – 438.

Hassanpour, H., Mesbah, M. & Boashash, B. (2004). Time-frequency based newborn EEG seizure detection using low and high frequency signatures, *Physiological Measurement* 25(4): 935–944.

M Tarvainen, J. Hiltunen, P. R.-a. & Karjalainen, P. (2004). Estimation of nonstationary eeg with Kalman smoother approach: An application to event-related synchronization, *IEEE Transactions On Biomedical Engineering* 51(3): 516–524.

Mallat, S. (2008). *A Wavelet Tour of Signal Processing*, 3rd edn, Academic Press.

Marchant, B. P. (2003). Time-frequency analysis for biosystems engineering, *Biosystems Engineering* 85(3): 261 – 281.

Michel, O., Baraniuk, R. & Flandrin, P. (64-67). Time-frequency based distance and divergence measures, *Proceedings of IEEE-SP International Symposium on Time-Frequency and Time-Scale Analysis*.

Poulimenos, A. & Fassois, S. (2006). Parametric time-domain methods for non-stationary random vibration modelling and analysis – A critical survey and comparison, *Mechanical Systems and Signal Processing* 20(4): 763–816.

Quiceno-Manrique, A., Godino-Llorente, J., Blanco-Velasco, M. & Castellanos-Dominguez, G. (2010). Selection of dynamic features based on timeâĂŞfrequency representations for heart murmur detection from phonocardiographic signals, *Annals of Biomedical Engineering* 38: 118–137. 10.1007/s10439-009-9838-3.

Sejdic, E., Djurovic, I. & Jiang, J. (2009). Time-frequency feature representation using energy concentration: An overview of recent advances, *Digital Signal Processing* 19(1): 153–183.

Sejdic, E. & Jiang, J. (2007). Selective Regional Correlation for Pattern Recognition, *IEEE Transactions on Systems, Man and Cybernetics* 37(1): 82–93.

Sepúlveda-Cano, L. M., Acosta-Medina, C. D. & Castellanos-Dominguez, G. (2011). Relevance analysis of stochastic biosignals for identification of pathologies, *EURASIP Journal on Advances on Signal Processing* 2011: 10.

Subasi, A. (2007). EEG signal classification using wavelet feature extraction and a mixture of expert model, *Expert Systems with Applications* 32(4): 1084–1093.

Tarvainen, M., Georgiadis, S., Lipponen, J., Hakkarainen, M. & Karjalainen, P. (2009). Time-varying spectrum estimation of heart rate variability signals with kalman smoother algorithm, *Engineering in Medicine and Biology Society, 2009. EMBC 2009. Annual International Conference of the IEEE*, pp. 1 –4.

Turk, M. & Pentland, A. (1991). Eigenfaces for recognition, *Journal of Cognitive Neurosicence* 3(1): 71–86.

Tzallas, A. T., Tsipouras, M. G., Fotiadis, D. I. & Member, S. (2008). Epileptic seizure detection in electroencephalograms using time-frequency analysis, *IEEE Transactions on Information Technology in Biomedicine* 13(5): 703—-710.

Yang, J., Zhang, D., Frangi, A. & Yang, J. (2004). Two-dimensional PCA: A new approach to appearance-based face representation and recognition, *IEEE Transactions on Pattern Analysis and Machine Intelligence* 26(1): 131–137.

Yu, L. & Liu, H. (2004). Efficient feature selection via analysis of relevance and redundancy, *Journal of Machine Learning Research* 5: 1205–1224.

Zhang, D. & Zhou, Z.-H. (2005). (2D)2PCA: Two-directional two-dimensional PCA for efficient face representation and recognition, *Neurocomputing* 69(1-3): 224 – 231. Neural Networks in Signal Processing.

14

Classification of Emotional Stress Using Brain Activity

Seyyed Abed Hosseini and Mohammad Bagher Naghibi-Sistani
Islamic Azad University-Mashhad Branch,
Ferdowsi University of Mashhad,
Iran

1. Introduction

Stress and Emotion are complex phenomena that play significant roles in the quality of human life. Emotion plays a major role in motivation, perception, cognition, creativity, attention, learning and decision-making (Seymour et al., 2008). A major problem in understanding emotion is the assessment of the definition of emotions. In fact, even psychologists have problem agreeing on what is considered an emotion and how many types of emotions exist. Kleinginna gathered and analyzed 92 definitions of emotion from literature present that day. He concludes that Emotion is a complex set of interactions among subjective and objective factors, mediated by neural/hormonal systems (Horlings, 2008). In fact, Emotion is a subcategory of stress.

A lot of research has been undertaken in assessment of stress and emotion over the last years. Most of researches in the domain of stress and emotional states use peripheral signals such as respiratory rate, Skin Conductance (SC), Blood Volume Pulse (BVP) (Zhai et al., 2006) and Temperature (McFarland, 1985). Most previous research, have investigated the use of EEG and peripheral signals separately, but little attention has been paid so far to the fusion between EEG and peripheral signals (Chanel, 2009; Chanel et al., 2009; Hosseini, 2009).

In one study, Aftanas et al. (2004) that showed significant differentiation of arousal based on EEG data collected from participants watching high, intermediate and low arousal images. Chanel (2009) asked the participants to remember past emotional episodes, and obtained the accuracy of 88% using EEG for 3 categories with Support Vector Machine (SVM) classifier. Hosseini et al. (2009) used the induction visual images based acquisition protocol for recording the EEG and peripheral signals under 2 categories of emotional stress states (Calm-neutral and Negatively-exited) of participants, and obtained the accuracy of 78.3% using EEG signals with SVM classifier. Kim et al. (2004) used the combination of music and story as stimuli and there were 50 participants, to introduce a user independent system, the results showed the accuracy of 78.4% and 61% for 3 and 4 categories of different emotions respectively. Takahashi (2004) used film clips to stimulate participants with five different emotions, resulting in 42% of correctly identified patterns. Schaaff & Schultz (2009) used pictures from the International Affective Picture System (IAPS) to induce three emotional states: pleasant, neutral, and unpleasant. They obtained the accuracy of 66.7% for three classes of emotion, solely based on EEG signals.

The aim of this chapter is to produce a new fusion between EEG and peripheral signals for emotional stress recognition. Since ElectroEncephaloGram (EEG) is the reflection of brain activity and is widely used in clinical diagnosis and biomedical research, it is used as the main signal. Brain waves occur during the activity of brain cells and have a frequency range of 1 to 100 Hz. Researchers have found that the following are the frequency bands of interest to interpret EEG signal: delta (1-4 Hz), theta (4-8 Hz), alpha (8-13 Hz), and beta (13-30 Hz) and gamma (> 30 Hz) (Ko et al., 2009).

One of the recent weaknesses, lack of proper channels selected brain signals are recorded. In this study, in order to choose the proper EEG channels, a cognitive model of the brain under emotional stress has been used (Hosseini et al., 2010a).

Every standard test in stress and emotion assessment has its own advantages and disadvantages (Hosseini, 2009). A efficient acquisition protocol was designed to acquire the EEG signals in five channels and peripheral signals such as Blood Volume Pulse (BVP), Skin Conductance (SC) and respiration, under images induction (calm-neutral and negatively excited) for the participants The visual stimuli images were selected from the subset IAPS database (Lang et al., 2005).

An important issue in every cognitive system is the correct labelling of the data. Here, labelling means the assessment of the data using a series of visual criteria used by psychologists and a proposed cognitive system for peripheral signals in order to verify the existence of a close correlation of the data and the psychological state of the subject. In this kind of research, putting the subject in the desired psychological state is very important. The process of labelling EEG signals consists of three stages: first self-assessment, second the qualitative analysis of peripheral signals and third the quantitative analysis of peripheral signals. Therefore, this new fusion link between EEG and peripheral signals are more robust in comparison to the separate signals.

2. Cognitive model of emotional stress

Cognitive models (also termed agent architectures) aim to emulate cognitive processing such as attention, learning, perception, and decision-making, and are used by cognitive scientists to advance understanding of the mechanisms and structures mediating cognition (Hudlicka, 2005). In the case of fear conditioning leading to emotional stress, several hypotheses have been proposed to explain how neural changes occur in the different components in a circuit leading to the observed behavioural responses. In mammalians, a part of the brain, called the limbic system, is mainly responsible for emotional processes (Xiang, 2007). We are going to describe developing a cognitive model of the limbic system based on these concepts. The main components of the limbic system involved in emotional stress processes are amygdala, orbito-frontal cortex, thalamus, sensory cortex, hypothalamus, hippocampus and some other of important areas. In this section, we are trying to briefly describe these components and their tasks. The amygdala, a small structure in the temporal lobes, plays a central role in emotion. It is generally accepted that the amygdala is crucial for the acquisition and expression of conditioned fear responses (for a review, see (LeDoux, 1996)). The amygdala and orbito-frontal cortex receive highly analyzed input from the sensory cortex. The amygdala, specifically its lateral nucleus, receives inputs from all the main sensory systems, as well as from higher-order association areas of the cortex and the hippocampus (Armony et al., 1997). Sensory information reaches the amygdala from the thalamus by the way of two parallel pathways: the direct pathways reach the amygdala quickly, but they are limited in their information content, as the thalamic cells of origin of the pathway are not very precise stimulus discriminators. The cortical pathway, on the other hand, is slower but capable of providing the amygdala with a much richer representation of the stimulus (Armony et al., 1997). The sensory cortex is the component next to the thalamus and receives its input through this component. The orbito-frontal cortex is another component, which interacts with the amygdala reciprocally. The orbito-frontal cortex also plays a role in reinforcement learning of emotions. The term prefrontal cortex refers to the very front of the brain, behind the forehead and above the eyes. It appears to play a critical role in the regulation of emotion and behaviour by anticipating the consequences of our actions. The prefrontal cortex may play an important role in delayed gratification by maintaining emotions over time and organizing behaviour toward specific goals (Xiang, 2007). The locus ceruleus contains a large proportion of the noradrenalin cell bodies found in the brain and it is a key brain stem region involved in arousal (Steimer, 2002). The Bed Nucleus of the Stria Terminalis (BNST) is considered part of the extended amygdala. It appears to be a centre for the integration of information originating from the amygdala and the hippocampus, and is clearly involved in the modulation of the neuroendocrine stress response (Steimer, 2002). The hypothalamus (ParaVentricular Nucleus (PVN) and Lateral Hypothalamus (LH)) lies below the Thalamus and it is believed to have various functions that regulate the endocrine system, the autonomous nervous system and primary behavioural surviving states (Steimer, 2002; Schachter, 1970). The Hypothalamic-Pituitary-Adrenal (HPA) axis ultimately regulates the secretion of glucocorticoids, which are adrenocortical steroids that act on target tissues throughout the body in order to preserve homeostasis during stress (Ramachandran, 2002). The hypothalamus also releases Corticotrophin-Releasing Hormone (CRH), which travels to the anterior pituitary gland, where it triggers the release of AdrenoCorticoTropic Hormone (ACTH), which, along with β-endorphin, is released into the bloodstream in response to stress. ACTH travels in the blood to the adrenal glands, where it stimulates the production and release of glucocorticoids such as cortisol. Cortisol feedback at the hypothalamus reduces CRF release. At the pituitary, it inhibits ACTH release, and at the adrenal gland, it inhibits further cortisol release. Cortisol feedback at the hippocampus inhibits CRF secretion from the hypothalamus. The release of all these chemicals causes important changes in the body's ability to respond to threats such as increased energy, heart rate and blood sugar resulting in increased arousal and pain relief (Carey, 2006). In order to choose the best channels for EEG signals, we implemented a new cognitive model (for a review of complete model, see (Hosseini et al., 2010a; Hosseini et al., 2010d)). The detail is shown in Fig. 1. (Hosseini et al., 2010a).

3. Acquisition protocol

3.1 Stimuli

Every standard test in stress and emotional states assessment has its own advantages and disadvantages (Hosseini, 2009). Most experiments that measure emotion from EEG signals use pictures from the International Affective Picture System (IAPS). The IAPS evaluated by several American participants on two dimensions of nine points each (1-9). The use of IAPS allows better control of emotional stimuli and simplifies the experimental design (Horlings, 2008).

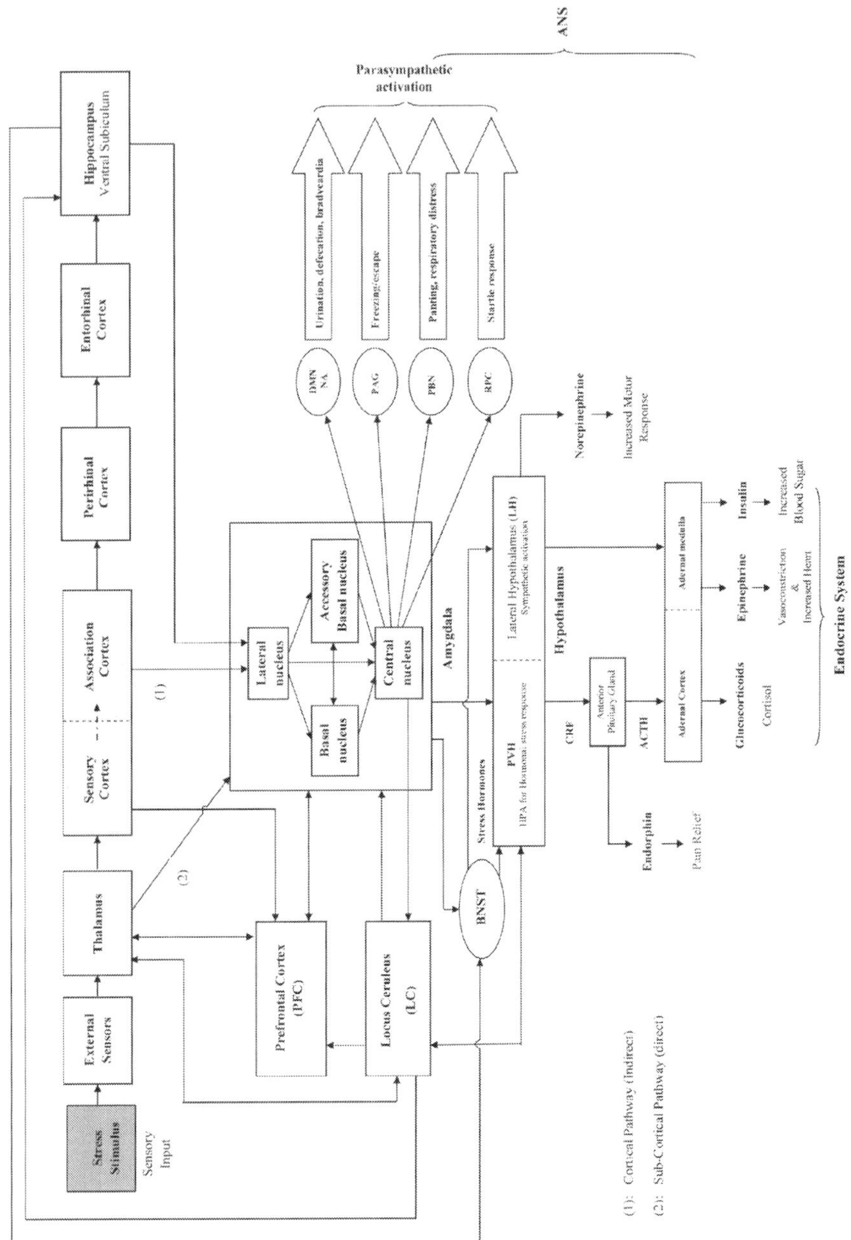

Fig. 1. A general cognitive map of brain for stress state

In this study, we chose the picture presentation test, base on the closeness of its assessment to our aims. The stimuli to elicit the target emotions (calm-neutral and negatively excited) were some of the pictures (http://www.unifesp.br/dpsicobio/adap/exemplos_fotos.htm). The valence dimension ranging from negative to positive and the arousal dimension, ranging from calm to excited. Information about both dimensions has been found to be present in EEG signals, which shows that emotion assessment from EEG signals should be possible.

The participant sits in front of a portable computer screen in a bare room relatively, the images to inform him about the specific emotional event he has to think of. Each experiment consists of 8 trials. Each stimulus consists of a block of 4 pictures, which ensures stability of the emotion over time. In addition, each picture is displayed for 3 seconds leading to a total 12 seconds per block. Prior to displaying images, a dark screen with an asterisk in the middle is shown for 10 seconds to separate each trial and to attract the participant's attention. The detail of each trial is shown in Fig. 2.

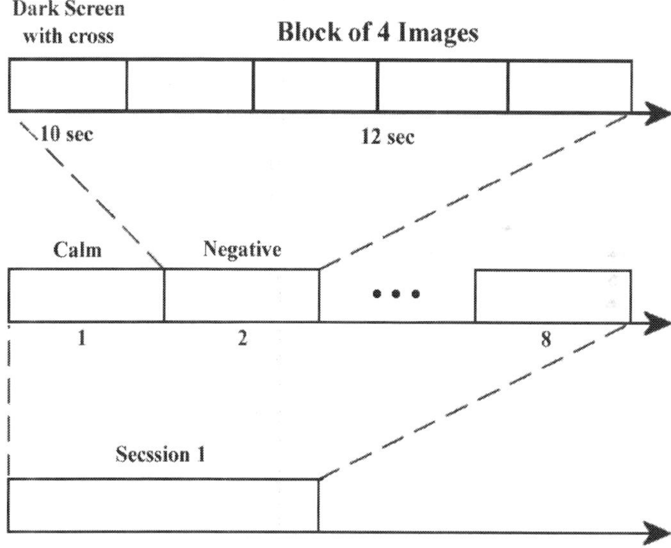

Fig. 2. The protocol of data acquisition

This epoch duration was chosen because to avoid participant fatigue. In Fig. 3, each presentation cycle started with a black fixation cross, which was shown for ten seconds. After that pictures were presented for twelve seconds.

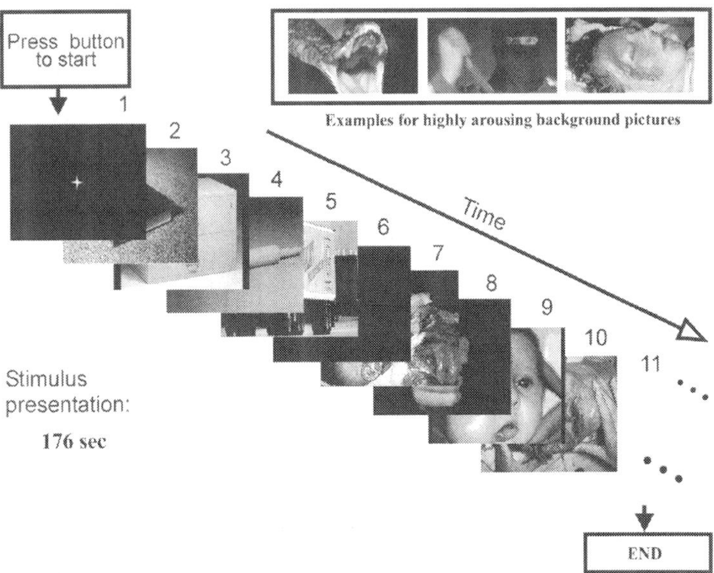

Fig. 3. Process of picture presentation

3.2 Subjects

Fifteen healthy volunteered subjects were right-handed males between the age of 20 and 24 years. Most subjects were students from biomedical engineering department of Islamic Azad University- Mashhad Branch. Each participant was examined by a dichotic listening test to identify the dominant hemisphere (Sadock, 1998; Hosseini, 2009). All subjects had normal or corrected vision; none of them had neurological disorders. These were done to eliminate any differences in subjects. All participants gave written informed consent. Then each participant was given a particulars questionnaire. During the pre-test, several questionnaires have been evaluated in order to check the best psychological input to start the protocol phase; this test is State-Trait Anxiety Inventory (STAI). At the end of the experiment, participants were asked to fill in a questionnaire about the experiment and give their opinions (Hosseini, 2009), because, it is possible that the emotion that a participant experiences differs from the expected value. For that reason, the participant is asked to rate his emotion on a self-assessment.

3.2 Procedure

We used a 10 channel Flexcom Infiniti device, with 14-bit resolution for data acquisition (http://www.thoughttechnology.com/flexinf.htm). It is connected to a PC using the USB port. An optical cable connects to device, to prevent any electrical charge from reaching the participant. The Flexcom Infiniti hardware only worked well with the accompanying software. Two programs were available, Biograph Infiniti Acquisition and ezscan. The central activity is monitored by recording EEGs. The peripheral activity is assessed by using the following sensors: a skin conductance sensor to measure sudation; a respiration belt to measure abdomen expansion; a plethysmograph to record blood volume pulse. We recorded SC by positioning two dedicated electrodes on the top of left index and middle fingers. The sample rate of the BVP and SC signals acquisition was 2048 Hz and then down-sampled to 128 Hz and respiration signal acquisition was 256 Hz and then down-sampled to 128 Hz. For reduce of calculation volume, were implemented the down sampling on BVP and SC signals. EEG was recorded using electrodes placed at 5 positions. The scalp EEG was obtained at location FP1, FP2, T3, T4 and Pz, as defined by the international 10-20 system and Ag/AgCl electrodes. In order to measure a reference signal that is (as much as possible) free from brain activity, we have two electrodes to attach to the participants earlobes. Average of A1 and A2 was used as reference. Impedance of all electrodes was kept below 5 KΩ. The sample rate of the EEG signal acquisition was 256 Hz. Each recording lasted about 3 minutes. More details of the data acquisition protocol can be found in (Hosseini, 2009).

4. Labeling process of EEG signals

An important issue in every cognitive system is the correct labelling of the data. In order to choose the best emotional stress correlated EEG signals, we implemented a new emotion-related signal recognition system, which has not been studied so far (Hosseini, 2009; Hosseini et al., 2010c). We recorded peripheral signals concomitantly in order to firstly recognize the correlated emotional stress state and then label the correlated EEG signals. In other words, we used the peripheral signals as a tutor for labeling system.

The process of labeling EEG signals consists of three stages: first self-assessment, second the qualitative analysis of peripheral signals and third the quantitative analysis of peripheral signals. Fig. 4 shows the different stages of the process. After the experiment, there was also a self-assessment stage, which is a good way to have an idea about the emotional stimulation "level" of the subject because emotions are known to be very subjective and dependent on previous experience (Savran et al., 2006). In this research, we will be able to get a general idea of the quality of the data, i.e. if the data are good or bad.

One kind of this data is respiration. Emotional stress processes influence respiration (Ritz et al., 2002; Wilhelm et al., 2006). Slow respiration, for example is linked to relaxation while irregular rhythm, quick variations, and cessation of respiration correspond to more aroused emotions like anger or fear. Another one is skin conductance, which measures the conductivity of the skin. Since sweat gland activity is known to be controlled by the sympathetic nervous system, Electro Dermal Activity (EDA) has become a common source of information to measure the Autonomic Nervous System. SC increases if the skin is sweaty, for example, when one is experimenting emotions such as stress. Moreover, blood pressure and Heart Rate Variability (HRV) are variables that correlate with defensive reactions, pleasantness of a stimulus, and basic emotions. We obtained Heart Rate (HR) signal using BVP signal recorded by a plethysmograph. A method to determine HR from a BVP signal is proposed in (Wan & Woo, 2004). Analysis of HRV provides an effective way to investigate the different activities of ANS, an increase of HR can be due to an increase of the sympathetic activity or a decrease of the parasympathetic activity. Two frequency bands (HR spectrum) are generally considered for HR signal, a Low Frequency (LF) band ranging from 0.05 Hz to 0.15 Hz and a High Frequency (HF) band including frequencies between 0.15 Hz and 1 Hz (Hosseini, 2009). In order to analyze the peripheral signals quantitatively, we need to pre-process them, to remove environmental noises by applying filters. The peripheral signals were filtered by moving average filters to remove noise.

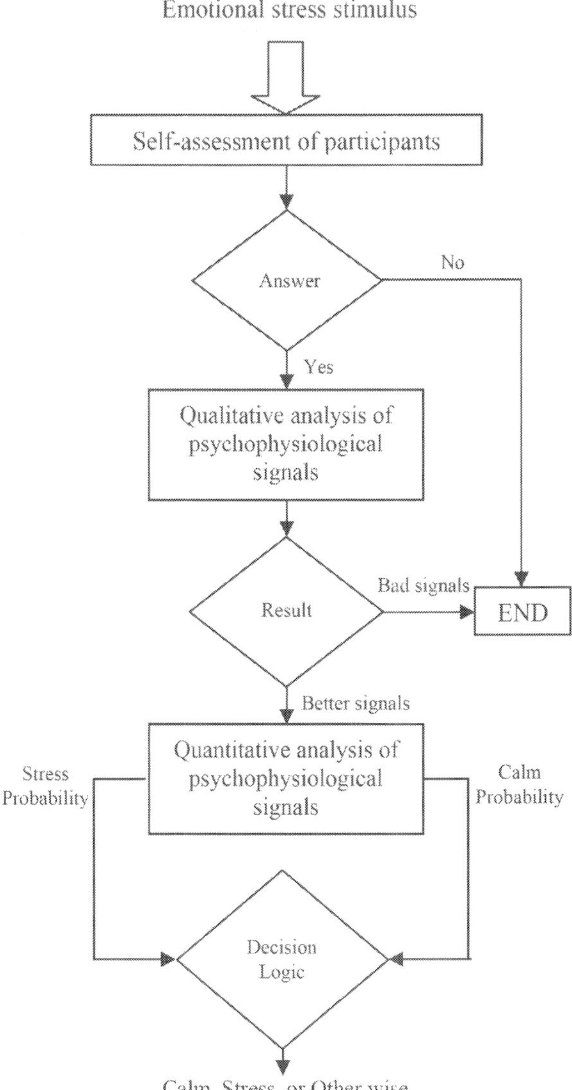

Fig. 4. Labeling process of EEG signals

We used a common set of feature values for analysis of the peripheral signals (Table 1) (Chanel et al., 2009; Hosseini, 2009). The respiration features are from time and frequency domains, the skin conductance features and the blood volume pulse features are from time domain, and the heart rate variability features are from time, frequency domains and fractal dimension.

Signal	Extracted features
Respiration	Mean, variance, Standard deviation, Kurtosis, Skewness, Maximum minus Minimum value, Power in the 0 to 2 Hz ($\Delta f=0.5$ Hz) bands.
Skin Conductance	Mean, variance, Standard deviation, Kurtosis, Skewness, Maximum, Mean of derivative, energy response and proportion of negative samples in the derivative vs. all samples.
Blood Volume Pulse	Mean, variance, Standard deviation, Kurtosis, Skewness, Mean of trough variability, Variance of trough variability, Mean of peak variability, Variance of peak variability, Mean of amplitude variability, Variance of amplitude variability, Mean value variability, Variance of mean value variability, Mean of baseline variability, Variance of baseline variability
Heart Rate Variability	Mean, variance, Standard deviation, Low power frequency of 0.05-0.15Hz, Proportion low power frequency vs. all power frequency, fractal dimension by Higuchi's algorithm

Table 1. Features Extracted from peripheral signals

The total number of features is: [10+9+15+6=40]. After extracting the features, we need to classify them using a classifier. There are several approaches to apply the SVM for multiclass classification (http://www.kernel-machines.org/software.html). The LibSVM MATLAB toolbox (Version 2.9) was used as an implementation of the SVM algorithms (Chang & Lin, 2009). In this study, the one-vs.-all method was implemented. Two SVMs that correspond to each of the two emotions were used. The ith SVM was trained with all of the training data in the ith class with calm labels, and the other training data with negative labels.

In the emotional stress recognition process, the feature vector was simultaneously fed into all SVMs and the output from each SVM was investigated in the decision logic algorithm to select the best emotional stress (Fig. 5). In the SVM classifier, was used a Gaussian Radial Basis function (RBF) as a kernel function. RBF projects the data to a higher dimension.

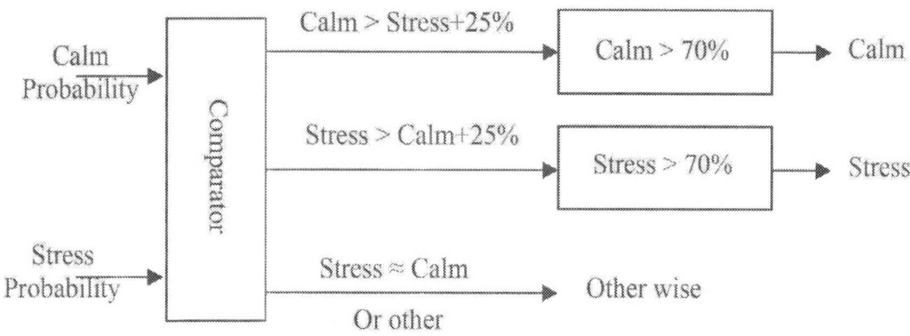

Fig. 5. Decision logic algorithm

A confusion matrix will also be used to determine how the samples are classified in the different classes. A confusion matrix gives the percentage of samples belonging to class ω_i and classified as class ω_j. The accuracy can be retrieved from the confusion matrix by summing its diagonal elements $P_{i,i}$ weighted by the prior probability $P(\omega_i)$ of occurrence of the class ω_i. The confusion matrices results of the SVM used for classification of the peripheral signals under two emotional stress states is given in Table 2.

Truth	Classified with SVM	
	Calm-neutral	*Negative excited*
Calm-neutral	65.4%	34.6%
Negative excited	11.5%	88.5%

Table 2. The confusion matrices across participants using peripheral signals using RBF kernel of SVM

The results show that, the classification accuracy with peripheral signals was 76.95% for the two categories, using SVM classifier with RBF kernel.

The numbers of rejected trials that are badly classified that is lower than the number of correctly classified. The percentage of rejected trials is 11%. Method at this stage it has been used to select suitable segments of EEG signal for improving accuracy of signal labeling according to emotional stress state. More details of the labeling process can be found in (Hosseini, 2009).

5. Analysis of EEG signals

5.1 Pre-processing

Before analysis, we first remove the data segment, which contains obvious eye blinking. We need to pre-process EEG signals in order to remove environmental noises and drifts. The data was filtered using a band pass filter in the frequency band of 0.5~60 Hz. Although we studied the EEG signals of up to 30 Hz, we included the 30 to 60 Hz bandwidth, because we need a double maximum frequency content when analyzing the data using HOS (Hosseini, 2009). The signals were filtered using the "filtfilt" function from the signal processing in MATLAB toolbox, which processes the input signal in both forward and reverse directions. This function allows performing a zero-phase filtering. Safety of signal phase information is very important in higher order spectra (Hosseini, 2009). In addition, a notch filter at 50 Hz was placed to discard the effect of power lines.

5.2 Quality aspect

First time, phase space introduced by W. Gibbs in 1901, that in this space all possible states of a system are represented, with each possible state of the system corresponding to one unique point in the phase space. In fact, all these unique points will make direction of trajectory. A sketch of the phase portrait may give qualitative information about the dynamics of the system. The method is based on the operated result numerically in the EEG dynamics system, the phase trajectory portrait is drawn out in the phase space with the time variance, and the course portrait of the state variables is drawn out with the time (Jiu-ming et al., 2004). The chaotic phenomena and the solution fraction are decided through comparison, analysis and integration. In the phase space, the close curve is corresponding to the periodical motion, while the chaotic motion is corresponding to the ever-non-close trajectory (strange attractor), which diverges randomly in some area, the corresponding figure is as following Fig. 6.

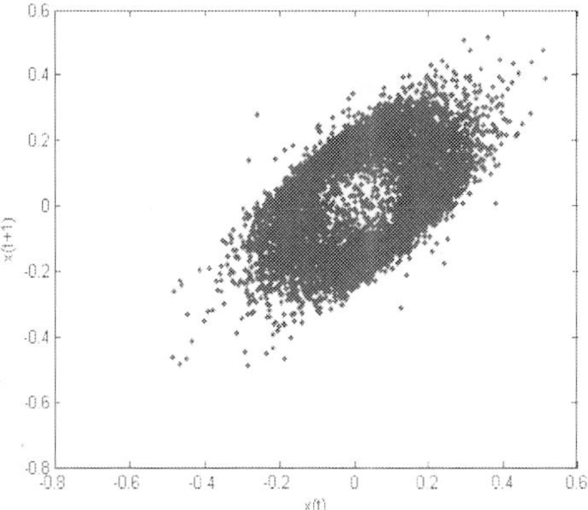

Fig. 6. Phase space state portraits for T3 channel of EEG signal for one participant in negative emotional stress state

5.3 Feature extraction

Feature extraction is the process of extracting useful information from the signal. We use a set of feature values for brain signals. Features are extracted for each channel of EEG signals. Since brain signals essentially have a chaotic and nonlinear behaviour, we performed emotional stress state assessment using both linear and nonlinear characteristics. Nonlinear measures have received the most attention in comparison with the measures mentioned before, for example time domain, frequency domain and other linear features. The nonlinear set of features used includes fractal dimension, approximate entropy and correlation dimension of the data.

5.3.1 Fractal dimension

Fractal dimension (FD) analysis is frequently used in biomedical signal processing, including EEG analysis. Higuchi's algorithm unlike many other methods requires only short time intervals to calculate fractal dimension. This is very advantageous, because EEG signal remains stationary during short intervals and because in EEG analysis it is often necessary to consider short, transient events.

In Higuchi's algorithm (Higuchi, 1988), k new time sequence are constructed from the signal $x(1)$, $x(2)$,..., $x(N)$ under study:

$$x_m^k = \{x(m), x(m+k),...,x(m+\left\lfloor \frac{N-m}{k} \right\rfloor k)\} \quad , \qquad m = 1,2,...k \tag{1}$$

Where m = 1, 2, ..., k and k indicate the initial time value, and the discrete time interval between points, respectively. For each of the k time series x^k_m, the length $L_m(k)$ is computed by:

$$L_m(k) = \frac{\sum_{i=1}^{\left\lfloor \frac{N-m}{k} \right\rfloor} |x(m+ik) - x(m+(i-1)k)|(N-1)}{\left\lfloor \frac{N-m}{k} \right\rfloor k} \tag{2}$$

Where N is the total length of the data sequence x, $(N-1)/[(N-m)/k]k$ is a normalization factor and k average length is computed as the mean of the k lengths $L_m(k)$ for $m =1,2,..., k$. This procedure is repeated for each k ranging from 1 to max k, obtaining an average length for each k. In the curve of $ln(L_m(k))$ versus $ln(1/k)$, the slope of the least-squares linear best fit is the estimate of the fractal dimension.

In this research, the best results were obtained for estimating the FD of the EEG; k_{max} = 10, rectangular window size, N = 512 samples (2 seconds) and window overlap = 0%.

5.3.2 Correlation dimension

Correlation dimension (D_2) is one of the most widely used measures of a chaotic process. In this reasearch, we used the Grassberger and Procaccia Algorithm (GPA) for estimating D_2 (Grassberger & Procaccia, 1983). The choice of an appropriate time delay τ and embedding dimension m is important for the success of reconstructing the attractor with finite data. The idea is to construct a function C(r) that is the probability that two arbitrary points on the orbit are closer together than r, where r is the radius of the sphere in the multidimensional space. This is done by calculating the separation between every pair of N data points and sorting them into bins of width dr proportionate to r. More precisely GPA computes the correlation integral C(r) given by,

$$C(r) = \frac{1}{N(N-1)} \sum_{i=1}^{N} \sum_{\substack{j=1 \\ i \neq j}}^{N} \theta(r - \|V(j) - V(i)\|) \qquad (3)$$

Where $\|V(j)-V(i)\|$ is the distance between the points V(j) and V(i) and $\Theta(.)$ is the heaviside function. D_2 is estimated as the slope of the log(C(r)) vs. log(r) graph as follows:

$$D_2 = \lim_{r \to 0} \frac{\log_2 C(N,r)}{\log_2(r)} \qquad (4)$$

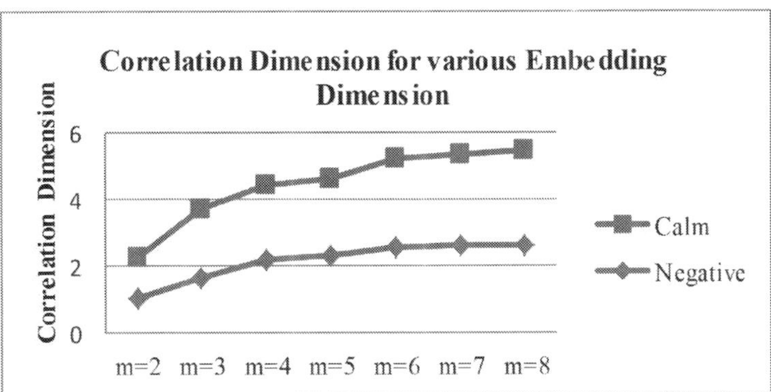

Fig. 7. A schematic graph of the correlation dimension plotted as a function of the embedding dimension. When the embedding dimension is equal to or greater than twice the dimension of the state space attractor (d_{sat}) the correlation dimension became independent of m. The correlation dimension of the attractor in this case is about 8.

We calculated D_2 with d_{sat} values varying from 2 to 10 for all the subjects. It can be seen that D_2 saturates after the embedding dimension of 7 (Fig. 7). Therefore, we have chosen d_{sat}=8 for constructing the embedding space and estimation of the invariants (In the test, m = 8 and τ = 6).

The determination is based on calculating the relative number of pairs of points in the phase-space set that is separated by a distance less than r. For a self-similar attractor, the local scaling exponent is constant, and this region is called a scaling region. This scaling exponent can be used as an estimate of the correlation dimension. If the d_{sat}=8 plots $C(N, r)$ vs. r on a *log-log* scale, the correlation dimension is given by the slope of the $log(C(r))$ vs. $log(r)$ curve over a selected range of r, and the slope of this curve in the scaling region is estimated by the least slope fitting (Fig. 8).

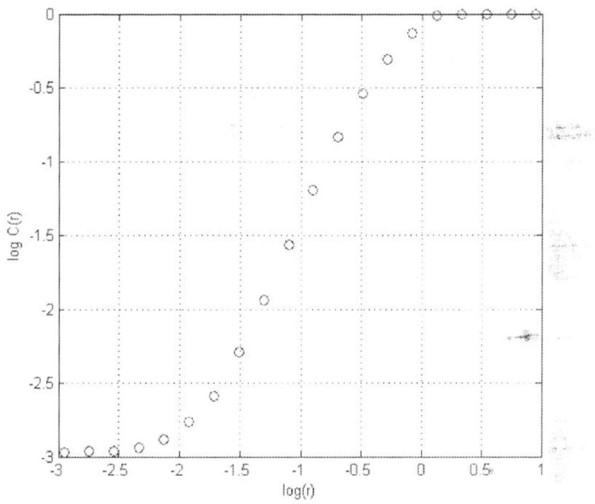

Fig. 8. A plot of log (C(r)) versus log(r) for logistic map data

5.3.3 Approximate entropy

Pincus introduced the first idea of approximate entropy (ApEn) in 1991, and it is a useful complexity measure for biological time series data (Pincus, 1991). ApEn is originated from nonlinear dynamics. ApEn is a statistical instrument initially designed to be applied to finite length and noisy time series data, it is scale invariant and model independent, evaluates both dominant and subordinate patterns in data, and discriminates series for which clear feature recognition is difficult. Notably it detects changes in underlying episodic behaviour not reflected in peak occurrences or amplitudes. To understand the concept of ApEn better, we describe the definition step by step as follows: Let the original data be $<X(n)> = x(1)$, $x(2),..., x(N)$, where N is the total number of data points. The calculation of ApEn of signal of finite length is performed as follows. First, fix a positive integer m and a positive real number r_f. Next, form the signal x the N-m+1 vector, defined by (5).

$$X_m(i) = \{x(i), x(i+1),..., x(i+m-1)\}$$
$$i = 1, 2,..., N - m + 1 \tag{5}$$

The quantity is calculated (6).

$$C_i^m(r_f) = \frac{number \ of \ such \ j \ that \ d[X_m(i), X_m(j)] \leq r_f}{N - m + 1}$$

$$i \neq j, j = 1, 2, ..., N - m + 1$$

(6)

Where the distance between the vectors and is defined as (7).

$$d[X_m(i), X_m(j)] = \max_{k=1,2,...,m+1} (|x(i+k) - x(j+k)|)$$

(7)

Next, the quantity is calculated as (8).

$$\varphi^m(r_f) = \frac{1}{N - m + 1} \sum_{i=1}^{N-m+1} Ln C_i^m(r_f)$$

(8)

Increase the dimension to m+1. Repeat steps (1)~(4) and find $\varphi^{m+1}(r_f)$. Finally, the ApEn is defined as (9).

$$ApEn(m, r_f) = \lim_{N \to \infty} (\varphi^m(r_f) - \varphi^{m+1}(r_f))$$

(9)

In actual operation, the number of data point is limited when the data length is N and the result obtained through the above steps is the estimate of ApEn, which can be denoted as (10)

$$ApEn(m, r_f, N) = \varphi^m(r_f) - \varphi^{m+1}(r_f)$$

(10)

Obviously, the value of the estimate depends on m and r_f. The parameter r_f corresponds to an a priori fixed distance between the neighboring trajectory points; therefore, r_f can be viewed as a filtering level and the parameter m is the embedding dimension determining the dimension of the phase space. As suggested by Pincus, r_f is chosen according to the signal's standard deviation (SD); in this paper we use the values r_f =0.2 SD and m=2 with SD taken over the signal segment under consideration.

5.3.4 Wavelet coefficients

Discrete Wavelet Transform (DWT) based feature extraction has been successfully applied with promising results in physiological pattern recognition applications (Murugappan et al., 2009). Choice of suitable wavelet and the number of levels of decomposition is very important in analysis of signals using DWT. In this study, we used Daubechies wavelet function with order db4 for extracting the statistical feature from the EEG signal (Murugappan et al., 2009). The number of levels of decomposition is chosen based on the dominant frequency components of the signal. The levels are chosen such that those parts of the signal that correlate well with the frequencies required for classification of the signal are retained in the wavelet coefficients. Since the EEG signals do not have any useful frequency components above 32 Hz, the number of levels was chosen to be 5. Thus the signal is decomposed into the details D1-D5 and one final approximation, A5. The range of various frequency bands are shown in Table 3.

Decomposition levels	Frequency Bandwidth (Hz)	Frequency bands
D1	64-128	Noises
D2	32-64	Noises (Gamma)
D3	16-32	Beta
D4	8-16	Alpha
D5	4-8	Theta
A5	0-4	Delta

Table 3. Frequencies corresponding to different levels of decomposition for "db4" wavelet with a sampling frequency of 256 Hz

The extracted wavelet coefficients provide a compact representation that shows the energy distribution of the EEG signal in time and frequency. Table 2 presents frequencies corresponding to different levels of decomposition for db4 wavelets with a sampling frequency of 256 Hz. It can be seen from table 2 that the components A5 are within the delta (0-4 Hz), D5 are within the Theta (4-8 Hz), D4 are within the alpha (8-13 Hz) and D3 are within the beta (13-30 Hz). Lower level decompositions related to higher frequencies have negligible magnitudes in a normal EEG. In order to, further diminish the dimensionality of the extracted feature vectors; statistics over the set of the wavelet coefficients was used.

- Mean of the absolute values of the wavelet coefficients in each sub-band
- Average power of the wavelet coefficients in each sub-band
- Standard deviation of the wavelet coefficients in each sub-band

These features are extracted for each channel, so the total number of features by this method is: $[3 \times 4] = 12$.

5.3.4 Higher order spectra parameters

We analyzed the EEG signal using higher order spectra that are spectral representations of higher order moments or cumulants of a signal (Hosseini et al., 2010b). In this part of paper, we studied features related to the third order statistics of the signal, namely the bispectrum. The bispectrum is a complex quantity, which has both magnitude and phase. The bispectrum is the Fourier transform of the third order correlation of the signal and is given by,

$$Bis(f_1, f_2) = E[X(f_1).X(f_2).X^*(f_1 + f_2)] \tag{11}$$

Where * denotes complex conjugate, $X(f)$ is the Fourier transform of the signal $x(nT)$ and $E[.]$ stands for the expectation operation. This method is known as direct Fast Fourier Transform (FFT) based method (Nikias & Mendel, 1993). There is also another indirect method, which is used in this study. For more details on this method please refer to (Hosseini et al., 2010b; Swami et al., 2000). If the bispectrum of a signal is zero, none of the wave components are coupled to each other.

Assuming that there is no bispectral aliasing, the bispectral of a real-valued signal is uniquely defined with the triangle $f_2 \geq 0$, $f_1 \geq f_2$ and $f_1 + f_2 \leq \pi$. For real processes, since discrete bispectrum has symmetric characteristics, it has 12 symmetry regions in the (f_1, f_2) plane (Swami et al., 2000). Some of these regions can be seen in (12):

$$Bis(f_1, f_2) = Bis(f_2, f_1) = Bis(-f_1 - f_2, f_2)$$
$$= Bis(-f_1 - f_2, f_1) = Bis(f_1, -f_1 - f_2) = Bis(f_2, -f_1 - f_2) \tag{12}$$

The normalized bispectrum (or bicoherence) is defined as

$$Bic(f_1, f_2) = \frac{Bis(f_1, f_2)}{\sqrt{P(f_1).P(f_2).P(f_1 + f_2)}} \tag{13}$$

Where $P(f_i)$ is the power spectrum.

Since bispectrum and bicoherence cannot fully help signal extraction, Hinich has developed algorithms to test for non-skewness (called Gaussianity) and linearity (Hinich, 1982). The basic idea is that if the third-order cumulants of a process are zero, then its bispectrum is zero, and hence its bicoherence is zero. If the bispectrum is not zero, then the process is non-Gaussian; if the process is linear and non-Gaussian, then the bicoherence is a non-zero constant (Hosseini et al., 2010b).

The Gaussianity test (actually zero-skewness test) involves deciding whether the expected value of the bicoherence is zero, that is, $E\{Bic(f_1, f_2)\}=0$. The test of Gaussianity is based on the mean bicoherence power,

$$S = \sum |Bic(f_1, f_2)|^2 \tag{14}$$

The squared bicoherence is chi-squared distributed (x2 distributed) with two degrees of freedom and non-centrality parameter Lambda (λ) (Swami et al., 2000). In (14) the squared bicoherence is the sum of P points in the non-redundant region, S is the estimated statistics for the Gaussianity test with chi-squared distributed and 2P degree of freedom, and Pfa is the probability of false alarm in rejecting the Gaussian hypothesis. More details can be found in (Hosseini et al., 2010b; Swami et al., 2000). In order to calculate these features, we used a 256 sample FFT with a default C parameter of 0.51. Based on these, the 2P degree of freedom will be 96. The analysis was done using the Higher Order Spectral Analysis (HOSA) toolbox (Swami et al., 2000). The bicoherence was computed using the direct FFT method in the toolbox.

For the whole bifrequency plane region, four quantities were calculated: sum of the bispectrum magnitudes, sum of the squares of the bispectrum magnitudes, sum of the bicoherence magnitudes, and sum of the squares of the bicoherence magnitudes.

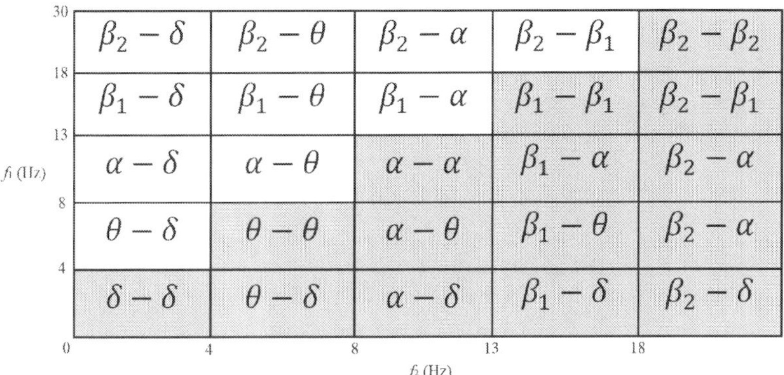

Fig. 9. The different regions used for analysis in bifrequency plane

Since bispectrum and bicoherence are functions of f_1 and f_2, in order to define the features, we will have five frequency intervals on each axis, as can be seen in Fig. 9. We will have 15 distinct regions. Then the defined features will be analyzed in each of these 15 regions and in the whole frequency range. These and the three other features obtained from Hinich's tests for Gaussian and linearity add up to make 7 features for each channel.

These seven features are extracted for each channel, so the total number of features by this method is: $[5 \times 4 \times (15+1)] + [5 \times 3] = 335$. The contour plots of the indirect estimate of the bispectrum are shown as examples for T3 channel in Figs. 10 and 11.

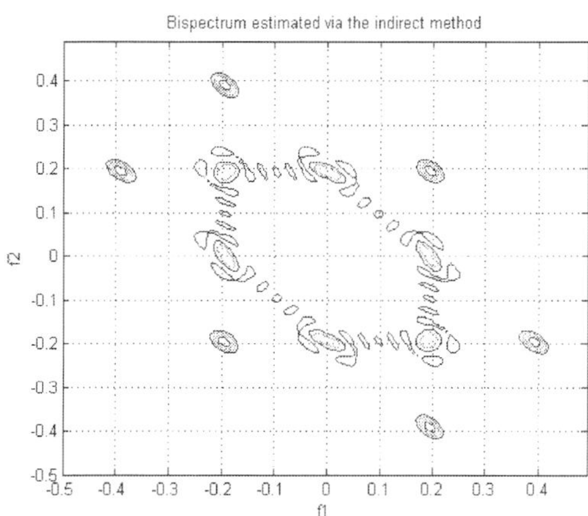

Fig. 10. A contour plot of the magnitude of the indirect estimated bispectrum on the bifrequency plane, for T3 in calm state

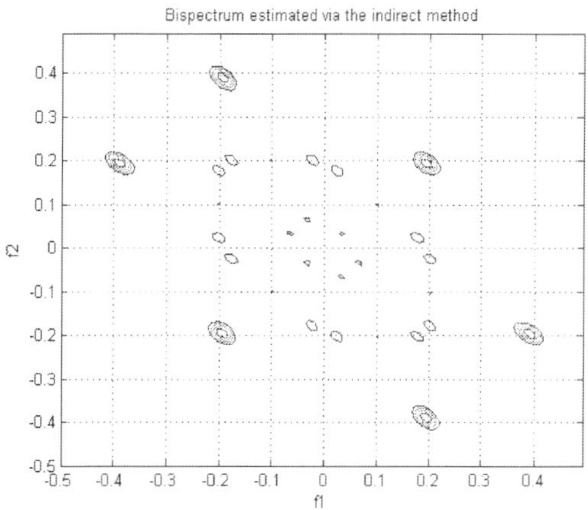

Fig. 11. A contour plot of the magnitude of the indirect estimated bispectrum on the bifrequency plane, for T3 in negative emotional stress state

5.4 Normalization

In order to normalize the features in the limits of [-1,1], we used (15).

$$Y_{norm} = \frac{-2Y_s' + Y_{smax}' + Y_{smin}'}{Y_{smin}' - Y_{smax}'} \tag{15}$$

Here Y_{norm} is the relative amplitude.

5.5 Feature selection

The feature vector presented contains 82 features for a channel EEG recorded over a period of 2 seconds. This leads to the problem of dimensionality, which is solved by in this section until some of the best features should be selected. This is of interest to improve the computational speed of the classification algorithm. Several methods of selecting appropriate features exist. One of the methods described is Genetic Algorithm (GA) (Haupt et al., 2004). The emphasis on using the genetic algorithm for feature selection is to reduce the computational load on the training system while still allowing near optimal results to be found relatively quickly. The GA uses populations of 100 sizes, starting with randomly generated genomes. The probability of mutation was set to 0.01 and the probability of crossover was set to 0.4. The classification performance of the trained network using the whole dataset was returned to the GA as the value of the fitness function, Fig. 12. We attempted to detect the feature sets related to negative/calm emotion response from EEG signal.

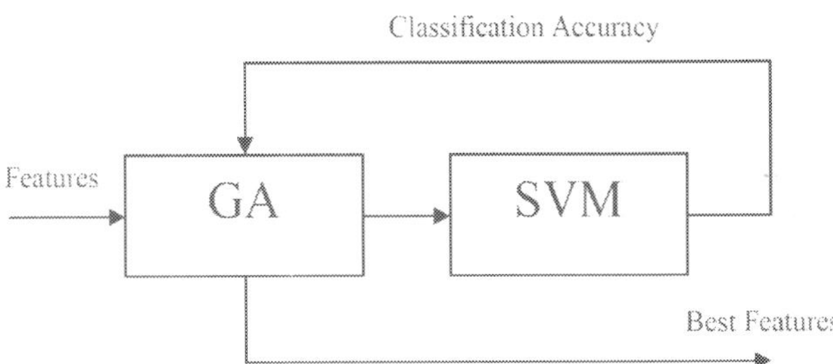

Fig. 12. Combination of GA and SVM to achieve the best features

We used genetic algorithm in assessment of all the features because a perfect feature group is not necessarily achievable by simply putting a few superior features since the data characteristics and features may have overlapping.

5.6 Classification

After extracting the desired good features, we still have to find the related emotional stress states in the EEG. A classifier will do this process. In this research, we have used both a static and a dynamic classifier and we will explain them.

5.6.1 Support vector machine

Support vector machines are maximum margin classifiers that try to maximize the distance between the decision surface and the nearest point to this surface. Nonlinear support vector machine, maps the input space to a high dimensional feature space, and then constructs a linear optimal hyper plane in the feature space, which relates to a nonlinear hyper plane in the input space. The major problem of training a learning machine to perform supervised classification is to find a function (kernel function) that can not only capture the essential properties of the data distribution, but also prevent the over-fitting problem. We used three kernel functions including linear, polynomial and radial basis function kernels. The C parameter that regulates the trade off between training error minimization and margin maximization is empirically set to1 in this study.

5.6.2 Elman Neural Network

Elman Neural Network (ENN) is a two-layer backpropagation network, with the addition of a feedback connection from the output of the hidden layer to its input. This feedback path allows Elman network to learn to recognize and generate temporal patterns, as well as spatial patterns. The Elman network has tansig neurons in its hidden (recurrent) layer, and purelin neurons in its output layer. This combination is special in that the two-layer networks with these transfer functions can approximate any function (with a finite number of discontinuities) with arbitrary accuracy. The only requirement is that the hidden layer must have enough neurons (Demuth et al., 2008). In this part, the numbers of input neurons are to number optimum features, the numbers of output neurons is 1 and empirically the numbers of hidden neurons is chosen 8. Hence, sigmoid function has been applied for the hidden and output layers, because the sigmoid function is nonlinear and differentiable. The Levenberg-Marquardt back-propagation algorithm is used for training. The Levenberg-Marquardt algorithm will have the fastest convergence compared with other training functions. The error ratio for stop training was considered 0.001.

6. Result

In this research, we used a 2 seconds time intervals rectangular window without overlap, corresponding to blocks of 512 samples of EEG signals for data segmentation. In classification is important that the training set contain enough samples (or instances). On the other hand, it also important that the test set contains enough samples to avoid a noisy estimate of the model performance. We used around 75% of the EEG signals for the training, and 15% of the data for testing whether the learned relationship between the data and emotional stress is correct and the last 10% was used for validating the data. The results show that, the average classification accuracy with EEG signals were 84.6% and 83.1% for the 2 categories (calm-neutral vs. negatively excited), using the SVM and ENN classifiers respectively. This is particularly true in our case since the number of emotional stimulations is limited by the duration of the protocols, which should not be too long to avoid participant fatigue as well as elicitation of undesired emotions. Cross-validation methods help to solve this problem by splitting the data in different training/test sets so that each sample will be used at least once for training and once for testing. The two well-known cross-validation methods are the k-fold and the leave-one-out. The system was tested using the 4-fold cross-validation method. This method reduces the possibility of deviations in the results due to some special distribution of training and test data, and ensures that the system is tested with different samples from those it has seen for training. By using this method, four accuracies are obtained from the four test sets so that it is possible to compute the average accuracy. The classification results of the EEG signals under two emotional stress states is given in Table 4.

Different kernel function	Linear	Poly	RBF
SVM classifier accuracy	71.1%	80%	84.6%
5-fold cross validation-error	29%	23.1%	22.6%

Table 4. Emotional stress classification accuracy on EEG signals using SVM for the three-kernel function

Table 5 gives the average classification accuracy in different five channels of EEG signals under two emotional stress states with using RBF kernel in SVM and ENN classifiers.

Classifier accuracy	Different channels of EEG signals				
	FP1	FP2	T3	T4	Pz
SVM	81.6%	76%	84.5%	81.5%	83.6%
ENN	75.1%	76.2%	81.7%	85.3%	83.2%

Table 5. The average classification accuracy in different channels using RBF kernel of SVM and ENN classifiers

Table 6 gives the average classification accuracy in different features set under two emotional stress states with using RBF kernel in SVM and ENN classifiers.

Classifier accuracy	Different features set		
	nonlinear	HOS	Wavelet
SVM	77.2%	82.4%	83%
ENN	81.7%	80.5%	78.2%

Table 6. The average classification accuracy in different features set using RBF kernel of SVM and ENN classifiers

7. Discussion and conclusion

In this research, we propose an approach to classify emotional stress in the two main areas of the valance-arousal space by using bio-signals. Several researchers have shown that, it is possible to measure emotional cues using EEG measurements, which is an important condition to be able to find emotional stress states from brain activity (Chanel, 2009; Horlings, 2008; Takahashi, 2004). We chose the picture presentation test, base on the closeness of its assessment to our aims. The reason we have chosen the brain signals over the pure peripheral signals is the fact that brain signals represent behaviour directly from their source but the peripheral signals are secondary manifestations of the autonomic nervous system in response to emotional stress.

With compare to the results analysis of peripheral signals, we will notice that the breathing and SC signals are less reliable in accuracy compared to BVP and HRV signals. The results showed that, the classification accuracy with peripheral signals was 76.95% for the two categories, using SVM classifier with RBF kernel. In order to choose the best channels for EEG signals, we implemented a new cognitive model (Hosseini et al., 2010a) and eventually used signals from frontal, temporal and occipital electrodes as the most important ones. The mere use of the personal moods and the subject's self-assessment to confirm the quality of the registered brain signals can cause many errors. As a result, we will need to use peripheral signals as a secondary trainer. In order to choose the best emotional stress state correlated EEG signals, we implemented a new emotion-related signal recognition system, which has not been studied so far (Hosseini & Khalilzadeh, 2010). We recorded peripheral signals concomitantly in order to firstly recognize the correlated emotional stress state and then label the correlated EEG signal. Recent researches on the EEG signals, revealed the chaotic nature of this signal. It is logical not to use conventional methods that assume emotion can be analyzed by linear models, because brain signals essentially have a chaotic nonlinear behaviour, we performed emotional stress state assessment using both linear and nonlinear features. Wavelet coefficients, higher order spectra and chaotic invariants like fractal dimension, approximate entropy and correlation dimension were used to extract the characteristics of the EEG signals. For most nonlinear measures a dimension should be defined to visualize the attractor in phase space, but the problem associated with all of them is that defined dimension for the phase space is not constant for all channels of recorded EEG signals or for different subjects, and depending on the conditions, the chosen dimension can be different. On the other hand, the performance of each measure can be dependent to the values of dimension, so by helping some equations and trial and error the optimum dimension for getting the best results can be discovered.

The results showed that, the correlation dimension of negative emotional stress state is less as compared to that of calm state, and be observed that Higuchi's algorithm indicates similar trend of reduction in FD value for negative emotional stress state compared to calm state. The reduction in FD values and D_2 characterizes the reduction in brain system complexity for participants with negative emotional stress state, therefore the number of the necessary dynamic equations for the description of the brain state in the negative emotional stress state decreases. A new approach to emotional stress states analysis by approximate entropy is described in this research. Approximate entropy is defined as a quantitative parameter to character the complexity (or irregularity) of EEG signals in different brain function status. The results of analysis of the nonlinear characteristics show that, if the parameters and the length of data are determined appropriately, the results can be a good representation of the brain behaviour in emotional stress states. Hence, the application of nonlinear time series analysis to EEG signals offers insight into the dynamical nature and variability of the brain signals. Therefore, those seem that nonlinear features would lead to better understanding of how emotional activities work.

In this research, for the first time in this investigational field, we had done a feature extraction using higher order spectra in emotional stress states assessment. The review of the contour plots in different channels of EEG signals as examples for in Figs. 10 and 11. This figures show that, most of the changes are amplification or diminish of the peaks or transfer of the peaks in the bifrequency plane. We concluded that HOS analysis could be an accurate tool in assessment of emotional stress states.

In this research, two of the advantages in this research, which confirm the credibility of our results, are using dichotic hearing test and using peripheral signals to label the brain signals. We have used both a static and a dynamic classifiers. The results show that, no meaningful different is not seen. Therefore, we can deduce that in short term data acquisition there is no specific dynamicity, which can be attributed to the short time intervals of 2 seconds. It is possible that by performing longer tests and using bigger intervals there is hope to identify some dynamics.

The results showed that, the importance of EEG signals for emotional stress assessment by classification as they have better time response than peripheral signals. We used 2 seconds time intervals with rectangular window without overlap, to analyze the brain signals, which resulted in a time resolution of 2 seconds in emotional stress states recognition. If we had used shorter time intervals with overlap, we could have achieved a greater but virtual time resolution, which, for example, can be useful in biofeedback applications. The problem of high dimensionality is solved by using Genetic Algorithm as a feature selection method. The results showed that, the average classification accuracy were 84.6% and 83.1% for two categories of emotional stress states using the SVM and ENN classifiers respectively. Therefore, each of two classifiers are same results in recognize of emotional stress state. In addition, the results showed that, this new fusion link, between EEG and peripheral signals are more robust in comparison to the separate signals. This is a great improvement in results compared to other similar published researches. We achieved a noticeable improvement of 6.3% and 10% in accuracy, using SVM and ENN classifiers respectively, in compared to our previous studies in the similar field (Hosseini et al., 2009).

Analyzing the results of previous researches is a difficult task, because to compare the results of the researches, which attempt to introduce emotion assessment systems as a classification problem, it is important to consider the way that emotions are elicited and the number of participants, the latter is important especially to introduce a user independent system. Due to these differences, we cannot exactly compare results with the results of the researches.

9. References

Aftanas, L.I.; Reva, N.V.; Varlamov, A.A.; Pavlov, S.V. & Makhnev, V.P. (2004). Analysis of Evoked EEG Synchronization and Desynchronization in Conditions of Emotional Activation in Humans: Temporal and Topographic Characteristics. *Neuroscience and Behavioral Physiology*, Vol. 34, No. 8, pp. 859-867.

Armony, J. L.; Schreiber, D. S.; Cohen, J. D. & LeDoux, J. E. (1997). Computational modeling of emotion: explorations through the anatomy and physiology of fear conditioning. *Review Paper, Elsevier Science*, Vol. 1, No. 1, pp. 28-34.

Carey, J. (2006). Brain Facts, a Primer on the Brain and Nervous System, *Society for Neuroscience*, USA.

Chanel, G. (2009). Emotion assessment for affective computing based on brain and peripheral signals, *Ph.D. Thesis Report, University of Geneve*.

Chanel, G.; Kierkels, J.J.M.; Soleymani, M. & Pun, T. (2009). Short-term emotion assessment in a recall paradigm, *International Journal Human-Computer Studies*, Vol. 67, pp. 607–627.

Chang, C.C. & Lin, C.J. (2009). LIBSVM: a Library for Support Vector Machines. Software Available from http://www.csie.ntu.edu.tw/~cjlin/libsvm/

Dedovic, K.; Renwick, R.; Khalili-Mahani, N.; Engert, V.; Lupien, S.J. & Pruessner, J.C. (2005). The Montreal Imaging Stress Task: using functional imaging to investigate the effects of perceiving and processing psychosocial stress in the human brain, *Journal Psychiatry Neurosci*, pp. 319-325.

Demuth, H.; Beale, M. & Hagan, M. (2008). Neural Network Toolbox™ 6 User's Guide, by The MathWorks, Inc.

Grassberger, P. & Procaccia, I. (1983). Characterization of strange attractors, Phys. Review Letter, Vol. 50, pp. 346-349.

Haupt, R.L. & Haupt, S.E. (2004). Practical Genetic Algorithms, *John Wiley & Sons*, Inc, (2th-Edition), pp. 189-190.

Higuchi, T. (1988). Approach to an irregular time series on the basis of the fractal theory, *Physica D*, Vol. 31, pp. 277-283.

Hinich, M.J. (1982). Testing for Gaussianity and Linearity of a Stationary Time Series, Time Series Analysis, pp. 169-176.

Horlings, R. (2008). Emotion recognition using brain activity, Delft University of Technology, Faculty of Electrical Engineering, Mathematics, and Computer Science, Man-Machine Interaction Group.

Hosseini, S.A. (2009). Quantification of EEG signals for evaluation of emotional stress level, *M.Sc. Thesis Report*, Biomedical Engineering, Islamic Azad University-Mashhad Branch. (Thesis in Persian).

Hosseini, S.A. & Khalilzadeh, M.A. (2010). Emotional stress recognition system using EEG and psychophysiological signals: Using new labelling process of EEG signals in emotional stress state, *Procssdings of IEEE, The International Conference on Biomedical Engineering and Computer Science* (ICBECS), pp. 90-95, Wuhan, China.

Hosseini, S.A.; Khalilzadeh, M.A.; Homam, S.M. & Azarnoosh, M. (2009). Emotional stress detection using nonlinear and higher order spectra features in EEG signal, *Journal of Electrical Engineering*, Vol. 39, No.2, pp. 13-24. (Article in Persian).

Hosseini, S.A., Khalilzadeh, M.A., Homam, S.M. & Azarnoosh M. (2010a). A Cognitive and Computational Model of Brain Activity during Emotional Stress, *Advances in cognitive science*, Vol. 12, No. 2, pp. 1-14. (Article in Persian).

Hosseini, S.A., Khalilzadeh, M.A., Naghibi-Sistani, M.B. & Niazmand V. (2010b). Higher Order Spectra Analysis of EEG Signals in Emotional Stress State, *Procssdings of IEEE The 2nd International conference on Information Technology and Computer science* (ITCS), pp. 60-63, Kiev, Ukraine.

Hosseini, S.A.; Khalilzadeh, M.A. & Changiz, S. (2010c). Emotional stress recognition system for affective computing based on bio-signals, *International Journal of Biological Systems* (JBS), *A Special Issue on Biomedical Engineering and Applied Computing*, Vol. 18, pp. 101-114.

Hosseini, S.A.; Homam, S.M.; Khalilzadeh, M.A. & Niazmand V. (2010d). Qualitative and quantitative evaluation of brain activity in emotional stress, *Iranian Journal of Neurology*, Vol. 8, No. 28.

Hudlicka, E. (2005). A Computational Model of Emotion and Personality: Applications to Psychotherapy Research and Practice, *Proceedings of the 10th Annual Cyber Therapy Conference: A Decade of Virtual Reality*, pp. 1-7, Basel, Switzerland.

Jiu-ming, L.; Jing-qing, L. & Xue-hua, Y. (2004). Application of chaos analytic methods based on normal EEG, *Proceedings of IEEE, The 3rd International Conference on Computational Electromagnetics and Its Applications*, pp. 426 – 429.

Kim, K.H.; Bang, S.W. & Kim, S.R. (2004). Emotion recognition system using short-term monitoring of physiological signals, *Medical and Biological engineering and Computing*, Vol. 42, pp. 419-427.

Ko, K.E.; Yang, H.C. & Sim K.B. (2009). Emotion Recognition using EEG Signals with Relative Power Values and Bayesian Network, *International Journal of Control, Automation, and Systems*, Vol. 7, No. 5, pp. 865-870.

Lang, P.J.; Bradley, M.M. & Cuthbert, B.N. (2005). International affective Picture System (IAPS): Affective ratings of pictures and instruction manual, *Technical Report A-6*, University of Florida, Gainesville, FL.

LeDoux, J. (1996). The Emotional Brain, Simon & Schuster, New York.

McFarland, R.A. (1985). Relationship of skin temperature changes to the emotions accompanying music, *Applied Psychophysiology and Biofeedback*, Vol. 10, No. 3, pp. 255-267.

Motie-Nasrabadi, A. (2004). Quantitative and Qualitative Evaluation of Consciousness Variation and Depth of Hypnosis through Intelligent Processing of EEG signals, *Ph.D. Thesis Report*, Amirkabir University, Tehran.

Murugappan, M.; Rizon, M.; Nagarajan, R. & Yaacob, S. (2009). FCM clustering of Human Emotions using Wavelet based Features from EEG, *International Journal of Biomedical Soft Computing and Human Sciences* (IJBSCHS), Vol. 14, No. 2, pp. 35-40.

Nikias, C.L. & Mendel, J.M. (1993). Signal Processing with Higher Order Spectra, *IEEE Signal Processing Magazine*, pp. 10-37.

Pincus, S.M. (1991). Approximate entropy as a measure of system complexity, Proc. Natl.Acad. Sci. USA, vol 88, pp: 2297-2301, 1991.

Ramachandran, V.S. (2002). Encyclopedia of the Human Brain, Elsevier, 4-Volume Set, Academic Press.

Ritz, T., Dahme; B., Dubois, A.B.; Folgering, H.; Fritz, G.K.; Harver, A.; Kotses, H.; Lehrer, P.M.; Ring, C.; Steptoe, A. & van-de-Woestijne, K.P. (2002). Guidelines for mechanical lung function measurements in psychophysiology, *International Journal of Psychophysiology*, Vol. 39, No. 5, pp. 546-567.

Sadock, B.J.; Kaplan, H. & Sadock, V.A. (1998). Synopsis of Psychiatry: Behavioral Sciences/Clinical Psychiatry, Lippincott Williams & Wilkins, 8th-Edition, 1998.

Savran, A.; Ciftci, K.; Chanel, G.; Mota, J.C.; Viet, L.H.; Sankur, B.; Akarun, L.; Caplier, A. & Rombaut, M. (2006). Emotion Detection in the Loop from Brain Signals and Facial Images, *Final Project Report*, eNTERFACE'06, Dubrovnik, Croatia.

Schaaff, K. & Schultz, T. (2009). Towards Emotion Recognition from Electroencephalographic Signals, *3rd International Conference on Affective Computing and Intelligent Interaction* (ACII) and Workshops, pp. 1-6.

Schachter, S. (1970). Some Extraordinary Facts about Obese Humans and Rats, American Psychologist, Vol. 26, pp.129-144.

Seymour, B. & Dolan, R. (2008). Emotion, Decision Making, and the Amygdala, *Review article*, *Journal of Neuron*, Vol. 58, pp.662-671.

Steimer, T. (2002). The biology of fear and anxiety related behaviors. Dialogues in clinical neurosciences, Vol. 4, No. 3, pp. 225-249.

Swami, A.; Mendel, J.M. & Nikias, C.L. (2000). Higher-Order Spectral Analysis (HOSA) Toolbox for Use with Matlab, Version. Available from
http://www.mathworks.com/matlabcentral/fileexchange/3013/

Takahashi, K. (2004). Remarks on Emotion Recognition from Bio-Potential Signals, *Proceedings of the 2nd International Conference on Autonomous Robots and Agents*, pp. 186-191, Palmerson North, New Zealand.

Wan, R.D. & Woo, L.J. (2004). Feature Extraction and Emotion Classification Using Bio-Signal, *Transactions on Engineering*, Computing and Technology V2, pp. 317-320, ISSN 1305-5313.

Wilhelm, F.H., Pfaltz, M.C. & Grossman, P. (2006). Continuous electronic data capture of physiology, behavior and experience in real life: towards ecological momentary assessment of emotion, *Interacting with Computers*, Vol. 18, No. 2, pp. 171-186.

Xiang, Y. & Tso, S.K. (2002). Detection and Classification of flows in Concrete Structure using Bispectra and neural networks, *NDT&E International*, Vol. 35, pp. 19-27.

Xiang, H. (2007). A Computational Model and Psychological Experiment Analysis on Affective Information Processing, *a doctoral dissertation submitted to the Graduate School of Engineering at the University of Tokushima*.

Zhai, J. & Barreto, A. (2006). Stress Detection in Computer Users Based on Digital Signal Processing of Noninvasive Physiological Variables, *Proceedings of IEEE, The 28th Annual International Conference Engineering in Medicine and Biology Society* (EMBS'06), pp. 1355-1358, New York, USA.

http://www.unifesp.br/dpsicobio/adap/exemplos_fotos.htm
http://www.thoughttechnology.com/flexinf.htm

15

Multiscale Modeling of Myocardial Electrical Activity: From Cell to Organ

Beatriz Trenor, Lucia Romero, Karen Cardona, Julio Gomis,
Javier Saiz and Jose Maria Ferrero (Jr.)
*Instituto Interunivesitario de Investigación en Bioingeniería y
Tecnología Orientada al Ser Humano, Universitat Politècnica de València*
Spain

1. Introduction

Cardiac arrhythmias represent a leading cause of morbidity and mortality in developed countries. In spite of intense research, the mechanisms of generation, maintenance and termination of theses arrhythmias are still not clearly understood. The ability to predict, prevent and treat these arrhythmias remains a major scientific challenge. In the last years, new technologies have produced a huge amount of information at different levels: subcellular, cellular, tissue, organ and system. However, the knowledge of each component is not sufficient by itself to understand its behavior and an integrative approach, which should take into account the complex interactions between all components is needed. This understanding is necessary to improve prevention and treatment of cardiac arrhythmias.

Traditionally, cardiac research has been based on experimental and clinical studies. However, in the last decades, a quantitative understanding of the biophysical and biochemical properties of individual cardiac myocytes and of the anatomical structure of the heart has permitted the development of computational models of single myocytes, portions of tissue and even the whole heart. These models have opened a new approach in studying the complex mechanisms underlying cardiac arrhythmias by means of computer simulations.

Integrated and multiscale models of the heart are improving very fast, as a large body of research is being made in this field. These models integrate, with a great degree of detail, the different levels of the organ, from the genetic characteristics of membrane ionic channels, to the electrophysiological characteristics of cardiac cells and to the anatomical structure of the different cardiac tissues. In this chapter, the basis of cardiac multiscale modeling will be reviewed and recent and specific case studies for the different levels will be described focusing on the understanding of cardiac arrhythmias during myocardial ischemia and drug treatment.

2. Modeling cardiac ion channels activity

Comprehensive models of the electrical activity of cardiac ion channels were formulated for the first time in 1952 (Hodgkin & Huxley, 1952). These models were based on the Hodgkin-

Huxley mathematical formalism, which allows the reproduction of macroscopic ionic currents. This approach computes the conductance of a certain ion channel as a function of the open probability of each gate of the channel and the maximum conductance of the membrane for that particular ion. In additon, gate transitions from closed to open and vice versa follow a first order voltage dependent behavior at a rate that is independent of the remaining gate states.

The improvements in the experimental techniques employed to measure and characterize the ionic currents responsible for the cardiac action potential have provoked a paralell evolution in the ion channel models, which have acquired an increasing complexity and realism. Two examples are the separation of certain currents into its components, like the slow and rapid delayed rectifier potassimum currents, and the discovery of ion current dependencies on electrolyte concentrations. Importantly, experimental data have evidenced the existence of state dependent transitions of ion channels that Hodgkin-Huxley formalism fails to reproduce. This fact has favored the development of Markov models for ion channels, which are based on the assumption that the transitions between channel states depend on the present conformation of the channel and not on its past history. Furthermore, recent developments in molecular biology and in the genetics of ion channels have made possible the characterization of the electrophysiological properties of a certain mutated ion channel (Tomaselli et al., 1995), allowing the development of its mathematical model using Markov models. Although Markov models can provide a more realistic formulation of ion channels, Hodgkin-Huxley models are also currently used because their computational requirements are significantly less demanding. Both formalisms are used to model ion channel-drug interactions and pathological situations.

2.1 Modeling myocardial ischemia at the ion channel level

The ionic current and action potential models developed in the last decades make it possible to simulate the electrical activity of cardiac cells both in normal and abnormal conditions. Among the latter, acute myocardial ischemia is one of the most threatening abnormalities that can occur in cardiac tissue because it can easily trigger malignant and potentially mortal reentrant tachyarrhythmias such as ventricular tachycardia (VT) and ventricular fibrillation (VF) (Janse & Wit, 1989). Indeed, VF subsequent to ischemia is considered as the first cause of mortality in Europe, the USA and a significant part of Asia (Ross, 1999).

Myocardial ischemia occurs when a coronary artery is occluded. When this happens, a certain zone of the myocardium (formed by the cells that depended on the occluded artery for their blood and nutrient supply) begins to suffer metabolic and electrophysiological changes. Specifically, K^+ ions begin to rapidly accumulate in the extracellular medium (a phenomemon termed hyperkalemia), the media (both intra and extracellular) become acidotic (with a drop in pH from 7.2-7.4 to 6.2-6.4 in 10-15 minutes), and oxygen levels decline (hypoxia). Hypoxia provokes in turn a depletion in intracellular ATP levels and a concomitant increase in ADP levels, which results in the partial activation of a specific type of K^+ current called ATP-sensitive potassium current ($I_{K(ATP)}$) (Noma, 1983).

To properly and predictively simulate the cardiac arrhythmias arising from myocardial ischemia, the model must be of a multi-scale nature and ischemia has to be modeled in the ion channel level, the cell level and the tissue level. While tissue modeling of ischemia will be adressed further in this chapter, ion channel ischemia modeling should be done as follows. First, hypoxia must be included in the model through its effects in $I_{K(ATP)}$ current activation (see below). Second, hyperkalemia must be simulated by increasing $[K^+]_o$ levels (Rodriguez et al., 2002). Elevated $[K^+]_o$ in turn alters the conductance of a number of sarcolemmal channels, such as I_{K1} or I_{Kr}, and these effects are included in most ion channel models published to date. Third, acidosis must be modeled through its effects in the maximum conductances and kinetic properties of the Na^+ and Ca^{2+} inward currents (Ferrero, Jr. et al., 2003; Shaw & Rudy, 1997a).

The $I_{K(ATP)}$ current, which is normally dormant in normoxic situations but is partially (though only slightly) activated in acute myocardial ischemia, is carried by K^+ ions (Noma, 1983), shows voltage-dependent inward rectification (but is otherwise non-voltage dependent) caused by Mg^{2+} and Na^+ ions (Horie et al., 1987), and is gated by intracellular ATP with intracellular ADP playing a modulating role in the ATP-mediated deactivation (Weiss et al., 1992). All these facts have to be present in an ion channel model of the current. In 1995, Ferrero et al. published the first comprehensive model for the myocardial $I_{K(ATP)}$ current (Ferrero, Jr. et al., 1996), which has been further improved more recently (Michailova et al., 2005).

The mathematical model for the $I_{K(ATP)}$ current includes all the aforementioned effects, which are represented in the following equation:

$$I_{K(ATP)} = \sigma \; g_0 \; p_o \; \gamma_{ir} \; f_{ATP} \left(V_m - E_K \right) \tag{1}$$

where σ is the channel density, g_0 the unitary conductance (which is $[K^+]_o$ dependent), γ_{ir} is a term that includes the inward rectification properties of the channels, f_{ATP} is a term that expresses the ATP and ADP dependence of the current, V_m is membrane potential and E_K the K^+ equilibrium (Nernst) potential. The inward rectification term is expressed as follows:

$$\gamma_{ir} = \frac{1}{1 + \left(\dfrac{[Mg^{2+}]_i}{K_{h,Mg}} \right)^2} \; \frac{1}{1 + \left(\dfrac{[Na^+]_i}{K_{h,Na}} \right)} \tag{2}$$

where $K_{h,Mg}$ and $K_{h,Mg}$ are voltage and $[K^+]_o$ dependent. Finally, the ATP-ADP dependence follows another Hill-type equation as follows:

$$f_{ATP} = \frac{1}{1 + \left(\dfrac{[ATP]_i}{K_{ATP}([ADP])} \right)^{H([ADP])}} \tag{3}$$

where both the semi-inhibition constant K_{ATP} and the Hill exponent H depend on the intracellular ADP concentration.

2.2 Modeling drug-ion channel interaction

Also at the ionic channel level, the effect of antiarrhythmic drugs can be mathematically formulated. Models that simulate effects of drugs and reproduce the associated clinical electrocardiography signal are highly relevant to assess and predict antiarrhythmic actions, and help to improve the efficacy and safety of pharmacologic therapy. Additionally, it starts to be considered as an important technological tool for helping the pharmaceutical industry to develop new antiarrhythmic drugs spending less time and money. In this field, Dr.

Starmer is one of the pioneers in modeling drug effects on sodium channels and an increasing number of research groups are developing 3D models of the heart to test drug actions. In the last years, our group has carried out different studies of antiarrhythmic and proarrhytmic effects of different drugs, such as pinacidil, dofetilide and lidocaine on cardiac arrhythmias.

To simulate the effects of drugs on ion channels, different kinds of models can be used (Brennan et al., 2009). Sometimes it is sufficient to change the conductance of ion channels by introducing the effect of the drug, but to be able to reproduce use- and frequency-dependent block it is necessary to use a state-dependent block model. In the state-dependent block model, drug interaction with ionic channels depends on the state of the channel. Drug-associated channels (blocked channels) do not conduct. The fraction of blocked non-conducting channels depends on the equilibrium between blocked and unblocked states. Two hypotheses have been proposed to reproduce the state-dependent block: the modulated receptor hypothesis and the guarded receptor hypothesis. The Modulated Receptor (MR) hypothesis (Hille, 1977; Hondeghem & Katzung, 1977) states that the affinity of a drug changes with the state of the channel. Additionally, the rate constants of state transitions are different for bound and unbound satates. This is the most general model to reproduce the effects of drugs; however a great number of parameters have to be estimated. The Guarded Receptor (GR) hypothesis (Starmer et al., 1984) assumes that the drug has a fixed and state-independent affinity for their receptor sites, but its access to the binding sites is controlled by the voltage-dependent channel gates. In this hypothesis, the rate constants for the state transitions do not change when the drug binds to the channel. The GR model is less complex than the MR model for the same drug-ion channel interaction as fewer parameters have to be estimated.

In the present section three different models of drugs: pinacidil, lidocaine, and dofetilide are described.

2.2.1 Modeling pinacidil effects

Pinacidil is a vasodilator drug and is known to increase $I_{K(ATP)}$ in cardiomyocytes, as well as in vascular smooth muscle and pancreatic Beta cells (Fan et al., 1990; Nakayama et al., 1990). The activation of ATP-sensitive potassium (K_{ATP}) channels in heart tissue, especially during myocardial ischemia, markedly changes action potential (AP) configuration by reducing AP duration (APD) (Nichols et al., 1991) and plays an important role in cardiac arrhythmogenesis (Janse & Kleber, 1981). To analyze the controversial effects of this drug through computer simulations, the first step is to build a model of the effects of pinacidil at the ion channel level. Pinacidil enhances the activity of $I_{K(ATP)}$ increasing the fraction of open K_{ATP} channels (f_{ATP}) (Fan et al., 1990). The equation of $I_{K(ATP)}$ formulated by Ferrero et al. (Ferrero, Jr. et al., 1996) was modified, as indicated in the following equations:

$$I_{K(ATP)} = \sigma\, g_0\, p_o\, f_{ATP}\, f_{PIN}\, (V_m - E_K) \tag{4}$$

$$f_{ATP} = 1 - \cfrac{[P]^H}{[A]^H + \cfrac{k_1 k_{11} k_{13} + [D]\, k_{11} k_{13} + k_1 k_{13}[P] + k_1[P][D]}{\dfrac{k_1 k_{11} k_{13}}{k_{d1}} + \dfrac{k_{11} k_{13}[D]}{k_{d2}} + \dfrac{k_1 k_{13}[P]}{k_{d3}} + \dfrac{k_1[P][D]}{k_{d4}}}} \tag{5}$$

The equation of f_{ATP} was based on the pharmacokinetic scheme depicted in Fig. 1. This scheme describes the mechanism of action by which ATP molecules close K_{ATP} channels, while pinacidil molecules open it. ATP, ADP and pinacidil molecules bind to different sites in the protein receptor (Nichols et al., 1991; Weiss et al., 1992). According to the open states when molecules of pinacidil and/or ADP are bound to the protein channel, the fraction of activated K_{ATP} channels was expressed in equation (5). Experimental data (Fan et al., 1990; Nakayama et al., 1990; Weiss et al., 1992) were fitted to equation (5) to determine the values of equilibrium dissociation constants and the Hill coefficient (H) (see Trenor et al. 2005 for details). A factor (f_{PIN}) addressing the voltage-dependent block of K_{ATP} channels by pinacidil was also included in $I_{K(ATP)}$ equation, as in Fan et al. (Fan et al., 1990).

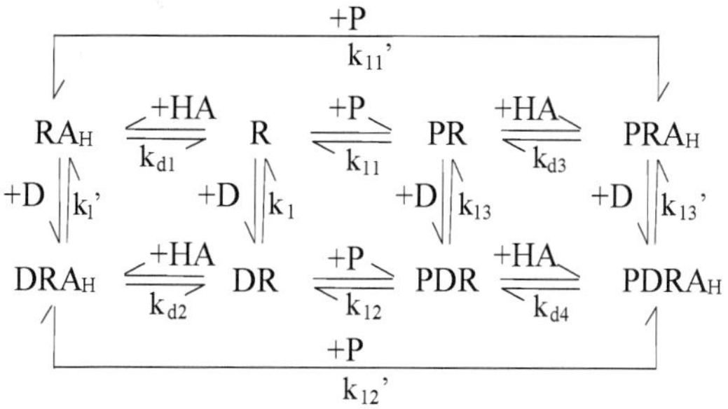

$$
\begin{array}{ccccccc}
 & & & +P \\
 & & & k_{11}{}' \\
RA_H & \underset{k_{d1}}{\overset{+HA}{\rightleftharpoons}} & R & \underset{k_{11}}{\overset{+P}{\rightleftharpoons}} & PR & \underset{k_{d3}}{\overset{+HA}{\rightleftharpoons}} & PRA_H \\
+D\,\big|k_I{}' & & +D\,\big|k_1 & & +D\,\big|k_{13} & & +D\,\big|k_{13}{}' \\
DRA_H & \underset{k_{d2}}{\overset{+HA}{\rightleftharpoons}} & DR & \underset{k_{12}}{\overset{+P}{\rightleftharpoons}} & PDR & \underset{k_{d4}}{\overset{+HA}{\rightleftharpoons}} & PDRA_H \\
 & & & +P \\
 & & & k_{12}{}'
\end{array}
$$

Fig. 1. Cyclic scheme representing different possibilities of binding to the channel receptor protein. R, P, A and D stand for the unoccupied receptor, pinacidil, ATP and ADP respectively. k_i are the overall equilibrium dissociation constants for the different steps of the cyclic reaction, and H is the Hill coefficient.

2.2.2 Modeling lidocaine effects

Lidocaine is a class I antiarrhythmic drug that exerts its effect by blocking inward sodium current (I_{Na}) in a use-dependent manner, and is more effective for high stimulation frequencies (Clarkson et al., 1988). The block of lidocaine exists both as neutral and charged forms at a physiological pH. The charged form predominates at low pH (6.4) due to the protonation of the neutral form with hydrogen molecules. Experimental data have confirmed that lidocaine is more effective and recovery from block is slowed (Broughton et al., 1984; Moorman et al., 1986; Wendt et al., 1993) under acidosis.

The formulated model of lidocaine-I_{Na} interaction takes into account the modulatory effect of pH on the Na^+ channel block and is based on the GR theory proposed by Starmer (Starmer & Courtney, 1986). Three main processes have been considered: the hydrophobic pathway, the hydrophilic pathway, and coupling between blocked channels by charged and neutral forms using a proton exchange process. Several experimental studies have suggested that the block of neutral drug takes place during the activated (O), inactivated (I) and resting (R) states (Bean et al., 1983; Clarkson et al., 1988), whereas the interaction between the charged form with the channel only takes place in the activated state (Liu et al., 2003; Moorman et al., 1986; Yeh & Tanguy, 1985). Fig. 2 represents the kinetic diagram of the complete model, and equations (6) and (7) mathematically describe the interaction of the neutral and charged form with Na^+ channels, respectively.

$$\frac{db_N}{dt} = \left[m^3 hj \cdot k_O + m^3 \left(1 - hj\right) \cdot k_I + \left(1 - m^3\right) \cdot k_R \right] \cdot \left[D_N\right] \cdot \left(1 - b_N - b_C\right) -$$

$$\left[m^3 hj \cdot l_O + m^3 \left(1 - hj\right) \cdot l_I + \left(1 - m^3\right) \cdot l_R \right] \cdot b_N + l_p \cdot b_C - k_p \left[H^+\right] \cdot b_N \tag{1}$$

$$\frac{db_C}{dt} = \left[m^3 hj \cdot k_C \right] \cdot \left[D_C\right] \cdot \left(1 - b_N - b_C\right) - \left[m^3 hj \cdot e^{-zV_m F / RT} \cdot l_C \right] \cdot b_C - l_p \cdot b_C + k_p \left[H^+\right] \cdot b_N \tag{2}$$

b_N and b_C stands for the fraction of channels blocked by the neutral and charged form. The association and dissociation rate constants for the different states (activated, inactivated, and resting) are k_O, k_I, k_R, l_O, l_I, and l_R, respectively. The activation channel gate is m and the inactivaction channel gates are h and j. Additionally, we have taken into account the rate constants k_p and l_p to determine the proton exchange process. In equation (7), the association and dissociation rate constants are k_C and l_C, respectively.

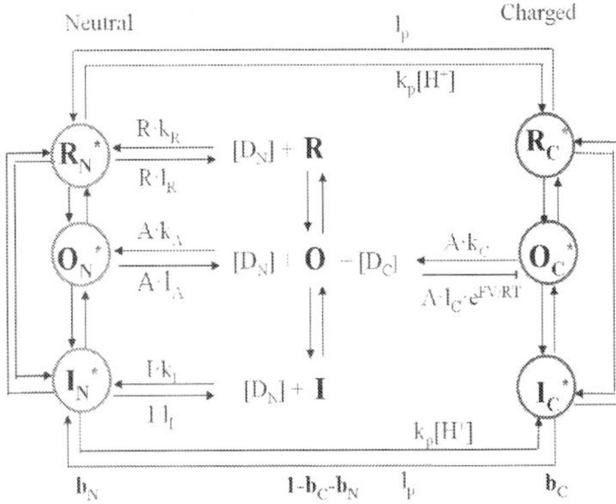

Fig. 2. Lidocaine interaction with Na^+ channels in both forms of the drug: neutral (b_N) and charged (b_C).

As stated in the GR hypothesis, we introduced the factor (1-b), where b is the sum of the b_N and b_C in the I_{Na} equation.

2.2.3 Modeling dofetilide effects

Dofetilide is a specific and potent blocker of the rapid component of the delayed rectifier K^+ current (I_{Kr}) with an IC_{50} in the nanomolar range (3.9-31 nmol/L) for ventricular myocytes (Carmeliet, 1992; Jurkiewicz & Sanguinetti, 1993; Weerapura et al., 2002b). Dofetilide is classified as a pure class III antiarrhythmic agent and provokes a prolongation of action potential duration (APD) without any effect on the resting membrane potential, action potential amplitude or maximum rate of depolarization (Jurkiewicz & Sanguinetti, 1993; Tande et al., 1990).

To model the effects of dofetilide on I_{Kr}, the formulation of I_{Kr} proposed by Zeng and Rudy (Zeng et al., 1995) for guinea pig ventricular cells was used. This formulation is based on experimental data obtained by Sanguinetti and Jurkiewicz (Sanguinetti & Jurkiewicz, 1990). In their model, I_{Kr} channels present three possible states: Closed (C), Open (O) and

Inactivated (I). The formulation of I_{Kr} in the ventricular cell model (Zeng et al., 1995) is expressed in equation (8).

$$I_{Kr} = G_{Kr\,max} X_r R (V_m - E_{Kr}) \qquad (3)$$

where V_m is the membrane potential, E_{Kr} is the reversal potential, G_{Krmax} is the maximum conductance of I_{Kr}, X_r is the activation gate and R is the time-independent inactivation gate. In our dofetilide-I_{Kr} model, the effect of dofetilide is represented by introducing the factor (1–b) in the I_{Kr} formulation (where b is the fraction of channels blocked by the drug). Thus, the new formulation of the rapid component of the delayed rectifier K$^+$ current taking into account the effect of dofetilide is

$$I_{Kr} = (1 - b) G_{Kr\,max} X_r R (V_m - E_{Kr}) \qquad (4)$$

The blocking activity (b) on I_{Kr} equation is modeled using the GR hypothesis (Starmer et al., 1984). Dofetilide experimental studies have shown drug-receptor interaction in open and inactivated states but not in closed states (Weerapura et al., 2002a; Yang et al., 1997). It has been also observed that the drug is trapped when the channel closes, thereby the transition between open and closed state is possible but dissociation of the drug does not occur at closed states (Carmeliet, 1992; Weerapura et al., 2002a). Taking into account these experimental evidences we suggest the model of I_{Kr} block by dofetilide shown in Fig. 3. Using this model, the blocking factor b for a concentration of dofetilide D can be calculated as:

$$\frac{db}{dt} = [X_r R k_O + X_r(1-R)k_I]D(1-b) - [X_r R r_O + X_r(1-R)r_I]b \qquad (5)$$

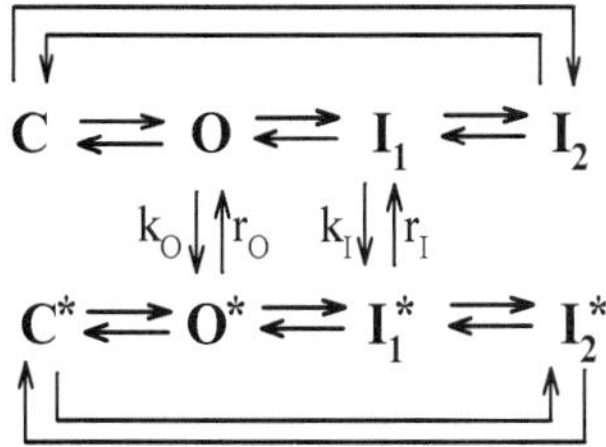

Fig. 3. Schematic model of dofetilide interaction with I_{Kr} channels in the different states: Closed (C), Open (O) and Inactivated (I_1 and I_2) potassium channels. k and r are the association and dissociation constants for the different states.

3. Modeling cardiac electrical cellular activity

The electrical activity of the cell is determined by the interaction of the multiple ionic channels and ion exchangers present in the cellular membrane. Their activity conditions the cardiac AP, which is intimately synchronized with the mechanical activity of the heart. Several computational models of cardiac cellular electrical activity have been developed, and characterize the activity of ventricular myocytes, atrial myocytes, sinus node and

Purkinje fibers for different animal species. The degree of complexity of these models increases going from heuristic models describing the physical process of cell excitation and propagation, such as Fitz-Hugh-Nagumo model (Fitzhugh, 1961), to phenomenological models (Bueno (Bueno-Orovio et al., 2008) model), and to extremely detailed ionic models. The most detailed ionic models for AP include transmembrane currents, ion transfer through transporters and dynamic changes of ion concentrations during the action potential. The ventricular AP models most extensively used in simulations because of their detailed and realistic formulation are Luo and Rudy model (Faber & Rudy, 2000; Luo & Rudy, 1994; Zeng et al., 1995) for guinea pig, Shannon (Shannon et al., 2005) and Mahajan (Mahajan et al., 2008) models for rabbit, and ten Tusscher (ten Tusscher & Panfilov, 2006) and Grandi (Grandi et al., 2010) models for human. As regards atrial myocytes, Nygren (Nygren et al., 1998) model and Courtemanche (Courtemanche et al., 1998) model have also had an important repercussion. Luo Rudy AP model was one of the first detailed models formulated and has been a fundamental base on which other models have been built. This model has been improved and extensively used to simulate the ventricular electrical activity. In these detailed AP models, the formulation of the ionic currents follow Hodgkin-Huxley, Goldmann-Hodgkin-Katz (GHK) or Markov formalisms, and the membrane potencial V_m is related to the ionic currents through equation (11).

$$I_m = C_m \frac{dV_m}{dt} + \sum_S I_S + \sum_p I_p \qquad (6)$$

where the total ionic current through the cell membrane (I_m) is expressed as the sum of all ionic currents (I_s through ionic channels and I_p through pumps and exchangers) plus the current through the membrane equivalent capacitor.

Fig. 4 shows a scheme of the main ionic currents of a ventricular myocyte (panel A) and the time course of membrane potential and some ionic currents (panel B) obtained by solving the non-linear differential equations system defined by equation (11) and the different ionic current equations in Luo and Rudy model (Faber & Rudy, 2000; Zeng et al., 1995).

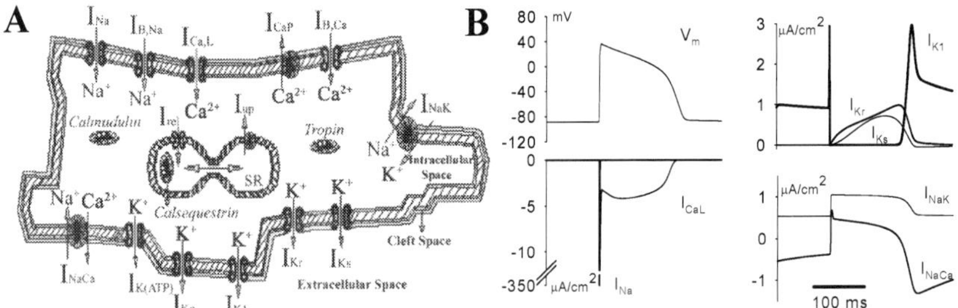

Fig. 4. Panel A: Schematic representation of a ventricular myocyte and the most significant ionic currents through the sarcolemma. Panel B: Temporal evolution of the membrane potential V_m, Ca^{2+}, Na^+ and K^+ currents, and currents through the Na^+/K^+ pump (I_{NaK}) and the Na^+/Ca^{2+} exchanger.

3.1 Modeling myocardial ischemia at cellular level

Acutely ischemic action potentials can be simulated using these AP models appropriately modified to represent ischemia-activated currents (such as $I_{K(ATP)}$) and ischemic-modified currents (e.g. the inward Na^+ and Ca^{2+} currents), as explained previously.

One of the main components of acute ischemia is hypoxia (i.e. lack of oxygen in the tissue), and the main change exerted by hypoxia to myocardial action potentials is a significant shortening in APD (Morena et al., 1980). The model proposed by Ferrero et al. for the ATP-sensitive K^+ current (Ferrero, Jr. et al., 1996) yielded the first theoretical proof of the determinant role of the $I_{K(ATP)}$ current in hypoxic action potential shortening (Ferrero, Jr. et al., 1996), which is an arrhythmic factor due to the APD dispersion it generates across the myocardium (Janse & Wit, 1989). Indeed, as shown in Fig. 5, although very few K_{ATP} channels do activate during acute myocardial ischemia (<1% in the first 15minutes), this degree of activation is enough to account for the >50% shortening in APD which is observed in experimental conditions (Morena et al., 1980).

When the simulated myocyte is subject to hyperkalemia and acidosis, as well as hypoxia, the main features of the ischemic AP waveforms are correctly reproduced (Ferrero, Jr. et al., 2003; Shaw & Rudy, 1997a). A shown in Fig. 6, ischemia produces APD shortening, resting potential elevation, upstroke phase division into two phases (the first one mediated by inward Na^+ current, the second one by inward Ca^{2+} current through the L-type channels). Moreover, acute ischemia changes important intrinsic AP properties which are pivotal in arrhythmogenesis (e.g., postrepolarization refractoriness). Overall, this ischemic AP simulations are the first level of the multi-scale ischemia simulations that will be described further in this chapter.

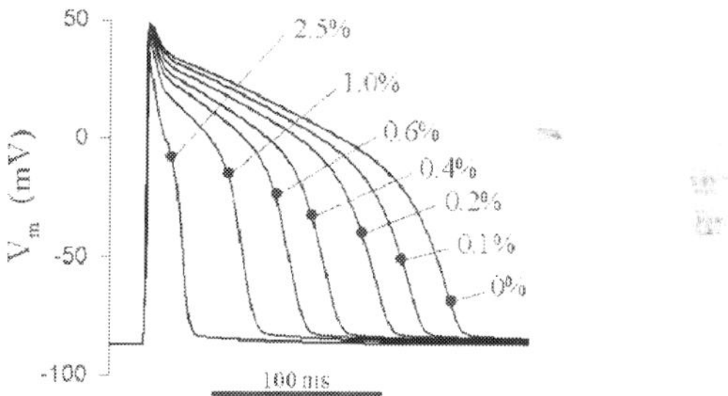

Fig. 5. Hypoxic action potentials simulated using a modified version of the dynamic Luo & Rudy model (Luo & Rudy, 1994) in which the $I_{K(ATP)}$ model formulated by Ferrero was included (Ferrero, Jr. et al., 1996). Numbers indicate percentage of K_{ATP} channel activation.

3.2 Effects of drugs at cellular level

As mentioned before, the electrical activity of the cell is altered under the effects of drugs. Once the effects of the drug have been formulated at the ionic channel level, the alterations of the electrical activity of the cell can be analyzed including the modified current in the AP model. In this way, the effects of pinacidil and lidocaine on ischemic cells are described. Also the effects of dofetilide on different types of ventricular cells will be analyzed.

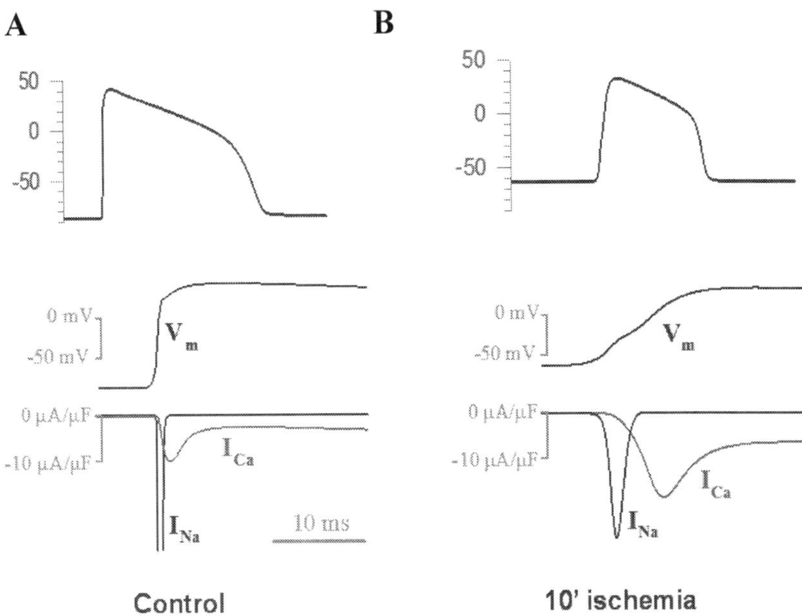

Fig. 6. Action potentials and inward ionic currents during control conditions (panel A) and 10 minutes of acute ischemia (panel B). The lower panels correspond to a zoomed view of the first 30 ms of the action potentials shown on the top panels. A significant decrease in inward Na+ current, together with an increase in Ca+2 current, is observed. The low I_{Na} in ischemia provoques the division of the upstroke phase of the action potential into two distinct phases, as seen experimentaly (Janse & Wit, 1989).

3.2.1 Effects of pinacidil on AP

As mentioned in section 2, pinacidil shortens the APD by the activation of K_{ATP} channels. To validate pinacidil model, the formulation of the effect of pinacidil (equations (4) and (5)) on $I_{K(ATP)}$ was introduced into the Luo and Rudy model (Luo & Rudy, 1994; Zeng et al., 1995). Simulations were carried out combining different concentrations of pinacidil with various [ATP]$_i$ and [ADP]$_i$ values corresponding to several stages of early acute ischemia (Cole et al., 1991; Nakayama et al., 1990; Weiss et al., 1992). The resulting APs are shown in Fig. 7. Consistent with experimental findings (Cole et al., 1991; Nakayama et al., 1990), our results show that increasing concentrations of pinacidil and/or decreasing intracellular ATP levels reduce APD. It is noteworthy that changes concerning intracellular ATP and ADP concentrations, occurring during acute ischemia, significantly enhance the effects of pinacidil. These changes in APD (and hence in cell refractoriness) could be key in determining the reentry probability in acute ischemia after the administration of the drug.

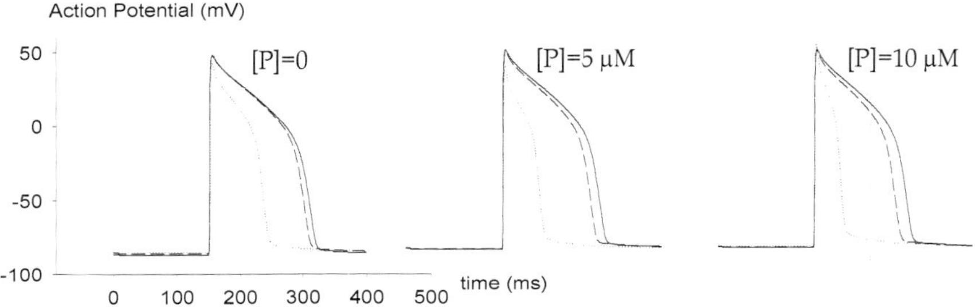

Fig. 7. Set of simulated single cell action potentials in the presence of different concentrations of pinacidil: 0, 5 and 10 µmol/L from left to right. Shortening of APD can be also observed under different concentrations of ATP: 6.8 mmol/L (solid line), 5 mmol/L (dashed line) and 2 mmol/L (discontinuous line).

3.2.2 Effects of lidocaine on AP

The block of I_{Na} by lidocaine leads to a decrease in the maximal AP upstroke (dV/dt_{max}). To simulate the effects of lidocaine on AP features, we incorporated the model of lidocaine into the Luo and Rudy AP model (Luo & Rudy, 1994). Specifically, we measured the reduction of the maximum AP upstroke for different stimulation frequencies and pH values when increasing concentrations of the drug. We examined the response of dV/dt_{max} to changes in pH from 7.4 to 6.4 for different concentrations of the drug (50 and 100 of µmol/L lidocaine) and at different stimulation frequencies. Panel A in Fig. 8, shows a decrease of 66% and 83% in dV/dt_{max} from the control value for 50 and 100 µmol/L lidocaine, respectively, at a basic cycle length (BCL) of 500 ms and pH 6.4. For a pH of 7.4 (see Fig. 8 panel B) , dV/dt_{max} was reduced in 45% and 61% for the same concentrations and BCL values. These data support the fact that lidocaine has a greater effect under lower pH. Furthermore, the use-dependent effect is more pronounced at lower pH, as the differences in the decrease of dV/dt_{max} for different stimulation frequencies are higher for low pH.

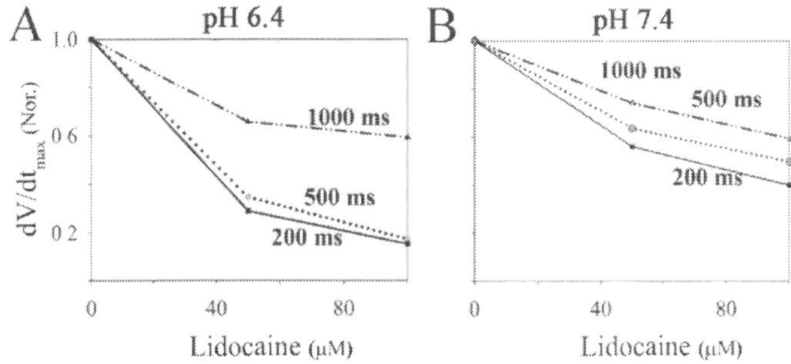

Fig. 8. The effects of lidocaine on dV/dt_{max} at pH values of 6.4 and 7.4 at different BCLs. The steady-state dV/dt_{max} was normalized (Nor) with respect to its value in the absence of the drug.

3.2.3 Effects of dofetilide on AP

The steady-state effects of dofetilide concentration on AP characteristics for the different kinds of guinea pig ventricular cells at different BCL values are shown in Fig. 9. In all simulations, once dofetilide was applied the cellular models were stimulated until steady- state was reached. Only magnitudes associated to the last stimulation pulse are shown. Fig. 9A shows that the prolongation of APD_{90}, for all tested dofetilide concentrations, significantly depends on the type of cell. APD_{90} of M-cells was markedly prolonged compared to endocardial and epicardial cells. For a concentration of 10 nmol/L, APD_{90} of endocardial cells was prolonged in 8.8%, 11.5% and 12.4% of control value (APD_{90} before the application of drug) for BCL of 300, 1000 and 2000 ms, respectively. For the same conditions, APD_{90} of epicardial cells was increased in 5.8%, 6.9% and 7.1% of control, respectively. However, under these conditions, APD_{90} of M-cells was substantially increased in 14.8%, 36.1% and 292.7% of control, respectively. The three types of cells present reverse use-dependency. Due to this effect, the prolongation of APD_{90} increased whith the BCL. Fig. 9B shows the relative increase of APD_{90} (ΔAPD_{90} in%) induced by different concentrations of dofetilide at different BCLs.

Fig. 9B shows that dofetilide presents reverse use-dependence in the range of tested concentrations (10 nmol/L to 1 µmol/L) with a much more pronounced effect in M-cells than endocardial or epicardial cells. Even more, when the concentration of dofetilide increased, the reverse use-dependency was enhanced.

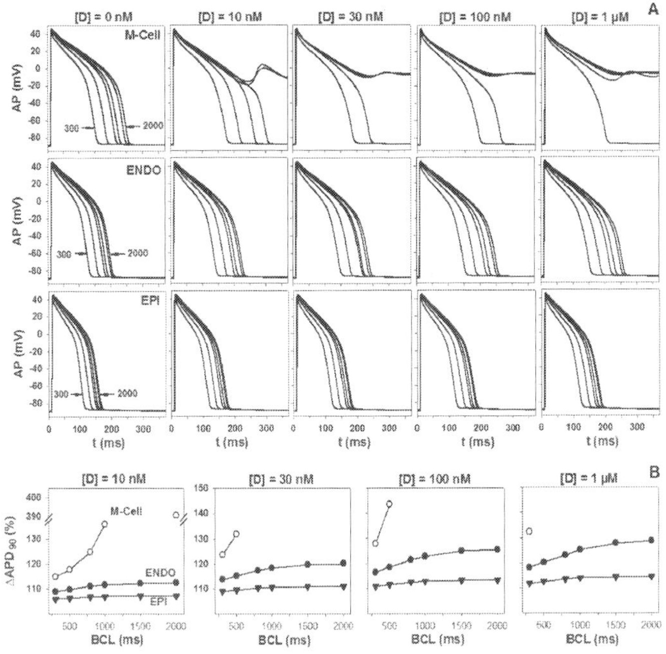

Fig. 9. Effects of different concentrations of dofetilide on steady-state AP waveform (panel A) and APD_{90} prolongation (panel B) from guinea pig endocardial, epicardial and M-cells at different BCL values.

4. Modeling cardiac tissue electrical activity

Abnormalities in impulse propagation are involved in the genesis and maintenance of cardiac arrhythmias and many experimental and theorical studies have analyzed action potential propagation both in normal and pathological situations. The electrical coupling between cells and the propagation process is described in the bidomain model (Tung, L., 1978). This model consists of two continuous domains, the intracellular and the extracellular domain, where electrical currents are governed by Ohm´s law. The following equations describe the bidomain model:

$$\nabla \cdot \left(D_i \nabla V_m \right) + \nabla \cdot \left(D_i \nabla V_e \right) = C_m \frac{\partial V_m}{\partial t} + I_{ion} + I_{st} \tag{7}$$

$$\nabla \cdot \left(D_i \nabla V_m \right) + \nabla \cdot \left(\left(D_i + D_e \right) \nabla V_e \right) = 0 \tag{8}$$

where D_i and D_e are the intracellular and extracellular conductivity tensors, respectively, V_e and V_m stand for the extracellular and the membrane potentials, respectively, C_m is membrane capacitance, I_{ion} represents the total ionic current density computed using AP models, and I_{st} is the stimulus current density.

Considering that anisotropy similarly affects the intracellular and the extracellular conductivity tensors ($D_i = \lambda D_e$, λ being a scalar variable), the bidomain model can be simplified into the monodomain model and the previous equations can be reduced to the following one:

$$\nabla \cdot \left(D \nabla V_m \right) = C_m \frac{\partial V_m}{\partial t} + I_{ion} + I_{st} \tag{9}$$

$$\text{where} \quad D = \frac{\lambda}{1 + \lambda} \cdot D_i \tag{10}$$

Subsequently, the monodomain model consists of an elliptic partial differential equation and a parabolic partial differential equation coupled to a system nonlinear ordinary differential equations describing the ionic current through the cellular membrane. As this model is mathematically simpler and less computational demanding than the bidomain model, it is widely used for cardiac electrophysiology simulations.

Heterogeneous structures of cardiac tissue can also be considered in tissue models allowing a wide use of cardiac models in the study of ionic mechanims of arrhythmias.

4.1 Tissue model of myocardial ischemia

In the case of pathological tissues, not only the altered AP models have to be considered but also the spatial inhomogeneities in the electrophysiological changes distributed within the tissue. If we consider the ischemic pathology, after coronary occlusion, the lack of oxygen and blood flow provokes important and heterogeneous electrophysiological changes in the affected ventricular cells defining an ischemic zone and a border zone, setting the stage for reentrant arrhythmias and VF. A large body of clinical and experimental studies try to unravel the mechanisms by which acute myocardial ischemia provokes life-threatening arrhythmias. However, the rapid changes arising during acute myocardial ischemia and the limitations in experimental techniques hamper the complete understanding of this pathology. In this way, computer simulations overcome these limitations providing a helpful tool to understand the electrophysiological changes arising during myocardial ischemia and the underlying mechanisms of reentrant arrhythmias observed during its acute phase. At the tissue level, our group has developed a regional model of ischemia, and the consideration of the temporal evolution of ischemia has allowed undertaking computational studies to assess the changes in the vulnerability of the ischemic tissue to reentry. Not only ionic currents have been analyzed to understand the process of reentry initiation but also the traditional indicator for reentry, i.e. dispersion of repolarization, and the safety factor (SF) for conduction (a parameter that quantifies the source-sink relationship of propagation) as an indicator for conduction block, have been evaluated.

A regional phase Ia ischemic 2D anisotropic monodomain tissue (Ferrero, Jr. et al., 2003; Romero et al., 2009; Trenor et al., 2007) was modeled with a high degree of electrophysiological detail. Changes in electrophysiological parameters were modeled according to experimental results (Coronel, 1994; Ferrero, Jr. et al., 1996; Irisawa & Sato, 1986; Weiss et al., 1992; Yatani et al., 1984). These changes are described in Fig. 10A, which shows the time-course of the three main components of acute ischemia: hypoxia, hyperkalemia and acidosis. Fig. 10B represents the distribution of a simulated cardiac 2D tissue comprising a normal zone (NZ), a circular central ischemic zone (CZ), and a ring-shaped ischemic border zone (BZ) surrounding the CZ. In the BZ all parameters affected by ischemia follow linear spatial gradients, as experimentally recorded (Coronel et al., 1988). Membrane kinetics was simulated by using a modified version of the Luo-Rudy dynamic AP model (LRd00) (Faber & Rudy, 2000) (see Romero et al. 2009 for details), which includes the mathematical formulation of $I_{K(ATP)}$ proposed by Ferrero et al. 1996 (Ferrero, Jr. et al., 1996).

A basic stimulus (S_1) followed by a prematures stimulus (S_2) at different coupling intervals (CIs) was applied on the edge of the tissue to quantify the vulnerable window (VW), an indicator of the vulnerability to reentry. The VW was defined as the interval of CIs that led to reentry. Fig. 10C shows gray-coded voltage snapshots of a figure-of-eight reentry developed after premature stimulation at minute 8.25 of ischemia. Our results demonstrated that during myocardial ischemia phase Ia, the VW of a bidimensional tissue had an asymmetric unimodal distribution, peaking at minute eight after coronary occlusion (see Fig. 10D), which is in close agreement with experimental observations (Cascio, 2001). We also analyzed the SF for conduction in the regional ischemic tissue using an improved version (Romero et al., 2009) of the formulation proposed by Shaw and Rudy (Shaw & Rudy, 1997c). Our results also indicate that, as ischemia progresses, the SF decreased and the heterogeneity of refractoriness grows. Therefore, a lack of correlation between dispersion of refractoriness and vulnerability to reentry was observed, although our results corroborate the fact that dispersion of refractoriness is essential to reentry generation. Moreover, we found that, in approximately half of the simulated reentries, the area where unidirectional block (UDB) took place was completely recovered from refractoriness when the AP propagation failed. However, the line where the SF dropped below unity matched very much the area where propagation failed in every simulation. Thus, it seemed that the reduction of the source-sink ratio is the ultimate cause of the UDB leading to reentry.

Reentrant patterns of activation during regional acute ischemia have been mechanistically analyzed also under the effects of pharmacologic agents, such as pinacidil or lidocaine.

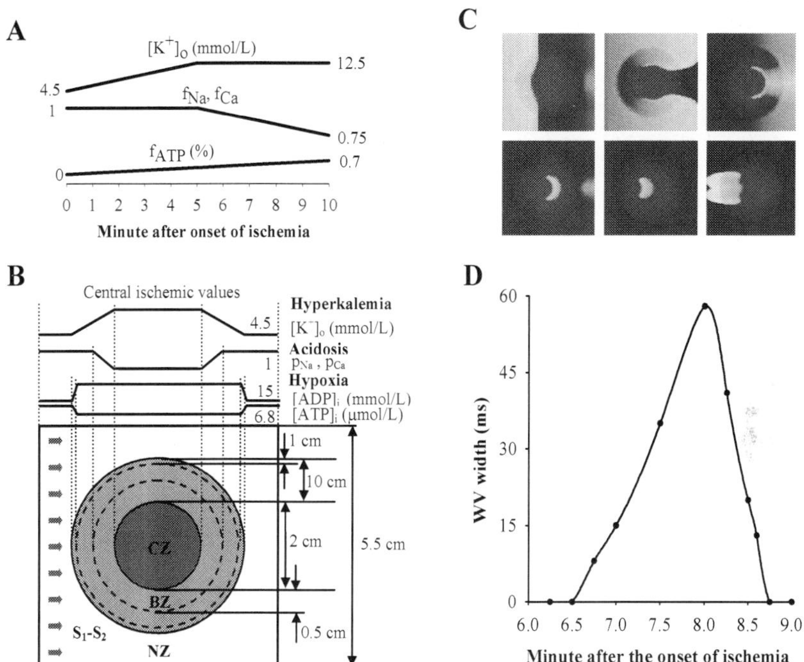

Fig. 10. Panel A: Evolution of electrophysiological parameters after the onset of myocardial ischemia in the CZ: $[K^+]_o$, f_{ATP}, and relative activation of I_{Na} (f_{Na}) and I_{CaL} (f_{Ca}). Panel B: Regional ischemic tissue layout comprising a NZ, a BZ, and a CZ. Spatial gradients of electrophysiological parameters are described above the tissue.

4.2 Drugs effects on reentry during myocardial ischemia

To analyze the arrhythmogenic effects of pinacidil, different sets of simulations were carried out using different concentrations of the drug. In each set the regionally ischemic 2D tissue described above was stimulated using the aforementioned S_1-S_2 protocol and the VW was evaluated. Table 1 shows that increasing the concentration of pinacidil had an interesting non-monotonic effect on the duration of the VW. Indeed, low concentrations of the drug increased the VW, until a maximum of 54 ms was reached for [P]=3 μm/L. If the concentration was further increased, the VW decreased, until the VW vanished for [P]=10 μm/L.

The simulations allowed to unravel the mechanisms underlying pinacidil-induced changes in vulnerability, through the analysis of the patterns of excitation in the tissue and the time evolution of ionic currents and membrane potential. Our results showed the existence of two opposite effects of pinacidil in terms of AP propagation, which modulate the biphasic effects on the VW. On the one hand, pinacidil enhances $I_{K(ATP)}$ (Ferrero, Jr. et al., 1996), which counteracts inward currents responsible for depolarization, mainly I_{Na} (which is depressed as a consequence of ischemia) and $I_{Ca(L)}$, so that AP reaches lower values of V_m during the depolarization phase. In this way, the potential gradient in the direction of propagation is also reduced, and less electrotonic current flows to downstream cells (Shaw & Rudy, 1997a), reducing axial current. In these conditions, the SF is reduced (Shaw & Rudy, 1997c) and propagation failure may develop. On the other hand, the $I_{K(ATP)}$ enhancement provoked by pinacidil reduces APD, which results in an earlier recovery of excitability (Shaw & Rudy, 1997b), favoring AP propagation. Both effects of pinacidil are related as follows: the earlier the cell recovers its excitability, the less axial current is needed to elicit an AP.

Pinacidil (mmol/L)	VW (ms)
0	45 [167-212]
0,001	49 [166-215]
0,003	54 [166-220]
0,005	46 [179-225]
0,007	14 [207-221]

Table 1. Width of the vulnerable window (VW) for different concentrations of pinacidil.

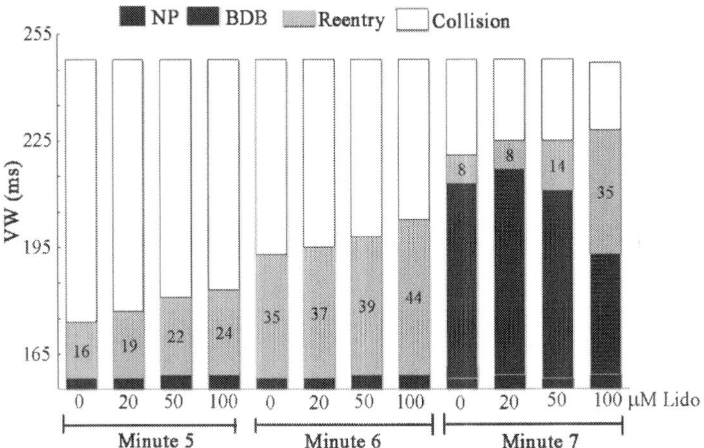

Fig. 11. Width of the VW in ms for different degrees of ischemia (5, 6, and 7 minutes after occlusion) and concentrations of lidocaine (20, 50, and 100 µmol/L).

We also simulated the effects of lidocaine on a regionally ischemic bidimensional tissue prone to reentrant circuits. Simulations were also carried out using an S_1-S_2 protocol applied on one edge of the tissue and the VW for reentry was calculated for various degrees of severity of ischemia and various concentrations of the drug (20, 50, and 100 µmol/L). The VWs for reentry are shown in Fig. 11, and follow an unimodal behavior with ischemia time course, peaking (35 ms) for 6 minutes after the onset of ischemia. When the concentration of lidocaine was increased, the VW became wider, indicating a higher vulnerability to reentry in the presence of the drug. This effect can be due in part to the heterogeneous action of the drug in the diverse zones of the tissue, contributing to the dispersion of CV and setting the stage for reentry.

4.3 Effects of dofetilide on 1D heterogeneous tissue

In the case of dofetilide, a class III antiarrhythmic drug recently approved by FDA (Food and Drug Administration) for the treatment of persistent atrial fibrillation and flutter, different studies have questioned the antiarrhythmic action of dofetilide in preventing and terminating ventricular tachycardias. Indeed, dofetilide promotes the prolongation of QT interval, which has been related to the trigger of a polymorphic ventricular tachycardia called *torsade de pointes*. The study of the proarrhythmic effects of dofetilide has also been undertaken with computer simulations at the tissue level, where pseudo ECGs have been evaluated, giving understanding about the mechanisms by which QT interval is altered by this drug.

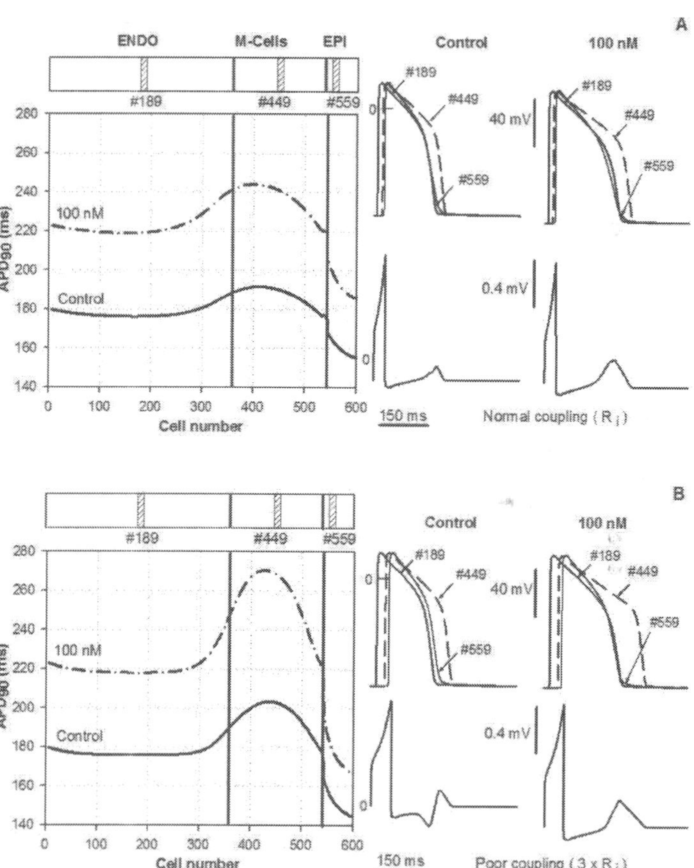

Fig. 12. APD$_{90}$ distribution in a heterogeneous linear strand, APs of three cells belonging to the different regions of the tissue and pseudoECG, in two different conditions: before the application of dofetilide (control) and when the steady-state in drug-binding was reached after the application of dofetilide 100 nmol/L (BCL= 1000 ms), for normal coupled fiber (panel A) and under poor coupling conditions (panel B).

To study the effect of dofetilide on transmural dispersion of repolarization (TDR), a linear strand including the three kinds of cells was used. Fig. 12A illustrates the steady-state APD_{90} distribution along a well-coupled heterogeneous fiber and the steady-state APs time-course of the three types of cells belonging to the different regions of the tissue (right side in Fig. 12) under two different conditions: before (control) and after the application of dofetilide 100 nmol/L. The pseudo ECGs are also represented before and after the application of the drug.

Our results show that in a well-coupled strand under control conditions, at a BCL of 1000 ms, M-cells present a maximum APD_{90} of 191 ms, which is 15 ms and 35 ms longer than the shortest APD of endocardial (176 ms) and epicardial (156 ms) cells, respectively. The application of dofetilide 100 nmol/L increased APD_{90} dispersion (difference between the maximum and the minimum APD_{90} in the fiber) from 35 ms to 58 ms, being the maximum APD_{90} recorded in the M-zone and the minimum in the epicardial zone. The electrograms show an increment in the QT interval induced by the application of dofetilide from 220.8 ms (control) to 274.6 ms for 100 nmol/L dofetilide.

The effect of decreasing the intercellular coupling (intercellular coupling resistance R_i multiplied by three) at a BCL of 1000 ms is shown in Fig. 12B. Poor coupling increased the APD_{90} dispersion from 35 ms (normal coupling) to 58 ms. Even more, under poor coupling conditions dofetilide induced a steeper distribution of APD along the fiber and the APD_{90} dispersion increased to 102 ms, for dofetilide concentration of 100 nmol/L. The QT intervals were higher than the ones observed in a well coupled fiber. The application of 100 nmol/L dofetilide induced a sharper increase of QT from a value of 251.8 ms in control, to 318 ms.

5. Modeling whole heart electrical activity

Whole heart models are needed to study arrhythmias that critically depend on the spatial organization of the heart. Some spatial physiological features may be localization dependent, such as regional ischemia or localized infarct scars. Furthermore, certain arrhythmias are uniquely encountered in the whole heart, such as large reentrant circuits in acute ischemia or initiation of atrial fibrillation by pulmonary venous foci. Other important considerations of the whole heart models are the cardiac fibers arrangement and transmural inhomogeneity in repolarization. Cardiac fibers are arranged as counter-wound helices encircling the ventricular cavities, and the local orientation of these fibers depends on transmural localization (Helm et al., 2005). On the other hand, the heterogeneous expression of I_{Ks}, I_{to}, and I_{NCX}, among others, leads to transmural inhomogeneity in repolarization (Antzelevitch & Fish, 2001; Antzelevitch et al., 1991). The vertiginous progress in medical images allows building realistic models of the heart including its highly complex anatomical structure of ventricles and/or atria (see Clayton et al. 2011 for review).

The mathematical problem associated to the resolution of the differential equations modeling the electrical propagation in a 3D heart model does not have an analytical solution. Indeed, electric conduction is described by a set of partial differential equations (PDEs) and ionic currents through the cell mambrane are described with a nonlinear stiff system of ordinary differential equations (ODEs). The numerical solution of the equations is very computationally demanding (Heidenreich et al., 2010b) and require the discretization in space and time of PDEs, as well as the integration of nonlinear systems of ODEs. The operator splitting technique for the time discretization (Qu & Garfinkel, 1999) is used to solve the equations system. The numerical methods used, such as finite differences method or finite elements method, are computationally demanding and require the use of high performance computing techniques.

Whole heart models also permit to relate the arrhythmic behavior with its manifestation in electrograms on the cardiac surface and in electrograms on the body surface, through a torso model (Weiss et al., 2009).

5.1 3D simulations of myocardial ischemia

The use of these ventricular 3D models has shed light into the mechanisms by which reentrant arrhythmias are initiated during regional myocardial ischemia. As an example, a 3D model of the human ventricles has been recently used to study the appearance of figure-of-eight reentry under regional acute ischemic conditions (Heidenreich et al., 2010a; Heidenreich et al., 2010b).

Fig. 13 shows different views of the simulated human ventricles. The detailed realistic local fiber orientation obtained from DTI images (diffusion tensor imaging) was introduced in the model and is key in determining the electrical propagation. An ischemic region was introduced in the left ventricle, following the same normal-border-central zone scheme explained in a previous section of this chapter. The central and right panels in Fig. 13 depict the values and gradients of the main ischemic parameters (namely $[K^+]_o$, $[ATP]_i$, I_{Na} maximum conductance and $I_{Ca(L)}$ maximum conductance).

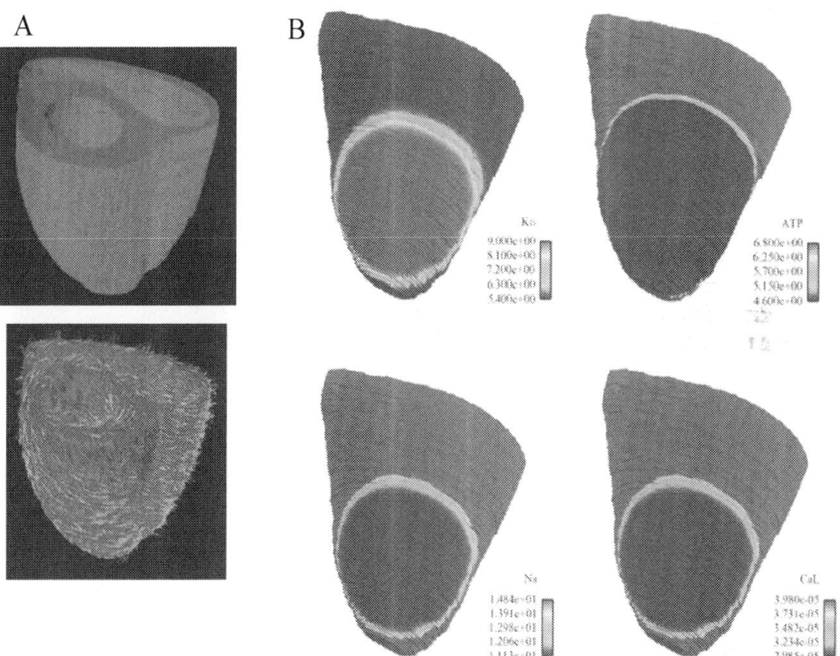

Fig. 13. Anatomically realistic human ventricles subject to regional acutely ischemic conditions (Heidenreich et al., 2010b). Top A panel: render image of the simulated ventricles. Bottom A panel: fiber orientation as obtained from DTI. Panel B: distribution of $[K^+]_o$, $[ATP]_i$, I_{Na} and $I_{Ca(L)}$ in the CZ, the NZ and the different epicardial BZs.

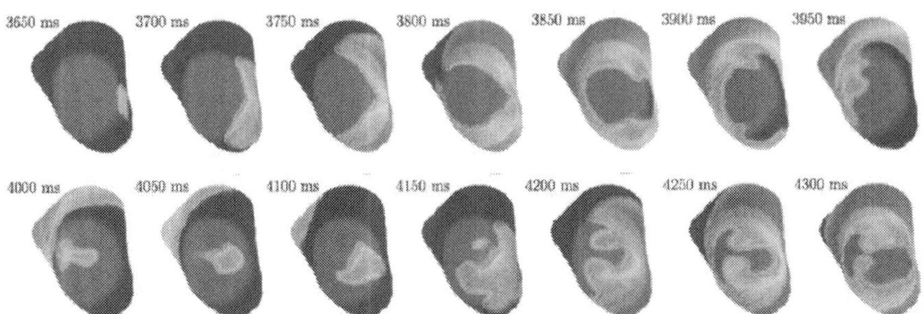

Fig. 14. Electrical activity in the simulated 3D human ventricles shown in Fig. 13 after the delivery of a premature extrastimuls in the BZ after a train of regular conditioning stimuli. A figure-of-eight reentry is initiated, which is very similar to experimentalty observed ischemic reentry (Janse & Wit, 1989).

As shown in Fig. 14, the model predicted the generation of figure-of-eight reentries, which cross the central ischemic zone formed in the epicardial surface due to the longer refractory period of the midmyocardial layers. Also, focal activity experimentally observed in the epicardium could be caused by re-entrant wavefronts propagating in the mid-myocardium that reemerge in the heart surface.

6. Conclusion

Multiscale modeling of the electrical cardiac activity represents nowadays a very valuable tool in cardiac disease research which complements experimental and clinical studies. Although significant progresses are made in this field, further improvements are required, such as the modeling of electromechanical coupling of the heart activity, which currently represents an important challenge for modelers. The vertiginous technical improvements in the obtention of medical images and genetic, molecular and ionic measurements, represent a great help to the modeling field, which is in the process of creating a virtual human.

7. Acknowledgment

This work was partially supported by the European Commission preDiCT grant (DG-INFSO-224381), by the Plan Nacional de Investigación Científica, Desarrollo e Innovación Tecnológica del Ministerio de Ciencia e Innovación of Spain (TEC2008-02090; TIN2004-03602; TEC 2005-04199/TCM; TIC 2001-2686), by the Programa de Apoyo a la Investigación y Desarrollo (PAID-06-09-2843) de la Universidad Politécnica de Valencia, by the Dirección General de Política Científica de la Generalitat Valenciana (GV/2010/078).

8. References

Antzelevitch, C. & Fish, J. (2001). Electrical heterogeneity within the ventricular wall. *Basic Res. Cardiol.*, Vol.96, No.6, pp. 517-527
Antzelevitch, C.; Sicouri, S.; Litovsky, S.H.; Lukas, A.; Krishnan, S.C.; Di Diego, J.M.; Gintant, G.A. & Liu, D.W. (1991). Heterogeneity within the ventricular wall. Electrophysiology

and pharmacology of epicardial, endocardial, and M cells. *Circ. Res.*, Vol.69, No.6, pp. 1427-1449

Bean, B.P.; Cohen, C.J. & Tsien, R.W. (1983). Lidocaine block of cardiac sodium channels. *J. Gen. Physiol*, Vol.81, No.5, pp. 613-642

Brennan, T.; Fink, M. & Rodriguez, B. (2009). Multiscale modelling of drug-induced effects on cardiac electrophysiological activity. *Eur. J. Pharm. Sci.*, Vol.36, No.1, pp. 62-77

Broughton, A.; Grant, A.O.; Starmer, C.F.; Klinger, J.K.; Stambler, B.S. & Strauss, H.C. (1984). Lipid solubility modulates pH potentiation of local anesthetic block of Vmax reactivation in guinea pig myocardium. *Circ. Res.*, Vol.55, No.4, pp. 513-523

Bueno-Orovio, A.; Cherry, E.M. & Fenton, F.H. (2008). Minimal model for human ventricular action potentials in tissue. *J. Theor. Biol.*, Vol.253, No.3, pp. 544-560

Carmeliet, E. (1992). Voltage- and time-dependent block of the delayed K+ current in cardiac myocytes by dofetilide. *J. Pharmacol. Exp. Ther.*, Vol.262, No.2, pp. 809-817

Cascio, W.E. (2001). Myocardial ischemia: what factors determine arrhythmogenesis? *J. Cardiovasc. Electrophysiol.*, Vol.12, No.6, pp. 726-729

Clarkson, C.W.; Matsubara, T. & Hondeghem, L.M. (1988). Evidence for voltage-dependent block of cardiac sodium channels by tetrodotoxin. *J. Mol. Cell Cardiol.*, Vol.20, No.12, pp. 1119-1131

Clayton, R.H.; Bernus, O.; Cherry, E.M.; Dierckx, H.; Fenton, F.H.; Mirabella, L.; Panfilov, A.V.; Sachse, F.B.; Seemann, G. & Zhang, H. (2011). Models of cardiac tissue electrophysiology: progress, challenges and open questions. *Prog. Biophys. Mol. Biol.*, Vol.104, No.1-3, pp. 22-48

Cole, W.C.; McPherson, C.D. & Sontag, D. (1991). ATP-regulated K+ channels protect the myocardium against ischemia/reperfusion damage. *Circ. Res.*, Vol.69, No.3, pp. 571-581

Coronel, R. (1994). Heterogeneity in extracellular potassium concentration during early myocardial ischaemia and reperfusion: implications for arrhythmogenesis. *Cardiovasc. Res.*, Vol.28, No.6, pp. 770-777

Coronel, R.; Fiolet, J.W.; Wilms-Schopman, F.J.; Schaapherder, A.F.; Johnson, T.A.; Gettes, L.S. & Janse, M.J. (1988). Distribution of extracellular potassium and its relation to electrophysiologic changes during acute myocardial ischemia in the isolated perfused porcine heart. *Circulation*, Vol.77, No.5, pp. 1125-1138

Courtemanche, M.; Ramirez, R.J. & Nattel, S. (1998). Ionic mechanisms underlying human atrial action potential properties: insights from a mathematical model. *Am. J. Physiol*, Vol.275, No.1, pp. H301-H321

Faber, G.M. & Rudy, Y. (2000). Action potential and contractility changes in [Na(+)](i) overloaded cardiac myocytes: a simulation study. *Biophys. J.*, Vol.78, No.5, pp. 2392-2404

Fan, Z.; Nakayama, K. & Hiraoka, M. (1990). Multiple actions of pinacidil on adenosine triphosphate-sensitive potassium channels in guinea-pig ventricular myocytes. *J. Physiol*, Vol.430, pp. 273-295

Ferrero, J.M., Jr.; Saiz, J.; Ferrero, J.M. & Thakor, N.V. (1996). Simulation of action potentials from metabolically impaired cardiac myocytes. Role of ATP-sensitive K+ current. *Circ. Res.*, Vol.79, No.2, pp. 208-221

Ferrero, J.M., Jr.; Trenor, B.; Rodriguez, B. & Saiz, J. (2003). Electrical activity and reentry during acute regional myocardial ischemia: insights from simulations. *International Journal of Bifurcation and Chaos*, Vol.13, No.7, pp. 67-78

Fitzhugh, R. (1961). Impulses and Physiological States in Theoretical Models of Nerve Membrane. *Biophys. J.*, Vol.1, No.6, pp. 445-466

Grandi, E.; Pasqualini, F.S. & Bers, D.M. (2010). A novel computational model of the human ventricular action potential and Ca transient. *J. Mol. Cell Cardiol.*, Vol.48, No.1, pp. 112-121

Heidenreich, E.; Gaspar, F.J.; Ferrero, J.M. & Rodriguez, J.F. (2010a). Compact schemes for anisotropic reaction-diffusion equations with adaptative time step. *International Journal for Numerical Methods Engineering*, Vol.82, No.8, pp. 1022-1043

Heidenreich, E.A.; Ferrero, J.M.; Doblare, M. & Rodriguez, J.F. (2010b). Adaptive Macro Finite Elements for the Numerical Solution of Monodomain Equations in Cardiac Electrophysiology. *Ann. Biomed. Eng*, Vol.38, No.7, pp. 2331-2345

Helm, P.; Beg, M.F.; Miller, M.I. & Winslow, R.L. (2005). Measuring and mapping cardiac fiber and laminar architecture using diffusion tensor MR imaging. *Ann. N. Y. Acad. Sci.*, Vol.1047, pp. 296-307

Hille, B. (1977). Local anesthetics: hydrophilic and hydrophobic pathways for the drug-receptor reaction. *J. Gen. Physiol*, Vol.69, No.4, pp. 497-515

Hodgkin, A.L. & Huxley, A.F. (1952). A quantitative description of membrane current and its application to conduction and excitation in nerve. *J. Physiol*, Vol.117, No.4, pp. 500-544

Hondeghem, L.M. & Katzung, B.G. (1977). Time- and voltage-dependent interactions of antiarrhythmic drugs with cardiac sodium channels. *Biochim. Biophys. Acta*, Vol.472, No.3-4, pp. 373-398

Horie, M.; Irisawa, H. & Noma, A. (1987). Voltage-dependent magnesium block of adenosine-triphosphate-sensitive potassium channel in guinea-pig ventricular cells. *J. Physiol*, Vol.387, pp. 251-272

Irisawa, H. & Sato, R. (1986). Intra- and extracellular actions of proton on the calcium current of isolated guinea pig ventricular cells. *Circ. Res.*, Vol.59, No.3, pp. 348-355

Janse, M.J. & Kleber, A.G. (1981). Electrophysiological changes and ventricular arrhythmias in the early phase of regional myocardial ischemia. *Circ. Res.*, Vol.49, No.5, pp. 1069-1081

Janse, M.J. & Wit, A.L. (1989). Electrophysiological mechanisms of ventricular arrhythmias resulting from myocardial ischemia and infarction. *Physiol Rev.*, Vol.69, No.4, pp. 1049-1169

Jurkiewicz, N.K. & Sanguinetti, M.C. (1993). Rate-dependent prolongation of cardiac action potentials by a methanesulfonanilide class III antiarrhythmic agent. Specific block of rapidly activating delayed rectifier K+ current by dofetilide. *Circ. Res.*, Vol.72, No.1, pp. 75-83

Liu, H.; Atkins, J. & Kass, R.S. (2003). Common molecular determinants of flecainide and lidocaine block of heart Na+ channels: evidence from experiments with neutral and quaternary flecainide analogues. *J. Gen. Physiol*, Vol.121, No.3, pp. 199-214

Luo, C.H. & Rudy, Y. (1994). A dynamic model of the cardiac ventricular action potential. I. Simulations of ionic currents and concentration changes. *Circ. Res.*, Vol.74, No.6, pp. 1071-1096

Mahajan, A.; Shiferaw, Y.; Sato, D.; Baher, A.; Olcese, R.; Xie, L.H.; Yang, M.J.; Chen, P.S.; Restrepo, J.G.; Karma, A.; Garfinkel, A.; Qu, Z. & Weiss, J.N. (2008). A rabbit ventricular action potential model replicating cardiac dynamics at rapid heart rates. *Biophys. J.*, Vol.94, No.2, pp. 392-410

Michailova, A.; Saucerman, J.; Belik, M.E. & McCulloch, A.D. (2005). Modeling regulation of cardiac KATP and L-type Ca2+ currents by ATP, ADP, and Mg2+. *Biophys. J.*, Vol.88, No.3, pp. 2234-2249

Moorman, J.R.; Yee, R.; Bjornsson, T.; Starmer, C.F.; Grant, A.O. & Strauss, H.C. (1986). pKa does not predict pH potentiation of sodium channel blockade by lidocaine and

W6211 in guinea pig ventricular myocardium. *J. Pharmacol. Exp. Ther.*, Vol.238, No.1, pp. 159-166

Morena, H.; Janse, M.J.; Fiolet, J.W.; Krieger, W.J.; Crijns, H. & Durrer, D. (1980). Comparison of the effects of regional ischemia, hypoxia, hyperkalemia, and acidosis on intracellular and extracellular potentials and metabolism in the isolated porcine heart. *Circ. Res.*, Vol.46, No.5, pp. 634-646

Nakayama, K.; Fan, Z.; Marumo, F. & Hiraoka, M. (1990). Interrelation between pinacidil and intracellular ATP concentrations on activation of the ATP-sensitive K+ current in guinea pig ventricular myocytes. *Circ. Res.*, Vol.67, No.5, pp. 1124-1133

Nichols, C.G.; Ripoll, C. & Lederer, W.J. (1991). ATP-sensitive potassium channel modulation of the guinea pig ventricular action potential and contraction. *Circ. Res.*, Vol.68, No.1, pp. 280-287

Noma, A. (1983). ATP-regulated K+ channels in cardiac muscle. *Nature*, Vol.305, No.5930, pp. 147-148

Nygren, A.; Fiset, C.; Firek, L.; Clark, J.W.; Lindblad, D.S.; Clark, R.B. & Giles, W.R. (1998). Mathematical model of an adult human atrial cell: the role of K+ currents in repolarization. *Circ. Res.*, Vol.82, No.1, pp. 63-81

Qu, Z. & Garfinkel, A. (1999). An advanced algorithm for solving partial differential equation in cardiac conduction. *IEEE Trans. Biomed. Eng*, Vol.46, No.9, pp. 1166-1168

Rodriguez, B.; Ferrero, J.M. & Trenor, B. (2002). Mechanistic investigation of extracellular K+ accumulation during acute myocardial ischemia: a simulation study. *American Journal of Physiology-Heart and Circulatory Physiology*, Vol.283, No.2, pp. H490-H500, 0363-6135

Romero, L.; Trenor, B.; Alonso, J.M.; Tobon, C.; Saiz, J. & Ferrero, J.M., Jr. (2009). The relative role of refractoriness and source-sink relationship in reentry generation during simulated acute ischemia. *Ann. Biomed. Eng*, Vol.37, No.8, pp. 1560-1571

Ross, R. (1999). Atherosclerosis--an inflammatory disease. *N. Engl. J. Med.*, Vol.340, No.2, pp. 115-126

Sanguinetti, M.C. & Jurkiewicz, N.K. (1990). Two components of cardiac delayed rectifier K+ current. Differential sensitivity to block by class III antiarrhythmic agents. *J. Gen. Physiol*, Vol.96, No.1, pp. 195-215

Shannon, T.R.; Wang, F. & Bers, D.M. (2005). Regulation of cardiac sarcoplasmic reticulum Ca release by luminal [Ca] and altered gating assessed with a mathematical model. *Biophys. J.*, Vol.89, No.6, pp. 4096-4110

Shaw, R.M. & Rudy, Y. (1997a). Electrophysiologic effects of acute myocardial ischemia. A mechanistic investigation of action potential conduction and conduction failure. *Circ. Res.*, Vol.80, No.1, pp. 124-138

Shaw, R.M. & Rudy, Y. (1997b). Electrophysiologic effects of acute myocardial ischemia: a theoretical study of altered cell excitability and action potential duration. *Cardiovasc. Res.*, Vol.35, No.2, pp. 256-272

Shaw, R.M. & Rudy, Y. (1997c). Ionic mechanisms of propagation in cardiac tissue. Roles of the sodium and L-type calcium currents during reduced excitability and decreased gap junction coupling. *Circ. Res.*, Vol.81, No.5, pp. 727-741

Starmer, C.F. & Courtney, K.R. (1986). Modeling ion channel blockade at guarded binding sites: application to tertiary drugs. *Am. J. Physiol*, Vol.251, No.4 Pt 2, pp. H848-H856

Starmer, C.F.; Grant, A.O. & Strauss, H.C. (1984). Mechanisms of use-dependent block of sodium channels in excitable membranes by local anesthetics. *Biophys. J.*, Vol.46, No.1, pp. 15-27

Tande, P.M.; Bjornstad, H.; Yang, T. & Refsum, H. (1990). Rate-dependent class III antiarrhythmic action, negative chronotropy, and positive inotropy of a novel Ik blocking drug, UK-68,798: potent in guinea pig but no effect in rat myocardium. *J. Cardiovasc. Pharmacol.*, Vol.16, No.3, pp. 401-410

ten Tusscher, K.H. & Panfilov, A.V. (2006). Alternans and spiral breakup in a human ventricular tissue model. *Am. J. Physiol Heart Circ. Physiol*, Vol.291, No.3, pp. H1088-H1100

Tomaselli, G.F.; Chiamvimonvat, N.; Nuss, H.B.; Balser, J.R.; Perez-Garcia, M.T.; Xu, R.H.; Orias, D.W.; Backx, P.H. & Marban, E. (1995). A mutation in the pore of the sodium channel alters gating. *Biophys. J.*, Vol.68, No.5, pp. 1814-1827

Trenor, B.; Ferrero, J.M., Jr.; Rodriguez, B. & Montilla, F. (2005). Effects of pinacidil on reentrant arrhythmias generated during acute regional ischemia: A simulation study. *Ann. Biomed. Eng*, Vol.33, No.7, pp. 897-906

Trenor, B.; Romero, L.; Ferrero, J.M., Jr.; Saiz, J.; Molto, G. & Alonso, J.M. (2007). Vulnerability to reentry in a regionally ischemic tissue: a simulation study. *Ann. Biomed. Eng*, Vol.35, No.10, pp. 1756-1770

Tung,L. (1978). A bi-domain model for describibg ischemic myocardial d-c potentials. Thesis/Dissertation. Massachussets Institute of Technology.

Weerapura, M.; Hebert, T.E. & Nattel, S. (2002a). Dofetilide block involves interactions with open and inactivated states of HERG channels. *Pflugers Arch.*, Vol.443, No.4, pp. 520-531

Weerapura, M.; Nattel, S.; Chartier, D.; Caballero, R. & Hebert, T.E. (2002b). A comparison of currents carried by HERG, with and without coexpression of MiRP1, and the native rapid delayed rectifier current. Is MiRP1 the missing link?. *J. Physiol*, Vol.540, No.Pt 1, pp. 15-27

Weiss, D.L.; Ifland, M.; Sachse, F.B.; Seemann, G. & Dossel, O. (2009). Modeling of cardiac ischemia in human myocytes and tissue including spatiotemporal electrophysiological variations. *Biomed. Tech. (Berl)*, Vol.54, No.3, pp. 107-125

Weiss, J.N.; Venkatesh, N. & Lamp, S.T. (1992). ATP-sensitive K+ channels and cellular K+ loss in hypoxic and ischaemic mammalian ventricle. *J. Physiol*, Vol.447, pp. 649-673

Wendt, D.J.; Starmer, C.F. & Grant, A.O. (1993). pH dependence of kinetics and steady-state block of cardiac sodium channels by lidocaine. *Am. J. Physiol*, Vol.264, No.5 Pt 2, pp. H1588. 3703-H1598

Yang, T.; Snyders, D.J. & Roden, D.M. (1997). Inhibition of cardiac potassium currents by the vesnarinone analog OPC-18790: comparison with quinidine and dofetilide. *J. Pharmacol. Exp. Ther.*, Vol.280, No.3, pp. 1170-1175

Yatani, A.; Brown, A.M. & Akaike, N. (1984). Effect of extracellular pH on sodium current in isolated, single rat ventricular cells. *J. Membr. Biol.*, Vol.78, No.2, pp. 163-168

Yeh, J.Z. & Tanguy, J. (1985). Na channel activation gate modulates slow recovery from use-dependent block by local anesthetics in squid giant axons. *Biophys. J.*, Vol.47, No.5, pp. 685-694

Zeng, J.; Laurita, K.R.; Rosenbaum, D.S. & Rudy, Y. (1995). Two components of the delayed rectifier K+ current in ventricular myocytes of the guinea pig type. Theoretical formulation and their role in repolarization. *Circ. Res.*, Vol.77, No.1, pp. 140-152

16

Methods of Weighted Averaging with Application to Biomedical Signals

Alina Momot
Silesian University of Technology, Institute of Computer Science
Poland

1. Introduction

During the analysis of real biomedical signals it can almost always be seen noise that distorts the image. The presence of interference is associated with the specific acquisition of these signals. For example in the case of bioelectric signals, disturbances may come from the hardware retrieves those signals, the powerline or the bioelectric activity of body cells. The bioelectric signals, which are widely used in most fields of biomedicine, are generated by nerve cells or muscle cells. The electric field propagates through the tissue and can be acquired from the body surface, eliminating the potential need to invade the biosystem. However, using surface electrodes results in high amplitude of noise and the noise should be suppressed to extract a priori desired information (Bruce, 2001).

There are many approaches to the noise reduction problem while preserving the variability of the desired signal morphology. One of the possible methods of noise attenuation is low-pass filtering such as arithmetic mean. The classical band-pass filtering is very simple method but also very ineffective because the frequency characteristics of signal and noise significantly overlap. Therefore there are developed other methods of noise attenuation based on transforming the input space of signal and creating a new space with the help of discrete cosine transform (Paul et al., 2000) or wavelets transform (Augustyniak, 2006), based on fuzzy nonlinear regression (Momot et al., 2005), nonlinear projective filtering (Kotas, 2009), higher-order statistics at different wavelet bands (Sharma et al., 2010) or extreme points determination by mean shift algorithm and dynamical model-based nonlinear filtering (Yan et al., 2010).

In the case of repeatable biomedical signals, another possible method of noise attenuation is the synchronized averaging (Jane et al., 1991). The method assumes that the biomedical signal is quasi-cyclic and the noise is additive, independent and with zero mean. Averaging could be performed by simple arithmetic mean or its generalization, namely weighted mean where the weights are tuned by some adaptive algorithm.

Recently there have been published several works concerning different approaches to the problem of determining the weights. The algorithm of adaptive estimation of the weights is described in (Bataillou et al., 1995). In (Leski, 2002) there is described method of estimation of the weights based on criterion function minimization. Application of Bayesian inference to the weights estimation problem is presented in (Momot et al., 2007a) and (Momot, 2008b). Weighted averaging method based on partition of input data set in time domain is described in (Momot et al, 2007b). The generalization of the method is presented in (Momot,

2008a). In (Momot, 2009a), there is presented comparative study of performance of weighted averaging methods using Bayesian inference and criterion function minimization. There were also published works describing algorithms based on fuzzy approaches to the problem of determining the weights. In (Momot, 2009b), there is presented the new weighted averaging method incorporating Bayesian and empirical Bayesian inference and its extension using fuzzy systems with fuzzy partitioning of the single repeatable input signal in the time domain. In (Momot & Momot, 2009c), there is described the weighted averaging method, where the weighting coefficients are fuzzy numbers instead of classical real numbers. Moreover in (Momot, 2010), there is presented an application of Bayesian weighted averaging to digital filtering 2D images.

Most of the mentioned above methods of weighted averaging were presented with application to noise suppression in ECG signal, the typical biomedical signal with a quasi-cyclical character. In the case of ECG signal the averaging in the time domain is only one of many methods of noise attenuation, but in some medical applications the averaging is the only method taken into account. For example in order to evaluate some clinical indexes based on the ST depression, such as ST versus HR (ST/HR) diagram or ST/HR hysteresis, the averaged ECG beats are necessary to compute (Bailon et al., 2002). Another example of biomedical repeatable signal in which noise attenuation can be performed using averaging methods is the high resolution electrocardiographic signal (HRECG). Methods of averaging help in detecting very low amplitude waves (which are called late potentials) originating in the ventricles of abnormal heart conditions patients (Laciar & Jane, 2001). Signal averaging methods are also required in the case of evoked potentials (EP), the electrical potentials recorded from the nervous system of patients, which are effects of a stimulation (in contrast to the spontaneous potentials as in the case of electroencephalography (EEG) or electromyography (EMG)) (Davila, 1992).

Traditional arithmetic averaging technique can be used when the noise is stationary (it is constant level of power noise) throughout the averaging period. If this condition is violated, increasing the input noise level during the averaging process results in increasing the residual noise and deteriorating quality of the averaged signal. Unfortunately, the physiological noise level often varies in tests, even if strict artifact rejection is applied (Elberling & Don, 2006). Thus, using methods of weighted averaging is motivated by the reason that most types of noise are not stationary and the variability of noise power can be observed.

The aim of this study is to reveal the fundamental differences among the mentioned versions of the weighted averaging methods and to present how these differences affect the quality of the averaged signal. In section 2, the necessary details of the compared methods are reminded. The differences among them and their applications are studied based on numerical experiments in section 3. The final conclusions are formulated in section 4.

2. Fundamental of weighted averaging

The biomedical signal with repetitive patterns can be (after segmentation and synchronization) represented by:

$$x_i(j) = s(j) + n_i(j), \quad i \in \{1, 2, \dots, N\}, j \in \{1, 2, \dots, L\} \tag{1}$$

where N is the number of cycles to be averaged, and L is the length of the single cycle. Typical assumption states that each signal cycle $x_i(j)$ is the sum of the signal $s(j)$, which is deterministic and invariant from cycle to cycle, and the random noise $n_i(j)$ with zero mean and variance cycle σ_i^2 (the noise remains stationary within each evolution, but its variance may vary from one cycle to the other). The assumptions and symbols are based on (Laciar & Jane, 2001).

The weighted averaged cycle can be expressed as:

$$\overline{x}(j) = \sum_{i=1}^{N} w_i x_i(j) \quad j \in \{1, 2, \ldots, L\},$$ (2)

where w_i is the weight for ith signal cycle. Usually, there is taken the assumption that the weights sum up to one ($\sum_{i=1}^{N} w_i = 1$), which leads to the unbiased estimation.

Depending on the choice of the weights, different types of the signal averaging methods can be defined. The simplest method is arithmetical averaging, where all weights are the same, equal to M^{-1}. The classical procedure assumes that the weights are proportional to the inverses of corresponding variances Johnson & Bhattacharyya (2009):

$$w_i = \sigma_i^{-2} \left(\sum_{k=1}^{N} \sigma_k^{-2} \right)^{-1} \quad i \in \{1, 2, \ldots, N\},$$ (3)

which leads to obtaining the arithmetical averaging weights if the noise power is the same in all cycles. However, in practice the variability of noise power is observed and it is impossible to measure the variances directly. Thus there are employed different methods to estimate the noise variances or to compute the optimal weights without direct estimation of the noise variance. These two approaches will be presented below. The Bayesian methods incorporate estimation of the noise variations and methods using criterion function minimization usually lead to direct computation of the weights.

2.1 Methods based on criterion function minimization

The noise variance, which appears in formula (3), can be estimated according to the formula (Laciar & Jane, 2001):

$$\hat{\sigma}_i = \frac{1}{L} \sum_{j=1}^{L} (\hat{n}_i(j) - \overline{n}_i)^2 \quad \text{with} \quad \overline{n}_i = \frac{1}{N} \sum_{j=1}^{L} \hat{n}_i(j),$$ (4)

where L is a length of the averaging window and $\overline{n}_i$ is the mean value of the estimated noise component of ith cycle in the averaging window.

Assuming that the signal is deterministic and invariant from cycle to cycle and the noise has zero mean, the estimated noise component can be described by:

$$\hat{n}_i(j) = x_i(j) - \overline{x}(j) \quad j \in \{1, 2, \ldots, L\}$$ (5)

and the formula (4) may be written in simplified form:

$$\hat{\sigma}_i^2 = \frac{1}{L} \sum_{j=1}^{L} (x_i(j) - \overline{x}(j))^2,$$ (6)

where $\overline{x}(j)$ is the averaged cycle in the analysis window.

It is worth noting that formula (6) contains $\overline{x}(j)$ defined by (2) and (3), thus the use an iterative determination of these values could improve the estimation. Generalization of this approach may lead to presented below Weighted Averaging method based on

Criterion Function Minimization (WACFM) (Leski, 2002). Another method described below is Weighted Averaging method based on Partition of input data set in time domain and using criterion function Minimization (WAPM) (Momot et al, 2007b) and generalization of the method (Momot, 2008a).

2.1.1 Weighted averaging method based on criterion function minimization

The main idea of the Weighted Averaging method based on Criterion Function Minimization (WACFM) (Leski, 2002) is minimization the following scalar criterion function:

$$I_m(\boldsymbol{w}, \overline{\boldsymbol{x}}) = \sum_{i=1}^{N} w_i^m \rho(\boldsymbol{x}_i - \overline{\boldsymbol{x}}), \tag{7}$$

where $m \in (1, \infty)$ is a weighting exponent parameter and $\rho(\cdot)$ is a measure of dissimilarity for vector arguments, i.e. $\boldsymbol{x}_i = [x_i(1), x_i(2), \dots, x_i(L)]^T$, and $\overline{\boldsymbol{x}} = [\overline{x}(1), \overline{x}(2), \dots, \overline{x}(L)]^T$. The measure of dissimilarity could be for example the quadratic function $\rho(\boldsymbol{t}) = \|\boldsymbol{t}\|^2 = \boldsymbol{t}^T \boldsymbol{t}$ and then the formula (7) can be expressed as:

$$I_m(\boldsymbol{w}, \overline{\boldsymbol{x}}) = \sum_{i=1}^{N} \left(w_i^m \sum_{j=1}^{L} (x_i(j) - \overline{x}(j))^2 \right). \tag{8}$$

Minimization the criterion function with respect to the weights vector $\boldsymbol{w} = [w_1, w_2, \dots, w_N]^T$ yields:

$$w_i = \frac{\rho(\boldsymbol{x}_i - \overline{\boldsymbol{x}})^{1/(1-m)}}{\sum_{k=1}^{N} \rho(\boldsymbol{x}_k - \overline{\boldsymbol{x}})^{1/(1-m)}} \quad i \in \{1, 2, \dots, N\}, \tag{9}$$

and for the quadratic function ρ it can be expressed as:

$$w_i = \frac{\left(\sum_{j=1}^{L} (x_i(j) - \overline{x}(j))^2 \right)^{1/(1-m)}}{\sum_{k=1}^{N} \left(\sum_{j=1}^{L} (x_k(j) - \overline{x}(j))^2 \right)^{1/(1-m)}}. \tag{10}$$

It is worth noting that for the parameter $m = 2$ this formula is equivalent to the formula (3) with variance estimated by the formula (6). However, the obtained for the quadratic function ρ averaged signal is given by:

$$\overline{\boldsymbol{x}} = \frac{\sum_{i=1}^{N} (w_i)^m \boldsymbol{x}_i}{\sum_{i=1}^{N} (w_i)^m}, \tag{11}$$

which is not exactly equivalent to the formula (2).

The optimal solution for minimization (7) with respect to $\boldsymbol{w}$ and $\overline{\boldsymbol{x}}$ is a fixed point of (10) and (11) and it could be obtained from the Picard iteration. Therefore the algorithm can be described as follows, where ε is a preset parameter.

1. Fix $m \in (0, \infty)$. Initialize $\bar{x}^{(0)}$ as the arithmetically averaged signal. Set the iteration index $k = 1$.

2. Calculate $w^{(k)}$ for the kth iteration using the formula (10).

3. Update the averaged signal for the kth iteration $\bar{x}^{(k)}$ using the formula (11) and $w^{(k)}$.

4. If $\| w^{(k-1)} - w^{(k)} \| > \varepsilon$ then $i \leftarrow i + 1$ and go to 2.

It is suggested to set parameter $m = 2$, because if parameter m tends to one, then the trivial solution is obtained where only one weight is equal to one and for large m the weights are similar to each other, like in arithmetic averaging (Leski, 2002).

2.1.2 Weighted averaging method based on partition of input data set

Below it is described the Weighted Averaging method based on Partition of input data set in time domain and using criterion function Minimization (WAPM) (Momot et al, 2007b) and generalization of the method (Momot, 2008a). The main idea of the WAPM is minimization the following scalar criterion function:

$$I(w_1, w_2) = \left\| x^1 w_1 - x^2 w_2 \right\|^2 = (x^1 w_1 - x^2 w_2)^T (x^1 w_1 - x^2 w_2), \qquad (12)$$

where the input set $x = [x_1, x_2, \ldots, x_N]$ $(x_i = [x_i(1), x_i(2), \ldots, x_i(L)]^T)$ is divided into two disjoint subsets x^1 and x^2 and w_1 and w_2 are the weights vectors, respectively.
Taking into account the constraints $w_1^T 1 = 1$ and $w_2^T 1 = 1$, which mean that sum of weights for each vector is equal to one, minimization (12) with respect to the weights vectors yields:

$$w_1 = \left((x^1)^T x^1\right)^{-1} (x^1)^T x^2 w_2 + \frac{1 - 1^T \left((x^1)^T x^1\right)^{-1} (x^1)^T x^2 w_2}{1^T \left((x^1)^T x^1\right)^{-1} 1} \left((x^1)^T x^1\right)^{-1} 1 \qquad (13)$$

and

$$w_2 = \left((x^2)^T x^2\right)^{-1} (x^2)^T x^1 w_1 + \frac{1 - 1^T \left((x^2)^T x^2\right)^{-1} (x^2)^T x^1 w_1}{1^T \left((x^2)^T x^2\right)^{-1} 1} \left((x^2)^T x^2\right)^{-1} 1. \qquad (14)$$

The optimal solution for minimization (12) with respect to w_1 and w_2 is a fixed point of (13) and (14) and it could be obtained from the Picard iteration, which leads to the averaged signal given by:

$$\bar{x} = \frac{N_1 x^1 w_1 + N_2 x^2 w_2}{N}, \qquad (15)$$

where N_1 and N_2 are the cardinalities of the two disjoint subsets x^1 and x^2, i.e. $N_1 + N_2 = N$. Although described above method involves partitioning of input set into two disjoint subsets, it can be generalized by increasing the number of disjoint subsets (Momot, 2008a). The generalized WAPM algorithm can be described as follows, where ε is a preset parameter.

1. Determine partition of input set x into disjoint subsets x^c with cardinalities N_c, where $c \in \{1, 2, \ldots, C\}$, $N_1 + N_2 + \ldots + N_C = N$ and $C \geq 2$. Calculate the following values, which remain constant during the whole iteration procedure:

$$
\begin{aligned}
X_{1,1}^{-1} &= \left((x^1)^T x^1\right)^{-1}, \\
X_{2,2}^{-1} &= \left((x^2)^T x^2\right)^{-1}, \\
&\cdots \\
X_{C,C}^{-1} &= \left((x^C)^T x^C\right)^{-1}, \\
X_{1,C} &= (x^1)^T x^C, \\
X_{2,1} &= (x^2)^T x^1, \\
&\cdots \\
X_{C,C-1} &= (x^C)^T x^{C-1}.
\end{aligned}
\tag{16}
$$

Initialize weights $w_C^{(0)}$ as in the case of arithmetical averaging (all the same and equal to N_C^{-1}). Set the iteration index $k = 1$.

2. Calculate $w_1^{(k)}$ for the kth iteration using

$$
w_1^{(k)} = X_{1,1}^{-1} X_{1,C} w_C^{(k-1)} + \frac{1 - 1^T X_{1,1}^{-1} X_{1,C} w_C^{(k-1)}}{1^T X_{1,1}^{-1} 1} X_{1,1}^{-1} 1.
\tag{17}
$$

3. Calculate $w_c^{(k)}$ for the kth iteration using

$$
w_c^{(k)} = X_{c,c}^{-1} X_{c,c-1} w_{c-1}^{(k)} + \frac{1 - 1^T X_{c,c}^{-1} X_{c,c-1} w_{c-1}^{(k)}}{1^T X_{c,c}^{-1} 1} X_{c,c}^{-1} 1,
\tag{18}
$$

for $c \in \{2, \ldots, C\}$.

4. If $\sum_{c=1}^{C} \| w_c^{(k-1)} - w_c^{(k)} \| > \varepsilon$ then $k \leftarrow k + 1$ and go to 2.

5. Calculate averaged signal

$$
\bar{x} = \frac{1}{N} \sum_{c=1}^{C} N_c x^c w_c.
\tag{19}
$$

It is suggested to use this method with equal in number of elements subsets and interlaced partitioning, i.e. to divide the input set into subsets with cardinalities equal N/C, where each of the subset indexes was equal to one plus remainder in division cycle index by C ($x^c = \{x_c, x_{c+C}, x_{c+2C}, \ldots, x_{c+N-C}\}$ for $c = 1, 2, \ldots, C$), to obtain the best performance (Momot, 2008a).

2.2 Methods based on statistical inference

Below there are presented weighted averaging methods, which incorporate Bayesian inference and the expectation-maximization technique: the Empirical Bayesian Weighted Averaging algorithm (EBWA) (Momot et al., 2007a) and the Empirical Bayesian Weighted Averaging using Cauchy distribution algorithm (EBWA.C) (Momot, 2008b). There is also presented the Simplified Empirical Bayesian Weighted Averaging algorithm (SEBWA) using method of moments to estimate the unknown parameters of signal and noise distributions (Momot, 2009b).

All the Bayesian methods are based on the assumption that the random noise $n_i(j)$, which appears in signal cycle $x_i(j)$ (see formula (1)), is zero-mean Gaussian with variance for the ith cycle σ_i^2 and the second component of the sum, i.e. the useful signal $s = [s(1), s(2), \ldots, s(L)]$, has also Gaussian distribution with zero mean and covariance matrix $B = \mathrm{diag}(\eta_1^2, \eta_2^2, \ldots, \eta_N^2)$. The zero-mean assumption for the useful signal expresses no prior knowledge about the real distance from the signal to the baseline.

From the Bayes rule it could be calculated the posterior distribution over the useful signal and the noise variance, which is proportional to

$$
p(s, \alpha | x, \beta) \propto \prod_{i=1}^{N} \alpha_i^{\frac{L}{2}} \exp\left(-\frac{1}{2} \sum_{i=1}^{N} \sum_{j=1}^{L} (x_i(j) - s(j))^2 \alpha_i \right)
$$
$$
\prod_{j=1}^{L} \beta_j^{\frac{1}{2}} \exp\left(-\frac{1}{2} \sum_{j=1}^{L} (s(j))^2 \beta_j \right),
\tag{20}
$$

where $\alpha_i = \sigma_i^{-2}$ and $\beta_j = \eta_j^{-2}$.

The main idea of the Bayesian method is to maximize this posterior distribution. The values s and α, which maximize it, can be calculated by setting the derivative of the logarithm of the posterior distribution to zero with respect to α_i and with respect to $s(j)$ respectively. The values can be expressed as:

$$
\alpha_i = \frac{L}{\sum\limits_{j=1}^{L} (x_i(j) - s(j))^2}, \quad i \in \{1, 2, \ldots, N\},
\tag{21}
$$

and

$$
s(j) = \frac{\sum\limits_{i=1}^{N} \alpha_i x_i(j)}{\beta_j + \sum\limits_{i=1}^{N} \alpha_i}, \quad j \in \{1, 2, \ldots, L\}.
\tag{22}
$$

Unfortunately it is impossible to measure β_j directly and the following methods estimate these values in different ways.

2.2.1 Empirical Bayesian weighted averaging algorithm

The Empirical Bayesian Weighted Averaging algorithm (EBWA) assumes the gamma prior for β_j with scale parameter λ and shape parameter p for all $j \in \{1, 2, \ldots, L\}$ and exploits the iterative expectation-maximization technique (Momot et al., 2007a). Conditional expected value of β_j is given by:

$$
E(\beta_j | s(j)) = \frac{2p + 1}{(s(j))^2 + 2\lambda}, \quad j \in \{1, 2, \ldots, L\}.
\tag{23}
$$

Assuming that p is a positive integer, the estimate $\hat{\lambda}$ of hyperparameter λ can be calculated based on first absolute sample moment:

$$
\hat{\lambda} = \left(\frac{\Gamma(p)(2p - 1)}{(2p - 1)!!} 2^{p - \frac{3}{2}} \frac{\sum\limits_{j=1}^{L} |s(j)|}{L} \right)^2,
\tag{24}
$$

where $(2p-1)!! = 1 \cdot 3 \cdot \ldots \cdot (2p-1)$, or based on third absolute sample moment:

$$\hat{\lambda} = \left(\frac{\Gamma(p)(2p-3)}{(2p-3)!!} 2^{p-\frac{7}{2}} \frac{\sum_{j=1}^{N} |x(j)|^3}{N} \right)^{\frac{2}{3}}, \tag{25}$$

however in this case assumption that p is greater than 1 is required.

Summarizing, the Empirical Bayesian Weighted Averaging (EBWA) algorithm can be described as follows, where ε and p are preset parameters.

1. Initialize $s^{(0)} \in R^L$ as in the case of arithmetical averaging (all the same and equal to N^{-1}) and set iteration index $k = 1$.

2. Calculate the hyperparameter $\lambda^{(k)}$ using (24) in the case of EBWA.1 (or using (25) in the case of EBWA.3, but only for $p > 1$), next $\beta_j^{(k)}$ using (23) for $j \in \{1, 2, \ldots, L\}$ and $\alpha_i^{(k)}$ using (21) for $i \in \{1, 2, \ldots, N\}$.

3. Update the signal $s^{(k)}$ using (22), $\beta_j^{(k)}$ and $\alpha_i^{(k)}$.

4. If $\|s^{(k)} - s^{(k-1)}\| > \varepsilon$ then $k \leftarrow k + 1$ and go to 2, else set the averaged signal $\bar{x} = s^{(k)}$ and stop.

It is suggested to use this method with parameter $p = 1$ (hence EBWA.1), because performed numerical experiments indicate that increasing values of p usually did not improve performance of the method (Momot, 2009a).

2.2.2 Empirical Bayesian weighted averaging using Cauchy distribution algorithm

The presented above EBWA method requires assumption that certain parameter p is a positive integer. The observation that increasing values of p usually did not improve performance of the method has become the motivation to extension of the algorithm for some values of $p < 1$. It can be observed that for $p = \frac{1}{2}$, function $p(s(j)|\lambda)$ is Cauchy probability distribution function:

$$p(s(j)|\lambda) = \frac{\sqrt{2\lambda}}{\pi \left(s(j)^2 + 2\lambda \right)} \tag{26}$$

with the scale parameter equal to $\sqrt{2\lambda}$ and the location parameter equal to 0. All absolute moments of the Cauchy distribution are infinite, but the first and third quartiles are the linear functions of scale parameter:

$$Q1 = -\sqrt{2\lambda}, \qquad Q3 = \sqrt{2\lambda}. \tag{27}$$

Thus the hyperparameter λ can be estimated based on sample interquartile range:

$$\hat{\lambda} = \frac{(\hat{Q}3 - \hat{Q}1)^2}{8}. \tag{28}$$

Therefore the Empirical Bayesian Weighted Averaging using Cauchy distribution algorithm (EBWA.C) can be described as follows, where ε is a preset parameter (Momot, 2008b).

1. Initialize $s^{(0)} \in R^L$ as in the case of arithmetical averaging (all the same and equal to N^{-1}) and set iteration index $k = 1$.

2. Calculate the hyperparameter $\lambda^{(k)}$ using (28), next $\beta_j^{(k)}$ using (23) for $j \in \{1, 2, \ldots, L\}$ and $\alpha_i^{(k)}$ using (21) for $i \in \{1, 2, \ldots, N\}$.

3. Update the signal $s^{(k)}$ using (22), $\beta_j^{(k)}$ and $\alpha_i^{(k)}$.

4. If $\|s^{(k)} - s^{(k-1)}\| > \varepsilon$ then $k \leftarrow k + 1$ and go to 2, else set the averaged signal $\bar{x} = s^{(k)}$ and stop.

2.2.3 Simplified empirical Bayesian weighted averaging algorithm

Below there is presented the Simplified Empirical Bayesian Weighted Averaging algorithm (SEBWA) which does not use hierarchical probabilistic model and does not require the determination of parameter p. In this method the unknown parameters of signal and noise distributions are estimated using method of moments (Momot, 2009b).

Giving assumption as described previously, but $\beta = \eta_1^{-2} = \eta_2^{-2} = \ldots = \eta_N^{-2}$, the posterior distribution of signal (see formula 20) can be calculated from the Bayes rule explicitly as Gaussian distribution with mean vector m:

$$\forall j \in \{1, 2, \ldots, L\} \quad m(j) = \frac{\sum_{i=1}^{N} \alpha_i x_i(j)}{\beta + \sum_{i=1}^{N} \alpha_i} \tag{29}$$

and covariance matrix equal to γ^{-1} multiplied by the identity matrix of dimension L, where

$$\gamma = \beta + \sum_{i=1}^{N} \alpha_i. \tag{30}$$

Therefore the original signal s can be estimated as $\hat{m}$ using (29) and the unknown parameters α_i for $i \in \{1, 2, \ldots, M\}$ and β can be estimated using method of moments (the estimated parameters of random distribution are expressed in terms of its moments which are substituted by the corresponding sample moments). Values α_i^{-1} are noise variations in each cycle and taking into account the mean equals zero

$$\hat{\alpha}_i = \frac{L}{\sum_{j=1}^{L} (x_i(j) - s(j))^2}, \quad i \in \{1, 2, \ldots, N\}. \tag{31}$$

Value β^{-1} is variation of the original signal and taking into account the zero-mean assumption

$$\hat{\beta} = \frac{L}{\sum_{j=1}^{L} (s(j))^2}. \tag{32}$$

Therefore the Simplified Empirical Bayesian Weighted Averaging algorithm (SEBWA) can be described as follows, where ε is a preset parameter.

1. Initialize $s^{(0)} \in R^L$ as in the case of arithmetical averaging (all the same and equal to N^{-1}) and set iteration index $k = 1$.

2. Calculate $\beta^{(k)}$ using (32) and $\alpha_i^{(k)}$ using (31) for $i \in \{1, 2, \ldots, M\}$.

3. Update the signal $s^{(k)}$ using (29), $\beta^{(k)}$ and $\alpha_i^{(k)}$, assuming $s^{(k)} = m$.

4. If $\|s^{(k)} - s^{(k-1)}\| > \varepsilon$ then $k \leftarrow k + 1$ and go to 2, else set the averaged signal $\bar{x} = s^{(k)}$ and stop.

It is suggested to use this method with fuzzy partition of signal cycle (this extension is presented in the next subsection), because the numerical experiments indicate that the simplified Bayesian method gives worse results with compare to the EBWA method, however using this method with fuzzy partition gives much better results with compare to the EBWA method (even EBWA with fuzzy partition) (Momot, 2009b).

2.3 Fuzzy extensions to weighted averaging methods

This subsection presents two aspects of possible fuzzy extensions applied to weighted averaging methods: fuzzy partition of signal cycle proposed in (Momot, 2009b) and using the fuzzy numbers as coefficients of weight vector instead of classical real numbers (applied to described above WACFM method in (Momot & Momot, 2009c)).

2.3.1 Fuzzy partition of signal cycle

The algorithms of weighted averaging can be extended by partition each signal cycle of the length L. The new idea of signal partition differs from previously presented in subsection 2.1.2 that earlier the set of N cycles was divided into disjoined subsets with cardinalities N_c and now the partition concerns each cycle separately, i.e. the length of averaging window changes.

The partition may be performed by using traditional (sharp) or fuzzy membership function. When the input signal is divided into K parts:

$$x_i^k(j) = \begin{cases} x_i(j), & j \in \{(k-1)L/K + 1, \ldots, kL/K\} \\ 0, & j \in \{1, \ldots, L\} - \{(k-1)L/K + 1, \ldots, kL/K\} \end{cases} \tag{33}$$

for $k \in \{1, 2, \ldots, K\}$, this partition will be called sharp. Taking into account Gaussian membership function with location parameter equal $a^k = (k - 0.5)L/K$ (for $k \in \{1, 2, \ldots, K\}$) and scale parameter $b = 0.25L/K$, defined by:

$$\mu_{(a^k,b)}(j) = \exp\left\{-\left(\frac{j - a^k}{b}\right)^2\right\}, \quad k \in \{1, 2, \ldots, K\}, \tag{34}$$

it is possible to divide the input signal into K fuzzy parts:

$$x_i^k(j) = \frac{x_i(j) \cdot \mu_{(a^k,b)}(j)}{\sum\limits_{k=1}^{K} \mu_{(a^k,b)}(j)}, \quad k \in \{1, 2, \ldots, K\}. \tag{35}$$

In both cases i is the cycle index $i \in \{1, 2, \ldots, N\}$ and j is the sample index in the single cycle $j \in \{1, 2, \ldots, L\}$ (all cycles have the same length L). The idea of this extension is to perform K times the averaging for $k \in \{1, 2, \ldots, K\}$ input data and then sum the weighted averages.

Although the partition may be performed by using traditional (sharp) or fuzzy membership function, the numerical experiments presented in (Momot, 2011) indicate that in the case of sharp partition incorrectly chosen number of parts may result in even worse results than the one obtained for the arithmetic averaging. Therefore it is suggested to use the fuzzy partition rather than the sharp partition (especially for the signals with unknown characteristics).

2.3.2 Using fuzzy numbers as coefficients of weight vector

Another aspect of possible fuzzy extensions applied to weighted averaging methods is using the fuzzy numbers as coefficients of weight vector instead of classical real numbers. This idea was presented for described above WACFM method in (Momot & Momot, 2009c), where the coefficients were replaced with symmetrical triangular fuzzy numbers. Consequently, the weighted average was a vector containing triangular fuzzy numbers and as the necessary to compute distance, between the input signal (vector of real numbers) and the averaged signal, was taken the distance between the real number and the α-cut of the corresponding fuzzy number.

The fuzzy membership function of a symmetrical triangular fuzzy number A can be expressed as:

$$\mu_A(x) = \max\left\{1 - \frac{|x - m_A|}{r_A}, 0\right\}, \tag{36}$$

where m_A is the center point of the fuzzy number and r_A is its radius. Thus, the α-cut of the fuzzy number A ($\alpha \in [0,1]$), defined as the ordinary subset $\{x \in \mathcal{R} : \mu_A(x) \geq \alpha\}$, is given by:

$$(A)_\alpha = [m_A - r_A(1 - \alpha), m_A + r_A(1 - \alpha)]. \tag{37}$$

The distance between a real number x and the α-cut of the symmetrical triangular fuzzy number A can be written explicitly as:

$$\rho_\alpha(x, A) = \max\left\{|x - m_A| - r_A, 0\right\} \tag{38}$$

and when the arguments of distance function $\rho_\alpha(\cdot, \cdot)$ are N-dimensional vectors, the formula can be expressed as:

$$\rho_\alpha(\boldsymbol{x}, \boldsymbol{A}) = \sum_{i=1}^{N} \left(\rho_\alpha(x_i, A_i)\right)^2. \tag{39}$$

Therefore, the Fuzzy Weighted Averaging algorithm based on Criterion Function Minimization (FWACFM) can be described as follows, where ε is a preset parameter (Momot & Momot, 2009c). It is assumed that values of parameters r (the radius of all symmetrical triangular fuzzy numbers) and α (the cutting level) remain constant during all iterations.

1. Determine parameters r and α. Initialize centers of fuzzy weights $\boldsymbol{w}^{(0)}$ setting all the same values equal to N^{-1}. Set the iteration index $k = 1$.

2. Calculate vector of centers of fuzzy weights $\boldsymbol{w}^{(k)}$ as:

$$w_i^{(k)} = \left(\rho_\alpha(\boldsymbol{x}_i, \overline{\boldsymbol{x}})^{\frac{1}{1-m}}\right) \Big/ \left(\sum_{k=1}^{N} \rho_\alpha(\boldsymbol{x}_k, \overline{\boldsymbol{x}})^{\frac{1}{1-m}}\right), \tag{40}$$

for $i \in \{1, 2, \dots, N\}$.

3. Calculate the averaged signal as:

$$\bar{x}^{(k)} = \left(\sum_{i=1}^{N} (W_i^{(k)})^m x_i \right) \Big/ \left(\sum_{i=1}^{N} (W_i^{(k)})^m \right), \tag{41}$$

where $W_i^{(k)}$ is a symmetrical triangular fuzzy number with center given by (40) and radius r.

4. If $\|w^{(k-1)} - w^{(k)}\| > \varepsilon$ then $k \leftarrow k+1$ and go to 2.

5. Calculate the final averaged signal as:

$$\bar{x} = \left(\sum_{i=1}^{N} (w_i^{(k)})^m x_i \right) \Big/ \left(\sum_{i=1}^{N} (w_i^{(k)})^m \right). \tag{42}$$

It is worth noting that during the iteration process both vectors: the averaged signal and the weights are treated as vectors of fuzzy numbers. At the end of the procedure the fuzzy averaged signal is defuzzified.

This algorithm is generalization of the original WACFM method because for radius equal zero both methods are equivalent. The numeric experiments presented in (Momot & Momot, 2009c) indicate that for some positive values of radius parameter such generalization of WACFM method can outperforms the original method. However, further research for method of automatic determinating this parameter is needed because even small increasing its value could rapidly increase the root mean square error.

Summarizing, taking into account higher computational complexity the Fuzzy WACFM algorithm than the original algorithm and difficulties in proper choosing the parameters r and α, usefulness of this method is rather limited. Therefore, the Fuzzy WACFM algorithm can be treated as an interesting theoretical study of the problem of using the fuzzy numbers as coefficients of weight vector instead of classical real numbers.

2.4 Adaptation of weighted averaging methods to 2D images

In the case of linear spatial filtering the response of the filter is given by a sum of products of the filter coefficients and the corresponding image pixels in the area spanned by the filter mask. For arithmetic mean filtering all the coefficients are the same and sum up to one. Mean filtering is often used to reduce noise in images due to its simplicity. It is an efficient method for reducing the amount of intensity variation between one pixel and the next. Mean filtering minimizes the influence of pixel values which are unrepresentative of their surroundings.

Like the mean filter, the median filter considers each pixel in the image, looking at its nearby neighbors, to decide whether or not it is representative of its surroundings. It replaces the pixel value with the median of neighboring pixel values instead of replacing it with the mean of those values. Mean filtering is special case of weighted averaging filtering where the filter mask coefficients are nonnegative and sum up to one (often the pixel at the center of the mask is multiplied by a higher value than any other, thus giving this pixel more importance in the calculation of the average). In this context, median filtering can be treated as an adaptive weighted averaging filtering. For median filtering the mask coefficients are not always constant, there is only one non-zero coefficient (equal one) and which coefficient is non-zero depends on result of the sorting operation.

When the mask coefficients are not constant there is a need of procedure how to compute the coefficients. Below there is presented a method for computing the values of the mask coefficient based on the described above weighted averaging method created originally for noise reduction in biomedical signal. The technique of adaptation of weighted averaging methods to digital filtering 2D images was introduced in (Momot, 2010) where the author used the Simplified Empirical Bayesian Weighted Averaging algorithm (SEBWA), which is described above in 2.2.3.

Given the radius R of the square mask and the input image f of $X \times Y$ dimension, the output image g dimension is $(X - 2R) \times (Y - 2R)$. For each pixel $f(x,y)$, i.e. $x \in \{R + 1, R + 2, \ldots, X - R\}$ and $y \in \{R + 1, R + 2, \ldots, Y - R\}$, there is computed sum based on the neighborhood of the pixel which determines the pixels $g(x,y)$ of the output image:

$$g(x,y) = \sum_{r=-R}^{R} \sum_{s=-R}^{R} w_{rs}\, f(x+r,y+s). \tag{43}$$

Each value $g(x,y)$ could be calculated by one of the described above iterative algorithms. In the case of SEBWA method the algorithm is given by following procedure:

1. Initialize $g(x,y)^{(0)}$ as the arithmetic average:

$$g(x,y)^{(0)} = \frac{1}{(2R+1)^2} \sum_{r=-R}^{R} \sum_{s=-R}^{R} f(x+r,y+s). \tag{44}$$

   If the sample variance of the neighborhood of the pixel:

$$\sigma^2(x,y) = \frac{1}{(2R+1)^2} \sum_{r=-R}^{R} \sum_{s=-R}^{R} \left(f(x+r,y+s) - g(x,y)^{(0)} \right)^2 \tag{45}$$

   is greater than zero, set the iteration index $k = 1$ else stop.

2. Calculate the hyperparameter $\alpha_{rs}^{(k)}$ as:

$$\alpha_{rs}^{(k)} = \left(f(x+r,y+s) - g(x,y)^{(k-1)} \right)^{-2}, \quad r,s \in \{1,2,\ldots,R\} \tag{46}$$

   and $\beta^{(k)}$ according to the formula:

$$\beta^{(k)} = \left(g(x,y)^{(k-1)} \right)^{-2}. \tag{47}$$

3. Update the average $g(x,y)^{(k)}$ for kth iteration as:

$$g(x,y)^{(k)} = \frac{\displaystyle\sum_{r=-R}^{R} \sum_{s=-R}^{R} \alpha_{rs}^{(k)} f(x+r,y+s)}{\beta^{(k)} + \displaystyle\sum_{r=-R}^{R} \sum_{s=-R}^{R} \alpha_{rs}^{(k)}}. \tag{48}$$

4. If $\left(g(x,y)^{(k)} - g(x,y)^{(k-1)} \right)^2 > \epsilon$ then $k \leftarrow k+1$ and go to 2, else stop.

The algorithm assumes that the values $f(x,y)$ are in interval $[0,1]$. Thus parameter $\beta^{(k)}$ is always positive, although for some values r and s the parameter $\alpha_{rs}^{(k)}$ could be undefined because of dividing by zero (the pixel represented by $(x+r, y+s)$ is equal the average $g(x,y)^{(k-1)}$ in kth iteration). In such case the parameter $\alpha_{r's'}^{(k)}$ should be set to a value significantly greater than other parameters $\alpha_{rs}^{(k)}$.

Numerical experiments presented in (Momot, 2010) evaluate this method with comparison to traditional arithmetic average filtering (mean filtering) and median filtering for synthetic and real images in presence of salt-and-pepper and Gaussian noise. Analyzing results of these methods in the case of salt-and-pepper noise (appearing as white and black dots superimposed on an image), it can be stated that using the new method gives results the same or slightly worse than the median filter. The mean filter for such type of noise gives poor results as expected, but the good results of the new method which originates from mean filtering is worth emphasizing. In the case of Gaussian noise analysis of the results shows that the best results are obtained for mean filtering as expected but the results for the new method are only slightly worse (median filter for such type of noise gives the worst results as expected).

Because in reality noise is often characterized by mixture of these two types, the hypothesis that the new method will give the best results in such cases was suggested. Nevertheless the conducted so far numerical experiments do not confirm such hypothesis and taking into account high computational complexity of this method its usefulness seems to be rather limited. Therefore, similarly as in the case of described above the Fuzzy WACFM algorithm in subsection 2.3.2, this method could be treated as an interesting theoretical study of the adaptation of weighted averaging methods to 2D images.

3. Numerical experiments

In this section there is presented performance of the described above methods. In all experiments, using weighted averaging, calculations were initialized as the means of disturbed signal cycles and the parameter ε was equal to 10^{-6}. For the computed averaged signal the performance of tested methods was evaluated by the root mean-square error (RMSE) between the deterministic component and the averaged signal. The maximal absolute difference between the deterministic component and the averaged signal (MAX) was also computed.

The simulated signal cycles were obtained as the same deterministic component with added independent realizations of random noise. As the deterministic component was taken ECG signal ANE20000, analytical signal compliant with the European Standard EN 60601-2-51 (2003). It is the standardized analytical ECG signal from the CTS database (Zywietz et al., 2001), designed to reproduce the typical ECG waveform with 60 bpm (beats per minute) heart rate.

This section contains results of several numerical experiments, which show the differences among the weighted averaging methods and the possibility of their applications. First subsection presents the influence of the number of cycles to be averaged on the results of the averaging procedure, next shows the impact of changes in the amplitude and type of noise on the performance of the investigated methods and last subsection describes results obtained when the fuzzy and sharp partition of the ECG signal is applied.

3.1 Influence of the averaged cycles number on the results of the averaging procedure

A series N of ECG cycles was generated with the same deterministic component and zero-mean white Gaussian noise with different standard deviations or real muscle noise with different amplitude. The amplitude of noise was constant during each cycle. The parameter N was equal 20, 40, 60, 80 or 100. For the first, second, third and fourth $N/4$ cycles, the noise standard deviations were respectively 0.1s, 0.5s, 1s, 2s, where s is the sample standard deviation of the deterministic component. Figure 1 presents the signal to be averaged for $N = 60$. The amplitude of the signal is expressed in μV and the length of the deterministic signal L is equal 1000.

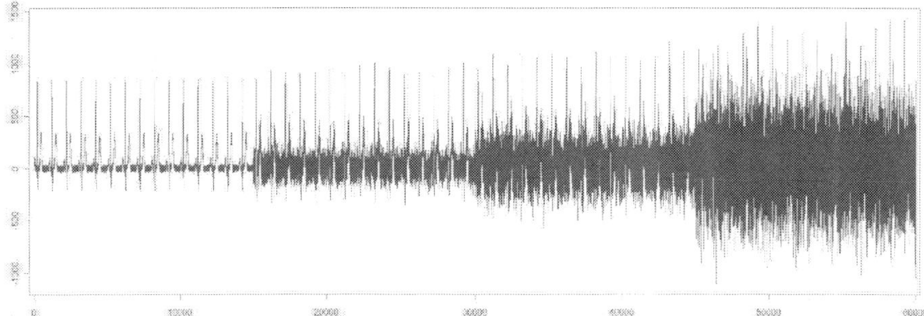

Fig. 1. ANE20000 with added Gaussian noise.

Table 1 presents the results of averaging 20 cycles obtained as the root mean-square error ($RMSE$) between the deterministic component and the averaged signal. The maximal absolute difference between the deterministic component and the averaged signal (MAX) is also shown in the table. The lower index G characterizes the results obtained for the Gaussian noise and the M indicates the muscle noise.

Method	$RMSE_G$	MAX_G	$RMSE_M$	MAX_M
AA	36.58372	107.12475	29.13075	91.23949
WACFM	13.76586	43.15516	17.73509	66.74813
WAPM.2	6.215809	23.274264	8.224947	27.706856
WAPM.3	6.472495	24.816161	7.955619	23.171022
WAPM.4	6.399116	22.656614	8.112725	23.318876
SEBWA	6.138603	22.835092	7.672932	24.281101
EBWA.1	6.084599	23.163887	7.542227	24.861945
EBWA.C	5.933567	23.092718	7.167177	24.713475

Table 1. Results for averaging 20 cycles.

The evaluated methods are described by following abbreviations:

AA – the traditional Arithmetic Averaging;

WACFM – the Weighted Averaging method based on Criterion Function Minimization (the required parameter m is set to 2, it is the value suggested by author of the method in (Leski, 2002));

WAPM – the Weighted Averaging method based on Partition of input data set in time domain and using criterion function Minimization (number after dot describes number of disjoint subsets of input data set);

SEBWA – the Simplified Empirical Bayesian Weighted Averaging method;

EBWA.1 – the Empirical Bayesian Weighted Averaging method with hyperparameter λ calculated based on first absolute sample moment (the required parameter p is set to 1, it is the value suggested by author of the method in (Momot, 2009a));

EBWA.C – the Empirical Bayesian Weighted Averaging method using Cauchy distribution.

The results presented in table 1 show that all the weighted averaging methods give the similar values of $RMSE$ or MAX except the WACFM method which gives the more than twice as worse results, although better than one obtained using traditional arithmetic averaging (AA). The best method in this case seems to be the EBWA.C and this applies to both Gaussian and muscle noise.

Method	$RMSE_G$	MAX_G	$RMSE_M$	MAX_M
AA	25.48282	90.57738	18.04031	53.39217
WACFM	4.459371	14.307712	12.65819	43.43847
WAPM.2	4.364517	14.906725	5.530065	18.993917
WAPM.3	4.347873	14.549218	4.775429	16.448935
WAPM.4	4.324780	14.256036	5.176974	16.936097
SEBWA	4.260886	14.473659	4.688686	14.488379
EBWA.1	4.228607	14.336413	4.646224	14.305369
EBWA.C	4.153096	13.956814	4.541089	13.865779

Table 2. Results for averaging 40 cycles.

The results of averaging 40 cycles contained in table 2 show that in the case of Gaussian noise all the weighted averaging methods give the similar values of $RMSE$ or MAX. Although in the case of muscle noise the WACFM method once again gives the more than twice as worse results, although still better than one obtained using traditional arithmetic averaging (AA). The best method in this case seems to be the EBWA.C and this applies to both Gaussian and muscle noise.

Method	$RMSE_G$	MAX_G	$RMSE_M$	MAX_M
AA	20.35780	71.61070	15.71738	48.69969
WACFM	3.825289	12.139730	12.44298	54.07430
WAPM.2	3.729522	12.222603	4.967362	14.089614
WAPM.3	3.684434	12.966805	4.198599	16.084199
WAPM.4	3.723764	12.982499	4.357827	15.039165
SEBWA	3.634302	12.292184	4.198425	16.198985
EBWA.1	3.61344	12.20644	4.168981	15.990323
EBWA.C	3.569731	11.982379	4.102664	15.675835

Table 3. Results for averaging 60 cycles.

The results of averaging 60 cycles contained in table 3 show that all the weighted averaging methods give the similar values of $RMSE$ or MAX both Gaussian and muscle noise (except of the WACFM method). Although the best method in this case seems to be the EBWA.C. As expected the results indicate that increasing number of cycles to be averaged decreasing the root mean square errors as well as the maximal absolute difference.

Method	$RMSE_G$	MAX_G	$RMSE_M$	MAX_M
AA	18.37609	77.90424	14.24187	47.40299
WACFM	3.281969	9.794294	4.030636	12.747331
WAPM.2	3.276318	10.421047	4.218003	12.839638
WAPM.3	3.232206	9.746258	3.691453	11.585205
WAPM.4	3.261982	9.962358	3.80167	10.47284
SEBWA	3.186362	9.657737	3.479337	11.553013
EBWA.1	3.177097	9.607379	3.460802	11.482392
EBWA.C	3.151826	9.463573	3.424195	11.293873

Table 4. Results for averaging 80 cycles.

The results of averaging 80 cycles contained in table 4 are similar to the ones in the table 3 (the 60 cycles averaging procedure). For Gaussian and muscle noise all the weighted averaging methods give the similar values of $RMSE$ or MAX and the slightly better method seems to be the EBWA.C. The same pattern can be observed in table 5 contained the results of averaging 100 cycles.

Method	$RMSE_G$	MAX_G	$RMSE_M$	MAX_M
AA	16.38897	57.06793	13.50228	39.93048
WACFM	2.829289	8.738847	3.726777	11.334553
WAPM.2	2.892244	8.895864	4.02018	12.07286
WAPM.3	2.806800	9.118727	3.561343	10.197009
WAPM.4	2.775190	8.569817	3.638291	11.357989
SEBWA	2.729694	8.378217	3.207977	9.226357
EBWA.1	2.721339	8.511705	3.193742	9.175142
EBWA.C	2.700835	8.544868	3.164265	9.031031

Table 5. Results for averaging 100 cycles.

The obtained results (tables 1 - 5), which can be compared because of the same the noise characteristics in all conducted experiments, indicate that increasing number of cycles to be averaged N decreases the root mean square errors as well as the maximal absolute difference. Thus it seems to be obvious that the better results will be obtained when the N is larger. Although in real application this conclusion may not be held because of problem of time alignment which is critical in the analysis of repetitive signals. Attempt of improvement of signal quality by increasing number of cycles to be averaged increases also the risk of misalignment caused by both noise and signal nonstationarity.

3.2 Influence of noise amplitude changes on the results of the averaging procedure

In the previous subsection the noise amplitude changes between the cycles (constant during each cycle) were described by the following function, where N is the number of cycles to be averaged:

$$A_0(i) = \begin{cases} 0.1, & i \in \{1,\ldots,N/4\} \\ 0.5, & i \in \{N/4+1,\ldots,N/2\} \\ 1, & i \in \{N/2+1,\ldots,3N/4\} \\ 2, & i \in \{3N/4+1,\ldots,N\} \end{cases} \tag{49}$$

multiplied by s, the sample standard deviation of the deterministic component. Now by changing the function A_0, which determines the noise amplitude changes within each cycle, the influence of noise level on the results of the averaging procedure is investigated. The number of cycles to be averaged is constant in the next experiments and equal 60.

Figure 2 presents the cycles of the signal with added nonstationary Gaussian noise. The noise amplitude is described by following function:

$$A_1(i) = \begin{cases} 0.1, & i \in \{1,\ldots,6\} \\ 0.1 + (i-6)/18, & i \in \{7,\ldots,42\} \\ 2, & i \in \{43,\ldots,54\} \\ (61-i)/3, & i \in \{55,\ldots,60\}. \end{cases} \tag{50}$$

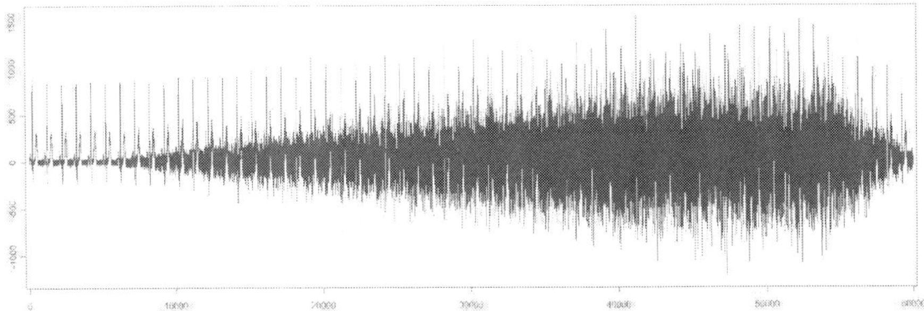

Fig. 2. ECG signal to be averaged with the noise amplitude described by function $A_1(\cdot)$.

Table 6 presents the results of averaging 60 cycles obtained as $RMSE$ (the root mean-square error between the deterministic component and the averaged signal) and MAX (the maximal absolute difference between the deterministic component and the averaged signal). Used abbreviations are the same as in the previous subsections. Comparing the results to the ones presented in table 3, it can be seen that despite the same range of noise amplitude level (from 0.1 to 2), now the results are worse in both cases: Gaussian and muscle noise. All the weighted averaging methods give the similar values of $RMSE$ or MAX except the WACFM method which gives the more than twice as worse results, although better than one obtained using traditional arithmetic averaging (AA). It is worth noting that the WACFM method in the case of rapidly changing the noise amplitude showed numerical instability.

Method	$RMSE_G$	MAX_G	$RMSE_M$	MAX_M
AA	26.64724	77.79896	19.75347	60.37421
WACFM	14.24589	49.80394	17.84805	80.87108
WAPM.2	5.443441	17.119353	8.052216	26.413713
WAPM.3	5.407122	16.690267	6.933108	20.198006
WAPM.4	5.391607	16.598576	7.314647	27.541761
SEBWA	5.338154	16.257010	6.849912	25.334237
EBWA.1	5.304617	16.036901	6.745417	25.654471
EBWA.C	5.190697	16.181674	6.506906	25.451207

Table 6. Results in the case of the noise amplitude described by function $A_1(\cdot)$.

All the presented above results show that all the weighted averaging methods give usually the similar values of $RMSE$ or MAX, the methods based on statistical inference are slightly better than the methods based on criterion function minimization and the EBWA.C method seems to be the best. The next experiment show that this conclusion may not be held. Figure 3 presents the cycles of the signal with added nonstationary Gaussian noise to be averaged where the noise amplitude is described by following function:

$$A_2(i) = \begin{cases} i/12, & i \in \{1,\dots,24\} \\ 2, & i \in \{25,\dots,36\} \\ (61-i)/12, & i \in \{37,\dots,60\}. \end{cases} \tag{51}$$

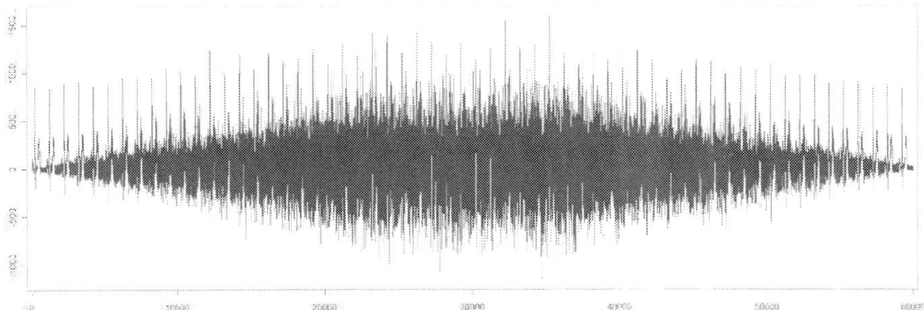

Fig. 3. ECG signal to be averaged with the noise amplitude described by function $A_2(\cdot)$.

Table 7 presents the results of averaging procedure and it can be seen that in this case the best seems to be the WAPM methods, especially WAPM.2 where the input set is divided into two disjoint subsets. In the case of Gaussian noise this method gives the best results both for $RMSE$ and MAX. In the case of real muscle noise this method gives the best result only for MAX and minimal $RMSE$ is obtained for WAPM.3.

Method	$RMSE_G$	MAX_G	$RMSE_M$	MAX_M
AA	24.95884	86.02304	22.18302	63.14914
WACFM	12.12508	47.95216	8.338565	51.949784
WAPM.2	6.97295	23.53681	7.664572	24.181065
WAPM.3	7.129491	25.233519	7.443705	30.669492
WAPM.4	7.566451	26.480298	7.986691	26.380763
SEBWA	12.12508	47.95216	8.338565	51.949784
EBWA.1	12.12508	47.95216	8.338565	51.949784
EBWA.C	12.12508	47.95216	8.338565	51.949784

Table 7. Results in the case of the noise amplitude described by function $A_2(\cdot)$.

Another interesting fact is equal results for WACFM and all the methods based on Bayesian inference caused the possibility of only one non-zero weight. In this case the methods find the least disturbed cycle and set the corresponding weight equal to 1. In the case of WAPM method the least number of non-zero weights is equal to the number of disjoined subsets. Here this property proved to be effective.

In the next experiment the cycles of the signal are contaminated by added nonstationary Gaussian noise with the amplitude described by following function:

$$A_3(i) = \begin{cases} (25-i)/12, & i \in \{1,\dots,24\} \\ 1/12, & i \in \{25,\dots,30\} \\ (i-30)/15, & i \in \{31,\dots,60\}. \end{cases} \tag{52}$$

Figure 4 presents the cycles of the signal and table 8 shows the results of averaging procedure in this case. Like previously all the weighted averaging methods give the similar values of $RMSE$ or MAX (except the WACFM method), the methods based on statistical inference are slightly better than the methods based on criterion function minimization and the EBWA.C method seems to be the best.

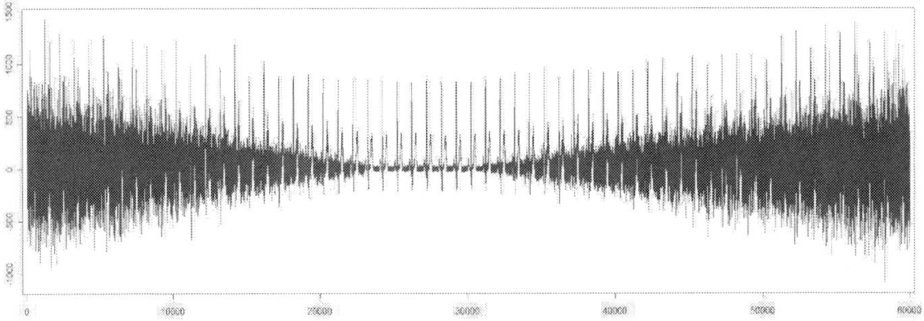

Fig. 4. ECG signal to be averaged with the noise amplitude described by function $A_3(\cdot)$.

Method	$RMSE_G$	MAX_G	$RMSE_M$	MAX_M
AA	22.18602	75.84577	20.08812	69.75064
WACFM	6.70973	21.06666	9.59511	30.20457
WAPM.2	3.530179	12.508598	3.84337	12.16353
WAPM.3	3.939755	12.860902	3.828325	12.001807
WAPM.4	3.393327	12.382687	3.773901	11.322390
SEBWA	3.048759	13.518930	3.747146	10.741282
EBWA.1	3.024732	13.315327	3.729486	10.967476
EBWA.C	2.993796	13.191613	3.686413	11.094574

Table 8. Results in the case of the noise amplitude described by function $A_3(\cdot)$.

The last experiment study the results with presence of noise with amplitude characteristics described by:

$$A_4(i) = i/30, \quad i \in \{1,\dots,60\}. \tag{53}$$

The signal to be averaged is presented in figure 5 and table 9 shows the results of averaging procedure. In this case the best seems to be the WAPM.2 method. All the weighted averaging methods give the similar values of $RMSE$ or MAX and equals for WACFM and all the methods based on Bayesian inference caused finding the least disturbed cycle and set the corresponding weight equal to 1.

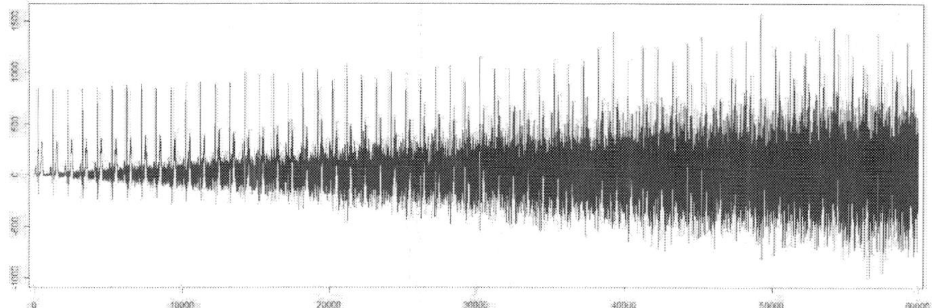

Fig. 5. ECG signal to be averaged with the noise amplitude described by function $A_4(\cdot)$.

Method	$RMSE_G$	MAX_G	$RMSE_M$	MAX_M
AA	22.19804	80.13893	16.19718	51.03785
WACFM	4.563198	15.679271	8.915569	28.417666
WAPM.2	4.220262	12.790181	6.802766	17.392957
WAPM.3	4.942776	17.736005	6.660585	23.792032
WAPM.4	5.453174	20.018136	7.315934	21.823084
SEBWA	4.563198	15.679271	8.915569	28.417666
EBWA.1	4.563198	15.679271	8.915569	28.417666
EBWA.C	4.563198	15.679271	8.915569	28.417666

Table 9. Results in the case of the noise amplitude described by function $A_4(\cdot)$.

3.3 Influence of the partition of the signal on the results of the averaging procedure

Below there are presented results of numerical experiments which investigate how partition of the input signal affects the results of the averaging procedure. In the experiments it is studies both sharp and fuzzy partitions described in subsection 2.3.1 and because of numerical instability of WACFM algorithm the method is omitted. The number of parts K is in $\{2, 3, 4, 5\}$ and for $K = 1$ the original method is used. Similarly to the previous subsection the number of cycles to be averaged is constant in the next experiments and equal 60.

First experiment studies influence of the partition on the root mean square error in the case presented in figure 1, where the signal is disturbed by zero-mean Gaussian noise with constant amplitude of noise during each cycle. For the first, second, third and fourth 15 cycles, the noise standard deviations were respectively 0.1, 0.5, 1, 2, multiplied by s, i.e. the sample standard deviation of the deterministic component. Results presented in table 3 show the RMSE equal 20.35780 in the case of the traditional arithmetic averaging method and the RMSE of the weighted averaging methods range from 3.569731 (EBWA.C) to 3.825289 (WACFM). This time the results are slightly different because of randomness of the noise and the RMSE for the traditional arithmetic averaging method is equal 22.09798. Detailed results for the weighted averaging methods are presented in table 10.

The root mean square errors presented in table 10 are computed in both type of partitions: sharp and fuzzy, with taking into consideration varying number of parts K. Obviously for $K = 1$ the results obtained for sharp and fuzzy partitions are equal (the signal in the single cycle is not divided). Analyzing the results presented in table 10 it is easy to conclude that without the partition all method gives similar RMSE although the methods based on Bayesian inference (SEBWA, EBWA.1, EBWA.C) are slightly better. The partition in the case of methods based on criterion function minimization (WAPM.2, WAPM.3, WAPM.4) results in deterioration of the RMSE (the same pattern may be seen for the WACFM method although the numerical instability of the algorithm makes it difficult and it is the reason that the results are not presented).

Method	type	$K=1$	$K=2$	$K=3$	$K=4$	$K=5$
WAPM.2	sharp	3.671434	3.735696	3.830139	3.981567	4.08268
	fuzzy		3.733926	3.808319	3.934622	4.046011
WAPM.3	sharp	3.588868	3.735696	3.830139	3.981567	4.08268
	fuzzy		3.733926	3.808319	3.934622	4.046011
WAPM.4	sharp	3.603876	3.624834	3.67803	3.706631	3.766816
	fuzzy		3.627341	3.665056	3.681049	3.757504
SEBWA	sharp	3.563763	3.570995	2.943464	3.112997	2.762172
	fuzzy		3.574001	2.884799	3.084993	2.777102
EBWA.1	sharp	3.547627	3.437116	3.022750	3.185023	3.024058
	fuzzy		3.478558	2.967808	3.166432	3.039432
EBWA.C	sharp	3.50404	2.823939	3.184680	3.562267	3.363044
	fuzzy		2.955845	3.110675	3.242250	3.655863

Table 10. RMSE for zero-mean Gaussian noise with amplitude described by function $A_0(\cdot)$.

Next experiment studies influence of the partition on the root mean square error in the case presented in figure 3, where the cycles of the signal were disturbed by nonstationary Gaussian noise with the noise amplitude described by function $A_2(\cdot)$. It is interesting case because here the best seems to be the WAPM method and using the Bayesian methods results in the same value of RMSE. In this experiment the RMSE for the traditional arithmetic averaging method is equal 25.25697 and detailed results for the weighted averaging methods are presented in table 11.

Method	type	$K=1$	$K=2$	$K=3$	$K=4$	$K=5$
WAPM.2	sharp	6.581978	6.878741	7.114349	7.615843	7.950328
	fuzzy		6.842354	7.083266	7.499244	7.751919
WAPM.3	sharp	6.913927	6.878741	7.114349	7.615843	7.950328
	fuzzy		6.842354	7.083266	7.499244	7.751919
WAPM.4	sharp	7.348039	7.425919	7.52601	7.751074	7.85626
	fuzzy		7.411294	7.532835	7.740782	7.784718
SEBWA	sharp	11.50770	11.66183	9.444625	10.08938	9.07164
	fuzzy		11.31708	9.30354	9.51357	8.564705
EBWA.1	sharp	11.50770	11.66183	9.555289	10.20881	9.443687
	fuzzy		11.31708	9.305964	9.642958	8.869182
EBWA.C	sharp	11.50770	8.726462	5.347378	5.509787	5.98894
	fuzzy		8.695319	5.481904	6.983782	6.328657

Table 11. RMSE for zero-mean Gaussian noise with amplitude described by function $A_2(\cdot)$.

The results presented in table 11 show that the partition in the case of methods based on statistical inference improves the results, even significantly for the EBWA.C method (the RMSE decreases more than twice).

The improvement or deterioration of results obtained using the partition are not expected in the cases when the amplitude of noise is constant within each cycle. The difference can be explained by randomness of the noise level in each part of the divided signal cycle despite the same value of standard deviation of random variable with Gaussian distribution which characterize the noise. Utility of the partition seems to be obvious in the cases when the assumption of noise amplitude constancy within each cycle is not hold. Presented below results of numerical experiments where the the amplitude of noise is not constant within each cycle show improvement of the root mean square errors for all tested methods.

Figure 6 presents the ECG signal to be averaged in this experiment, which is disturbed by Cauchy noise. The location parameter of Cauchy distribution is equal to 0 and the scale parameter is set to 0.01s, where s is the standard deviation of the deterministic component, i.e. the original ANE20000 signal.

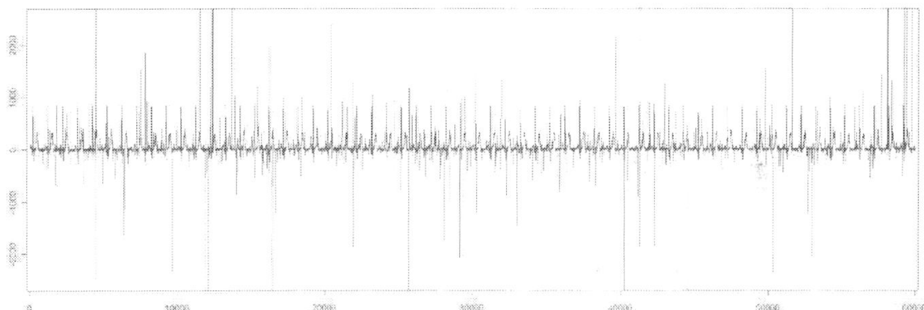

Fig. 6. ECG signal disturbed by Cauchy noise with scale parameter 0.01s.

The RMSE for the traditional arithmetic averaging method is equal 38.25505 and detailed results for the weighted averaging methods are presented in table 12.

Method	type	$K=1$	$K=2$	$K=3$	$K=4$	$K=5$
WAPM.2	sharp	4.293157	3.590644	5.802226	4.875072	3.05765
	fuzzy		3.782668	3.981781	3.457431	3.059209
WAPM.3	sharp	4.336904	3.590644	5.802226	4.875072	3.05765
	fuzzy		3.782668	3.981781	3.457431	3.059209
WAPM.4	sharp	4.124156	3.46319	2.910611	2.551464	2.364648
	fuzzy		3.560695	3.018473	2.807478	2.468142
SEBWA	sharp	4.044945	3.195667	2.195166	1.917149	1.644676
	fuzzy		3.396122	2.191550	2.215406	1.721535
EBWA.1	sharp	4.027516	3.093357	2.410249	2.033164	1.840781
	fuzzy		3.328734	2.384026	2.307351	1.923214
EBWA.C	sharp	3.970909	2.622315	2.405902	1.896787	1.818165
	fuzzy		2.966283	2.475908	2.14492	1.918657

Table 12. RMSE in the case of Cauchy noise with scale parameter 0.01s.

Analyzing the results it can be observed the improvement of the root mean square errors for all tested methods at least for some values of K. As was mentioned in the subsection 2.3.1 in the case of sharp partition incorrectly chosen number of parts may cause the deterioration of the results.

Figure 7 presents the ECG signal to be averaged in the last experiment, which is disturbed by Cauchy noise with the location parameter 0 and the scale parameter 0.05s, the standard deviation of ANE20000 signal. As can be seen the input signal is very distorted, particularly visible are many random impulse values. The RMSE for the traditional arithmetic averaging method is equal 2143.182 and detailed results for the weighted averaging methods are presented in table 13.

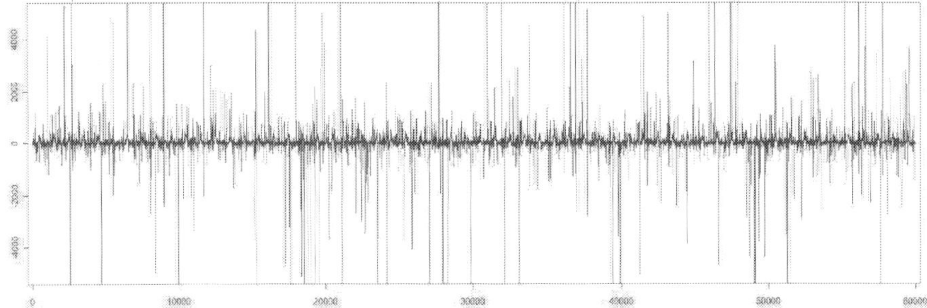

Fig. 7. ECG signal disturbed by Cauchy noise with scale parameter 0.05s.

Method	type	$K = 1$	$K = 2$	$K = 3$	$K = 4$	$K = 5$
WAPM.2	sharp	26.33396	23.59549	18.82174	16.77062	15.80005
	fuzzy		22.58925	19.25907	17.36819	15.80776
WAPM.3	sharp	23.19694	23.59549	18.82174	16.77062	15.80005
	fuzzy		22.58925	19.25907	17.36819	15.80776
WAPM.4	sharp	25.47250	20.02517	14.65732	13.77551	12.44631
	fuzzy		20.07785	15.25705	14.32465	12.49090
SEBWA	sharp	22.60814	17.82965	10.86278	10.33561	8.407054
	fuzzy		17.94750	10.86471	10.68507	8.42861
EBWA.1	sharp	21.00193	15.65491	10.68224	9.928945	8.798122
	fuzzy		16.40589	10.69901	10.31931	8.69519
EBWA.C	sharp	30.63047	24.34970	16.48281	12.77003	10.85225
	fuzzy		26.39931	16.21782	15.39638	11.52634

Table 13. RMSE in the case of Cauchy noise with scale parameter 0.05s.

Such great distortion of the signal in real cases obviously causes rejection of the disturbed signal, however this example shows that having the a priori information about the number of cycles and the length of the single cycle allows using some weighted averaging methods which recover the data with the relatively small error (compare the RMSE 2143.182, for the arithmetic averaging, and 8.407, for the SEBWA method with the sharp partition for $K = 5$).

4. Summary

This chapter presents several methods of weighted averaging: based on criterion function minimization (WACFM, WAPM) and on statistical inference (EBWA.1, EBWA.3, EBWA.C, SEBWA) together with fuzzy extensions, which use the fuzzy partition the signal cycle as well as using fuzzy numbers as coefficients of weight vector. The adaptation of SEBWA method to filtering of 2D images is also presented. This study reveals the fundamental differences among the weighted averaging methods and presents, through several numerical experiments, how these differences affect the quality of the averaged signal.

The most frequently used method, due to its simplicity, is the arithmetical averaging. The improvement of results obtained by the method can be reached rejecting the very noisy cycles. Averaging with rejecting very noisy cycles can be treated as weighted averaging method where the weights corresponding these cycles are set to zero. The crucial problem is how to find these cycles. The presented weighted averaging methods implement the automatic determining the weights, such that the most noisy cycles have the smallest weights (even zero in particular) and the least noisy ones receive the greatest weights, which increase their influence on the resulting averaged signal. Analyzing the presented results of performed numerical experiments, it is difficult to determine the best method, because for various power and type of noise accompanying the signal, different methods appear to give the best results.

This research was partially supported by Polish Ministry of Science and Higher Education as Research Project N N518 406438.

5. References

Augustyniak, P. (2006). Adaptive wavelet discrimination of muscular noise in the ECG, *Computers in Cardiology*, Vol. 33, pp. 481–484, ISSN: 0276-6574.

Bailon, R.; Olmos, S.; Serrano, P.; Garcia J. & Laguna P. (2002). Robust Measure of ST/HR Hysteresis in Stress Test ECG Recordings, *Computers in Cardiology*, Vol. 29, pp. 329–332, ISSN: 0276-6574.

Bataillou, E.; Thierry, E.;Rix, H. & Meste, O. (1995). Weighted averaging using adaptive estimation of the weights, *Signal Process.* Vol. 44, pp. 51–66, ISSN: 0165-1684.

Bruce, E.N. (2001). *Biomedical signal processing and signal modeling*, Wiley, ISBN: 0-471-34540-7, New York.

Davila, C.E. & Mobin M.S. (1992). Weighted averaging of evoked potentials. *IEEE Trans. Biomed. Eng.*, Vol. 39, No. 4, pp. 338–345, ISSN: 0018-9294.

Elberling, C. & Don, M. (2006). Detecting and assessing synchronous neural activity in the temporal domain, In: *Auditory Evoked Potentials - Basic principles and Clinical Application*, Burkard, R.F.; Eggermont,J.J; Don, M. (Eds.), pp. 102–123, Lippincott Williams & Wilkins, ISBN: 978-0-7817-5756-0, Philadelphia.

Jane, R.; Rix, H.; Caminal, P. & Laguna, P. (1991). Alignment methods for averaging of high-resolution cardiac signals: a comparative study of performance, *IEEE Trans. Biomed. Eng.*, Vol. 38, No. 6, pp. 571–579, ISSN: 0018-9294.

Johnson, R.A.; Bhattacharyya, G.K. (2009). *Statistics: Principles and Methods*, John Wiley & Sons, ISBN: 978-0-470-40927-5.

Kotas, M. (2009). Nonlinear projective filtering of ECG signals, In: *Biomedical engineering*. Mello C.A.B.,(Ed.), pp. 433–452, InTech, ISBN: 978-953-307-013-1.

Laciar, E. & Jane, R. (2001). An Improved Weighted Signal Averaging Method for High-Resolution ECG Signals, *Computers in Cardiology*, Vol. 28, pp. 69–72, ISSN: 0276-6574.

Leski, J. (2002). Robust weighted averaging, *IEEE Trans. Biomed. Eng.*, Vol. 49, No. 8, pp. 796–804, ISSN: 0018-9294.

Momot, A.; Momot M. & Leski J. (2005). The Fuzzy Relevance Vector Machine and its Application to Noise Reduction in ECG Signal, *J. Med. Inform. Technol.*, Vol. 9, pp. 99–106, ISSN: 1642-6037.

Momot, A.; Momot, M. & Leski, J. (2007a). Bayesian and empirical Bayesian approach to weighted averaging of ECG signal, *Bull. Pol. Acad. Sci., Technol. Sci.*, Vol. 55, No. 4, pp. 341–350, ISSN: 0239-7528.

Momot, A.; Momot, M. & Leski, J. (2007b). Weighted Averaging of ECG Signals Based on Partition of Input Set in Time Domain, *J. Med. Inform. Technol.*, Vol. 11, pp. 165–170, ISSN: 1642-6037.

Momot, A. (2008a). Weighted Averaging of ECG Signal Using Criterion Function Minimization, In: *Information Technologies in Biomedicine, Advances in Soft Computing*, Vol. 47, Pietka, E.; Kawa, J. (Eds.), pp. 267–274, Springer-Verlag, ISBN: 978-3-540-68167-0, Berlin Heidelberg.

Momot A., Momot M. (2008b). Empirical Bayesian Approach to Weighted Averaging of ECG Signal Using Cauchy Distribution. In: *Information Technologies in Biomedicine, Advances in Soft Computing*, Vol. 47, Pietka, E.; Kawa, J. (Eds.), pp. 275–282, Springer-Verlag, ISBN: 978-3-540-68167-0, Berlin Heidelberg.

Momot, A. (2009a). Methods of Weighted Averaging of ECG Signals Using Bayesian Inference and Criterion Function Minimization, *Biomed. Signal Process. Control*, Vol. 4, No. 2, pp. 162–169, ISSN: 1746-8094.

Momot, A. (2009b). Fuzzy Weighted Averaging of Biomedical Signal Using Bayesian Inference, In: *Man-Machine Interactions, Advances in Intelligent and Soft Computing*, Vol. 59, Cyran, K.A.; Kozielski, S.; Peters, J.F.; Stanczyk, U.; Wakulicz-Deja, A. (Eds.), pp. 133–140, Springer-Verlag, ISBN: 978-3-642-00562-6, Berlin Heidelberg.

Momot, A. & Momot, M. (2009c). Fuzzy Weighted Averaging Using Criterion Function Minimization, In: *Man-Machine Interactions, Advances in Intelligent and Soft Computing*, Vol. 59, Cyran, K.A.; Kozielski, S.; Peters, J.F.; Stanczyk, U.; Wakulicz-Deja, A. (Eds.), pp. 273–280, Springer-Verlag, ISBN: 978-3-642-00562-6, Berlin Heidelberg.

Momot, A. (2010). Application of Adaptive Weighed Averaging to Digital Filtering of 2D Images, In: *Information Technologies in Biomedicine (vol.2), Advances in Soft Computing*, Vol. 69, Pietka, E.; Kawa, J. (Eds.), pp. 33–44, Springer-Verlag, ISBN: 978-3-642-13104-2, Berlin Heidelberg.

Momot A. (2011). On Application of Input Data Partitioning to Bayesian Weighted Averaging of Biomedical Signals, *Expert Systems*, in press (accepted 28.01.2011).

Paul, J.S.; Reddy, M.R.; Kumar, V.J. (2000). A transform domain SVD filter for suppresion of muscle noise artefacts in exercise ECG's, *IEEE Trans. Bimed. Eng.*, Vol. 47, No. 5, pp.654–663, ISSN: 0018-9294.

Sharma, L. N.; Dandapat, S. & Mahanta, A. (2010). ECG signal denoising using higher order statistics in Wavelet subbands, *Biomed. Signal Process. Control*, Vol. 5, No. 3, pp. 214–222, ISSN: 1746-8094.

Yan, J.; Lu, Y.; Liu, J.; Wub, X. & Xu, Y. (2010). Self-adaptive model-based ECG denoising using features extracted by mean shift algorithm, *Biomed. Signal Process. Control*, Vol. 5, No. 2, pp. 103–113, ISSN: 1746-8094.

Zywietz, C.; Alraun, W. & Fischer, R. (2001). Quality assurance in biosignal processing - procedures and recommendations for evaluation for electrocardiological analysis systems, *Computers in Cardiology*, Vol. 28, pp. 201–204, ISSN: 0276-6574.

17

Development of a Neural Interface for PNS Motor Control

Christopher G. Langhammer, Melinda K. Kutzing,
Vincent Luo, Jeffrey D. Zahn and Bonnie L. Firestein
Rutgers, The State University of New Jersey
United States

1. Introduction

1.1 The design process

Engineering disciplines offer powerful analytical techniques which are applicable in a wide range of problem solving applications. As an emerging field, biomedical engineering draws on the tools of the classical engineering fields, such as mechanical, electrical, and chemical engineering, to address problems originating in complex biological or clinical systems. The real art of biomedical engineering comes in the creativity it takes to reframe these ill-defined biological or clinical problems into ones which can be addressed using the tools offered by classical engineering disciplines. Because the range of clinical and biological problems is so broad, it is impossible to give examples of every possible problem and their appropriate solution sets. However, developing a general framework in which complex, multilevel problems can be addressed can help formalize the process by which these problems are conceptualized and prevent them from becoming overwhelming in their complexity. This framework consists of the 5 following steps:

1. Identify a precise, well-defined problem (may be a sub-problem of a much larger problem)
2. Identify desired endpoint/solution to problem
3. Identify a set of reasonable assumptions based on current knowledge of the field
4. Based on the problem statement, desired endpoint, and assumptions, use engineering tools to design potential solutions
5. Identify optimal solution based on desired endpoint and the pros/cons associated with each solution
6. Repeat as necessary

By way of example, we will walk through these steps, demonstrating how it can be applied to neural prosthetics to see how it generates a new and promising approach to solving problems currently preventing progress in this field. The use of neural prosthetics is complex, involving many different therapeutic goals and technical approaches to achieving them. The above process will be repeated several times as we re-frame our biological problem and think through possible solutions, but it will differ slightly each time as it is used to address new problems arising at each decision point in the design process.

1.2 Defining the problem: Appropriately selecting a patient population and defining their clinical need

There are an estimated 1.7 million Americans living with limb loss [1] and many more suffering from peripheral nervous system (PNS) injury without expected motor recovery [2, 3]. Although these conditions result in significant loss of function, many patients do not take advantage of the powered prosthetics available to them, due mostly to the fact that the pros (restoration of partial function) do not outweigh the cons (cost and discomfort) [4-6]. The mechanical capabilities of prosthetic devices have become sophisticated, but motor tasks are generally driven by gross anatomic movements or low bandwidth myoelectric couplings, making them cumbersome [10-12]. For example, NASA has developed a robotic hand that approximates human dexterity, but commercially available prosthetic technology can currently control an extremely limited number of joints at a time. Amputees, therefore, are unable to benefit from the advanced hand [10]. For such prostheses, communication with the user is the weakest link in the chain of components that includes electronics, computing, and actuators, all of which are adequate for the application [10-12].

Neuroprosthetic devices aim to correct this deficiency by placing a prosthetic directly under neural control. Achieving this goal would give the user control over multiple joints simultaneously, restoring intuitive control over the prosthetic appendage. Restoration of real-time, dexterous control, however, requires high bandwidth communication between user and device. The neural interface is the point at which this communication occurs (reviewed recently in the popular press [13]). In the case of sensory prostheses, such as a cochlear implant [14, 15], the neural interface is designed to insert signals into the nervous system by stimulating the nervous tissue, while in the case of motor prosthetics [10, 16, 17], the purpose is to extract signals from the nervous system by recording the activity of the nervous tissue. Long-term efforts are aimed at creating hybrid systems capable of two-way communication with the nervous system for restoring full function to amputees as well as to other patient groups [18, 19].

While this technology has advanced rapidly, these devices have yet to perform at the level necessary to justify their use in large-scale clinical trials [8, 9]. The major hurdle to progress in the clinical advancement of neuroprosthetic devices is the development of neural interfaces capable of efficient communication with the nervous system [8, 11, 20]. In part, this is because neural interfaces are developed using performance objectives which do not have direct clinical corollaries. This rift between technological advancement and clinical advancement is exemplified by the examples of cochlear and cortical implants. Cochlear implants, using a neural interface with electrodes designed specifically for stimulating the cochlear nucleus, are widespread because they restore function and are relatively non-invasive. The size, positioning, and composition of the electrode contacts, however, make them unusable in recording applications. In comparison, other neural interface designs are used primarily in basic science research because they can both stimulate and record and can be used with multiple different tissue types from both the central nervous system (CNS) and PNS. However, they are not employed on a large scale clinically because it is difficult to justify their invasiveness relative to their clinical benefits.

Technologies exist that are capable of recording neural activity from both the PNS and CNS [21, 22], but they face problems acquiring large enough numbers of independent and appropriately tuned neural signals to provide reliable dexterous control. Current reviews of neural interface designs highlight the following functional criteria as primary bottlenecks [8, 20, 23, 24]:

- Obtaining stable, long-term recordings of large populations of neurons,
- Developing computationally efficient algorithms for translating neuronal activity into command signals capable of controlling a complex artificial actuator, and
- Determining how to use brain plasticity to incorporate prosthetics.

While it is nearly impossible to address each of these points optimally at the same time, it may be possible to address them within a single, clinical context by focusing design considerations on an appropriately selected patient base and a precisely identified clinical goal. For example, for the purpose of this case study, we will focus on amputees and others with severe PNS injury as our patient population and on restoring motor control through the use of neuroprosthetics as our clinical goal. Our subsequent design decisions can therefore be guided by the need to acquire neural information specifically about motor intention rather than simply acquiring neural signals generally.

1.3 Microelectrode arrays basics

The neurons of the PNS and CNS communicate using bioelectric events called action potentials (APs). To connect to the nervous system in a biologically relevant manner, we must integrate electronics and nervous tissue to transform these bioelectric signals into electronic signals which can be interpreted using computers. The gold-standard method to measure the activity of electrogenic cells uses electrodes pulled from metal wires and glass tubing and is not logistically adaptable to long-term or *in vivo* use. Although alternative methods, such as voltage-sensitive dyes, have been used, these methods are unsuitable for *in vivo* applications because of the infrastructure involved and the toxic side effects.

Microelectrode arrays (MEAs) were developed to overcome many of these problems by recording from multiple sites in a non-invasive way. Neuronal activity is recorded by placing a conductor, which is connected to a recording device, in the vicinity of a neuron's soma where neuronal APs create their largest transmembrane currents [25, 26]. This rapidly changing current creates voltage transients that can be transmitted along the conductor and subsequently recorded. A conductor will transmit all such activity along its length so that regional specificity is achieved by insulating the entire conductor except the points from which you want to record activity (Fig. 1 A).

MEAs are not, however, without limitations. Extracellular MEAs have been used with some success in recording from large populations of neurons, but they record only a fraction of the transmembrane voltage and record from the space surrounding the electrode rather than from the space inside of an individual neuron. Therefore, the extracellular voltage, referred to as the extracellular voltage trace (EVT), at any point is the sum of the activity of any neurons close enough that their APs can be detected (Fig. 1 B-C) [27] as well as background noise [28]. As a result, they suffer from poor signal fidelity, and single electrodes can wind up unintentionally recording from multiple neurons (Fig. 1 D). The interpretation of data from multiple neurons recorded on a single channel is a complex problem that has been likened to trying to understand the function of an orchestra without any knowledge that the final sound is generated by different instruments playing simultaneously [25]. Similarly, the most meaningful interpretations of neuronal activity depend on knowing the activity of single cells, due to the nature of information exchange through APs.

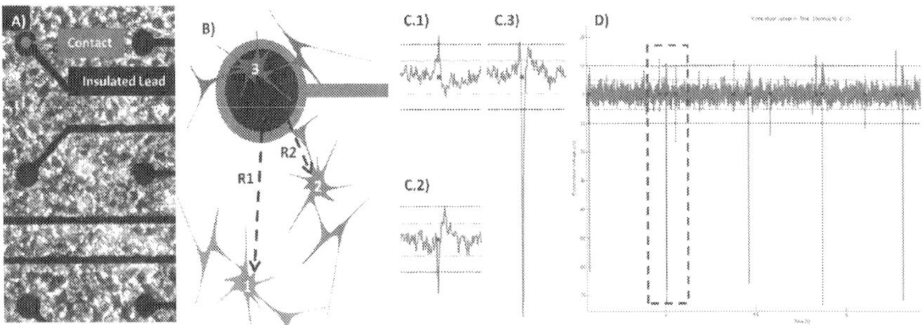

Fig. 1. Recording and interpretation of EVTs using an MEA. A) Phase microscopy of cortical neuron cell culture on commercially available MEA. B) Schematic representation of potential neuron locations relative to contact pad on MEA. C) Example segments of EVT recorded from a single electrode, showing three distinct spike morphologies (small-positive, small-negative, and large-negative), indicating the likely presence of three nearby neurons. Threshold levels used for spike detection are indicated by black dashes. D) Example EVT data recorded over 2 seconds, demonstrating temporal relationship of spike events.

MEAs are fabricated using standard integrated circuit (IC) and micro-electromechanical systems (MEMS) manufacturing techniques, which build MEAs on rigid substrates, such as glass or silicon [29]. In standard designs, a conducting layer of metal is deposited on top of the substrate and formed into the appropriate electrode contact and lead pattern using microlithography. Several layers of thin-film insulating material, usually silicone dioxide (SiO_2) or silicone nitride (Si_xN_y), are then deposited to insulate the conducting layer except at the sites of intended cell contact [30]. These electrodes can detect changes in voltage secondary to cellular depolarization at the conducting contact site, transmitting it along the conducting wires underneath the insulating layers to an amplifier and recording device [29]. As microfabrication technology has evolved, so have the means of generating features of varying size and shape. Standard lithographic techniques have reached new lower limits on the feature size they are able to create, and soft lithography has allowed the use of new materials and techniques to reduce cost. Such design decisions are eventually made based on the end use of the electrode, such as desired performance characteristics and the cell type or tissue type it is meant to interact with.

1.4 Cell-surface interactions

The first important interface is the cell-electrode interaction in which an electrogenic cell communicates with a substrate electrode. Fig. 2 A-B is a schematic of a neuron resting on top of an electrode in a planar electrode array [31]. Current can either be forced into the cell by the electrode, or cellular depolarizations can be detected by the electrode, depending on whether the electrode is stimulating or recording from the associated tissue. In Figure 2 the current originates in the cell and disperses into the culture environment and the electrode contact pad.

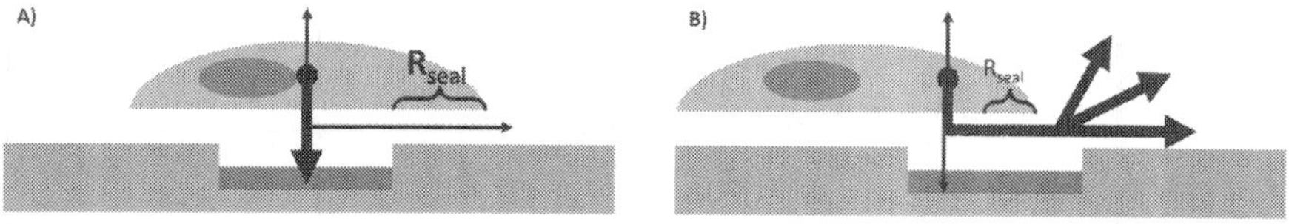

Fig. 2. Geometry of cell-electrode interactions. A) Good electrode coverage results in a high R_{seal} and more voltage observed at the electrode contact. B) Poor electrode coverage results in a low R_{seal}, greater dissipation of current into the culture environment and less voltage observed at the electrode contact.

The current in the sealing gap between cell and electrode arises from the lower cell membrane, and the resulting potential field is measured by the electrode. This current is divided into a portion that flows from the cell to the underlying electrode and a portion that leaks out around its boundaries (through the sealing gap) and into the medium. The relative amount of current traveling via each of these two paths is a function of the membrane characteristics of the cell, the material characteristics of the electrode, and the resistance of the sealing gap (R_{seal}) [31]. A high R_{seal} means that more of the current associated with the cellular depolarization is transmitted directly to the electrode (Fig. 2 A), while a low R_{seal} allows more of the current to leak from the sealing gap into the culture medium, escaping detection by the electrode (Fig. 2 B). R_{seal} is related to cell-electrode geometry (size, shape, and relative positions of the cell and electrode). Finite element solutions, based on a lumped RC-circuit model of the cell-electrode interface, identify two regions of R_{seal} based on this geometry: one in which the electrode is not entirely covered and R_{seal} is low, and one in which the electrode is completely covered and R_{seal} is high and dependent on the position of the electrode relative to the rest of the cell body [32]. The range of resistances is larger in the latter case, indicating that the relative positions of the electrode and cell body play an important role in determining R_{seal} regardless of whether the electrode is completely covered. High quality cell-electrode contacts, where quality is determined by electrode coverage and sealing, will permit selective and reliable recording [33]. Experiments have similarly demonstrated that the sealing resistance increases when the electrode is completely covered by the cell and drops off sharply when any portion is exposed directly to the medium [31].

Of the parameters in this model, R_{seal} is the only one related to mechanical design of the electrode. The practical implications of these findings are that maximizing recording fidelity means maximizing electrode area in such a way that electrode coverage, and therefore R_{seal}, is preserved. This is a goal easily accomplished using larger cells, as they can effectively cover larger electrodes, but which is very difficult for smaller structures such as axons.

1.5 Performance objectives

A complete neural interface should provide a control signal that restores natural movement to paralyzed body parts or prostheses without extensive learning. Most upper limb amputees want a prosthesis that requires less visual attention to operate, has sensory feedback, and can execute multiple movements simultaneously [34]. In other words, control should emerge from the voluntary intent to carry out an action, rather than the retraining of other actions. Researchers believe that with an efficient neural interface, efferent motor nerve signals carrying command information outward from the CNS could be used to control actuators in an artificial limb and to selectively stimulate afferent sensory neurons that carry sensory information towards the CNS, thus providing sensory feedback [34].

Because of the massive amounts of information exchanged between end organs and the brain during seemingly common tasks, future rehabilitative applications, like graded neuromuscular control or for prosthetic vision, will depend on the availability of large-scale, selective neural interfaces [33]. This requires that the neural interface record efferent nervous signaling with enough specificity to reproduce fine motor control [12]. Ideally, the device would acquire and distribute these signals in the least invasive way possible. At present, these are all major challenges. The design of the neural interface component of a neuroprosthetic device should be based on achieving the above by manipulating electrode design, material properties, surface chemistry, and implantation site.

Extracting motor control signals from the firing patterns of populations of neurons and using them to reproduce motor behaviors in artificial actuators are the two key operations that a clinically viable neuroprosthesis needs to perform [20]. It is easy to define success as simply improving the adhesion of nerve cells to an electrode array in order to improve signal acquisition *in vitro*; however, it is much more useful to set the endpoint for determining success as improved functionality by the end-users. Eventually, the goals of neural interfaces are for patients to use the system for restoring mobility and sensory functions associated with the activities of daily living and enhancing their quality of life and independence [21]. This means usability of the signal acquired by a neural interface, as well as signal fidelity, should be included in the definition of success.

Existing neural interface designs are as diverse as the nervous system itself, including multiple cortical, deep brain, spinal, non-invasive, and PNS-based approaches to stimulation and recording. Additional complexity is added by the exploding number of algorithms designed to analyze and decode the information recorded from neural interfaces. Consequently, there are essentially limitless pairings of technologies, nervous system targets, and disease states, which may potentially be addressed with technologies labeled as neural interfaces. The ultimate adoption of neuroprosthetic devices into mainstream clinical practice will depend on whether or not they improve significantly on current prosthetic designs' functionality. In this case, successful device function requires the integration of the nervous system, implantable device, and computational algorithm. In other words, the interface is one link in a chain of components that must work together to form a functional end product. As such, it should be designed with the links on either side in mind in order to facilitate these components integration into a whole.

Despite the speed with which computers execute complex algorithms, the human nervous system is far superior at tasks such as complex motor control [24]. The main processing task for algorithms associated with neural interfaces is decoding: deriving motor commands from neural impulses which can be used to drive prostheses. There are several approaches to decoding, including neural networks, pattern-recognition algorithms, and hybrid filters. None of these methods is clearly superior, as each carries an individual set of pros and cons, involving the amount of information that can be simultaneously processed, the amount of time it takes to do so, and the accuracy with which they can predict motor intention [10]. The types of algorithms employed to decode neural motor volition are an important constraint when designing a neural interface. Questions pertaining to the rate at which usable data can be acquired and the speed at which it can be translated into motor intention will drive decisions regarding implantation site and the target number of neural recordings, especially as more effort is put into including signal processing components on the implants themselves as a way of reducing the bandwidth required to transmit the acquired signal. As a means of illustrating the importance of having the appropriate amount of relevant data, imagine trying to read a computer screen with only a small number of pixels (Fig. 3). The more complex the message, the larger the number of pixels required to read it. Sadly, there is no exact answer to the question "how many independent neural signals are required to restore dexterous control?" because the answer is dependent on the nature of the signals and what type of device they are used to control. While small populations of highly tuned neurons can accurately predict movement parameters, highly tuned neurons are rare in a random sample of cortical cells. Because motor information is represented in this highly distributed way, large samples of recorded cortical neurons are preferred [20, 34, 35]. It has been estimated that recordings from 500 to 700 cortical neurons would be needed to achieve 95% accuracy in predicting one-dimensional hand movements [36]. The minimum number of recordings required to transform thoughts into a reasonable range of motions most likely exceeds 1000 [10], a number presently exceeding the capabilities of cortical probes.

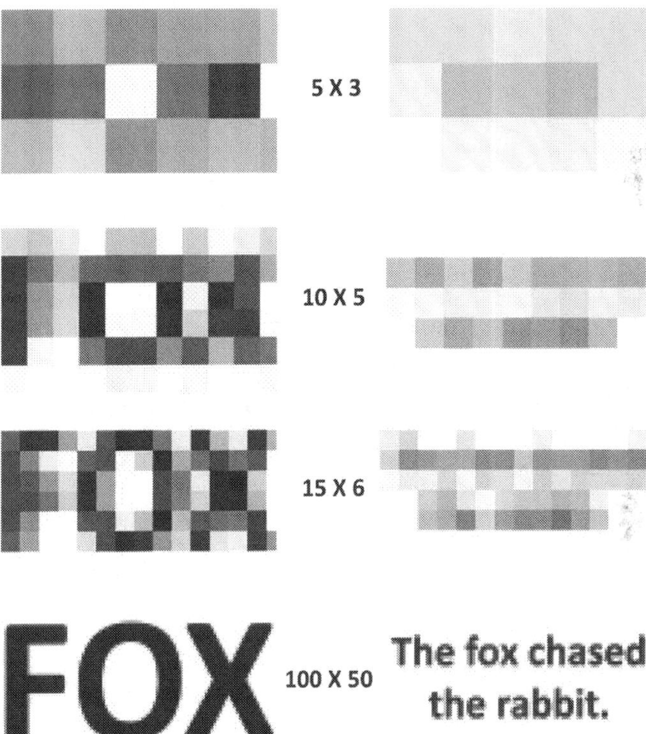

Fig. 3. More complex messages require a larger number of independent signal sources (in this case pixels) for proper decoding

The nervous system that handles this information consists of peripheral nervous structures and central nervous structures. Each region encodes, processes, and transmits information in a unique form, and therefore, has unique anatomic and physiologic characteristics which employ not only a highly dynamic and adaptive information structure, but also a highly dynamic physical environment. Recent findings suggest that the task of designing a device that acts in the same way and feels the same as the subjects' own limbs might be accomplished by designing devices which capitalize on the brain's ability to undergo experience-dependent plasticity and assimilates the prosthetic limb as if it were part of the subject's own body [20]. Electrode design and placement should aim to benefit from neural plasticity rather than combat it. Electrodes intended for use in a neural interface should be designed appropriately for their intended site of implantation, based on the characteristics of the target contact neural cell types and the coding structure of the neural information.

Due to the need for highly specialized algorithms to interpret the recorded neural signals, the design, size, material choice, and interface surface have to ensure temporally stable transducer properties of the neuron-electrode interface throughout the lifetime of the implant. Electrodes need to not only be non-destructive to the surrounding tissue and record from the same or similar set of neurons, but need to avoid encapsulation, inflammation, and other "foreign-object responses" which would alter its ability to record neural signals. Neural interfaces therefore have to fulfill high demands with respect to biostability and biofunctionality [21].

Finally, it is important to consider the attitudes of the end-users of neural interface technology. Fully paralyzed patients anxious to gain enhanced physical abilities may be willing to accept the risks of brain surgery and to live with hardware implanted in their brains, but most healthy people would probably not. Amputees and spinal cord injury patients are likely to fall along a range of attitudes regarding the concept of implanting devices in their brains. The key to success in restoring human capabilities will be gaining access to motor and sensory signals in an unobtrusive way [36].

1.6 Design decisions

As an exercise in engineering design, we are going to walk through a small amount of biological background and then discuss how this plays into designing a new interface. Because neuroprosthetic devices, and even neural interfaces specifically, involve multiple components, there is a hierarchical sequence to how design decisions need to be made. Every design decision made in the process comes with a set of benefits and drawbacks. While some aspects of our design are flexible, and the drawbacks they introduce can be minimized in the actual decision, others are more rigid and the drawbacks they introduce need to be mitigated in subsequent design decisions. Over the course of this chapter, we will see how each decision draws from those before it and affects those that follow.

Based on our goal of restoring dexterous control of powered prosthetic devices to our patient population, we need to answer the following questions: What type of information do we want from the nervous system? Where are we going to get that information from? How are we going to get it? To help us answer these questions, it helps to establish a conceptual framework by which to organize current approaches to interfacing with the nervous system. Based on the evolution of the field of neural interfaces so far, it is helpful to consider several different aspects of neural interface design:

- The intended function of the neural interface (signal recording or signal insertion)
- The site of implantation (CNS or PNS)
- Target electrogenic cell type (myotubes or neurons)
- The invasiveness of the implant (the degree to which it is destructive to the native tissue)

2. Design decision #1: Signal recording vs. signal insertion

The nervous system is a bidirectional communication system, with efferent signals carrying command information outward from the CNS and afferent signals carrying sensory information toward the CNS. Neural interfaces can be designed to restore function in instances where one or both of these transmission pathways have failed. Generally, "input prostheses" are designed to insert information into the nervous system (supplementing the afferent pathway), while "output prostheses" are designed to record information from the nervous system (supplementing the efferent pathway on the nervous side).

Input prostheses are designed to restore function in individuals with sensory disabilities by selectively stimulating nervous tissues to which natural nervous stimulation or response to environmental cues has been lost. The most advanced of these has brought the perception of sound to ~40,000 deaf individuals by means of electrodes implanted in the cochlea. Similar attempts are underway to provide images to the visual cortex [24], and the direct electrical stimulation of both cortical sensory areas and peripheral nerves has shown promising results in restoring the sensation of touch.

The major goal of output prostheses is recording neural signals with the intention of later translating them into meaningful command functions. These commands can then serve as a means to control disabled body parts or devices, such as computers or robotic limbs [37]. Current efforts to achieve this have been slowed by the need to record from large numbers of neurons (arguably thousands depending on the site of recording), which is a challenging biological problem, compounded by the need to analyze and interpret these neural signals in real time.

2.1 Decision summary

While simultaneous restoration of sensory and motor function in prosthetics is the ultimate goal, it is unclear that this is achievable using a single interface design. It is far more likely that this will ultimately be achieved using a combination of techniques (consider the earlier discussion of cochlear vs. cortical implants), due to the fact that electrode modifications made to optimize the recording or stimulating modality frequently come at the expense of the other modality. As such, we choose to limit our future design considerations according to our clinical goal of restoring motor control (Fig. 4).

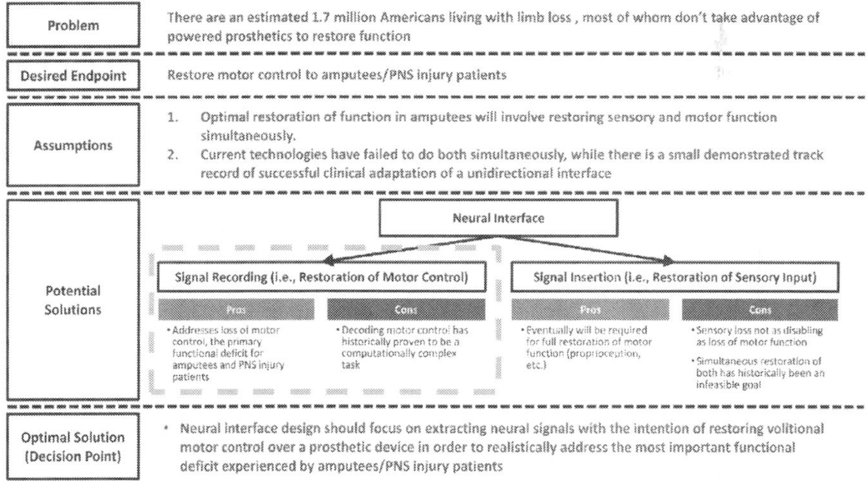

Fig. 4. Design process summary diagram after Decision #1

3. Design decision #2: Neural target (CNS vs. PNS)

The most important design constraint is the one over which we have the least control: the nature of the neural target our interface is designed to interact with. We can manipulate the rest of the components of the neuroprosthetic system, but the biology of the brain and nervous system is largely unalterable. The CNS typically refers to the nervous tissue contained within the skull and spinal column. The PNS refers to nervous tissue found outside of these locations which carry motor and sensory information to and from the CNS, such as the brachial and lumbar nerve plexuses or the radial and sciatic nerve trunks. The intention to perform an action is born in the cortex of the brain, is processed through multiple regions of the brain and spinal cord, and is transmitted along the axons of the PNS, finally arriving at the neuromuscular junction (NMJ) where it triggers the depolarization and contraction of the specific muscle cells required to perform the desired action. There is continual debate on where in this chain of transmission is the best location from which to derive a useful motor signal, and therefore, to target with a neural interface [8, 20, 22, 38-40].

3.1 Accessibility

One of the primary differences between the CNS and PNS has to do with accessibility of neural signals. With regards to the motor system, for example, the motor cortex of the CNS contains large cell bodies (upper motor neurons) while the portions of the PNS that are relevant to motor control consist mostly of axons from alpha motoneurons (lower motor neurons). The cell bodies in the motor cortex are large enough so that their depolarizations can be sensed using microelectrodes inserted into their vicinity, while the depolarizations occurring in lower motor axons are small enough so that they can only be sensed in aggregate (remember our earlier point about electrode sealing and cell size).

Historically, neural interfaces have been designed with the intention of communicating directly with cortical tissue [41]. Most of these efforts use penetrating MEAs to record the depolarization of cell bodies [11, 20-22]. With these designs, electrodes located at the end of micron scale spikes are inserted directly into the CNS, such as in the primary motor cortex or spinal cord [12]. While there are a number of benefits to this approach (most notably that it is technically simple to record a neural signal from a region where the large neuronal cell bodies may be accessed), progress is confounded by the complicated encoding of information in cortical brain regions [37] and by the highly invasive nature of implanting foreign devices in the CNS [41-46]. In the cases where these neural interfaces have been used *in vivo*, the surgical technique used for implantation strongly influences the long-term results. Most implantable microelectrode designs, which make direct contact with cortical tissue, enable good quality recordings to be made for several months, but recording quality deteriorates over time, due most likely to electrode encapsulation by fibrous tissue and cell death in the vicinity of the electrode [20]. Additionally, the size of electronic devices meant to be implanted inside of a living animal's skull is another design constraint that limits the functionality of cortical implants [10]. Thus, complicating issues for these electrodes include poor long-term recording due to fibrous encapsulation, inflammation, death of surrounding neurons, and insufficient data transfer and decoding ability to interpret signals recorded at the cortical implantation site [41, 45, 46].

The PNS may provide an especially useful point of access for neural interfaces in the case of restoring motor function to amputees and spinal cord injury patients. Amputation removes the structural elements of the limb, but the ends of lesioned nerves remain and continue to carry motor and sensory information from the removed limb. Even lesioned peripheral nerves that are not permitted to regenerate continue to demonstrate a normal pattern of discharge for the muscles that they originally innervated [47]. Both central and peripheral motor and somatosensory pathways retain significant residual connectivity long after limb amputation.

3.2 Encoding

Recent work has shown that motor information is represented in the cortex in a highly distributed way [20, 35]. Discoveries using fMRI indicate that cortical representations of different upper-limb regions are not demarcated into the discrete topographic areas of the classic homunculus. There are multiple foci representing a given limb movement and overlapping representations of disparate limb regions [34, 35]. What was thought at one time to be a simple topographical map superimposed on the cortex is far more complex. Each action originates with a few neurons in the motor cortex that trigger a large neural network that, in turn, coordinates the activities of several effector muscles. This neural network synthesizes input from thousands of tactile, positional, and visual sources with motor intention from the primary motor cortex to derive controlled motor output. Transforming this tangled mesh of millions of bioelectric signals into graceful movements is a routine accomplishment of our sensorimotor system but is not currently reproducible using computers [10]. As discussed previously, neurons which are highly tuned to motor intention are rare in a random sample of cortical cells. The farther synaptically removed from the periphery a neuron is, the more its activity is determined by its peers rather than by the environment, and the more it encodes cognitive abstractions rather than direct representations [25]. Because cortical motor information is represented in this highly distributed way, it may take recordings from hundreds to thousands of cortical cells to restore a reasonable range of motion [10, 20, 34-36].

In comparison to these complex CNS representations, PNS motor encoding is relatively simple. Peripheral nerves are organized somatotopically at both fascicular and subfascicular levels [34]. Each motoneuron synapses with many muscle fibers, constituting a motor unit. The neuromuscular junction is a one-to-one synapse, meaning that the excitation of a motoneuron produces the same frequency of action potentials in all muscle fibers in the motor unit. Graded contraction is produced by increasing the number of motor units activated and by increasing the frequency of action potentials [21]. Each muscle is controlled by up to a few hundred motor neurons [22], implying that each limb is supplied by several thousand. This high degree of organization in the neuromuscular system is achieved through the bidirectional interactions of myotubes and motoneurons. The final system architecture is the result of a highly interactive process between motoneurons and myotubes, involving the exchange of several known, and potentially more unknown, growth factors and cell adhesion molecules.

In the case of walking and other complex motor programs, complex signal processing occurs between the cortex and actuator muscles, and there is integration of sensory input from the visual and vestibular portions of the brain, which facilitate coordinated movement.

Recording from cortical sites may record movement intention but would not contain any information regarding the massive integration of environmental cues with motor intention that go into developing a useful motor signal. Recording or inputting signals in the PNS and allowing them to proceed through the many processing steps occurring naturally may result in improved communication. For example, cochlear implants are one of the most successful neural interfaces currently in clinical use. They restore hearing to the deaf by directly stimulating the nerve cells in the cochlea which fail to respond to normal sound stimuli. Attempts to stimulate more central areas of the cortex associated with hearing have been less successful, however, probably because of the loss of important signal processing in the periphery [24].

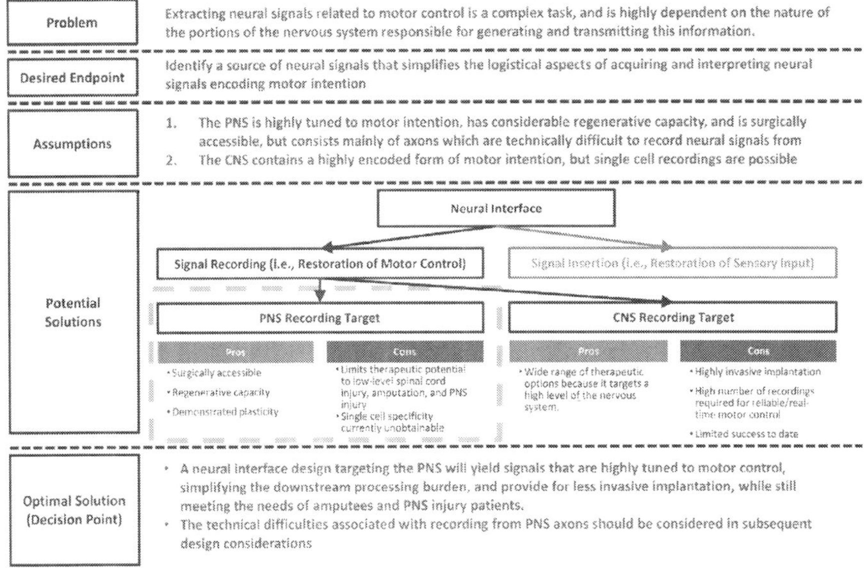

Fig. 5. Design process summary diagram after Decision #2

3.3 Decision summary

Many studies have centered around interfaces with the cerebral cortex because it was believed that motor intent and sensory percepts were more readily accessed there than elsewhere in the brain [37]. The benefits of a CNS interface include a more diverse set of applications, as it targets a higher region of the nervous system. However, recording from the CNS yields a highly encoded neural signal, as at that point the nervous impulses have not undergone the extensive processing performed in the cerebellum and spinal cord. The complicated nature of this encoding exacerbates the problems associated with decoding it and increases the number of signals required to establish reliable motor control. Due to its comparative physical accessibility, the discrete encoding of motor and sensory signals, and the regenerative capacity of peripheral axons [34, 47, 48], the PNS may represent a more convenient location for accessing neural signals.

Neural interfaces that target the PNS pose a good compromise between the benefits and drawbacks of many types of neural interfaces [38, 39]. Rather than placing microelectrodes into delicate nervous tissue, one could consider interfacing through the PNS and exploiting its capacity to "remap" motor and sensory functions, effectively outsourcing some of the requirements for efficient communication to the native neural structures. An MEA-based neural interface that targets the PNS improves on current technology by taking advantage of the specific nature of the PNS in managing motor control. Regenerating peripheral axons naturally re-innervate tissue different from their original locations. With training, patients are then able to assimilate the new axon distribution and regain limb function. Through rehabilitation, the patient may be able to learn to control particular motor functions directly by using the portions of the nervous system specifically designed for such a task. Taking advantage of naturally occurring neural plasticity in the PNS would reduce the need to interpret complex neural processing using computational tools from a small region of the brain or spinal cord, a process better handled by the CNS [12]. Essentially, based on what is known about motor coding in the periphery, by tapping into the PNS, there may be less need to decipher the "neural code." However, subsequent design decisions will have to be made which mitigate the technical difficulties of recording from axons due to their small size.

4. Design decision #3: Myotubes vs. neurons

4.1 Myotube signals as a proxy for neural signals

Attempts to use lesioned nerves directly as a source of information for prosthetic devices in human amputees have met with limited success, due in part to the low signal amplitude. In one set of experiments, the signals obtained from normal nerves via cuff electrodes during functional activity are in the range of 10-50 μV [47, 49]. However, the group also observed that larger motor signals can be obtained by allowing the lesioned nerves to innervate isolated slips of host muscle from which electromyographic (EMG) signals can be recorded by wire electrodes and that these larger EMG signals correlated with the smaller EMG signals in the nerves. This indicates that recording from a regenerated neuromuscular interface may allow the acquisition of stable, naturally amplified signals from lesioned nerves [47]. Furthermore, this is an excellent example of how motor neurons and myotubes communicate bidirectionally to promote each other's survival [50] and axonal regeneration. For example, denervated muscle strips attract the ingrowth of lesioned nerve fascicles. It has been shown that in the absence of neuromuscular synaptic transmission, nerve sprouts are generated as a form of self-repair and that both denervated and inactive muscle fibers release at least one sprouting factor. Three of the different proposed sprouting molecules, neuroleukin, insulin-like growth factor, and neural cell adhesion molecules, can be viewed as muscle-derived retrograde signaling molecules. These muscle-derived sprouting factors may be capable of diffusion for considerable distances [51]. Sprouts form in response to several stimuli but most notably in response to the sprouting factor secreted by partially denervated or paralyzed muscle [51].

Historically, the most clinically successful means of establishing a control signal for powered prosthetic devices has been recording the EMG activity of residual muscles [52,

53]. This is accomplished using residual muscles that were related to the activity of the prosthesis prior to amputation or by using EMG activity recorded from other unrelated muscles that have been retrained for prosthetic control [54]. More recently, a technique titled "targeted muscle reinnervation" (TMR) has been developed, in which the residual peripheral nerves left after an amputation are rerouted to muscles left useless by the loss of the limb [55]. These nerves regenerate onto the new musculature allowing the amputee to contract them by trying to perform actions with the missing limb, and providing a new EMG source from which more intuitive control over a powered prosthetic may be derived [56]. All currently available technologies depend on EMG recordings made at the skin's surface, and while muscle-implantable electrodes have been shown to be stable for long periods of time, such devices are almost exclusively used for functional electrical stimulation (FES) rather than EMG recording (with the notable exception of devices intended for diagnostic purposes) [22].

By using myotubes as the electrogenic cell type in a cultured probe approach, we may address several of the shortcomings of current neural interface designs. The increased size and depolarization amplitude of myotubes relative to neurons may make it easier to record depolarization events (Fig. 6 A-C). The favorable geometry and improved electrode sealing will relax some of the constraints on surface characteristics of the electrode itself, making it easier to design cell-favorable biointerfaces (Fig. 6).

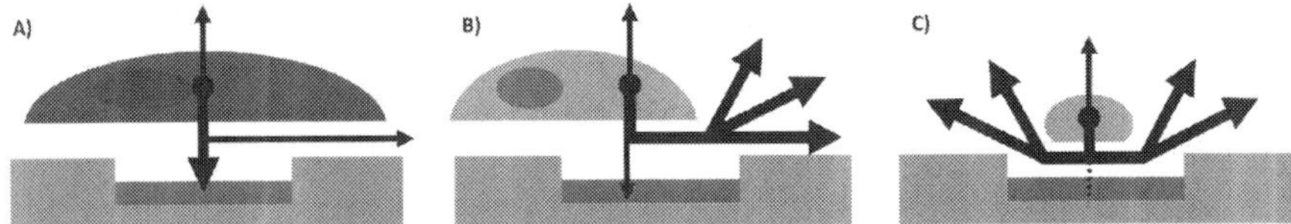

Fig. 6. Cell-electrode contacts shown in cross-section for A) myotube with good electrode coverage, B) neuronal cell body with reduced electrode coverage, and C) a neuronal axon, with minimal electrode coverage. The poor electrode coverage exhibited by the neuron and axon (B, C) allows current to leak into the surrounding environment. Complete sealing is more easily achieved using myotubes, due to their larger size.

4.2 Decision summary

There are three primary ways in which using myotubes rather than neurons and targeting the PNS rather than the CNS will improve on current neural interface designs: 1) the current understanding of cell-electrode contact suggests that the increased physical size and transmembrane current of myotubes will improve electrode sealing [31, 32, 57], 2) the bi-directional communication between myotubes and motoneurons may promote growth of axon collaterals from the native PNS into the cultured probe [34, 47], and 3) current knowledge about neural signaling suggests that targeting the PNS for neural interface implantation will simplify the algorithms involved in decoding motor intention by specifically targeting neural signals that are highly tuned to motor intention and targets a portion of the nervous system where motor intention has already undergone cerebellar processing [11, 21]. We will use cultured myotubes as a biological signal amplifier to record neural signals carried in α-motoneuron axons. Recording selectively from α-motoneuron axons is not feasible with traditional approaches since penetrating electrodes depend on proximity to the relatively large neuron cell bodies [30, 41] (Fig. 6 A-C). Neurites are much smaller and are correspondingly more difficult to record from [30] (Fig. 6 C). Using our approach, the myotube amplifies the signal traveling down the α-motoneuron axon by virtue of coupling through the neuromuscular junction (NMJ) in much the same way a loud speaker amplifies the voice of someone speaking into a microphone.

As discussed above, while the idea of using a myotube adaptor to amplify neural signals does use the regeneration of motoneuron axons onto denervated myotubes as a way of amplifying neural signals, the currently used techniques rely on recordings made on the surface of the skin. These recordings are therefore of large populations of myotubes in their native environment of functional muscle tissue. Recording from myotube populations in this manner may improve the signal acquisition by increasing the amplitude of neural signals, but it likely reduces the specificity of recording (i.e., it is no longer possible to precisely identify individual nerve fibers when they fire). Subsequent design decisions will need to mitigate this loss of specificity, and aim to increase the number of independent signals our device is likely to be able to record.

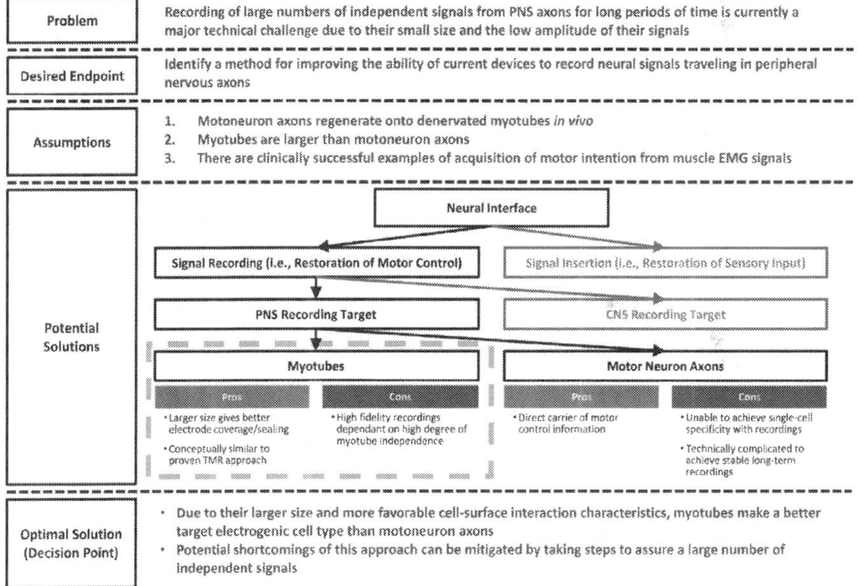

Fig. 7. Design process summary diagram after Decision #3

5. Design decision #4: Invasive vs. noninvasive

Some neural interfaces are designed to record from large populations of neurons in a completely non-invasive way, as in electroencephalography (EEG)-based and myoelectric neural interfaces. At the other end of the scale are neural interfaces designed to record from axons with single cell specificity which have regenerated through the electrode, requiring that the axons be transected prior to electrode implantation. The trade-off between the two is the degree of specificity of the neural recordings. Generally speaking, recording specificity increases with increasing invasiveness, where specificity refers to the ability of an electrode to differentiate between closely related signal sources and invasiveness refers to the extent of tissue damage the electrode is likely to cause. The benefit of specificity is that it increases the number of independent neural signals available from a given neural substrate. In general, a low number of signals and low specificity is acceptable for robust use and limited functionality, while high numbers and selectivity are required for improved spatial resolution and high functionality [21]. While highly specific recordings are believed to be required as a prerequisite for decoding fine motor control from neural signals, the risks associated with an invasive implantation procedure and potential tissue damage and loss of functionality in the long-term need to be considered in the design of any interface. There is some debate regarding the numbers of neuronal recordings necessary to resolve fine motor control, and the relative number will differ depending on the site of recording.

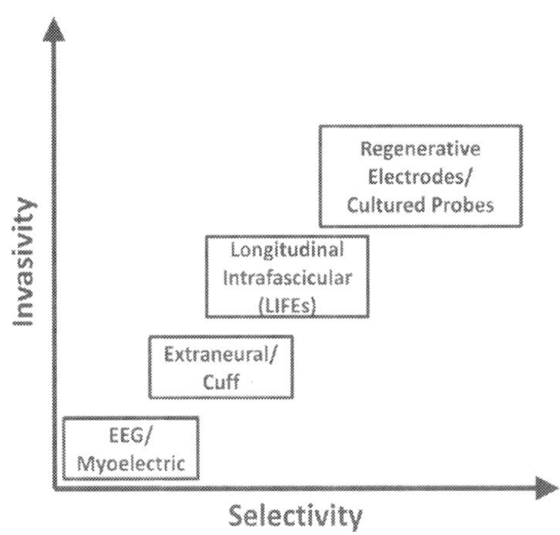

Fig. 8. Invasive PNS interfaces schematized by selectivity and invasiveness (Modified from [58])

Extraneural electrodes, which are relatively noninvasive and nonspecific, attach to the outside of peripheral nerves. The most popular current examples are cuff electrodes [21, 22, 49, 59], which attach to the outside of nerve bundles and record the electroneurgraphic signals of the impulses traveling down the enclosed fascicles (large, related axon clusters). Flat-interface nerve electrodes [21, 22] are a modified cuff designed to separate fascicles for improved recording from individual fascicles within the larger nerve bundle but are still only capable of recording a relatively low number of independent signals because the distance between the recording electrode surface and the axon precludes the identification of single spikes [21, 60]. Other notable problems with this technology are that the electroneurographic (ENG) activity recorded from a nerve with electrodes placed around its periphery is dominated by the excitation of large myelinated fibers and those located at superficial locations.

Intraneural electrodes, which are more invasive but more specific [21, 22], are inserted directly inside of the peripheral nerve where the recording sites can make nearly direct contact with the axons transmitting information. Notable examples include longitudinal intrafascicular electrodes [39], but also a number of other penetrating electrode designs have also been deployed in the PNS [61].

Regenerative electrodes, which are highly invasive and highly specific, are placed in the gap of peripheral nerves that have been fully transected and record from axons which regenerate through the electrode [62]. Problems with this type of interface are currently being addressed by redesigning the recording sites to be tubular rather than planar [63-66]. These tubular recording sites are frequently fabricated by rolling arrays of parallel microchannels, or microgrooves, with incorporated substrate-embedded MEAs into cylindrical constructs for implantation [67, 68]. Generally, axonal regrowth occurs from the proximal end of the transected nerve to the distal end, spanning the natural course of axonal regeneration. However, one group has recently speculated on the idea of a blind "endcap" design, in which regenerating axons would enter and not exit [66]. Furthermore, at least two groups are currently working to address the problem of enhancing such blind-ended axonal regeneration and stabilizing its long-term survival and viability by incorporating biological elements into the endcap, such as growth factors, as are frequently used within the context of artificial nerve conduits [69] [68], pools of living exogenous neurons [66], and even muscle cells [70-72].

Finally, *in vitro* designs have also been proposed, such as the "cultured probe" approach [21, 22, 33]. Cultured probes are a specific type of MEA in which electrogenic cells, typically neurons, are cultured on top of electrode arrays to promote the formation of an *in vitro* functional biointerface. These are electrodes on which nervous tissue has been cultured prior to implantation to develop a good seal with the electrode. The neurons are frequently grown in a way that one or a group of cells contacts only one electrode site. The hope is that upon implantation, the cultured neural tissue will functionally integrate with native neural tissue, establishing a link between electrode and the native nervous system. The theoretical advantage of this design is that the electrode-cell interface may be established and optimized in the laboratory, and because it is biologically active, it will actively promote the ingrowth of axon collaterals from the native nervous tissue. If both of these benefits prove possible, this technique may yield a very selective and efficient interface [22, 33].

5.1 Surface modifications and selectivity

The theoretical advantage of directly inserted probes is that they provide neural signals that are immediately available and do not depend on the variable ingrowth of axon collaterals from the native nervous system. By comparison, the benefit of a cultured probe is that it allows a custom environment to be made to achieve a wide range of desired cellular behavior. Deciding on an MEA design requires consideration of the intended function of the device, how this affects the manufacturing process, and in turn, the cost of the device. In our case, we are trying to create an interface that allows for acquisition of a large number of independent signals from a myotube culture.

One of the most unique aspects of skeletal muscle cells is the large morphological change that myoblast cultures undergo when fusing into contractile myotubes during development. As differentiation and maturation occurs, singly-nucleated myoblasts first adhere to the substrate, then align and fuse into multinucleated myostraps, and finally mature into contractile myotubes, which can be several orders of magnitude larger than their precursor myoblasts [73]. Each step of this process is instructed by each cell's genetic program, communication with neighboring cells [74], and interactions with the chemical [75], physical [76], and electrical [77, 78] extracellular environment. In skeletal myotube cultures, two basic morphologies are usually present: 1) branching multipolar and 2) spindle-shaped bipolar. Because the multipolar myotube is a single, continuous cell, it contracts as a single unit. In the case that two separate myotubes are next to each other but are not fused, they retain the ability to contract independently of one another. Great progress has been made in the field of skeletal muscle tissue engineering, and the wide range of potential applications is reflected in the wide range of tools employed to control myotube growth [79, 80].

Researchers have begun using a number of techniques to induce the formation of patterned neural circuits in order to study neural network function in this simplified context [30, 81-84]. Generally speaking, these techniques can be divided into two groups based on mechanism: 1) mechanically-based techniques, in which the topography of the electrode itself is in some way modified to cause directed cell adhesion or neurite outgrowth [81, 84] and 2) chemically-based techniques, in which chemical guidance cues are patterned onto the electrode surface [30, 82, 83]. The tendency of many cell types to respond in a predictable fashion to topographical features is well known [85]. The scale nature of the topographical modification is important in determining how different cell types will react to the feature or even what portion of the cell will react to the feature. If a feature is too small, the cell will exhibit only a very small reaction to it, while if a feature is too large, a cell may not interact with it enough to show any significant change in behavior.

5.2 Decision summary

We have determined that in order to use a neural interface to acquire motor intention, it must be able to perform the following tasks: 1) acquire a large number of independent signals and 2) remain stable over a wide range of times and mechanical conditions. We have determined that interfacing with myotubes, rather than neuronal cell bodies or axons, is the best way of doing this. Based on our selected cell type and the desired goal for the interface, the optimal interface design will likely be achieved using an implantable, cultured probe technique to maximize the number of potential independent signals that can be acquired. We aim to use tissue engineering tools to direct myotube formation to specific sites and to preserve the independence of individually formed myotubes. These two goals will be accomplished by using topographical cues to both improve cell adhesion to individual electrode contacts and to facilitate the ordered fusion of myocytes into myotubes, thereby creating a predictable pattern of cell-electrode contacts over the entire culture. Using myotubes as the electrogenic cell type alters how we approach electrode design. Because myotubes fuse in a linear pattern, longitudinal trenches will be used to guide myoblast alignment and fusion to specific electrode sites. Because the myotubes are large and have increased depolarization amplitudes relative to neurons, these topographical features can be larger than those used in strictly neuronal applications. Because of the increased size of skeletal muscle cells, the electrodes meant to interface with this cell type can have a larger feature size. This frees us to use a photoresist as our mask and insulator, significantly simplifying the manufacturing process.

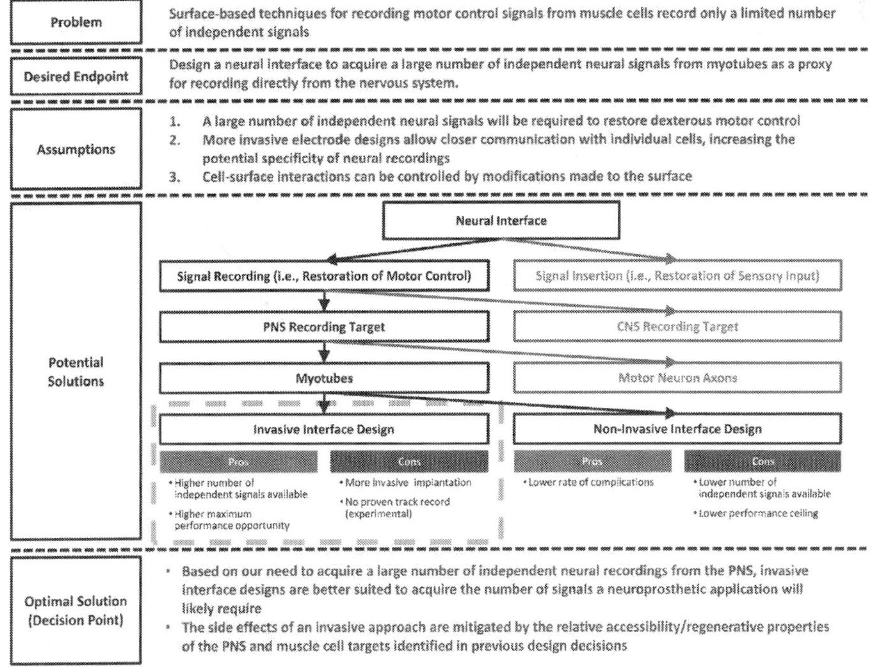

Fig. 9. Design process summary diagram after Decision #4

6. Experimental design

6.1 Proof of principal

In the preceding sections, we hypothesize that an MEA can be designed to guide myotube formation to specific electrode sites and can record myotube extracellular action potentials (EAPs) in a selective manner. It may, therefore, be possible to use this technology as a novel type of neural interface targeted to record from regenerating PNS axons, thereby recording motor intention along its final common pathway. Such an approach to neural interfaces would render the cultured probe effectively a cell-based biosensor [86]. Prior to being deployed in animal studies, these technologies are developed and tested *in vitro* in the form of modified planar MEAs [81, 87-92]. Much of the work done to date interfacing MEAs with cells *in vitro* has been performed with applications in two cell systems [86, 93]: 1) neurons, where the ability to identify the activity of single cells in spike trains through a process called "spike-sorting" is used to identify patterns of population activity and network dynamics and 2) cardiac myocytes, where spatial and temporal resolution allow the measurement of transduction velocity through sheets of linked cardiomyocytes. Although the design decisions we have made to this point have been based firmly on existing scientific knowledge, much of what we have proposed has never been demonstrated explicitly. Because restoring volitional motor control is such a complex clinical problem, the most appropriate next step is to use a highly reductionist system to provide *in vitro* proof of principal for the basic tenants underlying our proposal:

- Topographical cues can direct myotube formation and activity to specific sites
- This affects their electrical independence

6.1.1 Structured myotube cultures

The goal of producing large numbers of independently identifiable myotubes requires that myotube activity be guided to specific locations. Myotube morphology *in vivo* suggests the choice of topographical modifications in the form of parallel grooves as a means of inducing myotube alignment and directing formation to specific locations. Using a video analysis algorithm which analyzes myotube contraction and coordination from captured video files [94], we can analyze myotube contractile activity on unstructured and topographically patterned surfaces (Fig. 10 A-B), allowing us to be among the first researchers to investigate

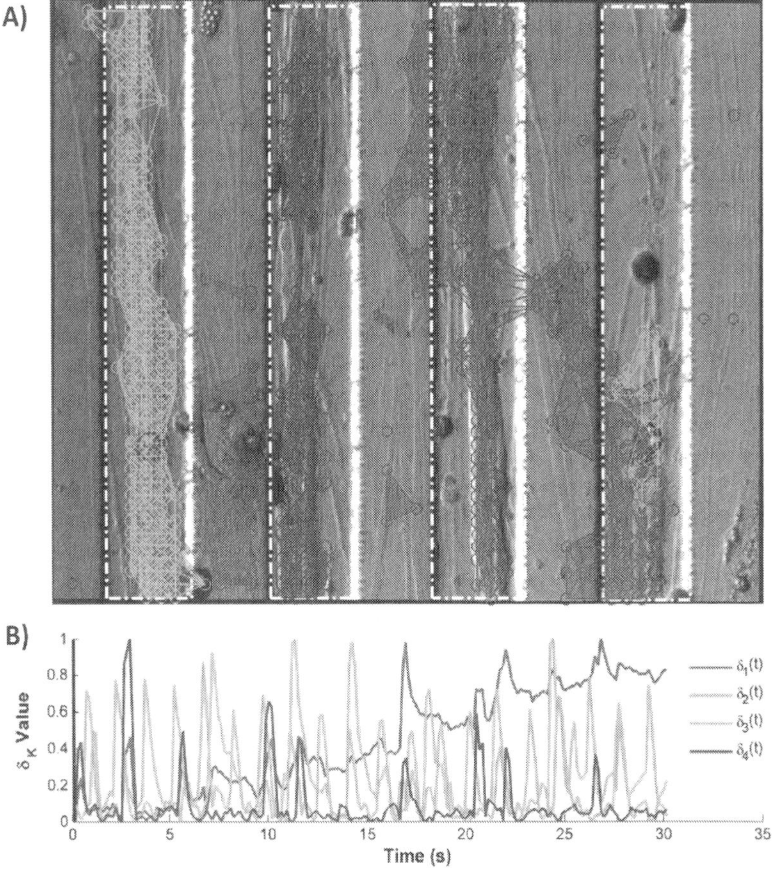

Fig. 10. The effects of microscale topographical trenches on myotube independence. (A) Example labeling of active myotubes in 100 μm trenches (each cell is color coded) (B) Cellular contraction activity tracked over time.

the effect of topography on myotube independence. We have found that rat myotube growth in microscale trenches causes a more rapid onset of spontaneous contractions and changes the spatial distribution of myotube activity compared to cells cultured on unstructured substrates. The percentage of total contractile activity increases within the trenches (Fig. 10 A), with few myotubes spanning multiple trenches. Overall, this indicates that the trenches successfully direct myotube formation to specific sites and facilitates the formation of 1:1 specificity between myotube contractile activity and trench location.

6.1.2 Detecting myotube and neuronal Extracellular Action Potentials (EAPs)

Work in this field to date has focused on neurons and cardiac myocytes [86, 93]. We have expanded on this foundation by successfully culturing primary rat skeletal myoblasts on MEA surfaces and differentiating them into spontaneously contractile myotubes (Fig. 11 A), which generate EAPs detectable with the underlying electrodes (Fig. 11 B). The shape of an EAP is a function of its spatial relationship with the electrode [26, 95], giving each bioelectrically active cell a unique EAP signature. Spike sorting is used to classify EAPs as coming from specific cells (or "units") and allows identification of the activity of several separate units recorded on the same electrode. Neurons have a stable interaction with surface electrodes (Fig. 11 C) and so have a stereotyped EAP morphology (Fig. 11 D). Myotubes are highly dynamic, and therefore, produce EAPs with arbitrary shapes, complicating detection (Fig. 11 B). Using commercially available MEAs and similar spike sorting algorithms, we find that the maximum and minimum µV deflection are on the same order of magnitude between cell types (Fig. 11 E) and that when this is normalized by electrode-specific recording characteristics, myotubes exhibit a slightly higher signal to noise ratio (SNR) (Fig. 11 F), indicating greater ease in identifying them over background. This may be due to their larger size facilitating electrode sealing [31, 96].

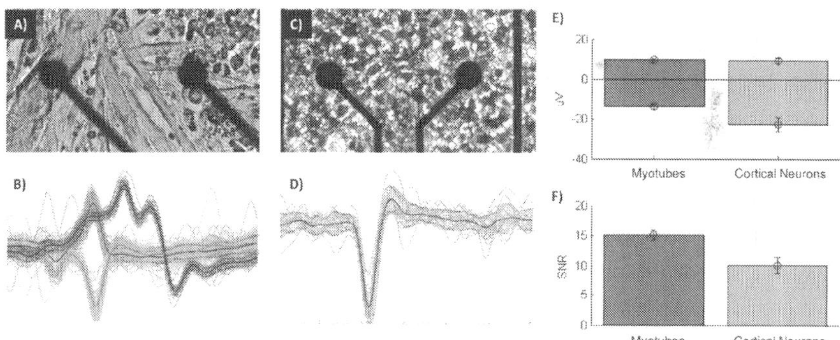

Fig. 11. Myotube vs. neuronal EAPs. Culture morphology and EAPs following spike sorting for (A-B) myotubes and (C-D) cortical neurons. (E) Quantification of EAP amplitude and (F) SNR for myotubes (red) and cortical neurons (blue). Myotube n=154, neuronal n=26, error bars represent the standard error of the mean. Reproduced with permission from [97].

6.1.3 Topographically modified MEA for structured explant and myotube cultures

The next step in our reductionist system is showing that the components above can be integrated on a single device. A prototype device was designed incorporating topographical modifications that direct myotube formation with a substrate embedded MEA. Specifically, two regions of trenches used to direct myotube formation to specific electrode sites are connected to a central field (Fig. 12 A). Two trench regions, oriented horizontally and vertically, consist of four grooves with a single electrode contact at the bottom. The central field contains five recording electrodes to record from multiple points. A large pad is included as an internal reference electrode (not shown). The electrodes are patterned to interface with a Multichannel Systems MEA recording headstage through external contact pads located around the periphery of the chip (Fig. 12 B). The electrode contact and lead pattern is produced by a lift-off technique [98] using standard optical lithography followed by sputtering of a 200/700 Å thick chromium/gold (Cr/Au) conducting electrode layer. A layer of SU-8 PR is then spin-coated onto the electrode-patterned surface and exposed and developed using a topographical feature mask to generate topographical trenches and a central confinement region, also selectively exposing the electrode contact pads located at the bottom of both while leaving the electrode leads electrically insulated from the culture environment. A PDMS ring is affixed to the surface creating a culture chamber around four recording fields, enabling multiple simultaneous experiments (Fig. 12 B). The fabrication process generates devices capable of recording myotubes and neuronal explant EAPs, which withstands repeated cycles through the sterilization-usage-regeneration processes involved in cell culture.

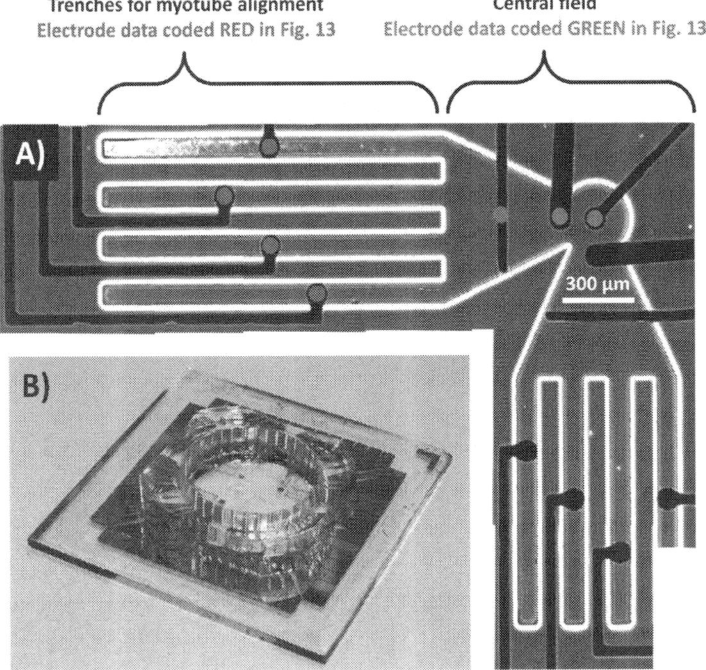

Fig. 12. Myo-MEA prototype. A) Microscopic view of 1 of the 4 recording fields. B) Full prototype including culture chamber.

6.1.4 Explant and myotube monoculture behavior on the myo-MEA

Rat myotubes have been cultured on the myo-MEA to characterize their activity. Myoblasts are seeded on the whole chip surface at 300,000 cells/cm² and allowed to differentiate into myotubes. Prior to seeding, the myo-MEA surface is treated overnight with laminin. Myotube formation is guided to the electrode contact sites by the trenches (Fig. 13 A), and contractility is directed by the topographical cues (Fig. 13 B). Because the entire chip surface was seeded, myotube EAP activity can be observed in the trench regions (red points) and the central regions (green points) (Fig. 13 C). Repeating electrode activation motifs, in which the same electrode activation pattern is repeated at multiple time points, are generated by single myotubes that span multiple electrodes. Total depolarization activity detected a combination of repeating vertical banding patterns (myotubes spanning multiple trenches and the central region) and units that fire in isolation (myotubes confined to a single trench). Obvious repeating activation motifs have been identified by hand (Fig. 13 C – colored rectangles).

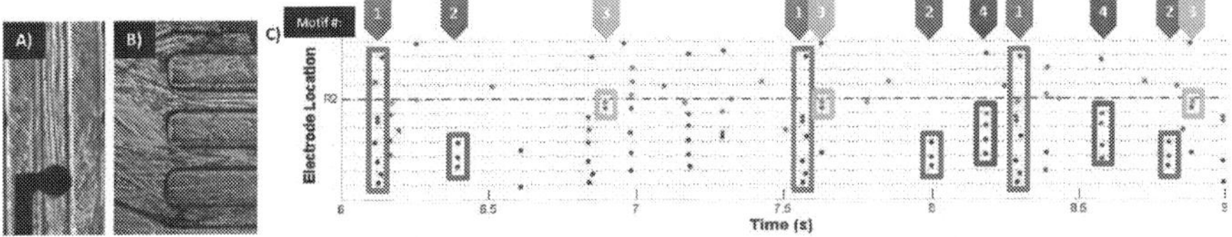

Fig. 13. Myotube formation (A) and contractility (B) guided by trenches. C) Myotube EAPs recorded from one of four fields of a myo-MEA as shown in Fig. 12 A, with example repeating activation motifs identified and labeled by hand (colored rectangles with labeled tags). Units are color-coded based on electrode location (central region = green, trench regions = red). Adjacent points represent adjacent electrodes within the myo-MEA.

Isolation of these activation motifs will ultimately allow us to identify how many independent myotubes are active on an electrode surface and their spatial distribution based on their EAPs. Within the context of the next-generation hybrid-biosensors and neural interfaces, this is an indicator of the number of independent signals the interface can record, and will enable us to optimize the myo-MEA geometry.

7. Clinical adaptations & future directions

The myo-MEA is a neural interface design meant to build on the success of EMG-based and PNS-based approaches to recording motor intent, taking advantage of the larger extracellular voltage changes caused by the depolarization of muscle cells relative to axons and the high degree of cellular specificity available using MEAs with a cultured probe approach (Fig. 14) [12, 81, 92]. The interface described herein (the myo-MEA) employs myotubes integrated with a topographically modified MEA to act as biological signal amplifiers for regenerated PNS motor axons. Using myotubes in this capacity represents a shift from current designs, which aim to record directly from neuronal sources (PNS axons) on a microscale, or from muscle tissue on a macroscale. In the proposed design, the myotubes are coupled to motoneuron axons through the NMJ, contracting in response to the EAPs they transmit. The myo-MEA records the activity of the myotubes as a proxy for recording from the axonal EAP directly. Because the myotube creates higher depolarization potentials, which are more easily detectable than those of a motor axon, this effectively amplifies the signal traveling from the motoneuron axon in the way a loud speaker amplifies the voice of someone speaking into a microphone.

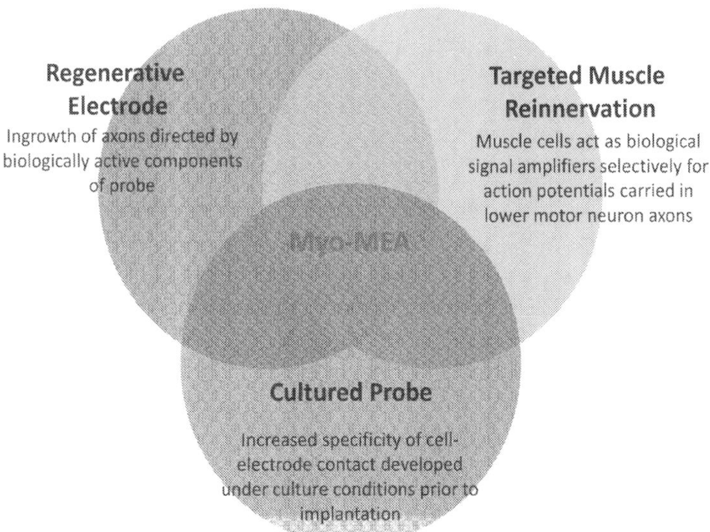

Fig. 14. Ven diagram of conceptual overlap of multiple approaches to neural interfacing and neuroprosthetics contributing to the myo-MEA design process

In the ultimate clinical adaptation of the idea (Fig. 15), we will culture myotubes on an electrode array in a modification of the traditional cultured probe concept [33], specifically employing microscale grooves to accomplish two goals: 1) to direct the formation of myotubes to specific electrode sites and 2) to preserve myotube independence from one another. Once the myotubes have formed and settled to electrode sites (Fig. 15 C), the array will be rolled into a cylinder [67, 68], trapping the myotubes in the resulting channels and putting the device in a conformation ready for implantation as a three dimensional peripheral nerve endcap [66] (Fig. 15 D). After attachment to the severed end of a peripheral nerve, motor axons would be encouraged to grow into the construct by the indwelling myotubes where they would synapse, forming functional neuromuscular junctions [70]. Action potentials carried along these regenerated motor axons would arrive at the myotubes, causing excitation and contraction and generating a microscopic EMG signal for each activated cell. When an individual neuron fires, each associated myotube depolarizes, causing voltage changes at a unique set of electrode contacts. Each neuron has a unique set of associated myotubes due to the synaptic pruning processes occurring at the NMJ, so each neuron will have a distinctive signature of activated electrodes. These EMG signals will therefore contain an encoded version of the motor intention carried along the peripheral nerve, which may be decoded in a similar fashion to the decoding involved in the TMR technique [56].

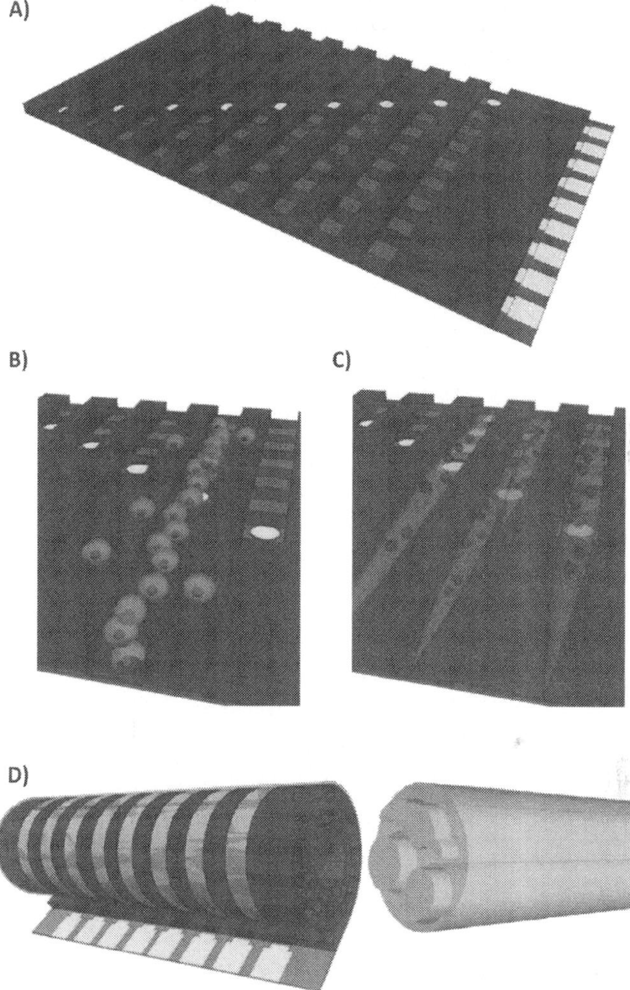

Fig. 15. Conceptual clinical implementation of the myo-MEA. A) A planar MEA is fabricated on a flexible substrate, and topographically modified with grooves. B) The myo-MEA is seeded with myoblasts or satellite cells taken from the patient. C) Myoblasts fuse into myotubes overlying the electrode sites located at the bottom of the grooves. D) The myo-MEA is rolled into a cylinder, trapping the myotubes inside and allowing axonal ingrowth from the open groove ends at the end of the device.

The crucial difference between this proposed device and existing regenerative electrodes is in the origin of the acquired signals. Traditional regenerative electrodes record signals directly from nerve cell axons, while the myo-MEA records signals generated by myotubes. Similarly, our technique relies on a similar re-wiring of the PNS as is involved in TMR. However, it differs substantially in that TMR relies on signals recorded at the skin's surface and which are therefore generated by muscle tissue, while the myo-MEA's recording sites are in direct contact with the myotubes and therefore reflect activity at a cellular level. It is our hope that by creating a neural interface based on a large array of isolated myotubes innervated by regenerated motor axons, we will be able to record a greater number of independent signals, and therefore, improve the efficiency of the interface. Eventual clinical adaptation of the myo-MEA would therefore bring with it the following benefits: **1)** selective regeneration of motor axons onto myotubes provides signals encoding primarily motor intention and largely excludes the sensory information and cognitive information carried by neurons that would not form NMJs with the myotubes, **2)** robust growth of myotubes and adhesion to the MEA surface relative to PNS axons provides a more stable long-term recording platform, and **3)** the neurotrophic activity of myotubes provides cues directing axonal ingrowth. The myo-MEA is uniquely designed to take advantage of myotube properties and their interaction with the PNS to specifically target neural signals that are highly tuned to motor intention, which have already undergone cerebellar processing. In so doing, the design addresses the specific needs of amputees and severe PNS injury patients in a way that other neural interfaces do not, and therefore, increases the chances of its clinical success in this patient base.

8. Acknowledgements

This work was funded by grants from National Science Foundation IBN-0919747; New Jersey Commission on Brain Injury Research, #09-3209-BIR-E-2. CGL and MKK were supported by Biotechnology Fellowship Grant 5T32GM008339 from National Institute of General Medical Sciences. CGL was also supported by a New Jersey Commission on Spinal Cord Injury Predoctoral Fellowship.

9. References

[1] Ziegler-Graham, K., et al., *Estimating the prevalence of limb loss in the United States: 2005 to 2050.* Archives of Physical Medicine and Rehabilitation, 2008. 89(3): p. 422-429.

[2] Noble, J., et al., *Analysis of upper and lower extremity peripheral nerve injuries in a population of patients with multiple injuries.* Journal of Trauma-Injury Infection and Critical Care, 1998. 45(1): p. 116-122.

[3] Robinson, L.R., *Traumatic injury to peripheral nerves.* Muscle & Nerve, 2000. 23(6): p. 863-873.

[4] Biddiss, E. and T. Chau, *Upper-limb prosthetics - Critical factors in device abandonment.* American Journal of Physical Medicine & Rehabilitation, 2007. 86(12): p. 977-987.

[5] Dudkiewicz, I., et al., *Evaluation of prosthetic usage in upper limb amputees.* Disability and Rehabilitation, 2004. 26(1): p. 60-63.

[6] Schultz, A.E., S.P. Baade, and T.A. Kuiken, *Expert opinions on success factors for upper-limb prostheses.* Journal of Rehabilitation Research and Development, 2007. 44(4): p. 483-489.

[7] NINDS. *Neural Interfaces Program: National Institute of Neurological Disorders and Stroke (NINDS):*. Wednesday, January 13, 2010 4:55:09 PM; Available from: http://www.ninds.nih.gov/research/npp/index.htm.

[8] Schwartz, A.B., et al., *Brain-controlled interfaces: Movement restoration with neural prosthetics.* Neuron, 2006. 52(1): p. 205-220.

[9] Hochberg, L.R., et al., *Neuronal ensemble control of prosthetic devices by a human with tetraplegia.* Nature, 2006. 442(7099): p. 164-171.

[10] Craelius, W., *The bionic man: Restoring mobility.* Science, 2002. 295(5557): p. 1018-+.

[11] Micera, S., et al., *Hybrid bionic systems for the replacement of hand function.* Proceedings of the Ieee, 2006. 94(9): p. 1752-1762.

[12] Pfister, B.J., et al., *Neural engineering to produce in vitro nerve constructs and neurointerface.* Neurosurgery, 2007. 60(1): p. 137-141.

[13] Grill, W.M., *Neural Interfaces.* American scientist, 2010. 98(1): p. 48.

[14] NINDS. *NIH Fact Sheet: Cochlear Implants.* 01-13-2010]; Available from: http://www.nih.gov/about/researchresultsforthepublic/CochlearImplants.pdf.

[15] NIDCD. *NIDCD - Cochlear Implants:*. [cited 2010 Wednesday, January 13, 2010 5:12:36 PM]; Available from: http://www.nidcd.nih.gov/health/hearing/coch.asp.

[16] Wang, S. and A. Regalado, *Harnessing Thought to Help the Injured,* in *The Wall Street Journal*2006.

[17] Fischman, J., *bi-on-ics; Etymology: from bi (as in "life") + onics (as in "electronics"); the study of mechanical systems that function like living organisms or parts of living organisms,* in *National Geographic Magazine*2010.

[18] Pelley, S., *The Pentagon's Bionic Arm: Pentagon Is Working To Develop A Life-Changing, High Tech Prosthetic Arm,* in *60 Minutes*:2009.

[19] DARPA, *REVOLUTIONIZING PROSTHETICS PROGRAM.* Fact Sheet - Defense Advanced Research Projects Agency: , 2008.

[20] Lebedev, M.A. and M.A.L. Nicolelis, *Brain-machine interfaces: past, present and future.* Trends in Neurosciences, 2006. 29(9): p. 536-546.

[21] Navarro, X., et al., *A critical review of interfaces with the peripheral nervous system for the control of neuroprostheses and hybrid bionic systems.* Journal of the Peripheral Nervous System, 2005. 10(3): p. 229-258.

[22] Rutten, W.L.C., *Selective electrical interfaces with the nervous system.* Annual Review of Biomedical Engineering, 2002. 4: p. 407-452.

[23] Fagg, A.H., et al., *Biomimetic brain machine interfaces for the control of movement.* Journal of Neuroscience, 2007. 27(44): p. 11842-11846.

[24] Mussa-Ivaldi, F.A. and L.E. Miller, *Brain-machine interfaces: computational demands and clinical needs meet basic neuroscience.* Trends in Neurosciences, 2003. 26(6): p. 329-334.

[25] Buzsaki, G., *Large-scale recording of neuronal ensembles.* Nature Neuroscience, 2004. 7(5): p. 446-451.

[26] Gold, C., et al., *On the origin of the extracellular action potential waveform: A modeling study.* Journal of Neurophysiology, 2006. 95(5): p. 3113-3128.

[27] Brown, E.N., R.E. Kass, and P.P. Mitra, *Multiple neural spike train data analysis: state-of-the-art and future challenges.* Nature Neuroscience, 2004. 7(5): p. 456-461.

[28] Martinez, J., et al., *Realistic simulation of extracellular recordings*. Journal of Neuroscience Methods, 2009. 184(2): p. 285-293.

[29] Madou, M., *Fundamentals of Microfabrication*. CRC Press, 2002.

[30] James, C.D., et al., *Extracellular recordings from patterned neuronal networks using planar microelectrode arrays*. Ieee Transactions on Biomedical Engineering, 2004. 51(9): p. 1640-1648.

[31] Buitenweg, J., et al., *Measurement of Sealing Resistance of Cell-Electrode Interfaces in Neuronal Cultures Using Impedance Spectroscopy*. Medical & Biological Engineering & Computing, 1998. 36: p. 630-637.

[32] Buitenweg, J., W. Rutten, and E. Marani, *Geometry-Based Finite-Element Modeling of the Electrical Contact Betwen a Cultured Neuron and a Microelectrode*. Ieee Transactions on Biomedical Engineering, 2003. 50(4): p. 501-509.

[33] Rutten, W., et al., *Neuroelectronic interfacing with cultured multielectrode arrays toward a cultured probe*. Proceedings of the Ieee, 2001. 89(7): p. 1013-1029.

[34] Dhillon, G.S., et al., *Residual function in peripheral nerve stumps of amputees: Implications for neural control of artificial limbs*. Journal of Hand Surgery-American Volume, 2004. 29A(4): p. 605-615.

[35] Schartz, A.B., *Useful signals from motor cortex*. The Journal of Physiology, 2007(579): p. 581-601.

[36] Brower, V., *When mind meets machine*. Embo Reports, 2005. 6(2): p. 108-110.

[37] Donoghue, J.P., *Connecting cortex to machines: recent advances in brain interfaces*. Nature Neuroscience, 2002. 5: p. 1085-1088.

[38] Di Pino, G., E. Guglielmelli, and P.M. Rossini, *Neuroplasticity in amputees: Main implications on bidirectional interfacing of cybernetic hand prostheses*. Progress in Neurobiology, 2009. 88(2): p. 114-126.

[39] Micera, S., et al., *On the Use of Longitudinal Intrafascicular Peripheral Interfaces for the Control of Cybernetic Hand Prostheses in Amputees*. Ieee Transactions on Neural Systems and Rehabilitation Engineering, 2008. 16(5): p. 453-472.

[40] Hatsopoulos, N.G. and J.P. Donoghue, *The Science of Neural Interface Systems*. Annual Review of Neuroscience, 2009. 32: p. 249-266.

[41] Schwartz, A.B., *Cortical neural prosthetics*. Annual Review of Neuroscience, 2004. 27: p. 487-507.

[42] Schwartz, A.B., *Useful signals from motor cortex*. Journal of Physiology-London, 2007. 579(3): p. 581-601.

[43] Polikov, V.S., P.A. Tresco, and W.M. Reichert, *Response of brain tissue to chronically implanted neural electrodes*. Journal of Neuroscience Methods, 2005. 148(1): p. 1-18.

[44] Szarowski, D.H., et al., *Brain responses to micro-machined silicon devices*. Brain Research, 2003. 983(1-2): p. 23-35.

[45] Ludwig, K.A., et al., *Chronic neural recordings using silicon microelectrode arrays electrochemically deposited with a poly(3,4-ethylenedioxythiophene) (PEDOT) film*. Journal of Neural Engineering, 2006. 3(1): p. 59-70.

[46] Seymour, J.P. and D.R. Kipke, *Neural probe design for reduced tissue encapsulation in CNS*. Biomaterials, 2007. 28(25): p. 3594-3607.

[47] Wells, M.R., et al., *A neuromuscular platform to extract electrophysiological signals from lesioned nerves: A technical note.* Journal of Rehabilitation Research and Development, 2001. 38(4): p. 385-390.

[48] Leuthardt, E.C., et al., *The emerging world of motor neuroprosthetics: A neurosurgical perspective.* Neurosurgery, 2006. 59(1): p. 1-13.

[49] Loeb, G.E. and R.A. Peck, *Cuff electrodes for chronic stimulation and recording of peripheral nerve activity.* Journal of Neuroscience Methods, 1996. 64(1): p. 95-103.

[50] Seniuk, N.A., *Neurotrophic Factors - Role in Peripheral Neuron Survival and Axonal Repair.* Journal of Reconstructive Microsurgery, 1992. 8(5): p. 399-404.

[51] English, A.W., *Cytokines, growth factors and sprouting at the neuromuscular junction.* Journal of Neurocytology, 2003. 32(5-8): p. 943-960.

[52] Parker, P., K. Englehart, and B. Hudgins, *Myoelectric signal processing for control of powered limb prostheses.* Journal of Electromyography and Kinesiology, 2006. 16(6): p. 541-548.

[53] Oskoei, M.A. and H.S. Hu, *Myoelectric control systems-A survey.* Biomedical Signal Processing and Control, 2007. 2(4): p. 275-294.

[54] Light, C.M., et al., *Intelligent multifunction myoelectric control of hand prostheses.* Journal of Medical Engineering & Technology, 2002. 26(4): p. 139-146.

[55] Kuiken, T.A., *Consideration of nerve-muscle grafts to improve the control of artificial arms.* Journal of Technology and Disability, 2003. 15(2): p. 105-111.

[56] Kuiken, T.A., et al., *Targeted Muscle Reinnervation for Real-time Myoelectric Control of Multifunction Artificial Arms.* Jama-Journal of the American Medical Association, 2009. 301(6): p. 619-628.

[57] Fromherz, P., *Sheet conductor model of brain slices for stimulation and recording with planar electronic contacts.* European Biophysics Journal with Biophysics Letters, 2002. 31(3): p. 228-231.

[58] Sergi, P.N., et al., *Biomechanical characterization of needle piercing into peripheral nervous tissue.* Ieee Transactions on Biomedical Engineering, 2006. 53(11): p. 2373-2386.

[59] Lertmanorat, Z., F.W. Montague, and D.M. Durand, *A Flat Interface Nerve Electrode With Integrated Multiplexer.* Ieee Transactions on Neural Systems and Rehabilitation Engineering, 2009. 17(2): p. 176-182.

[60] Wodlinger, B. and D.M. Durand, *Localization and Recovery of Peripheral Neural Sources With Beamforming Algorithms.* Ieee Transactions on Neural Systems and Rehabilitation Engineering, 2009. 17(5): p. 461-468.

[61] Branner, A., R.B. Stein, and R.A. Normann, *Selective stimulation of cat sciatic nerve using an array of varying-length microelectrodes.* Journal of Neurophysiology, 2001. 85(4): p. 1585-1594.

[62] Lago, N., et al., *Neurobiological assessment of regenerative electrodes for bidirectional interfacing injured peripheral nerves.* Ieee Transactions on Biomedical Engineering, 2007. 54(6): p. 1129-1137.

[63] Lacour, S.P., et al., *Long Micro-Channel Electrode Arrays: A Novel Type of Regenerative Peripheral Nerve Interface.* Ieee Transactions on Neural Systems and Rehabilitation Engineering, 2009. 17(5): p. 454-460.

[64] FitzGerald, J.J., et al., *Microchannels as axonal amplifiers*. Ieee Transactions on Biomedical Engineering, 2008. 55(3): p. 1136-1146.

[65] FitzGerald, J.J., et al., *Microchannel Electrodes for Recording and Stimulation: In Vitro Evaluation*. Ieee Transactions on Biomedical Engineering, 2009. 56(5): p. 1524-1534.

[66] Wieringa, P.A.W., R.W.F.; le Feber, J.; Rutten, W.L.C., *Neural growth into a microchannel network: Towards A regenerative neural interface*, in *Neural Engineering, 2009. NER '09. 4th International IEEE/EMBS Conference on*2009. p. 51-55.

[67] Lacour, S.P., et al., *Polyimide micro-channel arrays for peripheral nerve regenerative implants*. Sensors and Actuators a-Physical, 2008. 147(2): p. 456-463.

[68] Suzuki, T., et al., *Regeneration-Type Nerve Electrode Using Bundled Microfluidic Channels*. Electronics and Communications in Japan, 2009. 92(4): p. 29-34.

[69] Huang, Y.C. and Y.Y. Huang, *Biomaterials and strategies for nerve regeneration*. Artificial Organs, 2006. 30(7): p. 514-522.

[70] Egeland, B.M., et al., *Engineering and development of a stable, low-impedance, bioelectrical peripheral nerve interface*. Journal of the American College of Surgeons, 2009. 209(3): p. S76-S76.

[71] Kirkendoll, S., *Tissue engineering could improve hand use for wounded soldiers*, October 14, 2009, University of Michigan Health System Newsroom.

[72] Wells, M., M. Zanakis, and J. Ricci, *Efficacy of a Neural Interface for Potential Use in Limb Prosthetics*, 1996, NSF: NY.

[73] Sanes, J.R. and J.W. Lichtman, *Development of the vertebrate neuromuscular junction*. Annual Review of Neuroscience, 1999. 22: p. 389-442.

[74] Clark, P., et al., *Alignment of myoblasts on ultrafine gratings inhibits fusion in vitro*. International Journal of Biochemistry & Cell Biology, 2002. 34(7): p. 816-825.

[75] Molnar, P., et al., *Photolithographic patterning of C2C12 myotubes using vitronectin as growth substrate in serum-free medium*. Biotechnology Progress, 2007. 23(1): p. 265-268.

[76] Engler, A.J., et al., *Myotubes differentiate optimally on substrates with tissue-like stiffness: pathological implications for soft or stiff microenvironments*. Journal of Cell Biology, 2004. 166(6): p. 877-887.

[77] Liao, I.C., et al., *Effect of Electromechanical Stimulation on the Maturation of Myotubes on Aligned Electrospun Fibers*. Cellular and Molecular Bioengineering, 2008. 1(2-3): p. 133-145.

[78] Au, H.T.H., et al., *Interactive effects of surface topography and pulsatile electrical field stimulation on orientation and elongation of fibroblasts and cardiomyocytes*. Biomaterials, 2007. 28(29): p. 4277-4293.

[79] Koning, M., et al., *Current opportunities and challenges in skeletal muscle tissue engineering*. Journal of Tissue Engineering and Regenerative Medicine, 2009. 3(6): p. 407-415.

[80] Rowlands, A.S., J.E. Hudson, and J.J. Cooper-White, *From scrawny to brawny: the quest for neomusculogenesis; smart surfaces and scaffolds for muscle tissue engineering*. Expert Review of Medical Devices, 2007. 4(5): p. 709-728.

[81] Zeck, G. and P. Fromherz, *Noninvasive neuroelectronic interfacing with synaptically connected snail neurons immobilized on a semiconductor chip*. Proceedings of the

National Academy of Sciences of the United States of America, 2001. 98(18): p. 10457-10462.

[82] Chang, J.C., G.J. Brewer, and B.C. Wheeler, *Modulation of neural network activity by patterning*. Biosensors & Bioelectronics, 2001. 16(7-8): p. 527-533.

[83] Chang, J.C., G.J. Brewer, and B.C. Wheeler, *Neuronal network structuring induces greater neuronal activity through enhanced astroglial development*. Journal of Neural Engineering, 2006. 3(3): p. 217-226.

[84] Jimbo, Y., H.P. Robinson, and A. Kawana, *Simultaneous measurement of intracellular calcium and electrical activity from patterned neural networks in culture*. IEEE Trans Biomed Eng, 1993. 40(8): p. 804-10.

[85] Flemming, R.G., et al., *Effects of synthetic micro- and nano-structured surfaces on cell behavior*. Biomaterials, 1999. 20(6): p. 573-588.

[86] Kovacs, G.T.A., *Electronic sensors with living cellular components*. Proceedings of the Ieee, 2003. 91(6): p. 915-929.

[87] Zhang, J.Y., et al., *Combined topographical and chemical micropatterns for templating neuronal networks*. Biomaterials, 2006. 27(33): p. 5734-5739.

[88] Morin, F., et al., *Constraining the connectivity of neuronal networks cultured on microelectrode arrays with microfluidic techniques: A step towards neuron-based functional chips*. Biosensors & Bioelectronics, 2006. 21(7): p. 1093-1100.

[89] Ravula, S.K., et al., *A compartmented neuronal culture system in microdevice format*. Journal of Neuroscience Methods, 2007. 159(1): p. 78-85.

[90] Berdondini, L., et al., *A microelectrode array (MEA) integrated with clustering structures for investigating in vitro neurodynamics in confined interconnected sub-populations of neurons*. Sensors and Actuators B-Chemical, 2006. 114(1): p. 530-541.

[91] Nam, Y., K. Musick, and B.C. Wheeler, *Application of a PDMS microstencil as a replaceable insulator toward a single-use planar microelectrode array*. Biomedical Microdevices, 2006. 8(4): p. 375-381.

[92] Maher, M.P., et al., *The neurochip: a new multielectrode device for stimulating and recording from cultured neurons*. Journal of Neuroscience Methods, 1999. 87(1): p. 45-56.

[93] Stett, A., et al., *Biological application of microelectrode arrays in drug discovery and basic research*. Analytical and Bioanalytical Chemistry, 2003. 377(3): p. 486-495.

[94] Langhammer, C.G., J.D. Zahn, and B.L. Firestein, *Identification and Quantification of Skeletal Myotube Contraction and Association In Vitro by Video Microscopy*. Cytoskeleton, 2010.

[95] Bove, M., et al., *Interfacing Cultured Neurons to Planar Substrate Microelectrodes - Characterization of the Neuron-to-Microelectrode Junction*. Bioelectrochemistry and Bioenergetics, 1995. 38(2): p. 255-265.

[96] Buitenweg, J.R., W.L.C. Rutten, and E. Marani, *Extracellular stimulation window explained by a geometry-based model of the neuron-electrode contact*. Ieee Transactions on Biomedical Engineering, 2002. 49(12): p. 1591-1599.

[97] Langhammer, C.G., et al., *Skeletal myotube integration with planar microelectrode arrays in vitro for spatially selective recording and stimulation: A comparison of neuronal and myotube extracellular action potentials*. Biotechnology Progress, 2011. Accepted.

[98] Park, B.Y., R. Zaouk, and M.J. Madou, *Fabrication of Microelectrodes Using the Lift-Off Technique*, in *Methods in Molecular Biology*, S.D. Minteer, Editor, Humana Press Inc.: Totowa, NJ. p. 23-26.

18

A Case Study of Applying Weighted Least Squares to Calibrate a Digital Maximum Respiratory Pressures Measuring System

José L. Ferreira, Flávio H. Vasconcelos and Carlos J. Tierra-Criollo
Biomedical Engineering Laboratory
Universidade Federal de Minas Gerais, Belo Horizonte,
Brazil

1. Introduction

In recent years, technological advances in the area of medical equipments have allowed the use of these devices for different types of illness diagnosis and treatment of patients. Thereby, nowadays a lot of quantities and parameters related to the health state of the patient can be measured and used by clinicians to take a decision about the correct conduct to be adopted during the treatment.

However, despite the huge advances in the area, a question always must be arisen related to the use of medical equipments: the measurements are reliable? According to Lira (2002) and Parvis & Vallan (2002), such reliability is fundamental and a wrong evaluated value by the medical equipment can affect any decision and even compromise the condition of a patient at all. Therefore, the use of medical equipments requires periodical calibration and evaluation of measurement uncertainty.

All measuring instruments must be calibrated, to be considered adequate for use (Ferreira et al. 2010). VIM (2008) defines calibration as an operation that, under specified conditions, in a first step, establishes a relation between the quantity values with measurement uncertainties provided by measurement standards and corresponding indications with associated measurement uncertainties and in second step, uses this information to establish a relation for obtaining a measurement result from an indication.

This fact drew the attention of metrology and health organisms all around the world that have written a number of guides and technical recommendation for instrument calibration and determination of uncertainty for medical instrumentation before use in order to ensure high quality of the measurements. The Guide (GUM, 2003) is the result of a joint international committee whose aim was to publish a guide for uncertainty evaluation to be used as conventional guidelines in several different countries. That is the case of Brazil whose local NMI (National Measurement Institute), the INMETRO (Brazilian National Institute of Metrology, Standardization and Industrial Quality) has adopted the Guide to rule device calibration and its measurement uncertainty evaluation in the country.

In the Guide, the idea that the result of a measurement is only complete if the measured quantity value and the measured uncertainty are evaluated is reinforced. The Guide also presents the procedures that must be followed during this process, and indicates the weight least squares (WLS) method as a way to perform it.

The goals of this chapter is to present a case study of the application of weighted least squares to carry out the calibration and uncertainty evaluation of a digital maximum respiratory pressures measuring system: a prototype of manovacuometer developed at the *Biomedical Engineering Laboratory* (NEPEB) of Universidade Federal de Minas Gerais (UFMG).

In section 2, a description of the mathematical basis of the use of WLS for calibration is summarized. The measuring procedure employed in this work and the main features of the prototype are described in sections 3 and 4, where the calibration method is discussed as well. In sections 5, 6 and 7 the obtained results are presented, followed by the sections 8 and 9 in which presentation of discussion, conclusion and suggestion for future works is done.

2. The use of WLS for calibration

As aforementioned, the method of weighted least squares (Lira, 2002; GUM, 2003; Mathioulakis & Belessiotis, 2000; Press *et al.*, 1996) can be used for implementing calibration and uncertainty evaluation.

According to Mathioulakis & Belessiotis (2000), during the calibration process the J output values X_js measured by the equipment under calibration are compared to reference values Y_js applied on its input. In other words, a mathematical model with N parameters a_n is proposed in order to represent J calibration points (Y_j, X_j) as accurate as possible. To determine the values of a_n, the maximum likelihood estimator for the model parameters is calculated by minimizing the differences between measured and estimated data (Press *et al.*, 1996):

$$\sum_{j=1}^{J}\left[Y_j - y\left(X_j; a_1, a_2, \ldots a_N\right)\right]^2 \tag{1}$$

Equation (1) refers to the maximum likelihood estimator used for the least squares (LS) fitting whose name is derived from the fact that minimization is done taking into account the squares of the differences between measured and estimated data. In the case of the calibration points (Y_j, X_j), there are also standard deviations (or measurement uncertainties u_j) associated to the raw data that are not considered in (1). Because of this fact, an alternative maximum likelihood estimator, the chi-square function χ^2, is suggested by Mathioulakis & Belessiotis (2000), and this new approch is also known as *weighted least squares method* (WLS):

$$\chi^2 = \sum_{j=1}^{J}\frac{\left[Y_j - y\left(X_j; a_1, a_2, \ldots a_N\right)\right]^2}{u_j^2} \tag{2}$$

Therefore, by the WLS method, adjust uncertainties of the raw data are taken into account, situation that better describes the existing conditions at this work. Also as regarding as the case on focus, the proposed fit model is the bi-parametric curve:

$$y(X) = aX + b \tag{3}$$

where a is the slope and b is its intercept. Thus, considering this linear fitting of equation (3) the chi-squared function χ^2 becomes:

$$\chi^2(a,b) = \sum_{j=1}^{J} \frac{\left(Y_j - b - aX_j\right)^2}{u_{y,j}^2 + a^2 u_{x,j}^2} \tag{4}$$

Minimization of (4) over a and b is not trivial and requires the use of numerical techniques. As suggested by Press *et al.* (1996) and implemented at this work, the solution for (4) is obtained by scaling "the y_js so as to have variance equal to the x_j then to do a conventional linear fitting with weights derived from the (scaled) sum $u_{y,j}^2 + u_{x,j}^2$ ". Such a procedure is repeated until a determined limit for iterations can be reached.

To estimate the slope a, and the intercept b of (3) and the associated uncertainties, u_a e u_b, Mathioulakis & Belessiotis (2000) indicate the following equation:

$$\left(\mathbf{K}^T \cdot \mathbf{K}\right) \cdot \mathbf{C} = \mathbf{K}^T \cdot \mathbf{L} \tag{5}$$

where $\mathbf{C}$ is a vector whose elements are the fitted coefficients a and b; and $\mathbf{Q} = (\mathbf{K}^T . \mathbf{K})^{-1}$ is a matrix whose diagonal elements are the variances of a ($q_{2,2}$) and b ($q_{1,1}$). The off-diagonal elements $q_{1,2} = q_{2,1}$ are the covariances between these parameters. $\mathbf{K}$ is the matrix with $J \times 2$ components:

$$\mathbf{K} = \begin{bmatrix} k_{1,1} & k_{1,2} \\ \cdot & \cdot \\ \cdot & \cdot \\ \cdot & \cdot \\ k_{J,1} & k_{J,2} \end{bmatrix}, \tag{6}$$

with $k_{j,1} = \dfrac{1}{w_j}$ and $k_{j,2} = \dfrac{X_i}{w_j}$.

$\mathbf{L}$ is the vector:

$$\mathbf{L} = \begin{bmatrix} Y_1 / w_1 \\ \cdot \\ \cdot \\ \cdot \\ Y_J / w_J \end{bmatrix} \tag{7}$$

As can be seen from (6) and (7), $\mathbf{K}$ and $\mathbf{L}$ are weighted inversely by the pounds w_j. This fact suggests the name of the WLS calibration method.

3. The developed measuring system

Knowledge of maximum respiratory pressures, i.e., maximum inspiratory pressure (PImax) and maximum expiratory pressure (PEmax) exerted by muscles of respiratory system, can be used to a number of purposes, such as diagnosing of respiratory system diseases, convalescence of muscle strength during aging, the need to release mechanical ventilation and to evaluate the efficiency of a physiotherapeutic treatment. Furthermore, it is a simple, non-invasive way and reproducible for strength quantification of the respiratory system muscles (Black & Hyatt, 1969).

Maximum respiratory pressures can be measured with equipments so-called manovacuometers, designed for measuring supra-atmospheric (manometer) and sub-atmospheric pressures (vacuometer), and can be either analog or digital (Ferreira *et al.*, 2010). During the daily clinical and research practice, some problems are reported for those types of equipments. For instance, the former has complex calibration and is prone to reading errors. Both types of instruments have limitations associated to perform single reading and to allow tracing measurement curves. Due to these limits encountered for commercial manovacuometers, a digital manuovacuometer (DM) was designed at the NEPEB (Oliveira Júnior *et al.*, 2008) with some features whereby the drawbacks presented by the others existing manovacuometers could be overcome.

The prototype of digital measuring system includes two operating modules: a module for acquiring the analog pressure signal and a second one, responsible for A/D conversion that can be connected to a computer through a USB interface, as can be regarded in figure 1.

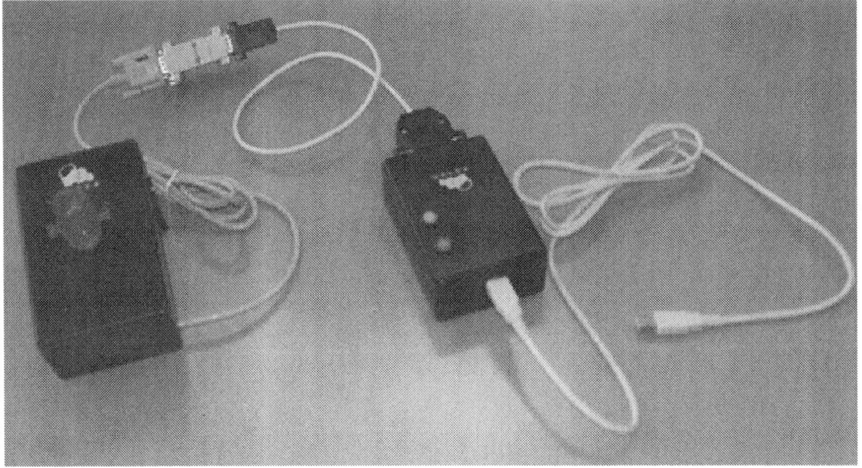

Fig. 1. The digital manovacuometer designed in our lab (NEPEB) and its operating modules. Adapted from Ferreira *et al.* (2010).

The analog pressure signals are collected by the acquisition module, within two piezoresistive differential sensors are employed (figure 2), one for measuring PImax and other for PEmax. The main operating characteristics of the sensor can be found in table 1 (Freescale, 2004). Another characteristic of this sensor which is important to be emphasized is that pressure on side P1 must be always higher than on P2. Thus, sensor 1 measures PEmax (PE applied on P1) and sensor 2 measures PImax (PI applied on P2). The sensors have a pressure range from 0 up to 50 kPa.

Characteristic	Symbol	Minimum	Typical	Maximum	Unit
Pressure Range	P_{CP}	0	-	50	kPa
Supply Voltage	V_F	4.75	5.00	5.25	Vdc
Supply Current	I_o	-	7.0	10.0	mAdc
Minimum Pressure Offset (0 to 85 °C) @ V_F = 5.0 Volts	V_{off}	0.088	0.20	0.313	Vdc
Full Scale Output (0 to 85 °C) @ V_F = 5.0 Volts	V_{FSO}	4.587	4.70	4.813	Vdc
Full Scale Span (0 to 85 °C) @ V_F = 5.0 Volts	V_{FSS}	-	4.5	-	Vdc
Accuracy	-	-	-	+/- 2.5%	V_{FSS}
Sensitivity	V/P	-	90	-	mV/kPa
Response Time	t_R	-	1.0	-	ms
Output Source Current at Full Scale Output	I_{o+}	-	0.1	-	mAdc
Warm-Up Time	-	-	20	-	ms
Offset Stability	-	-	+/- 0.5	-	%V_{FSS}

Table 1. Operating characteristics of the sensor MPX5050. Adapted from Freescale (2004).

According to Oliveira Júnior *et al.* (2008), the analog to digital conversion module has a built-in microcontroller that includes 13 channels, 10 bits A/D converter, and emulates the RS232 communication protocol that allows transferring data to a computer through an USB interface. The signal frequency of respiratory flow ranges from 0 to 40 Hz (Olson, 2010). Thus, a Butterworth low-pass, anti-aliasing filter, 40 Hz cutoff frequency (order 2) was used for a sampling frequency of 1 kHz (Oliveira Júnior *et al.*, 2008).

4. Protocols for collecting calibration points and uncertainty evaluation

For collecting the calibration points, the adopted procedures were in compliance with protocols described by INMETRO (INMETRO, 2008; INMETRO, 1997). According to such procedures, at first the pressure applied on the sensors is increased up to superior pressure range value and then decreased to 0 kPa. Each pressure value has to be applied during approximately five seconds and, after that, the average voltage is measured at the output of the manovacuometer.

The above procedure was performed four times for each sensor, and the average voltage, V_m, for both rising and fall curves were obtained for each sensor (table 2). Two extra points, whose pressure value is higher than superior range value (50 kPa), were inserted into the set of calibration points to check the starting region of non-linearity on the curve. In order to check for drifting two groups of data were collected in a time interval of six months from each other.

The calibration points for the sensor 2 (rising curve – first group of collected data) and its uncertainties are showed in table 2. P_r corresponds to the pressure values applied on the input of the sensors.

P_r (kPa)	u_{Pr} (kPa)	V_m (V)	u_{Vm} (V)
4.0	0.1	0.458	0.002
9.3	0.1	0.926	0.007
12.0	0.1	1.175	0.002
13.3	0.1	1.291	0.004
20.0	0.1	1.890	0.004
26.7	0.1	2.496	0.005
33.3	0.1	3.097	0.005
40.0	0.1	3.709	0.004
46.7	0.1	4.333	0.003
53.3	0.1	4.941	0.005

Table 2. Reference pressure, output voltage values and associated uncertainties – sensor 2 (rising curve – first group of collected data). Adapted from Ferreira *et al.* (2010).

To perform the measurements, the schematic implementation depicted in figure 2 was used as well.

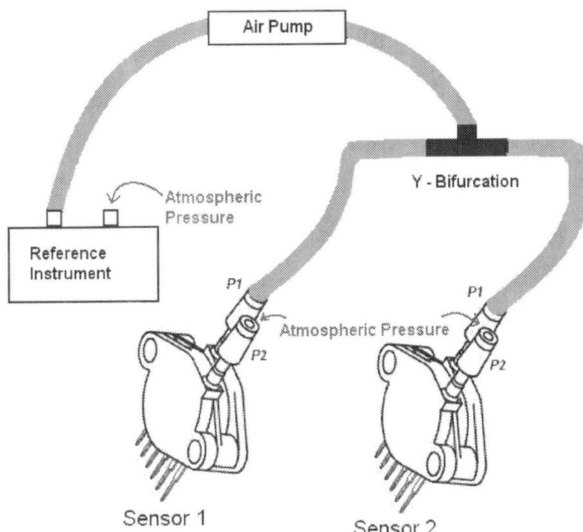

Fig. 2. Schematic implementation for prototype calibration (Adapted from Ferreira *et. al.*, 2010).

The methodology for prototype calibration employed the linear fitting using weighted least squares abovementioned. It was chosen to obtain curve fitting for the average rising and for the average fall curves for each sensor (Ferreira *et al.*, 2008). Concerning the measurement uncertainty for that prototype, it was determined according to the Guide (GUM, 2003).

The instrument used as standard (*Reference Instrument* – figure 2) during the calibration of the prototype was with 0.03% reported expanded uncertainty, for a coverage factor $k = 2$ and coverage probability of 95.45%.

5. Estimation of the calibration curves

Figures 3 and 4 depict the calibration points (V_m, P_r) and the associated mean transfer functions (increasing input pressure and decreasing input pressure – rising and fall) for both

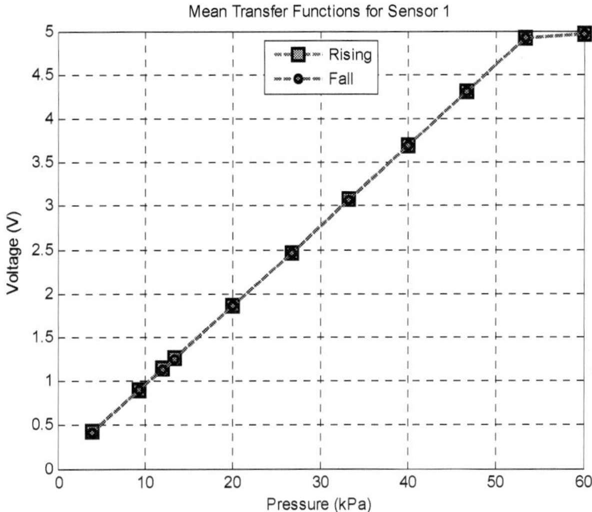

Fig. 3. Mean transfer functions for sensor 1 (first group of collected data) showing the calibration points (adapted from Ferreira *et. al.*, 2008).

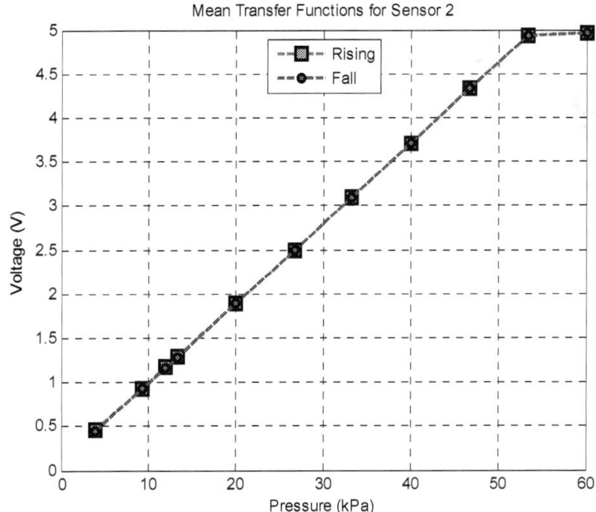

Fig. 4. Mean transfer functions for sensor 2 (first group of collected data) showing the calibration points (adapted from Ferreira *et. al.*, 2008).

sensors (first group of collected data) of the NEPEB manovacuometer. Regarding these figures, it can be noticed that linearity is present up to $P_r = 53.3$ kPa. Thus, calculations were carried out also considering the calibration point with this pressure value and the calibration point with pressure equal to 60 kPa was discarded.

As mentioned in secction 4, table 2 contains the calibration points for sensor 2 (rising curve – first group of collected data) and associated uncertaintes. Estimation of these uncertainties is in accordance with guidelines indicated in the Guide (2003). In the case of the uncertainty u_{Pr}, it was evaluated using the related standard expanded uncertainty and the resolution of the display device of the reference manovacuometer as follows:

$$u_{Pr} = \left(\frac{0.03\%}{2}\right) P_r . \tag{8}$$

In turn, the uncertainty u_{Vm} was estimated based on fluctuation of the repeated readings (prototype output voltage) around each calibration point (Mathioulakis & Belessiotis, 2000) correspondent to the standard deviation of the mean, u_V (type A uncertainty), that is:

$$u_{Vm} = \frac{s_V}{\sqrt{n}} . \tag{9}$$

where s_V corresponds to standard deviation of the voltage values for the four rising (falling) curves and n is the number of points ($n = 4$, in that case).

As discussed in section 2, the proposed model used for fitting the calibration points is described by equation (3). Thereby, considering the slope a and the intercept b, application of a reference pressure value on the input of the sensor results to a determined voltage V_m on its output, which, in turn, has to correspond to the pressure P_{rc}, measured by the prototype, i.e.:

$$P_{rc} = b + a V_m . \tag{10}$$

where P_{rc} is the pressure in kiloPascal that corresponds to the voltage V_m, indicated at the display of the prototype (Ferreira *et al.*, 2008a).

Solution of the expression (5) provides the values of the parameters of (10), their uncertainties and the covariance between the parameters, $Cov(a,b)$. In table 3, results calculated for both groups of experimental data (collected in between six month apart, as mentioned earlier) can be regarded.

Group of collected data	Curve		a (kPa/V)	u_a (kPa/V)	b (kPa)	u_b (kPa)	$Cov(a,b)$ (kPa)
1st	Sensor 1	Rising	10.9756	0.0230	-0.5570	0.0638	-1.25×10^{-3}
		Fall	10.9702	0.0221	-0.4865	0.0619	-1.16×10^{-3}
	Sensor 2	Rising	10.9994	0.0238	-0.8903	0.0668	-1.36×10^{-3}
		Fall	10.9913	0.0219	-0.8190	0.0621	-1.16×10^{-3}
2nd	Sensor 1	Rising	10.9820	0.0385	-0.6349	0.1074	-3.56×10^{-3}
		Fall	10.9991	0.0331	-0.8145	0.0909	-2.57×10^{-3}
	Sensor 2	Rising	10.9561	0.0384	-0.3471	0.1042	-3.42×10^{-3}
		Fall	10.9746	0.0347	-0,5133	0.0903	-2.65×10^{-3}

Table 3. Values for the parameters a and b, their uncertainties u_a and u_b and $Cov(a,b)$.

6. Consistency analysis

The importance for verifying the consistency analysis between the fitted model and experimental data which is implemented by using the so-called chi-squared test is highlighted by Lira (2002) and Cox & Harris (2006).

Lira (2002) mentions that the minimum value of the chi-squared function $\chi 2$, indicated by the expression (4) and denoted as $\chi^2_{\min}$ can be represented by a chi-squared distribution with $\upsilon = p - q$ degrees of freedom in such a way that $\chi^2_{\min}$ is close to $p - q$, where p is the number of calibration points and q is the number of model outputs. In other words, the Birge ratio represented in (11),

$$Bi = \left(\frac{\chi^2_{\min}}{p-q} \right)^{\!1/2}, \tag{11}$$

should be approximately equal to one. Hence, the closer to unity is the value of Bi, the better the model is adjusted to data.

Lira (2002) adds that a value for the Birge ratio close to the unity is not a proof that the model is correct. However, when Bi is significantly different from 1, it can be interpreted that something within the model is wrong.

The values of B_i for the adjusted models and both set of experimental data of the prototype manovacuometer are presented in table 4.

Birge Ratio	Group of collected data	Sensor 1		Sensor 2	
		Rising Curve	Fall Curve	Rising Curve	Fall Curve
Bi	1	1,0755	1,0716	1,0412	1,0869
	2	0,6949	0,6927	0,6877	0,8294

Table 4. Birge ratio for sensor 1 and sensor 2 curves and both groups of collect data with $p = 10$ points and $q = 1$ output.

7. Evaluation of measurement uncertainty

As mentioned earlier, the Guide (2003) mentions that any measurement result is composed by a numeric value indicating the quantity estimated value and by the measurement uncertainty. Frequently, the measurement uncertainty is estimated by using a mathematical measurement model which is a function which contains every quantity, including all corrections and correction factors that can contribute with a significant component of uncertainty to the measurement result (Ferreira et al., 2010).

The Guide also indicates the application of the *the law of propagation of uncertainties* to the mathematical measurement model mentioned above for estimation of the measurement uncertainty:

$$u_c^2(y) = \sum_{i=1}^{N} \left(\frac{\partial f}{\partial x_i} \right)^2 u^2(x_i) + 2 \sum_{i=1}^{N-1} \sum_{j=i+1}^{N} \frac{\partial f}{\partial x_i} \frac{\partial f}{\partial x_j} u(x_i, x_j) \tag{12}$$

According to Mathioulakis & Belessiotis (2000), the proposed model to estimate uncertainty, u_{Pc}, is derived from applying (12) to equation (10):

$$u_{Pc}^2 = \left(\frac{\partial P_{rc}}{\partial V_m}\right)^2 u^2(V_m) + \left(\frac{\partial P_{rc}}{\partial b}\right)^2 u^2(b) + \left(\frac{\partial P_{rc}}{\partial a}\right)^2 u^2(a) + 2\frac{\partial P_{rc}}{\partial b}\frac{\partial P_{rc}}{\partial xa}u(a,b) \qquad (13)$$

which results (Ferreira *et al.*, 2008):

$$u_{Pc} = \left(a^2 u_{Vm}^2 + u_b^2 + V_m^2 u_a^2 + 2V_m Cov(b,a)\right)^{1/2} \qquad (14)$$

where the uncertainty u_{Vm} is estimated considering the type A uncertainty, u_V, and the resolution of NEPEB manovacuometer, u_R. As example of estimation of the measurement uncertainty for the prototype, it was chosen the calibration point of the table 2 whose value of $P_r = 26.6$ kPa. Thereby:

$$u_V = \frac{s_V}{\sqrt{n}} = \frac{0.010}{\sqrt{4}} = 0.005V , \qquad (15)$$

$$u_R = \frac{0.001}{\sqrt{3}} = 0.0006V , \qquad (16)$$

$$u_{Vm}^2 = u_V^2 + u_R^2 \Rightarrow u_{Vm} = 0.005V . \qquad (17)$$

Taking account the values calculated by (15), (16) and (17) as well as those of the parameters, their uncertainties and covariance (table 3) and substituting in (14), results $u_{Pc} = 0.0654$ kPa. The standard combined uncertainty, in turn, was obtained by:

$$u_c^2 = u_{Pc}^2 + u_{Pr}^2 , \qquad (18)$$

where, again, $u_{Pr} = 0.1$ kPa is the uncertainty associated to reference instrument and is obtained from (8), resulting:

$$u_c = \sqrt{\left(\frac{0.03\%}{2} \times 26.7\right)^2 + 0.0654^2} = 0.1 kPa . \qquad (19)$$

Therefore, this is the calculated value for the standard combined uncertainty u_c.
Considering the coverage probability of 95.45% (Ferrero & Salicone, 2006), the effective number of degrees of freedom is $v_{eff} \to \infty$, indicating $k = 2$. Thus, the standard expanded uncertainty is estimated as $Up = 0.2$ kPa.
Calculated expanded uncertainty for the others calibrations points of the rising curve of the sensor 2 and remainder curves was estimated to range from 0.2 to 0.3 kPa for the first group of collected data. In figure 5, the obtained experimental data (calibration points) and estimated pressure curve for sensor 2 (rising), considering the first collected data set can be regarded.
The analysis implemented for calculating the measurement uncertainty of the data collected six month after the first group followed the same procedure carried out earlier, showed above. Great similarity to the first set of collected data was observed for the values concerning the evaluated uncertainty of the second group. In this case, calculated expanded uncertainty using WLS modeling was estimated to be around 0.3 to 0.5 kPa. Figure 6 depicts experimental data and estimated calibration curve for sensor 2 – rising curve (second group of collected).

8. Discussion

The linear model (3) showed itself a good approach for the available data since the mean transfer curves for the collected calibration data points for sensor 1 and 2 have a linear behavior (figure 3). This fact has already been indicated in Freescale (2004).

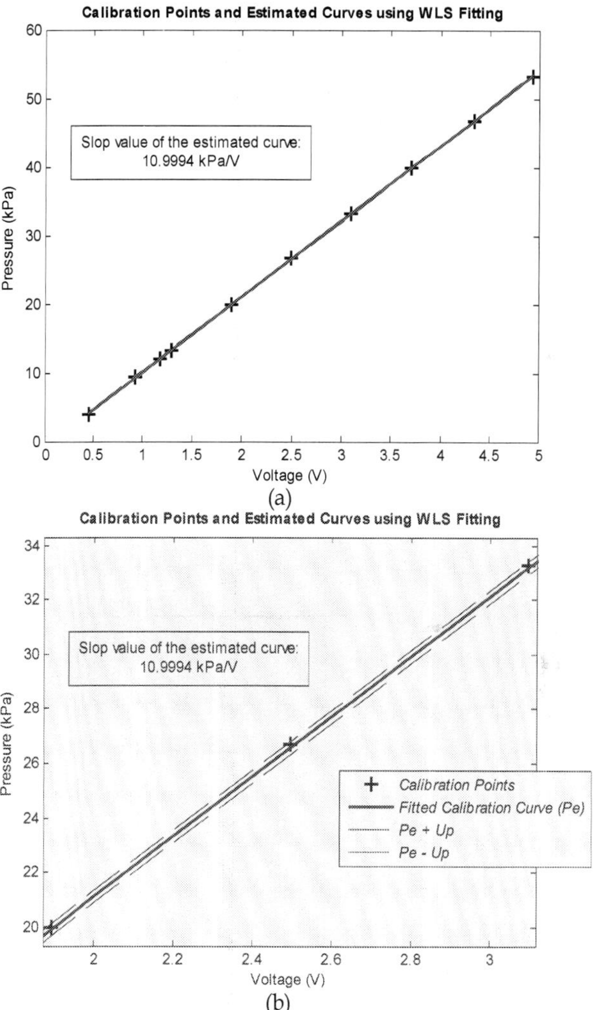

Fig. 5. (a) Calibration points and estimated curve by the model based on WLS and associated uncertainties for sensor 2 (rising) – considering the first group of collected data. (b) Zoom nearby $P_e = 26$ kPa: calibration points (+), estimated curve (P_e) resulting from linear adjustment and estimated curve associated to expanded uncertainty (P_e+U_p and P_e-U_p). Adapted from Ferreira *et. al.*, 2010.

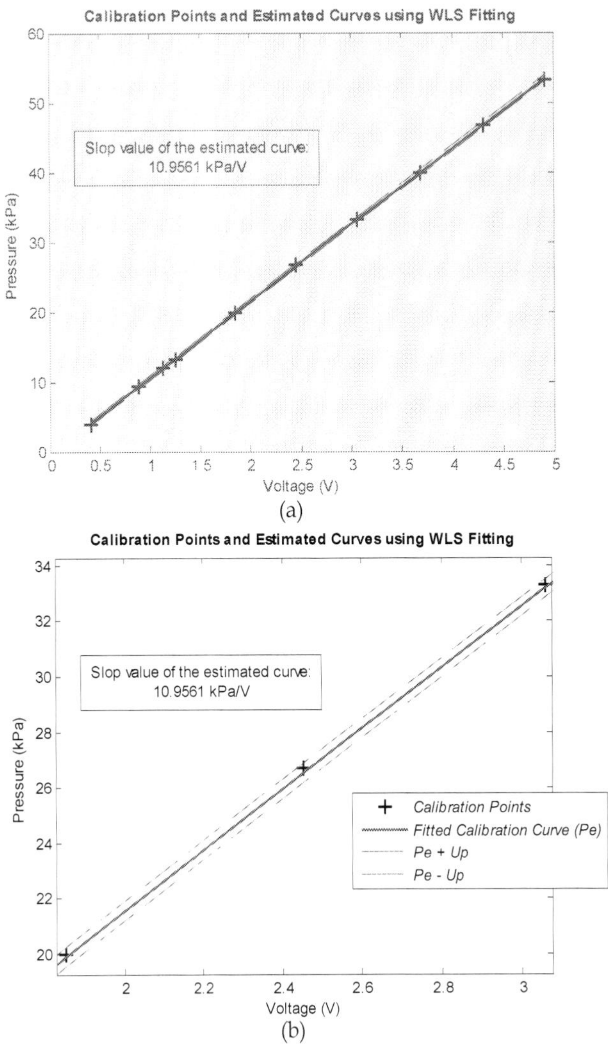

Fig. 6. (a) Calibration points and estimated curve by the model based on WLS and associated uncertainties for sensor 2 (rising) – considering the second group of collected data. (b) Zoom nearby P_e = 26 kPa: calibration points (+), estimated curve (P_e) resulting from linear adjustment and estimated curve associated to expanded uncertainty (P_e+U_p and P_e-U_p). Adapted from Ferreira *et. al.*, 2010.

As mentioned by Mathioulakis & Belessiotis (2000), the use of weight least squared (WLS) has the advantage not only to allow estimation of model parameters, but for also allowing calculation of the parameters uncertainties and covariance (table 3). Also as appointed by the Guide (GUM, 2003) and employed in this work for the digital manovacuometer (DM), such uncertainties and convariance can be just used for evalutation of measurement uncertainty of the prototype by the application of the law of propagation of uncertainties. Considering the calibration points and estimated calibration fitted curves presented in table 3, according to the consistency analysis indicated by Lira (2002) and Cox & Harris (2006), non-conformities between data and models were not observed: calculated values for the Birge ratio is near to unity (table 4).

As aforementioned, application of the law of progation of uncertainties on the linear model fitted to the calibration points (10) was employed for evaluating of measurement uncertaity for the prototype. The values for expanded uncertainty were estimated to range from 0.2 up to 0.5 kPa, considering all calibration points of the both groups of collected data by DM.

Comparison between pressure estimated using fitted calibration models and pressure values of calibration points (P_r) for both sensors and both group of data showed to have a rasonable coincidence as is depicted in figures 5 e 6. Noneless, as observed for the Birge ratio, a small difference is noticed when data collected six months apart are considered, which could appoints the need for verifying the periodicity of calibration for the prototype as well.

9. Conclusion and suggestions for future works

The calibration procedure has allowed to know about the reliability of the DM to measure maximum respiratory pressure. Calibration model using WLS proposed in this work was employed to obtain the calibration curves and to evaluate the measurement uncertainties for a digital manovacuometer prototype (developed at the NEPEB). The use of WLS for calibration showed itself to be appropriate for the avaiable data as well as a pratical way to evaluate the uncertainty since the proposed model itself can be used for evaluation of the measurement uncertainty by application of the law of propagation of uncertainties.

According to the model for evaluation of uncertainty, designed using weighted least squares adjustment (WLS) at the laboratory, the values for expanded uncertainty ranges from 0.2 up to 0.5 kPa. The small variation observed when comparing the two set of data acquired months apart for the values of ucertainty calculated by WLS modeling shows, clearly, the demand to perform periodic cheking. Such periodicity between calibrations has been checked, as mentioned by Fernandes *et al.* (2010).

The digital manovacuometer is already being used in clinical research application According to Montemezzo *et al.* (2010), it was checked that the results showed above are not influenced whether the used interface (mouthpiece and tube for respiratory pressure application on DM) is changed. As suggestions for future works, others uncertainty sources could be evaluated in the models to assess the impact on the results like those related to the low-pass filter, A/D converter and temperature variation.

10. Acknowledgments

To Fundação de Amparo à Pesquisa do Estado de Minas Gerais (FAPEMIG) for financial support.

11. References

Black, L. & Hyatt, R. (1969). Maximal respiratory pressures: normal values and relationship to age and sex. Am. Rev. Respir. Dis. 99 (5), pp. 696-702.

Cox, M. & Harris, P. (2006). Measurement uncertainty and traceability. *Meas. Sci. Technol.* (Jan.), 17, pp. 533-540, ISSN 1361-6501

Ferreira, J.; Pereira, N.; Oliveira Júnior, M.; Silva, J.; Britto, R.; Parreira, V.; Vasconcelos, F. & Tierra-Criollo, C. (2008). Application of weighted least squares to calibrate a digital system for measuring the respiratory pressures. *Proc. of Biodevices: 1st International Conference on Biomedical Electronics and Devices*, v. 1, pp. 220-223, ISBN 978-989-8111-17-3, Funchal, Portugal

Ferreira, J.; Pereira, N.; Oliveira Júnior, M.; Silva, J.; Britto, R.; Parreira, V.; Vasconcelos, F. & Tierra-Criollo, C. (2008a). Análise da calibração para um medidor digital de pressóes respiratórias. *Proc. of 21°. Congresso Brasileiro de Engenharia Biomédica*, pp. 741-744, ISBN 978-85-60064-13-7, Salvador, Brazil

Ferreira, J.; Pereira, N.; Oliveira Júnior, M.; Parreira, V.; Vasconcelos, F. & Tierra-Criollo, C. (2010). Maximum pressure measuring system: calibration and uncertainty evaluation. *Controle & Automação*. (Nov., Dec.), vol. 21, 6, pp. 588-597, ISSN 0103-1759

Ferrero, A., & Salicone, S. (2006). Measurement Uncertainty. *IEEE Instrum. Meas. Mag.*, (Jun.), pp. 44-51, ISSN 1094-6969

Freescale (2004). Integrated silicon pressure sensor on-chip signal conditioned, temperature compensated and calibrated. In: *Pressure sensors*. 03.11.2005. Available from: www.freescale.com

Fernandes, G.; Lage, F.; Montemezzo, D; Souza-Cruz, A.; Parreira, V. & Tierra-Criollo, C. (2010). Caracterização estática do protótipo para medição de pressões respiratórias máximas. *Proc. of 22°. Congresso Brasileiro de Engenharia Biomédica*, pp. 1403-1406, ISSN 2179-3220, Tiradentes, Brazil

GUM (2003). *Guide to the expression of uncertainty in measurement*, (3rd. Brazilian ed.), ABNT, INMETRO, ISBN 85-07-00251-X, Rio de Janeiro, Brazil

INMETRO (2008). DOQ-CGCRE-014 – Guide for carrying out calibration of digital measuring pressure systems (free translation). INMETRO, Rio de Janeiro, Brazil

INMETRO (1997). Procedure for verification of the sphygmomanometers with aneroid manometer (free translation). INMETRO, Rio de Janeiro, Brazil

Lira, I. (2002) *Evaluating the measurement uncertainty: fundamentals and practical guidance*, IoP, ISBN 0-7503-0840-0, Bristol and Philadelphia

Mathioulakis, E. & Belessiotis, V. (2000). Uncertainty and traceability in calibration by comparison. *Meas. Sci. Technol.* (Mar.), 11, pp. 771-775, ISSN 1361-6501

Montemezzo, D.; Fernandes, A.; Souza-Cruz, A.; Fernandes, G.; Lage, F.; Barbosa, M; Parreira, V. & Tierra-Criollo, C. (2010). Interferência de interfaces na mensuração das pressões respiratórias máximas. *Proc. of 22°. Congresso Brasileiro de Engenharia Biomédica*, pp. 1187-1190, ISSN 2179-3220, Tiradentes, Brazil

Oliveira Júnior, M.; Provenzano, F.; Moraes Xavier, P.; Pereira, N.; Montemezzo, D.; Tierra-Criollo, C.; Parreira, V. & Britto, R. (2008). Medidor digital de pressões respiratórias. *Proc. of 21°. Congresso Brasileiro de Engenharia Biomédica*, pp. 741-744, ISBN 978-85-60064-13-7, Salvador, Brazil

Olson, W. (2010). Basic concepts of medical instrumentation. In J. Webster (Ed.), *Medical instrumentation: application and design*, (4th. ed.), Wiley, ISBN 978-0471-67600-3, New York, U.S.A.

Parvis, M. & Vallan, A. (2002). Medical measurements and uncertainties. *IEEE Instrum. Meas. Mag.* (Jun.), pp. 12-17, ISSN 1094-6969

Press, W.; Teukolsky, S.; Vetterling, W. & Flannery, B. (1996). *Numerical recipes in C: the art of scientific computing*, (2nd. ed), University Press Cambridge, ISBN 0-521-43108-5, Cambridge, England

VIM (2008) - International vocabulary of metrology — Basic and general concepts and associated terms. [Online] Available < http://www.bipm.org/utils/common/documents/jcgm/JCGM_200_2008.pdf> ; Acess in April, 20, 2010.

Part 4

Bio-Imaging

19

Biomedical Image Volumes Denoising via the Wavelet Transform

Eva Jerhotová, Jan Švihlík and Aleš Procházka
Institute of Chemical Technology, Prague
The Czech Republic

1. Introduction

Image denoising represents a crucial initial step in biomedical image processing and analysis. Denoising belongs to the family of image enhancement methods (Bovik, 2009) which comprise also blur reduction, resolution enhancement, artefacts suppression, and edge enhancement. The motivation for enhancing the biomedical image quality is twofold. First, improving the visual quality may yield more accurate medical diagnostics, and second, analytical methods, such as segmentation and content recognition, require image preprocessing on the input.

Gradually, noise reduction methods developed in other research fields find their usage in biomedical applications. However, biomedical images, such as images obtained from computed tomography (CT) scanners, are quite specific. Modelling noise based on the first principles of image acquisition and transmission is a too complex task (Borsdorf et al., 2009), and moreover, the noise component characteristics depend on the measurement conditions (Bovik, 2009).

Additionally, noise reduction must be carried out with extreme care to avoid suppression of the important image content. For this reason, the results of biomedical image denoising should be consulted with medical experts.

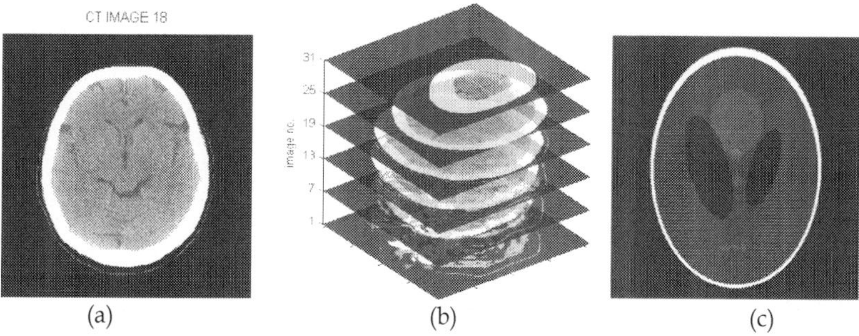

Fig. 1. A CT image of the brain (a), a subset of CT images (b) from the same examination, and the Shepp-Logan phantom image (c)

There is a range of noise reduction techniques applied to images either in the spatial domain or in a selected transform domain (Motwani et al., 2004). The former include linear or nonlinear low-pass filters, such as moving average filters, the Wiener filter or a variety of median filters. Left alone some recent developments of weighted median, the space domain techniques generally remove the majority of noise, but on the other hand, also blur sharp image edges. To overcome these problems, it is advantageous to use other domains for image representation and processing.

An optimal representation should capture key features of the signal in a relatively small number of large transform coefficients while the majority of the coefficients should be very small or zero. In other words, the representation should be sparse (Mallat, 2009). In this respect, the wavelet domain is a good choice. Both for signals with spatial transients and narrow-band frequency content, the wavelet transform represents a good compromise between the frequency and the spatial domain representations. Furthermore, for real-world images comprising both spatial transients such as edges and narrow-band components such as regular texture regions, the wavelet transform with the space-scale (or space-frequency) representation outperforms the other two (Percival & Walden, 2006).

Aiming at reducing noise in CT images, researchers focus on optimizing the filtered back-projection (FBP) algorithm used in CT-scanners for image reconstruction. For instance, You & Zeng (2007) propose an improved FBP algorithm, which incorporates the Hilbert transform, and Zhu & StarLack (2007) propose a method for predicting the noise variance and subsequently adapting weights and kernels of the FBP algorithm. Similar to other researches, they exploit a simple Shepp-Logan phantom image (Shepp & Logan, 1974) which is depicted in Fig. 1c. In their experiments, noise with various statistical properties is introduced into the projection data, and then the result reconstructed by the reconstruction algorithm is evaluated.

Some researchers study the possibilities of the wavelet transform in biomedical image denoising and compression. They most commonly use the critically sampled discrete wavelet transform (DWT). Khare & Shanker Tiwary (2005) utilise the dual-tree complex wavelet transform (DTCWT) for adaptive shrinkage. Bosdorf et al. (2008) propose a wavelet-based correlation analysis method applied to pairs of disjoint projections in dual-source CT-scanners in oder to extract and eliminate uncorrelated noise. The authors use both the DWT and undecimated DWT (UDWT) and in conclusion, indicate their preference for the computation efficiency of the DWT over the slightly better results quality produced by the UDWT. Wang & Huang (1996) and Wu & Qiu (2005) study the use of volumetric processing of biomedical image slices and its advantages in comparison with slice-by-slice processing.

In this chapter, we shall focus on wavelet-based techniques for noise reduction in image volumes produced by a standard CT-scanner (see Fig. 1). First, we shall describe the wavelet transform focusing on the DWT, the UDWT, the DTCWT, and their one-dimensional and multi-dimensional implementations. Second, we shall carry out the noise analysis on selected CT data sets. Final, we shall deal with wavelet-based denoising methods comprising wavelet coefficient thresholding methods (VisuShrink, SureShrink, and BayesShrink) and statistical modelling methods (the hidden Markov trees, the Gaussian mixture model, and the generalized Laplacian model) utilizing the Bayesian estimator.

2. Wavelet transform

The wavelet transform analyzes signals at multiple scales by changing the width of the analysis window, and produces their scale-space representation (Mallat, 2009). In contrast to the short-time Fourier transform, the wavelet transform deals with the limitations of uncertainty principle in a way that is more convenient for most real-world signals. This principle defines the trade-off between the length of the sliding window (i.e. the spatial resolution) and the distance between adjacent spectral lines (i.e. the frequency resolution). The wavelet transform exploits longer windows (i.e. better frequency resolution) for low frequency components of the signal, which are, nonetheless, usually of long duration, and shorter windows (i.e. better spatial resolution) for high frequency components of short duration. An important aspect of wavelet-based denoising is transform selection. In the following subsections, we shall discus the critically sampled DWT and two examples of a redundant wavelet transform with improved properties.

2.1 Discrete wavelet transform

The DWT is probably the most popular type of the wavelet transform in the signal and image processing field. This transform has become successful primarily in compression, as it became part of the JPEG2000 standard. This transform is computed via the subband coding algorithm designed by (Mallat, 2009). As displayed in Fig. 2, at each decomposition stage, the transform produces detail coefficients and approximation coefficients corresponding respectively to the upper half and the lower half of the input signal spectrum. The approximations then become an input of the next level.

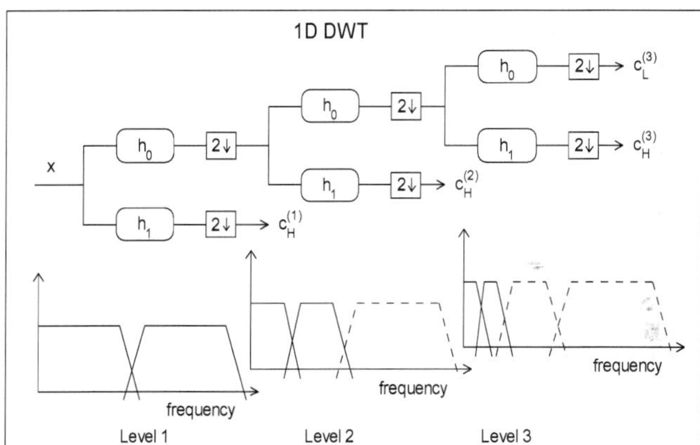

Fig. 2. The subband coding algorithm for computing the 1-dimensional DWT

The detail coefficients $c_H^{(j)}$ at stage j are produced through convolution of the approximations $c_L^{(j-1)}$ from the previous level (or the original signal when $j=1$) with the band-pass filter h_1 (derived from the wavelet function) and subsequent down-sampling by a factor of 2. The convolution is given as

$$c_H^{(j)}(k) = \sum_{k=-\infty}^{\infty} h_1(n - 2k) \cdot c_L^{(j-1)}(n). \tag{1}$$

Similarly, the low frequency approximations $c_L^{(j)}$ at level j are produced by the convolution with the low-pass filter h_0 (derived from the scaling function).

$$c_L^{(j)}(k) = \sum_{k=-\infty}^{\infty} h_0(n - 2k) \cdot c_L^{(j-1)}(n). \tag{2}$$

Due to down-sampling, the approximation vector is rescaled prior to entering the next decomposition level, while the filter taps are preserved unchanged.

We may also synthesize the original input signal from the decomposition coefficients. The inverse DWT is given as

$$c_L^{(j-1)}(k) = \sum_{n=-\infty}^{\infty} g_0(k - 2n) \cdot c_L^{(j)}(n) + \sum_{n=-\infty}^{\infty} g_1(k - 2n) \cdot c_H^{(j)}(n), \tag{3}$$

where $\boldsymbol{g}_0$ and $\boldsymbol{g}_1$ are respectively the low-pass and the band-pass reconstruction filters. Before computing the convolution, the subband coefficients are up-sampled by 2 by inserting zero-valued samples.

The decomposition and reconstruction filter banks are designed as orthogonal or bi-orthogonal (or dual) bases (Mallat, 2009). The limitation of the orthogonal solution is that the associated real-valued wavelet function cannot have compact support and be symmetrical at the same time, except the Haar wavelet. However, the Haar wavelet is not smooth. Bi-orthogonal solutions provide more construction freedom and allow for smoothness and symmetry. Symmetrical filters have a linear phase response, and hence do not cause phase distortion to which the human eye is particularly sensitive. Consequently, bi-orthogonal wavelets are nowadays probably the most widely used.

The DWT is the most computationally efficient of all wavelet transforms. However, critical sampling causes significant drawbacks. This transform lacks shift-invariance, zero-crossings often appear at the locations of signal singularities, and altering wavelet coefficients (for instance, during denoising) causes artefacts in reconstructed images. To overcome these problems, we may use a redundant wavelet representation.

2.2 Redundant wavelet transforms

In this section, we describe two redundant wavelet transforms: the undecimated discrete wavelet transform (UDWT) and the dual-tree complex wavelet transform (DTCWT) designed by Kingsbury & Selesnick (Selesnick et al., 2005). The former is calculated through the subband coding algorithm exploiting the same filters as the DWT. The distinction lies in omitting the down-sampling step in decomposition. Instead, the decomposition filters are up-sampled at each stage (Starck et al., 2007). As a result, the UDWT is shift invariant which means that a shift in the input signal corresponds to a shift in the transform output and does not cause any other changes in the coefficient values. On the other hand, leaving out the down-sampling step yields a significant computation burden. The redundancy of this transform depends on the number of decomposition levels L and is given as $[(2^d - 1) L + 1]:1$, where d denotes the number of dimensions. As a result, for 2-dimensional decomposition, the redundancy of this transform with respect to the DWT is 4:1 at stage 1, increases to 7:1 at stage 2, further increases to 10:1 at stage 3, etc.

In comparison with the UDWT, the DTCWT exhibits relatively moderate redundancy, which is $2^d:1$ with respect to the DWT. In contrast to the UDWT, this ratio does not increase with the number of stages. To illustrate the redundancy, the DTCWT produces twice as many coefficient values than the DWT in 1-dimensional space (i.e. 2 subbands of complex coefficients composed of the real and the imaginary parts).

The DTCWT is realized with FIR (finite impulse response) filters forming a tight frame, and is thus easily revertible (unlike, for instance, the Gabor transform). As displayed in Fig. 3, this transform employs two DWT-like trees a and b producing respectively the real parts c_a and the imaginary parts c_b of the complex wavelet coefficients $c = c_a + j \cdot c_b$, where $j = \sqrt{(-1)}$.

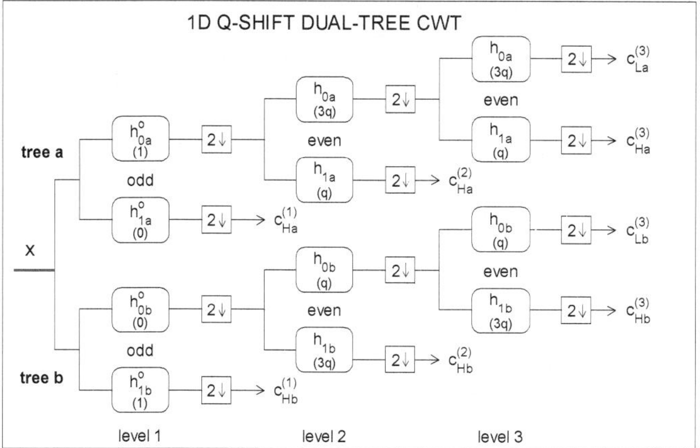

Fig. 3. The 1-dimensional DTCWT decomposition scheme

It may seem surprising that a real signal is converted into the complex wavelet representation by using real-valued filters. This is possible thanks to the Hilbert transform built into each transform stage. Ideally, the complex scaling function $\phi(t) = \phi_a(t) + j \cdot \phi_b(t)$ and the wavelet function $\psi(t) = \psi_a(t) + j \cdot \psi_b(t)$ should be analytic, which means that their respective real and imaginary parts constitute Hilbert transform pairs, so as $\phi_b(t) = \mathcal{H}\{\phi_a(t)\}$ and $\psi_b(t) = \mathcal{H}\{\psi_a(t)\}$. In the Fourier domain, this is equivalent to

$$\Psi_b(\omega) = -j \cdot \text{sign}(\omega) \cdot \Psi_a(\omega), \tag{4}$$

where sign denotes the sign function and ω the angular frequency. (The same relation applies also to the scaling function). As a consequence, the spectrum of the analytic wavelet is single-sided with zero magnitudes for negative frequencies. This property directly implies shift invariance, no aliasing, and the ability to isolate singularities of positive and negative directions in higher dimensions.

As the scaling and the wavelet function should be analytic, the filters associated with the real and the imaginary part of these functions must be delayed from each other by half a sample period

$$h_{0b}(n) = h_{0a}(n - 0.5), \tag{5}$$

where $\boldsymbol{h}_{0a}$ and $\boldsymbol{h}_{0b}$ are the low-pass filters of tree a and tree b, respectively. However, exact analycity cannot be achieved by functions with compact support. In other words, the Hilbert transformer is of infinite length and may not be exactly implemented with an FIR filter. Consequently, the wavelet and the scaling filters used in the DTCWT are only approximately analytic and shift-independent, and approximately fulfil condition (5).

In this chapter, we use the q-shift filter solution for the DTCWT by (Kingsbury, 2003). To achieve a higher degree of analycity at lower decomposition levels, this solution exploits different filters at level 1 than at higher levels. For level 1, it is possible to use the same filter set for both trees as long as it provides perfect reconstruction (for instance, one of the biorthogonal filter sets designed for the DWT). The only difference is that the filters in one tree are translated by one sample from the corresponding filters in the other tree

$$h_{0b}^o(n) = h_{0a}^o(n-1), \tag{6}$$

and also each to the other within the same tree (as indicated by the value in brackets in Fig. 3). Beyond level 1, we employ the approximately analytic q-shift filters, for which the low-pass (and also the high-pass) filters from opposite trees are time-reversed versions of each other

$$h_{0b}(n) = h_{0a}(N-1-n). \tag{7}$$

A similar relation applies also to the analysis and synthesis filters. These filters are of even length and approximately symmetrical, as their point of symmetry is ¼-sample away (i.e. q-shifted) from the centre. Hence, the filters exhibit a q-sample group delay and their individual phase response is not exactly linear. On the other hand, the assymmetry makes the orthonormal perfect reconstruction feasible. For the overall complex wavelet and also the scaling function, the conjugate phase response is exactly linear and the magnitude is approximately shift-invariant. In addition to the shift-invariance property, the DTCWT provides better directional selectivity than both the DWT and UDWT in multiple dimensions.

2.3 Multidimensional wavelet transform

Computing the multidimensional wavelet transform is straightforward due to its separability. This property implies that the n-dimensional (nD) transform may be implemented as n consecutive 1D transform in different directions as illustrated in Fig. 4 for the DWT. For $n=3$, we may proceed for instance in the following order. First, each slice of the image volume is processed in the row direction resulting into the low frequency coefficients (i.e. the approximations c_L) and the high frequency coefficients (i.e. the details c_H). The resulting 1D decomposed slices are then processed in the column direction yielding the 2D transform of 4 coefficients subbands (c_{LL}, c_{LH}, c_{HL}, and c_{HH}) for each image slice. Finally, the set of the 2D transform coefficients matrices is processed in the between-slice direction producing 8 subbands (c_{LLL}, c_{LLH}, c_{HLL}, ..., and c_{HHH}). The coefficients c_{LLL} constitute an input to the next level of the 3D transform (Hošťálková, Vyšata, & Procházka, 2007).

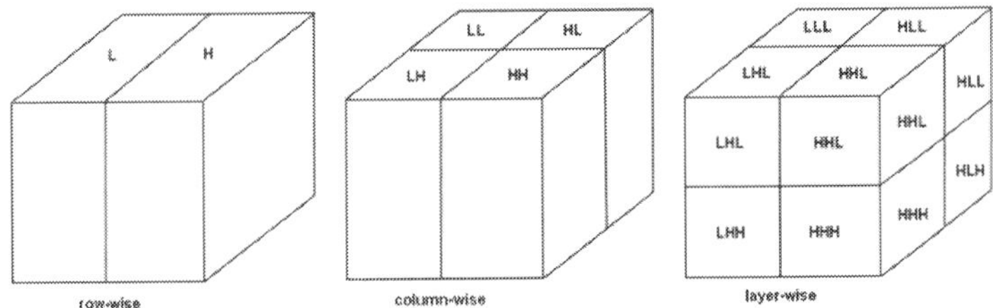

Fig. 4. The 3-dimensional DWT computation steps for a single decomposition level

Please note that for the UDWT, the procedure is identical except that the size of the 3-dimensional cube depicted in Fig. 4 doubles its size in the respective direction at each step. For the DTCWT, the multidimensional decomposition procedure is similar except producing a different number of subbands. For instance, the 2D DTCWT produces 8 subbands of complex-valued coefficients which correspond to 4:1 redundancy w.r.t. the 2D DWT of 4 subbands of real-valued coefficients. Despite being separable, the 2D DTCWT is truly directional. Its 6 directional subbands separate positive and negative singularity orientations (-75°, -45°, -15°, +15°, +45°, +75°). In contrast, the separable DWT mixes the negative and positive orientations together in its 3 subbands (0°, ±45°, ±90°). The improved directional selectivity in higher dimensions represents another advantage over both the critically sampled DWT and UDWT.

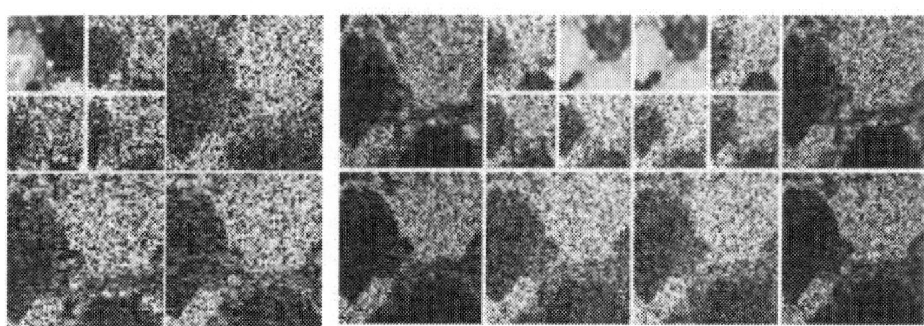

Fig. 5. The 2-diomensional DWT (left) and DTCWT (right) decomposition up to level 2 for a cropped biomedical image

The volumetric wavelet transform does not necessarily need be uniform in all three directions. We may for instance use longer filters within the slices and shorter filters in the direction between slices (Wang & Huang, 1996). The rationale behind this lies in the variance of the spatial resolution in different directions. In the between-slice direction, the resolution is coarser than in the intra-slice directions (depending on the slice thickness and spacing).

3. Wavelet-based denoising methods

As proved in a range of signal processing research areas, the wavelet transform is a suitable representation for estimating noise free images from their noisy observations owing to its sparsity and multiscale nature. As outlined in Fig. 6, denoising is based on image

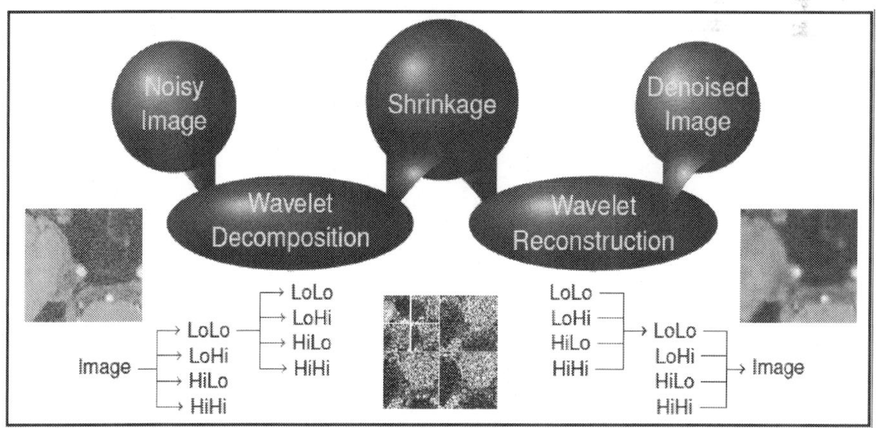

Fig. 6. The wavelet shrinkage procedure demonstrated on a cropped biomedical image decomposed by the DWT to the second level

transformation into the wavelet domain and subsequent reconstruction from the altered detail coefficients and unchanged approximation coefficients from the last decomposition level. This procedure is called wavelet shrinkage and is associated with two main-stream approaches, which are discussed in this section: coefficient thresholding and probabilistic coefficient modelling.

3.1 Noise analysis

The quality of CT images depends directly on the radiation dose from an examination. The dose is influenced by the following quantities (McNitt-Gray, 2006): X-ray tube current, exposure time, beam energy, slice thickness, table speed, type of the reconstruction algorithm, focal-spot-to-isocenter distance, detector efficiency, etc. Overall, CT image acquisition is a complex process affected many factors, such as the post-processing algorithm and nonlinearities of several parts of the device. By minimizing the radiation exposure of the patient, the amount of noise and artefacts increases.

Noise analysis represents a fundamental initial step of advanced noise suppression algorithms. In common devices, such as cameras with CCD (charged coupled device) or CMOS (complementary metal-oxide-semiconductor) sensors, noise analysis is based on acquisition of a testing pattern, which contains several patches with constant greyscale levels ranging from black to white (Gonzalez & Woods, 2002). However, CT image volumes are a specific case and more realizations of the same acquisition process cannot be obtained so simply. One option would be to use phantoms (for instance water phantoms), which mimic the consistence of the human body (basically - bone, tissue, water, and air). It is then possible to analyze the noise component by using several images generated by scanning the phantom. Another option of obtaining the data for noise analysis would be to acquire the same volumetric slice twice during a regular examination. However, this would increase the radiation dose for the patient and the noise would be still impacted by motion-generated artefacts (e.g. from breathing). To prevent from any motion, the patient head would have to be tightly fixed which is not applicable.

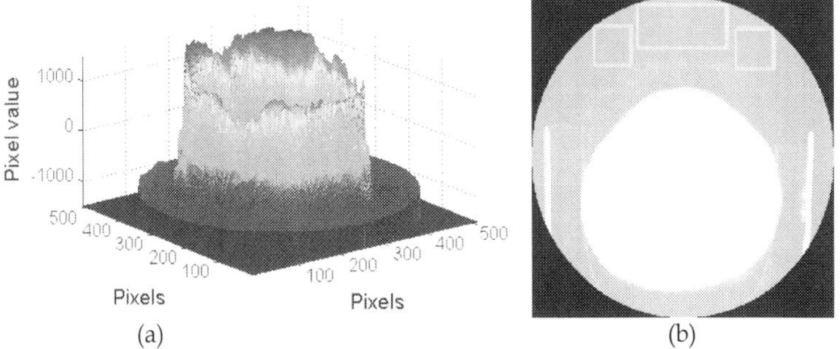

Fig. 7. The intensity profile of a typical CT slice (a) and examples of selected background patches (marked by the three rectangles at the top of the image) (b)

New interesting possibilities arise with introduction of multi-detector scanners. Bosdorf et al. (2008) analyse noise in images from the latest generation dual-source CT-scanners, which produce two images of the same slice (one from each detector). The authors propose to extract the uncorrelated noise component via wavelet-based correlation analysis of the corresponding images. According to their findings, the noise in CT images is non-white, usually of an unknown distribution, and not stationary.

In our experiments, we analyzed images from a standard CT-scanner and without possessing the corresponding phantom images for noise analysis. In order to analyze noise characteristics, we selected patches of the background, i.e. the part of the image capturing no part of the patient's head or the bed as apparent from Fig. 7b with an altered histogram. Nevertheless, this type of analysis does not reveal whether the noise is signal-dependent or not.

Even though we are aware that the noise is not strictly additive, we assume the additive noise model

$$y = x + n \tag{8}$$

for the sake of simplicity (y denotes the observed signal, x the noise-free signal, and n independent noise). We analyze the noise for each image of the volume individually, since the noise variance changes considerably from slice to slice. Fig. 7a shows a typical intensity profile of a CT image.

As we demonstrate below, the noise obtained from the background patches as well as the observed signal may be modelled using the GLM (generalized Laplacian model) or the GMM (Gaussian mixture model) in the spatial domain. The parameters of these models may be estimated exploiting the method of moments. This method is based on comparing the sample moments with the theoretical moments (Simoncelli & Adelson, 1996). Let us consider samples $\{y_i\}_{i=1}^{I}$ of the observed signal and define the kth sample moment

$$M_k = \frac{1}{I}\Sigma_{i=1}^{I} y_i^k, 1 \leq k \tag{9}$$

and the theoretical moment

$$m_k = \int_{-\infty}^{\infty} y^k \, p(y; \theta_1, \theta_2, \ldots, \theta_m) dy, \tag{10}$$

where $p(y)$ denotes the probability density function of y. The parameters $\theta_1, \theta_2, \ldots, \theta_m$ of the probability distribution are estimated through the following system of equations

$$M_k = m_k, 1 \leq k \leq m. \tag{11}$$

3.1.1 Generalized Laplacian model of the noise

Every background patch is analyzed in the following way. We compute an optimized histogram to obtain the PDF (probability density function) of the noise, which is then tested for normality. The quality of the histogram shape depends greatly on the bin width B_W. There is a range of approaches for bin width optimization, such as those described in (Scott, 1979) and (Izenman, 1991). The bin width originally proposed by Freedman & Diaconis can be written as

$$B_W = 2(n_{0.75} - n_{0.25})I^{-\frac{1}{3}}, \tag{12}$$

where the term in the parentheses denotes a so-called interquartile range between the 75th percentile n_(0.75) and the 25th percentile n_(0.25). In our experiments, the Kolmogorov-

Smirnov test rejected the null hypothesis that the samples come from the Gaussian distribution at the significance level $\alpha = 0.05$ in most of the tested images.

Hence, it is necessary to employ a more general model. We choose a model with heavy tails given by

$$p_n(n; \mu, s, \nu) = \frac{e^{-\left|\frac{n-\mu}{s}\right|^\nu}}{Z(s,\nu)}, n \in (-\infty; \infty), \tag{13}$$

where μ denotes the mean value, the parameter ν presents generalization in the sense of the PDF shape, and the parameter s controls the PDF width. The function $Z(s,\nu) = \frac{2s}{\nu}\Gamma\left(\frac{1}{\nu}\right)$, where $\Gamma(r) = \int_0^\infty t^{r-1} e^{-t} dt$ is the gamma function, normalizes the exponential to a unit area. The PDF parameters may be estimated by using the system of moment equations. For simplicity we consider noise n with $\mu = 0$. The second and the fourth moment of the noise n are given as

$$m_2(n) = \frac{s^2 \Gamma\left(\frac{3}{\nu}\right)}{\Gamma\left(\frac{1}{\nu}\right)}, \quad m_4(n) = \frac{s^4 \Gamma\left(\frac{5}{\nu}\right)}{\Gamma\left(\frac{1}{\nu}\right)}, \tag{14}$$

As proposed by Simoncelli & Adelson (1996), parameters estimation may be simplified using the kurtosis

$$\kappa_n = \frac{m_4(n)}{m_2^2(n)} = \frac{\Gamma\left(\frac{5}{\nu}\right)\Gamma\left(\frac{1}{\nu}\right)}{\Gamma^2\left(\frac{3}{\nu}\right)}. \tag{15}$$

The above described model is widely known as the generalized Laplacian model (GLM). This model is commonly used to model filtered images, such as the wavelet coefficients of high frequency bands. The histogram and the modelled PDF for a selected background patch are depicted in Fig. 8a using the logarithmic scale, which clearly illustrates the quality of the fit.

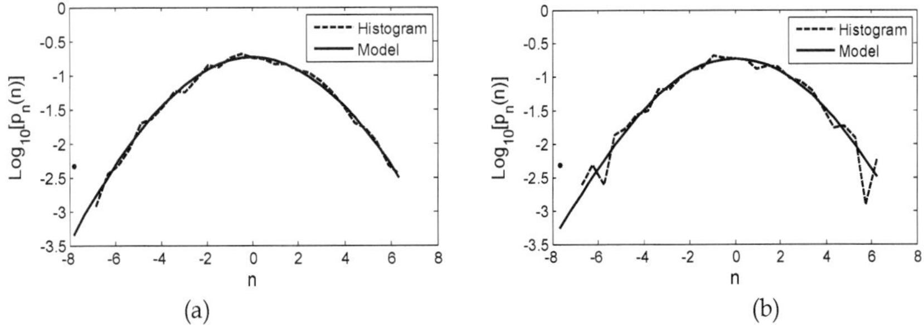

Fig. 8. The normalized histogram of the analyzed noise fitted with the GLM ($\nu = 1.89$, $s = 3.02$, $\mu = -0.34$) (a) and the GMM ($\sigma_{1n} = 2.10$, $\sigma_{2n} = 2.77$, $a = 0.89$) (b)

For denoising, we transform images into the wavelet domain. In case of the Gaussian-distributed noise, the noise parameters are preserved unaffected by the transformation. In contrast, for the non-Gaussian noise, the parameters change and thus need be re-estimated. We may either estimate the parameters directly in the wavelet domain (e.g. via the method of moments), or alternatively, transform the moments into the wavelet domain (Davenport, 1970).

3.1.2 Gaussian mixture model of the noise

Another possibility of modelling noise in the selected background patches is the Gaussian mixture model (GMM). This model is generally given by a mixture of a certain number of Gaussians with the variances σ_{kn} and the mean values μ_{kn} (Samé & al., 2007)

$$p(n) = \sum_{k=1}^{K} \alpha_{kn} \, \mathcal{N}(n; \mu_{kn}, \sigma_{kn}^2), \tag{16}$$

where α_{kn} are the proportions of the mixture satisfying the constraint $\sum_{k=1}^{K} \alpha_{kn} = 1$. As a compromise between solvability of the moment equations system and quality of the fit, we set $K = 2$. The GMM is than given by

$$p(n) = \alpha_n \mathcal{N}(n; \mu_{1n}, \sigma_{1n}^2) + (1 - \alpha_n)\mathcal{N}(n; \mu_{2n}, \sigma_{2n}^2), \tag{17}$$

where the mean values μ_{kn} are assumed to equal zero.

To estimate the model parameters in the wavelet domain, we may use the system of moment equations employing the second and the fourth central moment derived in (Švihlík, 2009). The noise parameters (the variances σ_{1N}, σ_{2N} and the mixture proportion α_N) may be directly estimated from the wavelet coefficients $N = WT\{n\}$ as follows. First, the variance σ_{1N} is estimated as $\sigma_{1N} = N_{0.999}/3$, where $N_{0.999}$ denotes the 99.9th percentile. Second, the proportion α_N is estimated from kurtosis

$$\kappa_N = \frac{m_4(N)}{m_2^2(N)} \approx \frac{3}{\alpha_N}, for \; \alpha_N - 1 \to 0, \tag{18}$$

where $m_4(N)$ and $m_2(N)$ are the central moments of N. And final, the remaining model parameter σ_{2N} is then given as (Švihlík, 2009)

$$\sigma_{2N}^2 = \frac{m_2(N) - \alpha_N \sigma_{1N}^2}{1 - \alpha_N}. \tag{19}$$

Using the logarithmic scale, Fig. 8b displays the result of fitting the model to the histogram of the selected background patch.

3.2 Wavelet coefficient thresholding

The method of wavelet coefficients thresholding is based on suppressing low-energy detail coefficients which are presumed to noise-dominated. To do this, we may choose different thresholding functions. The basic two thresholding function types are the hard thresholding and the soft thresholding function. For the former, the coefficients generated by altering the observed real-valued coefficients $\{Y_i\}_{i=1}^{I}$ are given by

$$Y_i^{(thr)} = \hat{X}_\iota = \begin{cases} Y_i & \text{for } |Y_i| > \delta^{(h)} \\ 0 & \text{otherwise} \end{cases} \tag{20}$$

where $\delta^{(h)} \in \mathbb{R} \geq 0$ stands for the hard threshold limit and $\hat{X}_\iota$ denotes the estimated coefficients of the noise-free signal. For soft thresholding, the thresholded coefficients are given as

$$Y_i^{(thr)} = \hat{X}_\iota = \begin{cases} sign(Y_i) \cdot (|Y_i| - \delta^{(s)}) & \text{for } |Y_i| > \delta^{(s)} \\ 0 & \text{otherwise} \end{cases} \tag{21}$$

where $\delta^{(s)} \in \mathbb{R} \geq 0$ stands for the soft threshold limit. In case of complex-valued coefficients, we threshold the magnitudes and keep the phase $\angle Y_i$ unchanged. For instance, the soft thresholding formula remains almost the same except that the magnitude $|Y_i| = \sqrt{Y_{i_a}^2 + Y_{ib}^2}$ replaces Y_i and as a result, the sign function may be omitted. We then use the thresholded magnitudes to obtain the complex thresholded coefficient

$$Y_i^{(thr)} = \widehat{X}_i = |Y_i| \cdot e^{j \cdot \angle Y_i} \tag{22}$$

Hard thresholding preserves the coefficient with the values greater than the threshold. This may, however, introduce discontinuities in the coefficients values, which may result in artefacts. In contrast, the soft thresholding function does not introduce artefacts owing to being continuous. This function complies with the assumption that noise is distributed evenly in all coefficients. However, when this is not the case, this technique reduces also the values of the coefficients corresponding to the underlying noise-free signal, which results in edge blurring (Percival & Walden, 2006).

3.2.1 Threshold estimation methods for the Gaussian noise

Threshold estimation methods vary in the assumption of the noise variance uniformity for different scales and subbands and in the threshold value estimation methods which they employ(Percival & Walden, 2006). In general, orthonormal transforms preserve the statistics of the i.i.d. (independent identically distributed) Gaussian noise. That is the reason why the most widely used methods are derived with this assumption.

The VisuShrink method (Donoho & Johnstone, 1994) assumes the noise variance the same for all thresholded subbands. The noise variance is estimated using the median absolute deviation (MAD) of the coefficients from the highest-frequency subband which is presumed to be noise-dominated.

$$\hat{\sigma}_{MAD} = \frac{median(|c^{hh1}|)}{0.6745}, \tag{23}$$

where the constant in the denominator corresponds to the Gaussian distribution. The primary advantage of this variance estimation method is its robustness to outliers. The estimated noise variance is than exploited for computing the universal threshold with the same value for all levels and subbands

$$\delta = \sigma_n \sqrt{2 \cdot \log L}, \tag{24}$$

where σ_n is the noise standard deviation, L is the number of signal samples and log is the natural logarithm. This threshold computation formula is derived by minimizing the probability that any noise sample will exceed the threshold limit. The resulting threshold is applied to the wavelet coefficients via the soft thresholding technique defined in (21). VisuShrink removes the vast majority of noise from the image, but also tends to over-smooth the image since common signals are not sparse enough to comply with the minmax theory. In response to these findings, Donoho & Johnstone proposed another method called SureShrink (Stein's Unbiased Risk Estimate Shrinkage), which produces subband-adaptive thresholds and is optimal in the mean-squared error sense. They further proposed a hybrid scheme combining the above approaches, since SureShrink does not perform well for situations of extreme sparsity.

In literature, SureShrink is often compared with BayesShrink (Chang, Yu, & Vetterli, 2000) for different types of data and the two methods. BayesShrink derives the threshold within the Bayesian framework assuming a generalized Gaussian distribution of the wavelet coefficients (Percival & Walden, 2006) and the additive noise model of the observed coefficients

$$Y = X + N, \tag{25}$$

where $N = WT\{n\}$ denotes the noise coefficients and $X = WT\{x\}$ the noise-free signal coefficients. Hence for the corresponding variances we may write

$$\sigma_Y^2 = \sigma_X^2 + \sigma_N^2. \tag{26}$$

The mean square error in a subband may be approximated by the corresponding Bayesian squared error risk with the generalized Gaussian as the prior. The threshold which minimizes the Bayesian risk (is nearly optimal) is produced as

$$\delta = \frac{\sigma_N^2}{\sigma_X}, \tag{27}$$

These parameters are estimated from the data for each subband. The noise variance σ_N is estimated via (23), and by exploiting (26), the variance of the noise-free signal σ_X is estimated as

$$\widehat{\sigma}_X^2 = \sqrt{\max(\widehat{\sigma}_Y^2 - \widehat{\sigma}_N^2, 0)}, \tag{28}$$

where the estimate of the observed coefficients variance is computed from each subband given as

$$\widehat{\sigma}_Y^2 = \frac{1}{I} \sum_{i=1}^{I} Y_i^2, \tag{29}$$

while assuming the zero mean.

3.2.2 Wavelet coefficients thresholding for the non-Gaussian noise

In case that the noise analysis identifies noise to be non-Gaussian and the moment equation systems for GMM and GLM models are not well satisfied, the thresholding method must be modified. The threshold value is usually derived for the noise with the Gaussian distribution. In accordance with the outcomes of the noise analysis we proposed a simple equation for the evaluation of the threshold value of the GLM. For the universal threshold from (24), the threshold value δ is given by the weighted standard deviation of a given distribution (e.g. parameter σ for the Gaussian distribution). When considering the GLM from (13) with $\mu = 0$ in the wavelet domain, the thresholding value is given by the square root of second central moment

$$\delta = w\sqrt{m_2(s, v)} = w\sqrt{\frac{s^2 \Gamma\left(\frac{3}{v}\right)}{\Gamma\left(\frac{1}{v}\right)}} = w\sqrt{\frac{1}{I}\sum_{i=1}^{I} N_i^2} \tag{30}$$

where N_i denotes the wavelet coefficients of noise n, w denotes the weight, which can be approximately in the range between 1 to 6 and it should be optimized for the acquired data.

Now let us consider the DTCWT. In case of complex-valued coefficients, we threshold the magnitudes while keeping the phase unchanged as described in (22). It is evident that the

PDF of the wavelet coefficients magnitudes is asymmetric, and its mean is not zero. We consider the real and imaginary components of the complex coefficients to be i.i.d. Gaussian. Hence, the magnitude is Rayleigh-distributed. The Rayleigh PDF is given by

$$p_N(N; \sigma) = \frac{N}{\sigma^2} e^{\frac{-N^2}{2\sigma^2}}, N \geq 0 \tag{31}$$

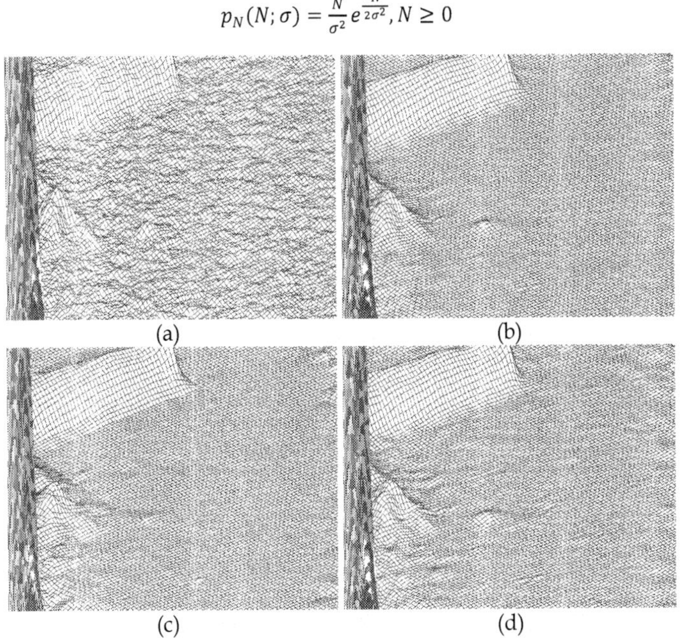

Fig. 9. A selection of the intensity profile of a selected CT slice presenting the noisy image ($D(n)$ = 14.42) (a), the result of denoising using the UDWT ($D(n)$ = 0.69; Daubechies 6) (b), using the DWT ($D(n)$ = 1.11; Le Gall biorthogonal filters) (c), and using the DTCWT ($D(n)$ = 0.94; Le Gall biorthogonal filters at level 1 and qshift filters beyond level 1) (d)

where $\sigma > 0$. Similarly as in (30), we define the threshold value as the weighted square root of second raw moment

$$\delta = w\sqrt{m_2(\sigma)} = w\sqrt{2\sigma^2\Gamma(2)}, \tag{32}$$

where parameter σ can be estimated using maximum likelihood as follows

$$\hat{\sigma} = \sqrt{\frac{1}{2I}\Sigma_{i=1}^{I} |N|_i^2}, \tag{33}$$

where N are the complex wavelet coefficients of noise n. It is worthwhile to mention that we use the second raw moment $m_2(\sigma) = 2\sigma^2\Gamma(2)$ instead of second central moment $m_2(\sigma) = \frac{4-\pi}{2}\sigma^2$ for the threshold value evaluation. The reason is that the optimal value of δ is found by changing the weight w and the mentioned two moments are both a function of parameter σ. The example of the estimated PDFs computed from the magnitudes of the complex wavelet coefficients at decomposition level 1 are depicted in Fig. 10. The threshold value evaluated for this case is $\delta = 3.4$. Hence, only a negligible part of PDF of Y are thresholded.

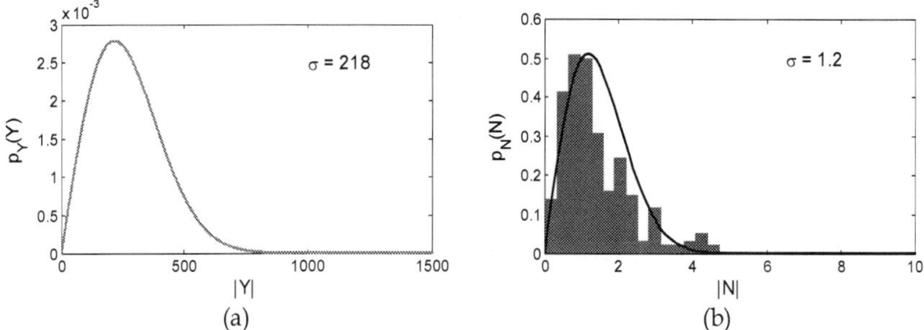

Fig. 10. The PDFs of the complex wavelet coefficients magnitudes for the noisy observation (a) and the noise (b) including the noise histogram

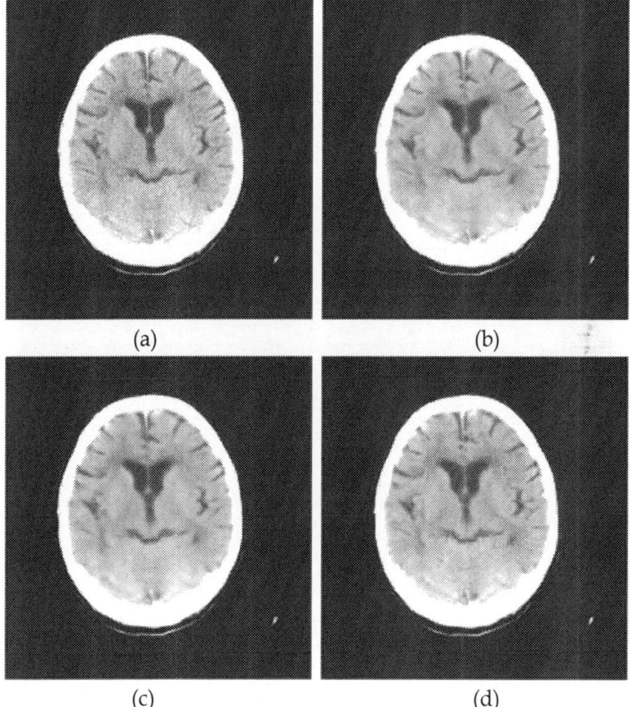

Fig. 11. Denoising using soft thresholding of a selected CT slice presenting the noisy image slice ($D(n) = 14.42$) (a), the result of denoising using the UDWT ($D(n) = 0.69$; Daubechies 6) (b), using the DWT ($D(n) = 1.11$; Le Gall biorthogonal filters) (c), and using the DTCWT ($D(n) = 0.94$; Le Gall biorthogonal filters and qshift filters) (d)

A selected CT slice from our image database thresholded assuming a non-Gaussian noise by using various wavelet transforms is depicted in Fig. 11. The results appear similar, except that in case of the DWT, the image is slightly over-smoothed. Fig. 9 shows the same image using the intensity profiles, whose sample variances $D(n) = \frac{1}{I-1}\sum_{i=1}^{I}(n_i - E(n))^2$ considerably decreased for all three implemented wavelet transforms.

Additionally, we produced another set of denoising results using the BayesShrink method described in subsection 3.2.1. As depicted in Fig. 12, we performed BayesShrink using the DTCWT and the DWT. In case of the DTCWT, we used equation (33) for computing the parameter σ of the Rayleigh distribution and also the second central moment for both the observed signal and the noise extracted from the background patches. Similarly for the DWT, we assumed the GLM and evaluated its parameters both for the noise model and the observation in the wavelet doman. In this experiment, the BayesShrink method produced a too small threshold for the DWT. For the DTCWT, the threshold seems appropriate, since the difference image appears to contain primarily noise.

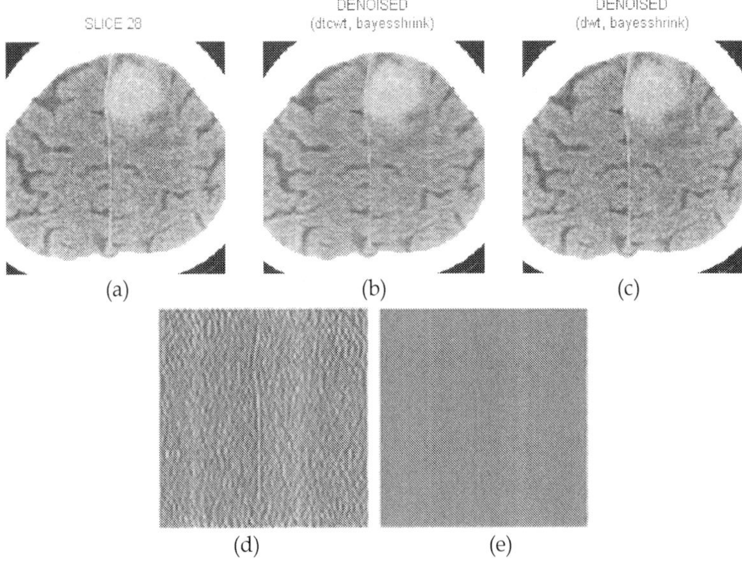

Fig. 12. The results of the BayesShrink method using the non-Gaussian noise models and soft thresholding presenting the noisy image (a), the result of using the DTCWT (b) and the DWT (c) and the corresponding difference images of $D(n)$ = 2.87 (d) and $D(n)$ = 0.6 (e) of the normalized intensities between [-10; 10]

3.3 Statistical modelling of the wavelet coefficients

The other broad family of wavelet-based noise reduction methods is based on **statistical modelling** of the wavelet coefficients. As demonstrated in numerous publications (Romber et al., 2001), these methods usually outperform the thresholding techniques with respect to the result quality. On the other hand, they also yield greater computational complexity. In this subsection, we discuss two different methods: the hidden Markov trees (HMT) and two types of the marginal probabilistic models discussed above - the GMM and the GLM.

3.3.1 Bayesian estimator

The probabilistic methods utilize the Bayesian estimator (Hammond & Simoncelli, 2008) to estimate the underlying signal from its noisy observation based on the a priori information. There are two basic variants of this estimator, depending on whether the estimator is designed to optimize the minimum mean square error (MMSE) or the maximum a posterior (MAP) risk function.

Once again, we assume the additive noise model of the noisy wavelet coefficients observations in (25). The conditional mean of the posterior PDF $p_{X|Y}(x|y)$ produces the least square estimation of X. The MMSE estimator (Simoncelli & Adelson, 1996) (Izenman, 1991)is given as

$$\hat{X}(Y) = \int_{-\infty}^{+\infty} p_{X|Y}(x|y)x\,dx = \frac{\int_{-\infty}^{+\infty} p_{Y|X}(y|x)p_X(x)x\,dx}{\int_{-\infty}^{+\infty} p_{Y|X}(y|x)p_X(x)\,dx} = \frac{\int_{-\infty}^{+\infty} p_N(y-x)p_X(x)x\,dx}{\int_{-\infty}^{+\infty} p_N(y-x)p_X(x)\,dx}, \tag{34}$$

where $p_{Y|X}(y|x)$ denotes a likelihood function, $p_X(x)$ represents the a priori model, and $p_N(x)$ stands for the noise model.

The MAP estimator is given by the following formula

$$\hat{X}(Y) = \arg\min_x p_{X|Y}(x|y) = \arg\min_x p_{Y|X}(y|x)p_X(x) = \arg\min_x p_N(y-x)p_X(x). \tag{35}$$

Bayesian statistics represent a powerful signal estimation tool (Rowe, 2003). In contrast to the classical Fisher approach, which exploits only the observed data, the Bayesian approach allows subsuming the prior information into the solution and thus produces useful results even for small datasets.

3.3.2 Wavelet-based a priori models

The above described marginal models (the GMM and the GLM) are suitable for modelling noise in tBayesian estimators, as discussed in subsections 3.1.2 and 3.1.1, and also as the a priori model of the noise-free signal. Assuming additive noise in the wavelet domain from (25), the observed coefficients Y are given as a summation of two GMM distributions. Hence, its second and fourth theoretical central moments are given by

$$m_2(Y) = m_2(X) + m_2(N), \tag{36}$$

$$m_4(Y) = m_4(X) + 6\,m_2(X)\,m_2(N) + m_4(N), \tag{37}$$

where the moments of Y and N are evaluated using the sample moments. The kth central sample moments of a random variable R is given by

$$M_k(R) = \frac{1}{I}\sum_{i=1}^{I}(R_i - E(R))^k. \tag{38}$$

From (36) and (37), it is possible to compute the moments $m_2(X)$ and $m_4(X)$ of the useful signal X. Finally, the signal parameters may be estimated using the same equations as for the noise N (i.e. (18) and (19)). The parameters estimation results highly depend on the estimation quality of the sample moments.

For the wavelet-based GLM, equations (36) and (37) are also valid. The GLM of the noise-free signal is given as

$$p_X(X; \varepsilon, \lambda) = \frac{e^{-\left|\frac{X}{\lambda}\right|^{\varepsilon}}}{Z(\lambda, \varepsilon)}, X \in (-\infty; \infty) \tag{39}$$

where ε denotes the shape parameter and λ is the variance parameter. Similarly to noise estimation in (15), the parameters of the signal may be easily estimated through the kurtosis

$$\kappa_X = \frac{m_4(X)}{m_2^2(X)} = \frac{\Gamma\left(\frac{5}{\varepsilon}\right)\Gamma\left(\frac{1}{\varepsilon}\right)}{\Gamma^2\left(\frac{3}{\varepsilon}\right)}. \tag{40}$$

Using equations (36) and (37), we obtain

$$\kappa_X = \frac{m_4(Y) - m_4(N) - 6m_2(N)(m_2(Y) - m_2(N))}{(m_2(Y) - m_2(N))^2}. \tag{41}$$

And from the second central moment we derive

$$\lambda = \sqrt{(m_2(Y) - m_2(N))\frac{\Gamma\left(\frac{1}{\varepsilon}\right)}{\Gamma\left(\frac{3}{\varepsilon}\right)}}. \tag{42}$$

Again, the values of the moments for Y and N may be estimated from the data using the sample moments exploiting (38).

Noise suppression methods based on Bayesian estimation are generally more efficient than the thresholding methods, mainly in case of considerable noise contamination. Fig. 13 shows the Shepp-Logan phantom contaminated by generalized Laplacian noise ($s = 30.0$, $v = 1.78$, $\mu = 0$) and subsequently denoised by the MMSE estimator. The quality improvement after denoising was assessed using Root Mean Square Error (RMSE)

$$RMSE = \sqrt{\frac{1}{I}\Sigma_{i=1}^{I}(x_i - \hat{x}_i)^2}, \tag{43}$$

which was computed for the original image x and the denoised image $\hat{x}$ and also for the the original image x and the noisy image y. The generalized Laplacian noise was generated by high-pass convolution filtering of a real-world image.

The described Bayesian estimation represents a powerful tool for image denoising. However, we presume that one of the following factors is in conflict with solvability of the denoising task: the analyzed noise is not strictly Additive and/or signal-independent, or the derived equation systems for the GMM and the GLM (originally derived for astronomical data (Švihlík & Páta, 2008)) are not well satisfied.

3.3.3 Wavelet-based hidden Markov trees

Wavelet coefficients thresholding methods assume the wavelet transform to de-correlate the signal thoroughly. However, this is not a correct assumption. The wavelet coefficients are interrelated and exhibit persistence across scale and clustering within scale. Both these properties are captured by the hidden Markov tree (HMT) models (Baraniuk, 1999). Acording to the persistency property, the coefficient values propagate across scale from parent to child within the tree. This means that a large parent coefficient corresponding to a signal singularity should have large children coefficients, while a parent coefficient associated with a noise-related singularities should not. Clustering within scale signifies that a large (small) coefficient value is expected in the vicinity of a large (small) coefficient.

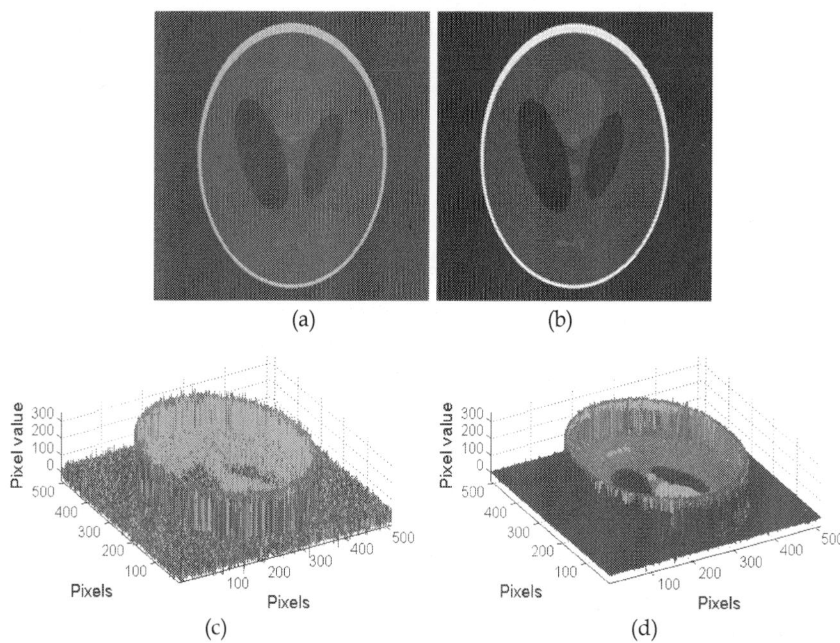

Fig. 13. The Shepp-Logan phantom with added noise (RMSE = 22.7) (a) and the denoised image using the UDWT with the Daubechies 6 wavelet (RMSE = 5.5) (b) and the respective intensity profiles (c) and (d)

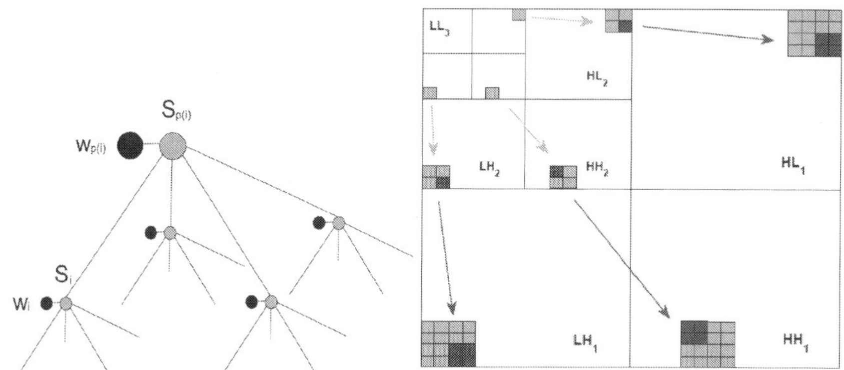

Fig. 14. The wavelet-based HMT hierarchy for 2-dimensional DWT, where each parent node $p(i)$ has four children i

As depicted in Fig. 14, the HMT connects the hidden states of a child node S_i and a parent node $S_{p(i)}$ and not the actual coefficients values Y_i, $Y_{p(i)}$ associated with these states. For modelling the inter-scale dependencies, the HMT uses an M-component mixture of conditional Gaussian distributions $N(\mu_{i,m}, \sigma_{i,m}^2)$ associated with hidden states $S_i = m$, since the PDF of the wavelet coefficients is peaky and heavy-tailed. The overall PDF is given by

$$f(Y_i) = p(S_i = m)f(Y_i|S_i = m) \tag{44}$$

where $p(S_i = m)$ is the probability mass function (PMF) of the hidden state S_i of the node i satisfying $\sum_{m=1}^{M} p(S_i = m) = 1$ and $f(Y_i|S_i = m)$ is the conditional probability that the observed coefficients value y_i given the state S_i corresponds to $G(\mu_{i,m}, \sigma_{i,m}^2)$. For simplicity, we use the mixture of two Gaussians $(M = 2)$.

The intra-scale dependencies are captured by the transition probabilities. For M=2, the transition probability matrix connecting the children hidden states S_i given the parent state $S_{p(i)}$ is given as

$$f\left(S_i = m|S_{p(i)} = n\right) = \begin{pmatrix} f\left(S_i = 1|S_{p(i)} = 1\right) & f\left(S_i = 1|S_{p(i)} = 2\right) \\ f\left(S_i = 2|S_{p(i)} = 1\right) & f\left(S_i = 2|S_{p(i)} = 2\right) \end{pmatrix}. \tag{45}$$

The persistence property implies that $f_{1,1} \gg f_{2,1}$, $f_{2,2} \gg f_{1,2}$.

The HMT are used for denoising in the following fashion (Crouse et al., 1998). First, the model is fitted to the noise observation coefficients using the expectation maximization (EM) algorithm. This training algorithm comprises the E-step, in which the state information propagates upwards and downwards through the tree, and the M-step, in which the model parameters θ are recalculated and then input into the next iteration. We do not have multiple realizations of the same process. Hence, to prevent over-fitting of the model to the data, we tie the tries within subbands so as to obtain 3 independent HMT models for the 3 subbands of the 2-dimensional DWT. The results of model fitting for the first decomposition level of the DWT are shown in Fig. 15.

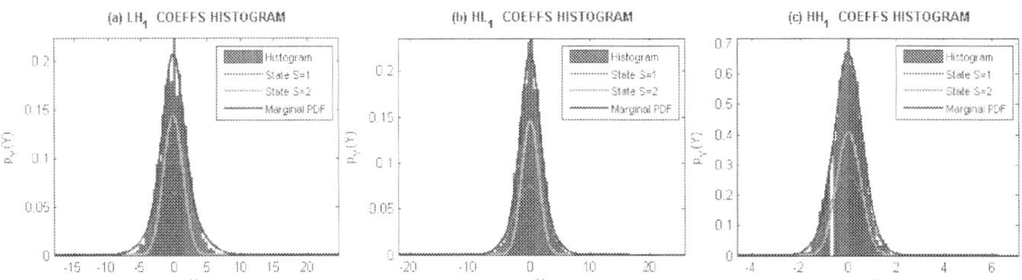

Fig. 15. The results of the HMT training for the CT image in Fig. 16 presenting histograms of the detail coefficients subbands from level 1 LH_1 (a), HL_1 (b), and HH_1 (c), respectively and the GMM of conditional probabilities

Second, the trained model is exploited as the a priori signal PDF in order to compute the conditional mean estimates of the noisy observations given the noise-free signal coefficients.

Again, we assume the additive nose model in (25), where N is the independent identically distributed Gaussian noise. The conditional mean estimate of X_i, given the observed coefficients Y and the HMT model parameters θ is given by

$$E[X_i|Y,\theta] = \sum_{m=1}^{M} p(S_i = m) \cdot \frac{\sigma_{i,m}^2}{\sigma_n^2 + \sigma_{i,m}^2} \cdot Y_i \qquad (46)$$

where $p(S_i = m)$ and $\sigma_{i,m}$ are obtained from the HMT model and σ_n is the noise standard deviation which may be estimated from the background patch or using the MAD in (23).

As example of HMT-based image denoising is displayed in Fig. 16. The wavelet-based HMTs (Romberg et al., 2001) capture dependencies between the wavelet coefficients across scales, since image singularities, such as edges, persist across scales, while the noise-dominated coefficients lack such intra-scale consistence. This approach yields very good denoising results, however requires a computationally expensive training.

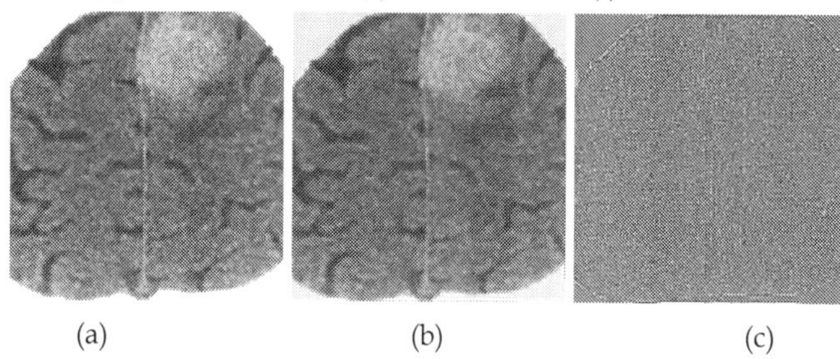

(a)   (b)   (c)

Fig. 16. 2 Denoising a selected CT image using the 2-level DWT with the LeGall biorthogonal filters depicting the observed image (a), its denoised equivalent, and the difference image (c) of the intensity range [-10,10]

4. Conclusion

In this chapter, we described different types of the wavelet transform including both non-redundant (the DWT) and redundant representations (the DTCWT and the UDWT). In general, the DTCWT and the UDWT outperform the DWT due to their shift-invariance; however, at the expense of redundancy. The DTCWT is less redundant than the UDWT and provides better directional selectivity.

We carried out preliminary noise analysis on 2 CT-datasets. The noise component in CT images is very complex and, presumably, also non-stationary. However, for simplicity, we assumed that the noise is stationary within the image and used the additive noise model. In order to model the noise, we selected a few background patches and modelled their distributions using the generalized Laplacian model or the Gaussian mixture model. The noise models were then exploited for wavelet coefficients thresholding. This required deriving threshold estimation equations corresponding to these models and also for the assumed Rayleigh distribution of the DTCWT coefficients magnitudes. The denoising results by using each of the three described wavelet transform were demonstrated on the CT-image data.

Since the threshold-based methods tend to blur edges and cause artefacts (the extent of this problem depends based on the used wavelet transform and thresholding method), we decided to implement the probabilistic methods. In general, these methods outperform the thresholding methods in the resulting image quality (mainly in case of considerable noise contamination); however, at the expense of greater computation cost. The described Bayesian estimation represents a powerful tool for image denoising. However, we presume that one of the following factors is in conflict with solvability of the denoising task: the analyzed noise is not strictly additive and/or signal-independent, or the derived equation systems for the GMM and the GLM are not well satisfied. In this perspective, the thresholding methods due to their relative simplicity revealed greater robustness towards non-fulfilment of the assumptions of the noise characteristics. On the other hand, the hidden Markov trees (HMT) of wavelet coefficients performed well and produced good quality image results with reduced noise and unblurred edges.

In future work, we shall focus on experiments in a larger scale. We shall carry out a thorough noise analysis on more datasets (on different CT-scanners if applicable) and also compare different denoising methods both by interviewing medical experts and by designing and evaluating appropriate quality metrics. Regarding methods development, we will further focus on the probabilistic methods experimenting with the use of more than two components in the Gaussian mixture model, the DTCWT instead of the DWT, and possibly also volumetric denoising techniques.

5. Acknowledgment

This work was funded by the research grant MSM 6046137306 of the Ministry of Education, Youth and Sports of the Czech Republic.

6. References

Baraniuk, R. G. (1999). Optimal tree approximation with wavelets. *SPIE Tech. Conf.Wavelet Applications Signal Processing VII, vol. 3813*, (pp. 196-207). Denver, CO.

Borsdorf, A., Kappler, S., Raupach, R., Noo, F., & Hornegger, J. (2009). Local Orientation-Dependent Noise Propagation for Anisotropic Denoising of CT-Images. IEEE Nuclear Science Symposium Conference Record (NSS/MIC).

Bosdorf, A., Raupach, R., Flohr, T., & Hornegger, J. (2008). Wavelet Based Noise Reduction in CT-Images Using Correlation Analysis. *IEEE Transactions on Medical Imaging , 27* (12), 1685-1703.

Bovik, A. (2009). *The Essential Guide to Image Processing*. Academic Press, U.S.A.

Chang, G., Yu, B., & Vetterli, M. (2000). Adaptive Wavelet Thresholding for Image Denoising and Compression. *9* (9), 1532-1546.

Crouse, M. S., Nowak, R. D., & Baraniuk, R. G. (1998). Wavelet-Based Statistical Signal Processing Using Hidden Markov Models. *IEEE Trans. on Signal Processing , 46* (4), 886-902.

Davenport, W. B. (1970). *Probability and Random Processes: An Introduction for Applied Scientists and Engineers* (1st ed.). New York: Prentice Hall, Inc.

Donoho, D. L., & Johnstone, I. M. (1994). Ideal spatial adaptation by wavelet shrinkage. *Biometrika , 3* (81).

Gonzalez, R. C., & Woods, R. E. (2002). *Digital Image Processing* (2nd ed.). (Bovik, Ed.) Elsevier Academic Press.

Hammond, D. K., & Simoncelli, E. P. (2008). Image Modeling and Denoising With Orientation-Adapted Gaussian Scale Mixtures. *IEEE Transactions on Image Processing , 17* (11).

Hošťálková, E., Vyšata, O., & Procházka, A. (2007). Multi-Dimensional Biomedical Image De-Noising Using Haar Transform. *In Proc. of 15th Int.l Conf. on Digital Signal Processing*, (pp. 175-178). Cardiff.

Izenman, A. J. (1991). Recent Developments in Nonparametric Density Estimation. *Journal of the American Statistical Association , 86* (413), 205-224.

Khare, A., & Shanker Tiwary, U. (2005). A New Method for Deblurring and Denoising of Medical Images using Complex Wavelet Transform. *27th Annual Int. Conf. of the Engineering in Medicine and Biology Society* (pp. 1897 - 1900). Shanghai : IEEE-EMBS.

Kingsbury, N. G. (2003). Design of Q-shift Complex Wavelets for Image Processing Using Frequency Domain Energy Minimisation. *International Conference on Image Processing* (pp. NK1--4). Vancouver: IEEE.

Mallat, S. (2009). *A Wavelet Tour of Signal Processing* (3rd ed.). Academic Press, Elsevier.

McNitt-Gray, M. F. (2006). Tradeoffs in CT Image Quality and Dose. *33* (6), 2154–2162.

Motwani, M. C., Gadiya, M. C., & Motwani, R. C. (2004). Survey of Image Denoising Techniques. *Global Signal Processing Expo and Conference.* Santa Clara, CA.

Percival, D. B., & Walden, A. T. (2006). *Wavelet Methods for Time Series Analysis. Cambridge Series in Statistical and Probabilistic Mathematics.* New York, U.S.A.: Cambridge University Press.

Romberg, J., Choi, H., & Baraniuk, R. G. (2001). Bayesian Tree-Structured Image Modeling Using Wavelet-Domain Hidden Markov Models. *IEEE Transactions on Image Processing , 10* (7).

Rowe, D. B. (2003). *Multivariate Bayesian Statistics: Models for Source Separation and Signal Unmixing.* Chapman and Hall/CRC.

Samé, A., & al., e. (2007). Mixture Model-Based Signal Denoising. *Advances in Data Anal. and Classification , 1* (1), 39-51.

Scott, D. W. (1979). On Optimal and Data-Based Histograms. *Biometrika , 66* (3), 605-610.

Selesnick, W., Baraniuk, R. G., & Kingsbury, N. G. (2005). The Dual-Tree Complex Wavelet Transform. *IEEE Signal Processing Magazine , 22* (6).

Shepp, L. A., & Logan, B. F. (1974). The Fourier Reconstruction of a Head Section. *Transactions on Nuclear Science , NS-21,* ;NS-21:21–43.

Simoncelli, E. P., & Adelson, E. H. (1996). Noise Removal via Bayesian Wavelet Coring. *3rd IEEE International Conference on Image Processing*, (pp. 379 - 382). Lausanne (Switzerland).

Starck, J. L., Fadili, J., & Murtagh, F. (2007). The Undecimated Wavelet Decomposition and its Reconstruction. *IEEE Transactions on Image Processing , 16* (2), 297-309.

Švihlík, J. (2009). Modeling of Scientific Images Using GMM. *Radioengineering , 18* (4), 579-586.

Švihlík, J., & Páta, P. (2008). Elimination of Thermally Generated Charge in Charged Coupled Devices Using Bayesian Estimator. *Radioengineering , 17* (2), 119-124.

Thavavel, v., & Murugesan, R. (2007). Regularized Computed Tomography using Complex Wavelets. *Int. Journal of Magnetic Resonance Imaging , 1* (1), 27-32.

Wang, J., & Huang, H. K. (1996). Medical Image Compression by Using Three-Dimensional Wavelet Transformation. *IEEE Trans. on Medical Imaging* , 15 (4), 547-554.

Wu, X., & Qiu, T. (2005). Wavelet Coding of Volumetric Medical Images for High Throughput and Operability. *IEEE Transactions on Medical Imaging* , 24 (6).

You, J., & Zeng, G. L. (2007). Hilbert Transform Based FBP Algorithm for Fan-Beam CT Full and Partial Scans. *IEEE Transactions on Medical Imaging* , 26 (2), 190-199.

Zhu, L., & StarLack, J. (2007). A Practical Reconstruction Algorithm for CT Noise Variance Maps Using FBP Reconstruction. *Proc. of SPIE: Medical Imaging 2007: Physics of Medical Imaging. 6510*, p. 651023. SPIE.

20

Determination of Optimal Parameters and Feasibility for Imaging of Epileptic Seizures by Electrical Impedance Tomography: A Modelling Study Using a Realistic Finite Element Model of the Head

L. Fabrizi[1], L. Horesh[1], J. F. Perez-Juste Abascal, A. McEwan[3],
O. Gilad[1], R. Bayford[2] and D. S. Holder[1]

[1]*Department of Medical Physics and Bioengineering, University College London,*
[2]*Department of Natural Science, Middlesex University, London,*
[3]*School of Electrical and Information Engineering, The University of Sydney,*
[1,2]*UK*
[3]*Australia*

1. Introduction

One potentially powerful application of Electrical Impedance Tomography (EIT) lies in the detection of the source of epileptic seizures in the brain (Holder, 2005). Many patients with epilepsy can be treated with drugs, but surgical resection of the abnormal region which produces seizures may be the only option in severe cases (Engel, Jr., 1993; Rosenow and Luders, 2001). For these, EIT could be used to provide continuous imaging over days while the subject is observed on a ward and so could, uniquely, provide images of conductivity changes related to increased blood volume or cell swelling in the onset zone of the brain where the seizure starts. If successful, this would provide imaging evidence not possible with any other method and would obviate the need in some difficult cases for invasive investigation with intracranial electrodes (Fabrizi et al., 2006).

It has already been shown that impedance increases locally in the brain by 3-12% at 1kHz up to 22% at 50 Hz during induced epileptic seizures (Elazar et al., 1966; Fox et al., 2004; VAN HARREVELD and Shade, 1962). Resistance changes of 5.5-7.1% associated with focal and generalized seizures have been imaged with EIT using a ring of electrodes placed on the exposed cortex of rabbits at 51 kHz (Rao, 2000). It therefore seems plausible that these changes are large enough to enable EIT to produce images of conductivity variations of clinical interest. Nevertheless, in a first pilot study in humans, it was not possible to measure reproducible boundary voltage changes during seizures as they were reaching 1-54% (Fabrizi et al., 2006). The most probable explanation was that true scalp voltage changes due to cerebral seizure were obscured by movement artefacts. However it was not clear whether even in ideal conditions it would have been possible to obtain informative tomographic images.

Therefore it is important to understand what are the EIT hardware and recording system requirements that would maximise the chance of detecting reliable changes associated with an epileptic seizure. In this chapter, computer simulations of the problem are used to suggest the best recording parameters, set a specification for hardware accuracy, and, finally, assess whether EIT imaging of seizures appears feasible with the suggested optimal arrangement in ideal conditions.

1.1 Experimental design

The complex boundary voltages on the scalp were calculated by solving the forward problem for a realistic 3D Finite Element Model (FEM) of the human head under normal conditions and during focal epileptic seizures. The FEM comprised regions of grey and white matter, cerebrospinal fluid (CSF), skull, scalp and eyes. The complex conductivities were extrapolated from the literature at 7 frequencies between 5Hz and 4MHz, as this is the available range in present EIT systems (McEwan et al., 2006; Oh et al., 2005). Four brain regions, which are common sources of epileptic activity, were chosen as the epileptic onset areas. The detection from scalp measurements was of increasing difficulty, as they decreased in volume and increased in depth. For simplicity, the tissues were all assumed to be isotropic.

Two different current level patterns with respect to frequency were considered, in order to choose the best measuring combination of frequencies or single frequency: (i) a uniform level of 100µA across the whole spectrum; (ii) an increasing pattern with frequency, as the International Electrotechnical Commission IEC601 standard specifies a 'patient auxiliary current' limit of 100µA from 0.1 Hz to 1 kHz; then $100*f$ µA from 1 kHz to 100 kHz where f is the frequency in kHz; then 10 mA above 100 kHz.

To assess whether the voltage changes obtained in the simulation were large enough to provide clinically useful EIT images, images after adding random noise of 0.3-0.4% to the simulated boundary voltages were reconstructed. For the reconstruction, 50 kHz simulated current was adopted, as findings from the previous section predicted that it would give the highest signal-to-noise ratio (SNR).

Because a temporal resolution of 1 sec is needed to record epileptic seizures, temporal averaging could be considered in order to enhance the SNR.. Different EIT data recording strategies allow different acquisition speeds and therefore time averaging capabilities. The recording strategies to consider are: a) Serial – a single impedance measuring circuit with a multiplexer; b) Semi-parallel – multiple parallel recording but a single current source which is multiplexed between different electrode pairs or c) Fully-parallel – multiple simultaneous current injection and record. The degree of averaging can be estimated as follows: for 31 electrodes, the reconstruction algorithm usually employed in EIT brain imaging has 258 electrode combinations, with 21 different injection pairs. If two periods are sufficient for each measurement and 1 µs is need for the combination switching, the number of frames n which can be averaged in 1 second is $1/(2*258*(1/f+1e-6))$ for a serial system, $1/(2*21*(1/f+1e-6))$ for a semi-parallel system and $f/2$ for a fully-parallel system, where f is the measuring frequency (Table 1). The noise reduction is given by $\sqrt{n}$.

System Type	Current Frequency	
	50 Hz	50 kHz
Serial	no (no)	185 (10x)
Semi-parallel	2.4 (no)	2268 (34x)
Fully-parallel	50 (5x)	50k (158x)

Table 1. Number of frames which can be averaged in 1 second with serial, semi-parallel and fully-parallel systems (resulting noise reduction factor)

2. Methods

2. Impedance properties of tissues in the head
2.1 Impedance values for resting conditions

The conductivity values were obtained with a cubic interpolation between data points taken from the literature at available frequencies. Data collected from tissues as close as possible to living human tissue in the frequency range 5Hz-4MHz were considered. If the frequency range was only partially covered, data from different studies were integrated. Data obtained at body temperature were used when available, otherwise a linear correction of +2 %/oC was applied (Foster and Schwan, 1989). Four-terminal measurements were preferred over two-terminal measurements.

The model used in this chapter was isotropic and homogeneous. Mean representative conductivity values for anisotropic tissues such as scalp, skull and white matter were adopted.

2.2 Scalp

The scalp is the soft tissue that envelops the skull. It comprises skin, connective tissue (superficial fascia), epicranial aponeurosis and epicranius. During EIT experiments, the stratum corneum of the skin is often removed by abrasion. As the authors were not aware of any validated direct measurements of scalp conductivity at the time of writing, they approximated it as a homogenous layer of skeletal muscle. Conductivity was therefore estimated from values for excised bovine paravertebral muscle at body temperature, taking into account muscle anisotropy at 10 Hz-10 MHz (Gabriel et al., 1996a). Considering that muscle fibres in the scalp are parallel to the head surface and to the skull, the final representative scalp conductivity was considered as 2/3 transverse and 1/3 longitudinal that of the muscle, as the current may cross the fibres in the longitudinal or transverse direction (Horesh, 2006).

2.3 Skull

The skull comprises a trabecular layer embedded in two cortical layers. The representative skull conductivity was considered as 2/3 that of cortical bone and 1/3 that of trabecular to represent this composition. Cortical and trabecular bone are anisotropic; unfortunately, no studies which account for this appear to have been performed over the frequency range of interest. Cortical bone admittivity has been measured on rat femur freshly excised over a frequency range of 10 Hz-100 MHz at body temperature without considering anisotropy (Kosterich et al., 1983). Trabecular bone was represented using measurements on frozen cancellous bovine femur samples (Sierpowska et al., 2003) defrosted at room temperature just before the measurements, which were conducted between 20 Hz and 5 MHz. Human trabecular bone was found to be about twice more conductive than bovine under similar experiment conditions (Sierpowska et al., 2005), so the real part of the conductivity was doubled and increased by 30% to adjust a recording temperature of 22 to 37 °C.

2.4 Cerebrospinal fluid (CSF)

CSF is an ionic fluid with high conductivity and null permittivity. The former was almost constant between 10 Hz and 10 kHz for human CSF at body temperature (Baumann et al., 1997). As CSF is a purely resistive medium, the mean of the values below 10 kHz was taken to be constant up to 4 MHz.

2.5 Grey matter

Grey matter mainly comprises nerve cell bodies and their branches, a small proportion of myelinated axons and glial cells; its structure is essentially isotropic. In-vivo measurement in humans have been conducted at 50 kHz (Latikka et al., 2001), but the admittivity of bovine tissue in-vitro was measured between 10 Hz and 20 MHz (Gabriel et al., 1996a). These data were translated according to the Lattika recordings at 50 kHz.

2.6 White matter

White matter mainly comprises myelinated nerve axons, which have different longitudinal and transverse conductivity, and is anisotropic. Since the nerve fibres are randomly oriented, the white matter has been considered to have an equivalent volume of 1/3 of fibres longitudinal to the current path and 2/3 transverse (Ranck, Jr., 1963). The conductivity of a bundle of parallel axons was measured in the two directions in-vivo in the dorsal column of cats between 5 Hz and 50 kHz (Ranck, Jr. and BEMENT, 1965). An averaged conductivity (1/3 longitudinal + 2/3 transverse) was calculated as representative of the white matter. The conductivity of in-vitro bovine tissue has been measured between 10 Hz and 20 MHz (Gabriel et al., 1996a). These data were translated according to the mean difference from the spectrum obtained from Ranck and Bement recordings for the overlapping frequency range and employed in the model.

2.7 Eyes

The eye is a complex ensemble of structures, whose admittivities have been measured separately. Only the cornea, lens, retina, sclera, vitreous and aqueous humours compartments were considered; the other parts of the eye are physically small and their contribution was discounted. The volume of each compartment was estimated from the images on http://www.discoveryfund.org/anatomyoftheeye.html. Due to lack of information through our frequency range, the admittivities extrapolated between 10 Hz and 100 GHz with a model simulating four Cole-Cole type dispersions were employed in the model (Gabriel et al., 1996b). The admittivity of retina was assumed to be equal to that of cornea, since they were similar between 1 MHz and 10 MHz (Gabriel et al., 1996a) and that of aqueous humour was assumed equal to that of vitreous humour, since they were similar between 5 Hz and 2 kHz (Lindenblatt and Silny, 2001).

2.8 Values employed in the model

The real part of the conductivities of the tissues is about 1 order of magnitude larger than the imaginary part (Fig. 1; Table 2).

2.9 Conductivity changes due to focal epilepsy

Published data on impedance changes during seizures are discontinuous over the frequency range considered in this chapter. Impedance changes during spreading depression (SD) were therefore considered to integrate these data. SD has already been used as a model for epilepsy since it has similar impedance characteristics (Boone et al., 1994) and probably is due to the same cell processes (Leao, 1944).

The real and imaginary component of the resistivity have been measured separately in anesthetized rabbits during SD at frequencies between 5Hz and 50kHz (Ranck Jr, 1964). The change in conductivity and dielectric constant have also been recorded in anesthetized rats at frequencies between 300 kHz and 100 MHz (Yoon et al., 1999). These measurements were converted in specific conductivity and scaled to take into account differences between epilepsy and SD, such as lower extracellular space shrinkage (Lux et al., 1986). Resistance changes of 9.5±1.4% during focal epileptic seizures at 47 kHz were measured locally in anesthetized rabbits (Rao, 2000). The ratio between this change and the change in the real part of the resistivity in SD at 50 kHz (Ranck's measurement closer to 47 kHz) was used to transform changes due to SD to changes due to epilepsy. Since the basic mechanisms underlying both SD and epilepsy are likely to be identical (VAN HARREVELD and Shade, 1962) the changes in cell membrane could be considered the same in both conditions. The main difference between them is then the different extent of cell swelling. When the extracellular space shrinks, more current is likely to go through the cells (Ranck Jr, 1964). Since cell swelling is less in epilepsy, the variation in the real and imaginary component of the resistivity would be reduced to the same extent in epilepsy with respect to SD; the same conversion was used also at frequencies different from 50 kHz. The predictions from these assumptions were similar to those found experimentally by Elazar et al. (Elazar et al., 1966) and Fox et al. (Fox et al., 2004).

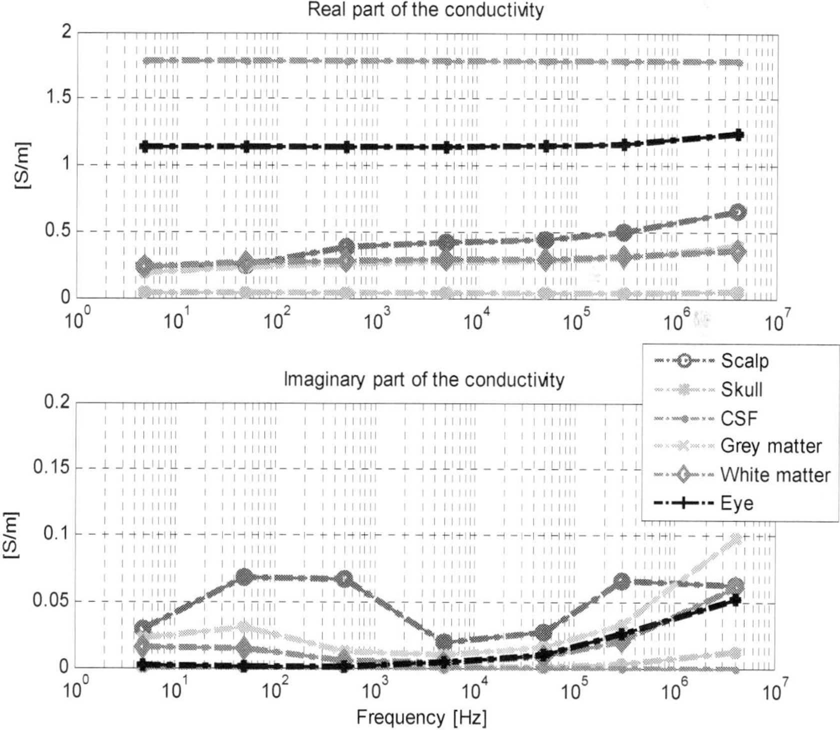

Fig. 1. Estimated conductivity spectra of the tissues in the adult human head employed in this study.

Tissue		Frequency						
		5Hz	50Hz	500Hz	5kHz	50kHz	300kHz	4MHz
Scalp	Re (S/m)	0.235	0.247	0.382	0.419	0.437	0.503	0.653
	Im (S/m)	0.029	0.067	0.067	0.019	0.027	0.066	0.062
Skull	Re (S/m)	0.037	0.037	0.038	0.038	0.039	0.041	0.047
	Im (S/m)	5e-4	4e-4	1e-4	2e-4	0.001	0.002	0.012
CSF	Re (S/m)	1.793	1.793	1.793	1.793	1.793	1.793	1.793
	Im (S/m)	0	0	0	0	0	0	0
Grey matter	Re (S/m)	0.185	0.232	0.259	0.270	0.285	0.306	0.391
	Im (S/m)	0.023	0.030	0.012	0.009	0.016	0.033	0.098
White matter	Re (S/m)	0.238	0.273	0.283	0.288	0.296	0.309	0.361
	Im (S/m)	0.016	0.014	0.005	0.004	0.009	0.019	0.062
Eyes	Re (S/m)	1.136	1.139	1.139	1.142	1.150	1.163	1.238
	Im (S/m)	0.002	0.001	0.001	0.004	0.009	0.026	0.052

Table 2. Estimated values of the real (Re) and imaginary (Im) part of the conductivity spectra of the tissues in the adult human head employed in this study in the frequency range 5Hz-4MHz.

The imaginary part of the conductivity of the grey matter has a larger proportional change than the real part, but its absolute change is smaller (Fig. 2).

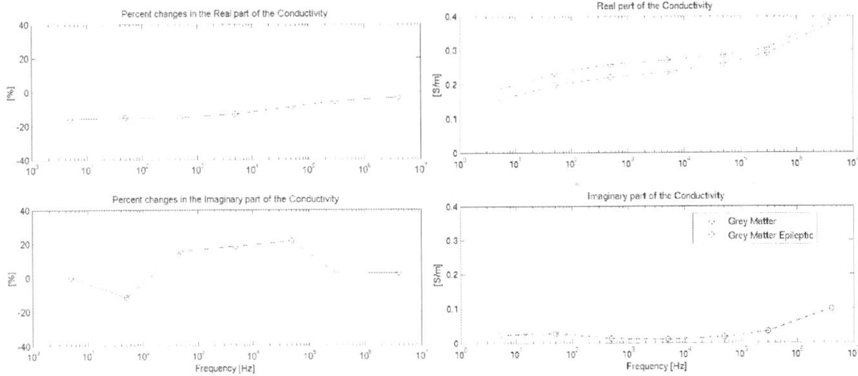

Fig. 2. Estimated conductivity proportional (left) and absolute (right) changes due to focal epilepsy.

3. Methods

3.1 Forward problem and 3D Finite Element Model

In order to determine the boundary voltage changes, the complex forward problem was solved for a realistic 3D Finite Element Model of the human head. The model was obtained using a modified version of EIDORS-3D Toolkit, which includes a finite element field solver (Polydorides and Lionheart, 2002) and a realistic head shaped multi-compartment mesh of 53000 elements generated with I-DEAS software (Tizzard et al., 2005). The compartments included scalp, skull, CSF, white and grey matter and eyes. Thirty-one electrodes and one ground, 10 mm in diameter, were placed in a modified 10-20 system on the scalp. A frequency-dependent contact resistance, obtained experimentally, was included in the model; it decreased from 3 kΩ at 5 Hz to 250Ω at 4 MHz.

The forward problem was solved at 5 Hz, 50 Hz, 500 Hz, 5 kHz, 50 kHz, 300 kHz, and 4 MHz. In each case, the value of the complex conductivity at that frequency was assigned to each compartment. The forward problem was first solved for brain under normal conditions. Then it was solved using the same mesh with modification of the grey matter conductivity for four possible epileptic regions: the lateral temporal lobe, the parahippocampus and hippocampus together, the parahippocampus alone and the hippocampus alone (Fig. 3). The temporal lobe was represented as a disc of 18 cm3 close to the surface, the parahippocampus as a prism with triangular base of 6 cm3 and the hippocampus as a cylinder of 2.5 cm3 deep in the brain. Data from the simulations were obtained from all 94395 possible non-equivalent electrode combinations, according to symmetry and reciprocity principles. No potential differences were calculated from electrode pairs containing current carrying electrodes.

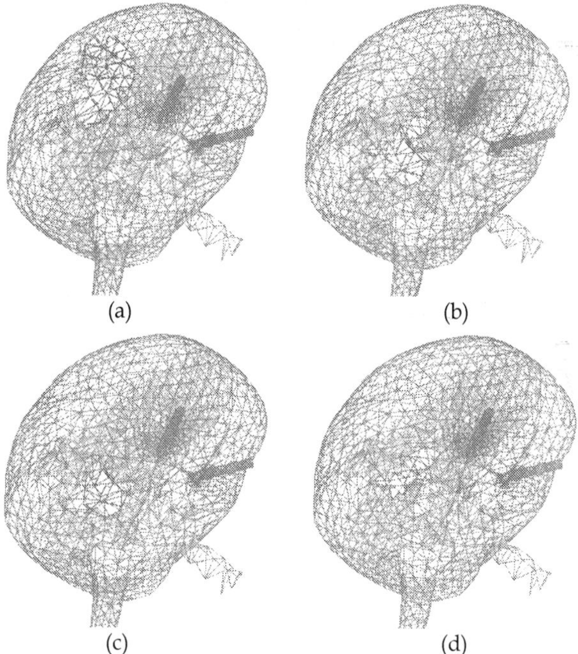

(a)   (b)

(c)   (d)

Fig. 3. Focal seizure areas: (a) right lateral temporal lobe; (b) right hippocampus and parahippocampus; (c) right parahippocampus; (d) right hippocampus.

3.2 Boundary voltage analysis method

The complex boundary voltages obtained from all the electrode combinations with a current of 100 µA were considered and the same analysis was conducted separately on the real and imaginary part. Combinations with a low amplitude which could not be accurately measured or likely to be obscured by noise – less than 0.1 μV for changes during seizures or 100 μV for standing boundary voltages under normal conditions – were eliminated from further investigation for each frequency. The average of the highest 1% of these changes was taken as a representative index together with the corresponding mean absolute change across frequencies. A theoretical advantage existed if greater currents were injected at higher frequencies according to safety standards. To examine this, the effect of greater injected current was simulated by multiplication of boundary voltages, since these are linearly related to injected current with the employed forward problem. The boundary voltages at 5 kHz and 50 kHz were multiplied by $(100*f)\mu A/100\mu A$ and the boundary voltages at 300 kHz and 4 MHz by 10mA/100μA. Since the measured voltages would be greater, the gain of the measuring amplifiers would have needed to be decreased to avoid saturation. To take this into account, combinations with less than 1 μV on the boundary voltage changes during seizures or 1 mV on the standing boundary voltages under normal conditions were eliminated from further investigation for each frequency.

3.3 Image reconstruction

Reporting of the greatest 1% of voltage changes is a simple guide to peak changes. In order to examine whether the predicted changes would translate into clinically useful images, images of the above perturbations were reconstructed using the potential changes obtained from the simulation of a polar injection protocol of 258 electrode combinations with a current of 5 mA at 50 kHz. Random noise with RMS of 0.35% and of 20% was added respectively to the real and imaginary part of the boundary voltages before reconstruction. This noise level was that present on the boundary voltages measured on a cylindrical saline tank with stainless steel electrodes (McEwan et al., 2006). To simulate the possibility of noise reduction with averaging, the noise was decreased 10, 34 or 158 times for serial, semi-parallel or fully parallel systems respectively (Table 1). The linear inverse problem was solved using a complex sensitivity matrix pseudo-inverted by truncated singular value decomposition (Bagshaw et al., 2003), with a fixed truncation level of 10^{-3} of the magnitude of the largest singular value, employing the same mesh of the forward problem.

4. Results

4.1 Simulated boundary voltage changes during seizures with 100μA applied at all frequencies

4.1.1 Real part

The top 1% of changes was 0.77%(1.45μV) at 5-50 Hz falling to 0.12%(0.2μV) at 4 MHz for a seizure in the temporal lobe. It decreased with depth of seizure site to 0.05%(0.13μV) at 5 Hz for a seizure in the hippocampus falling to 0%(0μV) at 4 MHz (Fig. 4, Table 3).

Seizure Focus	Voltage Changes	
	Real	Imaginary
Temporal	0.77%(1.45μV) - 0.77%(1.35μV)	0.48%(0.56μV) - 0.44%(0.57μV)
Para+Hippo	0.15%(0.25μV) - 0.16%(0.24μV)	0.12%(0.15μV) - 0.1%(0.14μV)
Parahippocampus	0.1%(0.16μV) - 0.1%(0.16μV)	0.03%(0.05μV) - 0.03%(0.05μV)
Hippocampus	0.05%(0.13μV) - 0.05%(0.13μV)	0% - 0%

Table 3. Averages of the highest 1% changes at 5Hz - 50Hz when the current level is kept constant across frequency

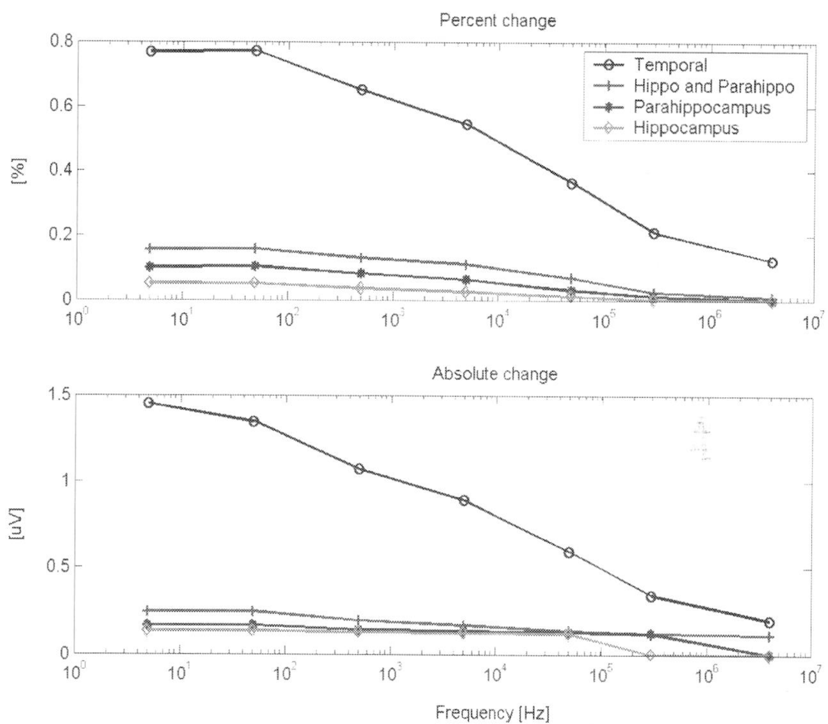

Fig. 4. Average of the largest 1% percent changes

The proportion of electrode combinations with measurable signal increased with the increase of the size of the epileptic region and its proximity to the surface (Table 4).

Seizure Focus	Current Frequency						
	5 Hz	50 Hz	500 Hz	5 kHz	50 kHz	300 kHz	4 MHz
Temporal	79.00	78.70	76.66	74.00	66.75	53.19	35.16
Para+Hippo	56.37	56.34	51.28	45.47	31.61	13.15	1.37
Parahippocampus	41.63	41.68	35.55	29.36	16.18	3.60	0.00
Hippocampus	23.84	23.59	17.90	12.79	4.03	0.02	0.00

Table 4. Percentage of electrode combinations which measure a voltage under normal conditions larger than 100 µV and a change larger 0.1 µV during seizures.

4.1.2 Imaginary part

The top 1% of changes was 0.48-0.44%(0.56-0.54µV) at 5-50 Hz falling to 0%(0µV) at 5 kHz for a seizure in the temporal lobe. It fell to 0%(0µV) at all frequencies for a seizure in the hippocampus (Fig. 5, Table 3).

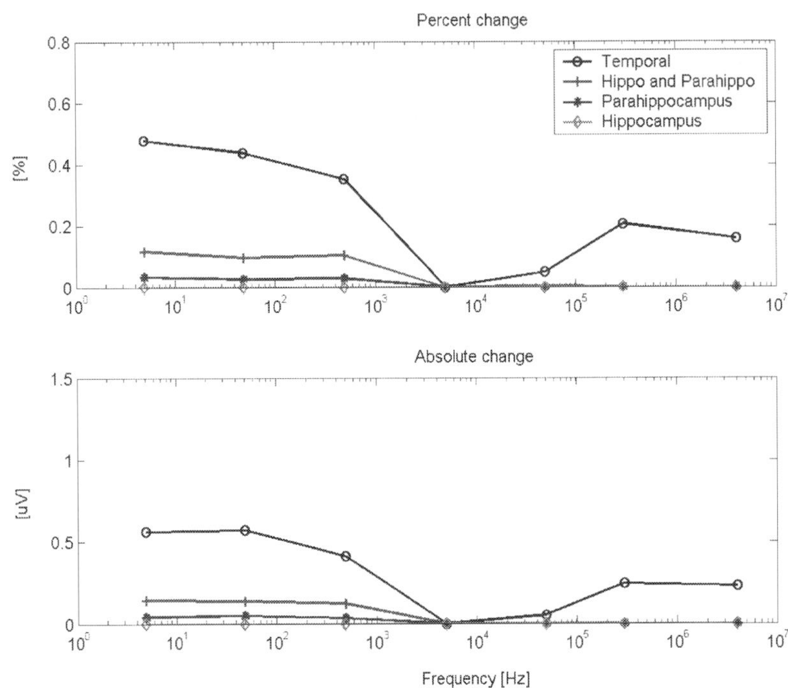

Fig. 5. Average of the largest 1% percent changes

The proportion of electrode combinations with measurable signal was lower than in the real part (Table 5).

Seizure Focus	Current Frequency						
	5 Hz	50 Hz	500 Hz	5 kHz	50 kHz	300 kHz	4 MHz
Temporal	2.36	3.63	1.50	0.00	0.19	4.22	11.40
Para+Hippo	1.03	1.45	0.91	0.00	0.01	0.00	0.00
Parahippocampus	0.39	0.45	0.32	0.00	0.00	0.00	0.00
Hippocampus	0.00	0.00	0.00	0.00	0.00	0.00	0.00

Table 5. Percentage of electrode combinations which measure a voltage under normal conditions larger than 100 µV and a change larger 0.1 µV during seizures.

4.2 Boundary voltage changes during seizures using higher current at high frequencies
4.2.1 Real part
The top 1% of changes was 0.26%(3.4µV) at 500 Hz increasing to 0.97%(21µV) at 50 kHz for a seizure in the temporal lobe. It was 0% (0µV) at 500 Hz increasing to 0.06%(1.8µV) at 50 kHz for a seizure in the hippocampus (Fig. 6, Table 6).

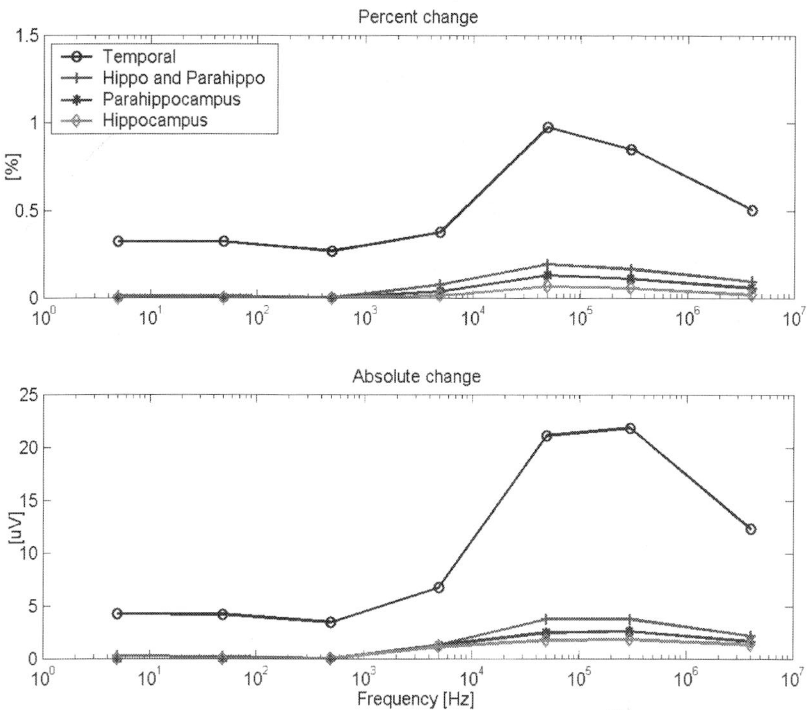

Fig. 6. Average of the largest 1% percent changes

The proportion of electrode combinations with measurable signal increased with the increase of the size of the epileptic region, its proximity to the surface and generally with the increase of the measuring frequency peaking between 50 and 300 kHz before falling at 4MHz (Table 7).

Seizure Focus	Voltage Changes	
	Real	Imaginary
Temporal	0.97%(21.1μV)	1.4%(19.8μV)
Para+Hippo	0.19%(3.75μV)	0.23%(2.9μV)
Parahippocampus	0.12%(2.5μV)	0.15%(1.9μV)
Hippocampus	0.06%(1.75μV)	0.08%(1.2μV)

Table 6. Averages of the highest 1% changes at 50 kHz when the current level conformed to the IEC601 standard

Seizure Focus	Current Frequency						
	5 Hz	50 Hz	500 Hz	5 kHz	50 kHz	300 kHz	4 MHz
Temporal	15.74	15.08	12.89	55.65	92.31	93.94	89.50
Para+Hippo	0.26	0.19	0.00	21.60	79.30	82.12	68.75
Parahippocampus	0.00	0.00	0.00	8.57	69.39	72.88	54.38
Hippocampus	0.00	0.00	0.00	1.09	53.75	58.42	36.02

Table 7. Percentage of electrode combinations which measure a voltage under normal conditions larger than 1 mV and a change larger 1 µV during seizures.

4.2.2 Imaginary part

The top 1% of changes was 0%(0µV) at 500 Hz and below increasing to 1.39%(20µV) at 50 kHz for a seizure in the temporal lobe. It was 0% (0µV) at 500 Hz and below increasing to 0.08%(1.2µV) at 50 kHz for a seizure in the hippocampus (Fig. 7, Table 6).

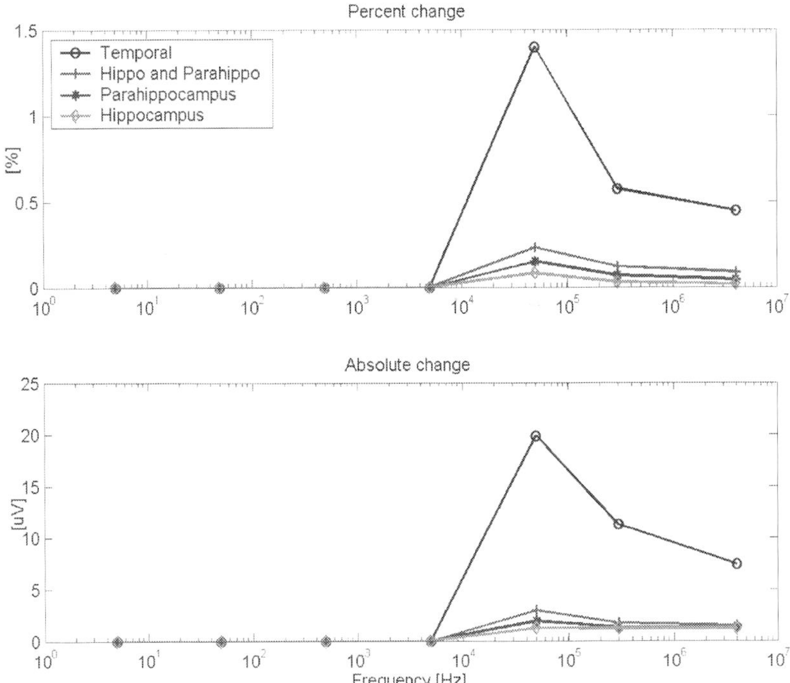

Fig. 7. Average of the largest 1% percent changes

At low frequencies, no electrode combinations had a measurable signal and the overall amount increases with the increase of the frequency (Table 8).

Seizure Focus	Current Frequency						
	5 Hz	50 Hz	500 Hz	5 kHz	50 kHz	300 kHz	4 MHz
Temporal	0.00	0.00	0.00	0.00	35.52	64.93	74.20
Para+Hippo	0.00	0.00	0.00	0.00	23.61	37.72	43.28
Parahippocampus	0.00	0.00	.0.00	0.00	15.46	22.22	26.27
Hippocampus	0.00	0.00	0.00	0.00	5.56	8.14	10.42

Table 8. Percentage of electrode combinations which measure a voltage under normal conditions larger than 1 mV and a change larger 1 µV during seizures.

4.3 Images reconstructed after addition of noise to simulated boundary voltages

Images of the real part in which a clear change occurred at the site of simulated seizure could be observed for all averaging cases for temporal lobe seizures. For the other three regions, this was only the case for fully parallel systems, which permitted the greatest degree of averaging. For imaginary component images, such accurate images could only be observed for temporal and combined hippocampal and parahippocampal seizure regions for the parallel injection and recording case (Fig. 8-Fig. 11).

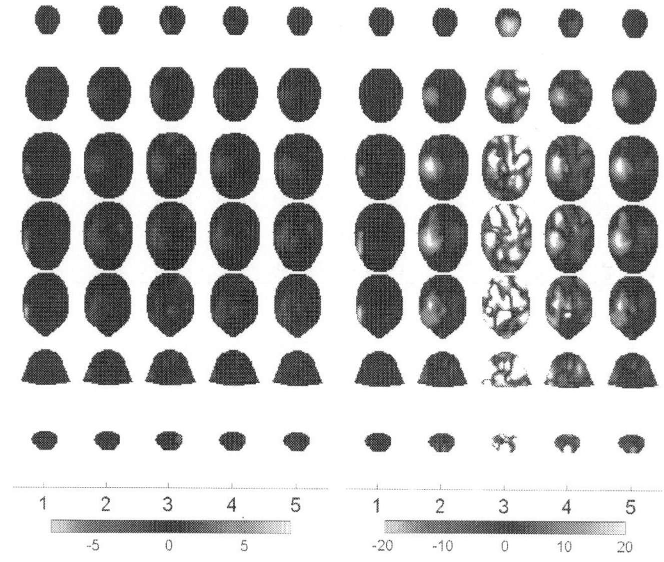

Fig. 8. Temporal lobe seizure. In this and the following figures, columns indicate simulated seizure region (1), reconstruction without noise (2), reconstruction with noise for serial (3), semi-parallel (4) and fully parallel (5) systems. Slices are shown from top of the head (top) to bottom (bottom). The colour bar indicates percentage impedance change. Real and imaginary changes are shown on the left and right respectively.

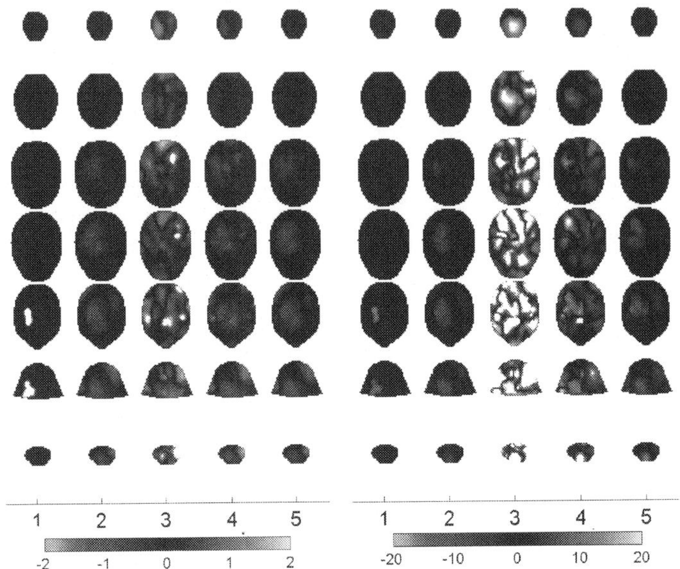

Fig. 9. Parahippocampus and hippocampus together.

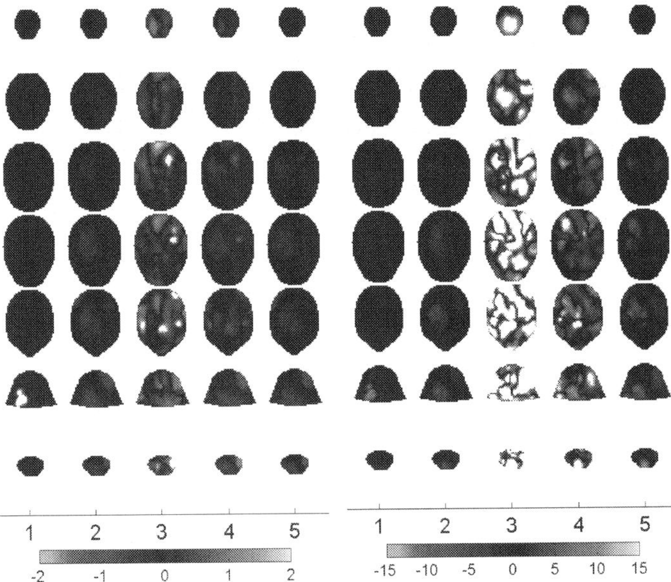

Fig. 10. Parahippocampus.

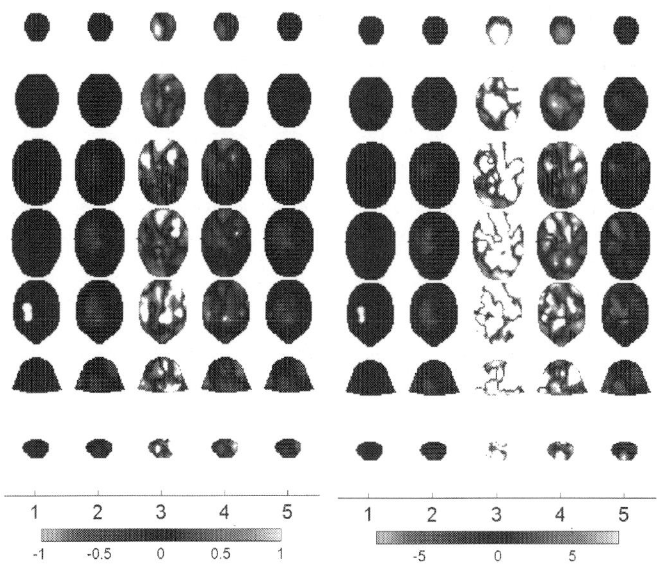

Fig. 11. Hippocampus.

5. Discussion

5.1 Summary of results

For a current level of 100 μA at all frequencies, the top 1% of the changes of the boundary voltage was almost 0.8% (1.5 μV) and 0.5% (0.6 μV) for the real and imaginary part respectively for lateral temporal lobe perturbation at 5-50 Hz. The same changes for seizures in parahippocampus and hippocampus together or separate were up to 10 times smaller. With higher current for high frequency, the top 1% of the changes of the boundary voltages was almost 1% (21 μV) and 1.4% (20 μV) for the real and imaginary part respectively for lateral temporal lobe perturbation at 50 kHz. The same changes were still up to 10 times smaller for seizures in smaller and deeper regions of the grey matter. In comparison, noise was estimated as 0.035, 0.01 or 0.002% for serial, semi-parallel or fully parallel systems respectively. With these settings, reasonably accurate images of the real component could be obtained during temporal lobe seizure for all averaging cases, and for the other three regions only for imaging with a parallel recording and injection system which permitted the most averaging. Images of the imaginary component were noisier but appeared reasonably accurate for parallel injection and recording only, and for the larger and more superficial cases of temporal lobe or combined parahippocampal and hippocampal seizures.

5.2 Technical issues

Advanced methodologies for 3D meshing, and in particular, to handle complex geometrical structures as those in the human head have been developed (Tizzard et al., 2005). These are based on segmentation of a MRI, extrapolation and smoothing of surfaces and then meshing of the different regions of the head. This has been validated in comparison to analytical solution for a homogenous sphere (Bagshaw et al., 2003) and with experimental measurements in a homogenous spherical saline tank and humans for low frequencies (Gilad et al., 2009).

The required mesh density for modelling is affected by the following factors:

1. PDE;
2. continuity / discontinuity of the conductivity;
3. smoothness of the volume;
4. measurement error;
5. mesh quality measures;
6. linear solver and preconditioner used;
7. machine precision.

The mesh resolution adopted in the modelling presented in this chapter was chosen (by means of progressive refinement) to provide modelling errors that were below typical measurement errors. It is important to note, that the price of overly refined model is in computation and conditioning of the resulting system.

Further improvements to the accuracy of the modelling could probably be achieved by overcoming a number of other simplifications in the method presented. The conductivities of the skull, white matter, scalp and eye were represented by a unique value for each frequency. In reality they comprise more types of tissue, are not homogenously distributed, and have a different conductivity in different directions (anisotropic). The values of the conductivities of the head tissue were approximated. Considering the anisotropy of the tissues, especially for scalp and skull, may decrease the boundary voltage changes estimated up to 5 folds, as 50% more current would be shunt through the scalp (Abascal et al. 2008). Assessing the influence of anisotropy in the reconstructed images would be ideal but validation of anisotropy is mayor work in itself and was beyond the purpose of this chapter. The literature does not provide the ideal data for human head modelling, which would be given by human in-vivo 4 terminal measurements on the considered frequency range. For this reason studies that were as close as possible to this standard had to be considered and reasonable corrections and integrations between information applied. The conductivity spectra finally adopted can be considered the best approximation of the real ones within the confinements of the approximations adopted in the model and current knowledge.

The noise included in the simulated data before reconstruction was given by preliminary results and was assumed to be random. This may be worse in the case of real measurement on patients on the ward (Meeson et al., 1996) and it may not be random, and therefore not possible to reduce with averaging. This chapter presents an estimate of the minimum SNR necessary to obtain a clinically useful EIT image, but a rigorous noise characterisation is necessary.

Simulation based feasibility analysis is a powerful method as the setup of the study can be almost completely controlled and quantified. Nevertheless, modelling is obviously limited, as it is often impossible to capture adequately all the possible factors that influence the measurements. Yet, this chapter provides a general guidance for the level of hardware accuracy that is needed for application in imaging epilepsy.

5.3 Best measuring frequencies

Using the same current of 100 μA at all frequencies (in a measuring set-up where all the frequencies are injected together), recordings at the lower frequencies of 5 and 50 Hz have the highest changes in percent and absolute values. This appears physiologically reasonable, as the greatest change in conductivity during seizures occurs at these frequencies. This is because the greatest distinction between extra- and intra-cellular space occurs at these low frequencies, being the current mostly confined outside the cell membrane.

Increasing the current according to the IEC601, the frequency with the highest changes is 50 kHz. This is because the benefit from injection of increased current appears to outweigh the larger intrinsic changes at low frequencies. This is self-evident for the criterion of absolute voltages, which may be expected to be higher as a result of the larger current injected. However, the explanation for proportional cases is not immediately apparent, as these might be expected to be independent of injected current – the standing and changed voltages during seizures might be expected to scale proportionately. The explanation is presumably because fewer voltages fall below the exclusion threshold for voltages too low to be significant, and these include those with the larger changes.

The RMS noise in the boundary voltages is about 0.3-0.4% for the real part in frequencies up to 100 kHz and it varies between 100-350% at 50 Hz and 15-25% at 50 kHz for the imaginary component. For a seizure in the temporal lobe, this translates to a signal-to-noise ratio of 2:1-3:1 for the real part measurement at 5-50 Hz with a current of 100 µA and at 50 kHz with a current of 5 mA; while for the imaginary part would be below 1:1.

Reducing the noise with averaging, it is likely that the signal-to-noise ratio could be increased 10 times at 50 kHz with a serial system or ideally more than 150 times with a fully parallel system. At this frequency the absolute value of the signal measured would be reaching tens of µV in temporal lobe epilepsy.

5.4 Noise influence on the image reconstruction

With the level of noise which is likely to be present with systems such as the UCH Mark 2.5 after averaging, only changes in the real part of the conductivity of the temporal lobe can be recognised in the reconstructed images. When the changes happen in deeper parts of the brain, the SNR is too low to give a clinically useful image. The noise is too large in the imaginary part and obscures the signal in any situation. This also suggests that if movement artefacts, which are of the order of few percent (Fabrizi et al., 2006), are present it would be not feasible to reconstruct any image. Even in the best case, the spatial resolution of the obtained EIT images is presently not alone good enough to guide the surgeon as to where to perform tissue resection. However this is likely to be at least as good as the spatial resolution of the EEG inverse source modelling (Merlet and Gotman, 2001), with which epileptic foci were identified within the resection borders in 90% of cases (Michel et al., 2004).

The SNR may be enhanced averaging more frames, but with a penalty in temporal resolution, using other signal processing tools or a different EIT system. A semi-parallel system seems to be able to image the real part of the perturbation in an area as small as the parahippocampus, but only the imaginary part of a perturbation in the temporal lobe. A fully-parallel system seems to be able to image everything, except the imaginary part for a perturbation in the hippocampus.

5.5 Future work

Sensitivity improvements rely on the possibility of reducing the baseline noise and on the intrinsic EIT instrumentation sensitivity. It may also be possible to average across different seizures in the same subject, assuming that those arising from the same onset zone can be identified clinically. Now that figures for the boundary voltage changes expected during seizures have been estimated, researchers need to ascertain that baseline noise can be kept well below the signal under controlled and clinical conditions.

The baseline variability in previous experiments was of the order of a few percent using standard EEG electrodes and it was mostly related to movement, and was presumably due changes in contact impedance (Fabrizi et al., 2006). Alternative electrode designs, such as hydrogel electrodes, have been explored (Tidswell et al., 2003) and should be reconsidered for reducing movement artefacts under ambulatory condition. As it is already common practice in long term EEG monitoring, electrodes could also be secured with collodion, which is a kind of medical glue. Future work may include the use of signal processing tools, such as principal component analysis, already implemented in EEG, to enhance EIT sensitivity, which may separate the voltage changes of interest from the noise (Perez-Juste Abascal, 2007).

It seems possible that baseline variability can be reduced below the signal expected, especially when the seizure occurs in the temporal lobe, as this has been possible in animal studies. The first useful experiment that could be carried out in the telemetry ward would be similar to that conducted by Gilad (Gilad and Holder, 2009). Employing patients with known epileptic conditions, an array of electrodes could be placed on the side of the head where the epilepsy onset area is expected, inject current from the best current injection pair and record potential from all the other electrodes combinations without involving current injection switching. This would be the optimal set-up to measure seizure-related boundary voltage changes, whose detection would lead to a future application of EIT as new method for neuroimaging in epilepsy.

The current EIT systems designed for brain imaging are the UCH Mk 2.5 (McEwan et al., 2006) and UCH Mk1b (Yerworth et al., 2002) serial systems and the KHU Mk1, which has parallel recording capabilities (Oh et al., 2007). However the possibility of using fully-parallel EIT systems originally designed for other applications could be considered. The Dartmouth group developed a fully parallel multifrequency 64-channel system for breast imaging (10kHz to 10MHz) which has an acquisition rate of 30 fps, that could possibly be raised to 60 fps adopting only 32 channels (Halter et al., 2008). The OXBACT 5 has been developed for thoracic imaging, it has a frequency range between 26 - 56 kHz, 16 current sources, 64 voltage measurement and could acquire 25 fps (Yue and McLeod, 2008). Another system developed for thoracic imaging is the Rensselaer ACT4, which measures between 300Hz - 1MHz and has 72 channels and a slower acquisition rate of 2 fps (Liu et al., 2005). So it appears that with already available systems a noise reduction between 5 and 8 times could be obtained.

On the basis of the predictions reported in this chapter, it seems plausible that neocortical seizures could be imaged if movement artefact could be kept to a minimum. This could be achieved by recording in the quiet interval of a few seconds before clonic or tonic movement occurs. It may also be possible to improve signal-to-noise by averaging across seizures and by recording at different frequencies and employing signal processing tools which separate the signal of interest from background activities. With these manoeuvres, it may also be possible to image deeper seizures from the mesial temporal lobe or deeper sources from other regions of the brain.

6. Appendix A. Derivation of complex conductivity changes during seizures

In the following discussion these symbols were adopted:
- ρ^{*r}_n $(= \rho'^r_n + j\rho''^r_n)$ the resistivity before the onset of the spreading depression at frequencies between 5 Hz and 50 kHz, where the superscript r indicates data recorded by Ranck (Ranck, 1963; Rank, 1964; Ranck and Bement, 1965);

- ρ^{*r}_{sd} $(= \rho'^{r}_{sd} + j\rho''^{r}_{sd})$ the average of the resistivity over the 30 sec with the highest changes at frequencies between 5 Hz and 50 kHz, where the superscript r indicates data recorded by Ranck (Ranck, 1963; Rank, 1964; Ranck and Bement, 1965);

- $\Delta\sigma'^{y}_{sd}$ the percent change in conductivity at frequencies between 300 kHz and 100 MHz, where the superscript y indicates data recorded by Yoon (Yoon et al., 1999);

- $\Delta\varepsilon^{y}_{sd}$ the percent change in dielectric constant at frequencies between 300 kHz and 100 MHz, where the superscript y represents Yoon measurements;

- $\Delta\rho_{ep}$ the resistivity change due to epilepsy measured at 47 kHz by Rao (Rao, 2000).

The subscript n stays indicates "normal", sd for "spreading depression" and ep for "epilepsy". The correction factor to account for the differences between spreading depression and epilepsy is calculated as:

$$R_{\rho} = \frac{\Delta\rho_{ep}}{\Delta\rho''^{r}_{sd}} \quad \text{where} \quad \Delta\rho''^{r}_{sd} = \frac{\rho''^{r}_{sd}(50kHz) - \rho''^{r}_{n}(50kHz)}{\rho''^{r}_{n}(50kHz)}$$

The resistivity during epilepsy at frequencies between 5 Hz and 50 kHz can be estimated as:

$$\rho'^{r}_{ep} = (\rho'^{r}_{sd} - \rho'^{r}_{n})R_{\rho} + \rho'^{r}_{n}$$

$$\rho''^{r}_{ep} = (\rho''^{r}_{sd} - \rho''^{r}_{n})R_{\rho} + \rho''^{r}_{n}$$

And the conductivity for normal, spreading depression and epileptic conditions as:

$$\sigma'^{r}_{n} = \frac{\rho'^{r}_{n}}{\rho'^{r2}_{n} + \rho''^{r2}_{n}} \quad \sigma'^{r}_{ep} = \frac{\rho'^{r}_{ep}}{\rho'^{r2}_{ep} + \rho''^{r2}_{ep}}$$

$$\sigma''^{r}_{n} = \frac{\rho''^{r}_{n}}{\rho'^{r2}_{n} + \rho''^{r2}_{n}} \quad \sigma''^{r}_{ep} = \frac{\rho''^{r}_{ep}}{\rho'^{r2}_{ep} + \rho''^{r2}_{ep}}$$

The percentage changes in conductivity at frequencies between 5 Hz and 50 kHz are then:

$$\Delta\sigma'^{r}_{ep} = \frac{\sigma'^{r}_{ep} - \sigma'^{r}_{n}}{\sigma'^{r}_{n}}$$

$$\Delta\sigma''^{r}_{ep} = \frac{\sigma''^{r}_{ep} - \sigma''^{r}_{n}}{\sigma''^{r}_{n}}$$

To translate the percent change of the conductivity at frequencies between 300 kHz and 100 MHz due to spreading depression in percent change due to epilepsy another conversion factor has to be calculated:

$$R_{\sigma} = \frac{\Delta\sigma'^{r}_{ep}(50kHz)}{\Delta\sigma'^{r}_{sd}(50kHz)}$$

Therefore the conductivity changes due to epilepsy at frequencies between 300 kHz and 100 MHz are:

$$\Delta\sigma'^{y}_{ep} = R_{\sigma}\Delta\sigma'^{y}_{sd}$$

A percent change in the dielectric constant corresponds with a percent change in the quadrature component of the conductivity, therefore:

$$\Delta\sigma''^{y}_{ep} = R_{\sigma}\Delta\varepsilon^{y}_{sd}$$

The overall spectrum of the percent conductivity change was obtained by joining $\Delta\sigma'^{r}_{ep}$ with $\Delta\sigma'^{y}_{ep}$ and $\Delta\sigma''^{r}_{ep}$ with $\Delta\sigma''^{y}_{ep}$ and used to modify the grey matter conductivity to simulate epileptic conditions (Fig. 2).

7. References

Bagshaw, A.P., Liston, A.D., Bayford, R.H., Tizzard, A., Gibson, A.P., Tidswell, A.T., Sparkes, M.K., Dehghani, H., Binnie, C.D., Holder, D.S., 2003. Electrical impedance tomography of human brain function using reconstruction algorithms based on the finite element method. Neuroimage. 20, 752-764.

Baumann, S.B., Wozny, D.R., Kelly, S.K., Meno, F.M., 1997. The electrical conductivity of human cerebrospinal fluid at body temperature. IEEE Trans.Biomed.Eng 44, 220-223.

Boone, K., Lewis, A.M., Holder, D.S., 1994. Imaging of cortical spreading depression by EIT: implications for localization of epileptic foci. Physiol Meas. 15 Suppl 2a, A189-A198.

Elazar, Z., KADO, R.T., Adey, W.R., 1966. Impedance changes during epileptic seizures. Epilepsia 7, 291-307.

Engel, J., Jr., 1993. Update on surgical treatment of the epilepsies. Summary of the Second International Palm Desert Conference on the Surgical Treatment of the Epilepsies (1992). Neurology 43, 1612-1617.

Fabrizi, L., Sparkes, M., Horesh, L., Perez-Juste Abascal, J.F., McEwan, A., Bayford, R.H., Elwes, R., Binnie, C.D., Holder, D.S., 2006. Factors limiting the application of Electrical Impedance Tomography for identification of regional conductivity changes using scalp electrodes during epileptic seizures in humans. Physiol.Meas. 27, 163-174.

Foster, K.R., Schwan, H.P., 1989. Dielectric properties of tissues and biological materials: a critical review. Crit Rev.Biomed.Eng 17, 25-104.

Fox, J.E., Bikson, M., Jefferys, J.G., 2004. Tissue resistance changes and the profile of synchronized neuronal activity during ictal events in the low-calcium model of epilepsy. J.Neurophysiol. 92, 181-188.

Gabriel, S., Lau, R.W., Gabriel, C., 1996a. The dielectric properties of biological tissues: II. Measurements in the frequency range 10 Hz to 20 GHz. Phys.Med.Biol. 41, 2251-2269.

Gabriel, S., Lau, R.W., Gabriel, C., 1996b. The dielectric properties of biological tissues: III. Parametric models for the dielectric spectrum of tissues. Phys.Med.Biol. 41, 2271-2293.

Gilad, O., Holder, D.S., 2009. Impedance changes recorded with scalp electrodes during visual evoked responses: implications for Electrical Impedance Tomography of fast neural activity. Neuroimage. 47, 514-522.

Gilad, O., Horesh, L., Holder, D.S., 2009. A modelling study to inform specification and optimal electrode placement for imaging of neuronal depolarization during visual evoked responses by electrical and magnetic detection impedance tomography. Physiol Meas. 30, S201-S224.

Halter, R.J., Hartov, A., Paulsen, K.D., 2008. A broadband high-frequency electrical impedance tomography system for breast imaging. IEEE Trans.Biomed.Eng 55, 650-659.

Holder, D.S., 2005. Electrical Impedance Tomography. Insitute of Physics Publishing, Bristol and Philadelphia.

Horesh, L., 2006. Some novel approaches in modelling and image reconstruction for multi-frequency electrical impedance tomography of the human brain. University College London, London.

Kosterich, J.D., Foster, K.R., Pollack, S.R., 1983. Dielectric permittivity and electrical conductivity of fluid saturated bone. IEEE Trans.Biomed.Eng 30, 81-86.

Latikka, J., Kuurne, T., Eskola, H., 2001. Conductivity of living intracranial tissues. Phys.Med.Biol. 46, 1611-1616.

Leao, A.A.P., 1944. Spreading depression of activity in cerebral cortex. J.Neurophysiol. 7, 359-390.

Lindenblatt, G., Silny, J., 2001. A model of the electrical volume conductor in the region of the eye in the ELF range. Phys.Med Biol 46, 3051-3059.

Liu, N., Saulnier, G.J., Newell, J.C., Kao, T.J., 2005. ACT 4: A high-precision, multi-frequency Electrical Impedance Tomograph. XI Conf. on Biomedical application of EIT (London, UK).

Lux, H.D., Heinemann, U., Dietzel, I., 1986. Ionic changes and alterations in the size of the extracellular space during epileptic activity. Adv.Neurol. 44, 619-639.

McEwan, A., Romsauerova, A., Yerworth, R., Horesh, L., Bayford, R., Holder, D., 2006. Design and calibration of a compact multi-frequency EIT system for acute stroke imaging. Physiol Meas. 27, S199-S210.

Meeson, S., Blott, B.H., Killingback, A.L., 1996. EIT data noise evaluation in the clinical environment. Physiol Meas. 17 Suppl 4A, A33-A38.

Merlet, I., Gotman, J., 2001. Dipole modeling of scalp electroencephalogram epileptic discharges: correlation with intracerebral fields. Clin.Neurophysiol. 112, 414-430.

Michel, C.M., Murray, M.M., Lantz, G., Gonzalez, S., Spinelli, L., Grave de, P.R., 2004. EEG source imaging. Clin.Neurophysiol. 115, 2195-2222.

Oh, T.I., Lee, E.J., Woo, E.J., Kwon, O., Seo, J.K., 2005. Multi-frequency EIT and TAS hardware development. XI Conf. on Biomedical application of EIT (London, UK).

Oh, T.I., Woo, E.J., Holder, D., 2007. Multi-frequency EIT system with radially symmetric architecture: KHU Mark1. Physiol Meas. 28, S183-S196.

Perez-Juste Abascal, J.F., 2007. Improvement in reconstruction algorithms for electrical impedance tomography of brain function. University College London.

Polydorides, N., Lionheart, W.R.B., 2002. Toolkit for three-dimensional Electrical Impedance Tomography: a contribution to the Electrical Impedance Tomography and Diffuse Optical Reconstruction software project. Mea.Sci.Technol. 13, 1871-1883.

Ranck Jr, J.B., 1964. Specific impedance of cerebral cortex during spreading depression, and an analysis of neuronal, neuroglial, and interstitial contributions. Exp.Neurol. 9, 1-16.

Ranck, J.B., Jr., 1963. Analysis of specific impedance of rabbit cerebral cortex. Exp.Neurol. 7, 153-174.

Ranck, J.B., Jr., BEMENT, S.L., 1965. The specific impedance of the dorsal columns of cat: an anisotropic medium. Exp.Neurol. 11, 451-463.

Rao, A., 2000. Electrical Impedance Tomography of brain activity: studies into its accuracy and physiological mechanisms. London: University College London.

Rosenow, F., Luders, H., 2001. Presurgical evaluation of epilepsy. Brain 124, 1683-1700.

Sierpowska, J., Hakulinen, M.A., Toyras, J., Day, J.S., Weinans, H., Jurvelin, J.S., Lappalainen, R., 2005. Prediction of mechanical properties of human trabecular bone by electrical measurements. Physiol Meas. 26, S119-S131.

Sierpowska, J., Toyras, J., Hakulinen, M.A., Saarakkala, S., Jurvelin, J.S., Lappalainen, R., 2003. Electrical and dielectric properties of bovine trabecular bone--relationships with mechanical properties and mineral density. Phys.Med.Biol. 48, 775-786.

Soni, N.K., Paulsen, K.D., Dehghani, H., Hartov, A., 2006. Finite element implementation of Maxwell's equations for image reconstruction in electrical impedance tomography. IEEE Trans.Med Imaging 25, 55-61.

Tidswell, A.T., Bagshaw, A.P., Holder, D.S., Yerworth, R.J., Eadie, L., Murray, S., Morgan, L., Bayford, R.H., 2003. A comparison of headnet electrode arrays for electrical impedance tomography of the human head. Physiol Meas. 24, 527-544.

Tizzard, A., Horesh, L., Yerworth, R.J., Holder, D.S., Bayford, R.H., 2005. Generating accurate finite element meshes for the forward model of the human head in EIT. Physiol Meas. 26, S251-S261.

Van Harreveld, A., Shade, J.P., 1962. Changes in the electrical conductivity of cerebral cortex during seizure activity. Exp.Neurol. 5, 383-400.

Yerworth, R.J., Bayford, R.H., Cusick, G., Conway, M., Holder, D.S., 2002. Design and performance of the UCLH mark 1b 64 channel electrical impedance tomography (EIT) system, optimized for imaging brain function. Physiol Meas. 23, 149-158.

Yoon, R.S., Czaya, A., Kwan, H.C., Joy, M.L., 1999. Changes in the complex permittivity during spreading depression in rat cortex. IEEE Trans.Biomed.Eng 46, 1330-1338.

Yue, X., McLeod, C., 2008. FPGA design and implementation for EIT data acquisition. Physiol Meas. 29, 1233-1246.

21

General Adaptive Neighborhood Image Processing for Biomedical Applications

Johan Debayle and Jean-Charles Pinoli
Ecole Nationale Supérieure des Mines de Saint-Etienne, CIS/LPMG-CNRS
France

1. Introduction

In biomedical imaging, the image processing techniques using spatially invariant transformations, with fixed operational windows, give efficient and compact computing structures, with the conventional separation between data and operations. Nevertheless, these operators have several strong drawbacks, such as removing significant details, changing some meaningful parts of large objects, and creating artificial patterns. This kind of approaches is generally not sufficiently relevant for helping the biomedical professionals to perform accurate diagnosis and therapy by using image processing techniques. Alternative approaches addressing context-dependent processing have been proposed with the introduction of spatially-adaptive operators (Bouannaya & Schonfeld, 2008; Ciuc et al., 2000; Gordon & Rangayyan, 1984; Maragos & Vachier, 2009; Roerdink, 2009; Salembier, 1992), where the adaptive concept results from the spatial adjustment of the sliding operational window. A spatially-adaptive image processing approach implies that operators will no longer be spatially invariant, but must vary over the whole image with adaptive windows, taking locally into account the image context by involving the geometrical, morphological or radiometric aspects. Nevertheless, most of the adaptive approaches require a priori or extrinsic informations on the image for efficient processing and analysis. An original approach, called General Adaptive Neighborhood Image Processing (GANIP), has been introduced and applied in the past few years by Debayle & Pinoli (2006a;b); Pinoli & Debayle (2007). This approach allows the building of multiscale and spatially adaptive image processing transforms using context-dependent intrinsic operational windows. With the help of a specified analyzing criterion (such as luminance, contrast...) and of the General Linear Image Processing (GLIP) (Oppenheim, 1967; Pinoli, 1997a), such transforms perform a more significant spatial and radiometric analysis. Indeed, they take intrinsically into account the local radiometric, morphological or geometrical characteristics of an image, and are consistent with the physical (transmitted or reflected light or electromagnetic radiation) and/or physiological (human visual perception) settings underlying the image formation processes. The proposed GAN-based transforms are very useful and outperforms several classical or modern techniques (Gonzalez & Woods, 2008) - such as linear spatial transforms, frequency noise filtering, anisotropic diffusion, thresholding, region-based transforms - used for image filtering and segmentation (Debayle & Pinoli, 2006b; 2009a; Pinoli & Debayle, 2007). This book chapter aims to first expose the fundamentals of the GANIP approach (Section 2) by introducing the GLIP frameworks, the General Adaptive Neighborhood (GAN) sets and two kinds of GAN-based image transforms: the GAN morphological filters and the GAN Choquet filters. Therefater in Section 3, several GANIP processes are illustrated in the fields of image restoration, image enhancement and image segmentation on practical biomedical application examples. Finally, Section 4 gives some conclusions and prospects of the proposed GANIP approach.

2. Fundamentals of the General Adaptive Neighborhood Image Processing (GANIP) approach

2.1 GLIP frameworks

In order to develop powerful image processing operators, it is necessary to represent intensity images within mathematical frameworks (most of the time of a vectorial nature) based on a physically and/or psychophysically relevant image formation process. In addition, their mathematical structures and operations (the vector addition and then the scalar multiplication) have to be consistent with the physical nature of the images and/or the human visual system, and computationally effective. Thus, although the Classical Linear Image Processing Framework (CLIP), based on the usual vectorial operations, has played a central role in image processing, it is not necessarily the best choice. Indeed, it was claimed (Rosenfeld, 1969) that the usual addition is not a satisfactory solution in some non-linear physical settings, such as that based on multiplicative or convolutive image formation model (Oppenheim, 1967; Stockham, 1972). The reasons are that the classical addition operation and consequently the usual scalar multiplication are not consistent with the combination and amplification laws to which such physical settings obey. However, using the power of abstract linear algebra, it is possible to go up to the abstract level and to explore General Linear Image Processing (GLIP) frameworks (Oppenheim, 1967; Pinoli, 1997a), in order to include situations in which images are combined by processes other than the usual vector addition. Consequently, operators based on such intensity-based image processing frameworks should be consistent with the physical and/or physiological settings of the images to be processed. For instance, the Logarithmic Image Processing (LIP) framework of intensity images $(f, g, \dots)$ has been introduced (Jourlin & Pinoli, 1988; 2001; Pinoli, 1987) with its vector addition $\triangle$ and its scalar multiplication $\triangle$ defined respectively as following:

$$f \triangle g = f + g - \frac{fg}{M} \tag{1}$$

$$\alpha \triangle f = M - M \left(1 - \frac{f}{M} \right)^{\alpha}, \quad \alpha \in \mathbb{R} \tag{2}$$

where $M \in \mathbb{R}^{+}$ denotes the upper bound of the range where intensity images are valued. The LIP framework has been proved to be consistent with the transmittance image formation model, the multiplicative reflectance image formation model, the multiplicative transmittance image formation model, and with several laws and characteristics of human brightness perception (Pinoli, 1997a;b). For example, the figure 1 shows an illustration of X-ray image enhancement in the CLIP and LIP frameworks.

2.2 GAN sets

The space of image (resp. criterion) mappings, defined on the spatial support $D \subseteq \mathbb{R}^2$ and valued in a real numbers interval $\tilde{E}$ (resp. E), is represented in a GLIP framework, denoted $\mathcal{I}$ (resp. $\mathcal{C}$). The GLIP framework $\mathcal{I}$ (resp. $\mathcal{C}$) is then supplied with an ordered vectorial

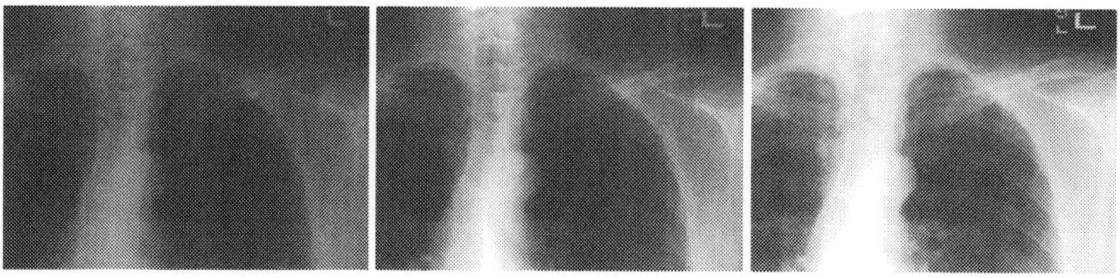

(a) original image   (b) CLIP enhancement   (c) LIP enhancement

Fig. 1. Example of thorax X-ray image enhancement in the CLIP and LIP frameworks. The LIP framework provides the best results from a visual point of view.

structure, using the formal vector addition $\tilde{\oplus}$ (resp. $\ominus$), the formal scalar multiplication $\tilde{\otimes}$ (resp. $\otimes$) and the classical partial order relation $\geq$ defined directly from those of real numbers. Two kinds of General Adaptive Neighborhoods can be introduced: the weak GANs and the strong GANs, defined in the following.

2.2.1 Weak GANs

For each pixel $x \in D$ and for an image $f \in \mathcal{I}$, its associated weak GAN, denoted $V_{m_O}^h(x)$, is included as subset in D. The GANs are built upon a criterion mapping $h \in \mathcal{C}$ (based on a local measurement such as luminance, contrast, thickness, ... related to f), in relation with an homogeneity tolerance m_O belonging to the positive intensity value range $E^{\oplus}$. The weak GANs are mathematically defined as following:

$$\forall (m_O, h, x) \in E^{\oplus} \times \mathcal{C} \times D, \quad V_{m_O}^h(x) = C_{h^{-1}([h(x)\ominus m_O, h(x)\oplus m_O])}(x) \tag{3}$$

where $C_X(x)$ denotes the path-connected component (with the usual Euclidean topology on $D \subseteq \mathbb{R}^2$) of the subset $X \subseteq D$ containing $x \in D$ and $h^{-1}(Y) = \{x \in D; h(x) \in Y\}$ for $Y \subseteq E$. The weak GANs satisfy several properties (Debayle & Pinoli, 2006a) such as reflexivity, increasing with respect to m_O, equality between iso-valued points, $\oplus$-translation invariance and $\otimes$-multiplication compatibility.

To much more understand the definition of the weak GANs, a one-dimensional example is presented in Figure 2, with the CLIP framework selected for the space of criterion mappings. Figure 3 illustrates on a real human retina image the GANs of two pixels computed with the luminance criterion in the CLIP framework with the homogeneity tolerance value $m = 20$. The GANs are self-determined and fit with the local spatial structures of the image. Indeed, the GAN of the pixel within a retinal vessel is only made up of a part of the vascular tree while the other GAN is restricted to the retinal fovea.

2.2.2 Strong GANs

A new collection of GANs, namely the strong GANs, denoted $N_{m_O}^h(x)$, is introduced:

$$\forall (m_O, h, x) \in E^{\oplus} \times \mathcal{C} \times D, \quad N_{m_O}^h(x) = \bigcup_{z \in D} \{V_{m_O}^h(z) | x \in V_{m_O}^h(z)\} \tag{4}$$

Obviously :

$$V_{m_O}^h(x) \subseteq N_{m_O}^h(x) \tag{5}$$

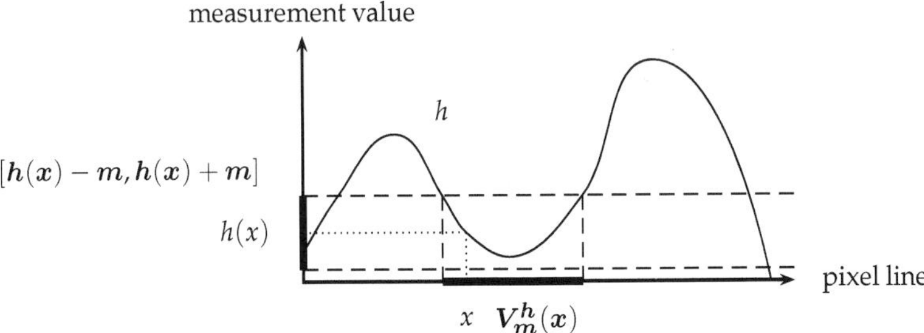

Fig. 2. One-dimensional representation of a weak GAN in the CLIP framework selected for the space of criterion mappings: for a pixel $x \in D$, its associated GAN, $V_m^h(x)$, is computed in relation with the considered criterion mapping $h \in C$ and a specified homogeneity tolerance value $m \in \mathbb{R}^+$.

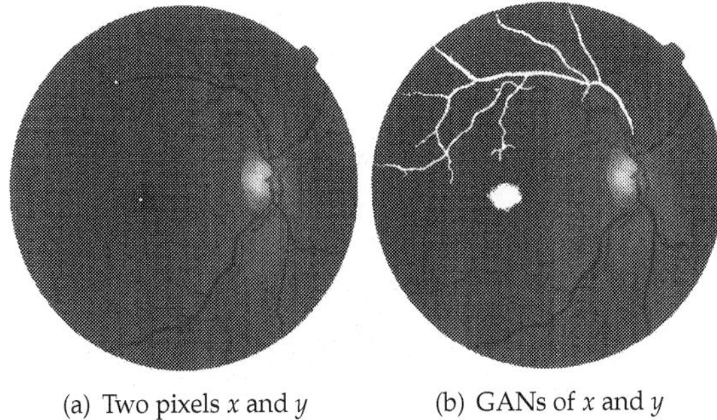

(a) Two pixels x and y (b) GANs of x and y

Fig. 3. Example of two weak GANs (b) on a human retina image (a) acquired by optical microscopy. The GANs are determined by the image itself.

The strong GANs $N_{m_\bigcirc}^h(x)$ satisfy similar properties as weak GANs. In addition, they satisfy the symmetry property:

$$x \in N_{m_\bigcirc}^h(y) \Leftrightarrow y \in N_{m_\bigcirc}^h(x) \tag{6}$$

The symmetry condition is relevant for topological and visual reasons (Debayle & Pinoli, 2005b) and allows to simplify the mathematical expressions of adaptive operators without increasing the computational complexity of the algorithms.
These GANs (weak and strong) are now used for defining adaptive morphological and Choquet filters.

2.3 GAN mathematical morphology

The origin of mathematical morphology stems from the study of the geometry of porous media by Matheron (1967). The mathematical analysis is based on set theory and lattice algebra. Its development is characterized by a crossfertilization between applications, methodologies, theories, and algorithms. It leads to several processing tools in the aim of image filtering, image segmentation, image classification, image measurement, pattern recognition, or texture analysis.

2.3.1 Classical morphological operators

The two fundamental operators of Mathematical Morphology (Serra, 1982) are mappings that commute with the infimun and supremum operations, called respectively erosion and dilation. To each morphological dilation there corresponds a unique morphological erosion, through a duality relation, and vice versa. Two operators ψ and ϕ defines an adjunction or a morphological duality Serra (1982) if and only if: $\forall (f, g) \in \mathcal{I} \quad \psi(f) \leq g \Leftrightarrow f \leq \phi(g)$.

The dilation and erosion of an image $f \in \mathcal{I}$ by a Structuring Element (SE) of size r, denoted B_r, are respectively defined as:

$$D_r(f) : \begin{cases} D \to \tilde{E} \\ x \mapsto \sup_{w \in \check{B}_r(x)} f(w) \end{cases} \tag{7}$$

$$E_r(f) : \begin{cases} D \to \tilde{E} \\ x \mapsto \inf_{w \in B_r(x)} f(w) \end{cases} \tag{8}$$

where $B_r(x)$ denotes the SE located at pixel x, and $\check{B}_r(x)$ is the reflected subset of $B_r(x)$.

The basic idea in the General Adaptive Neighborhood Mathematical Morphology (GANMM) (Debayle & Pinoli, 2006a; Pinoli & Debayle, 2009) is to replace the usual structuring element by GANs, providing adaptive operators and filters.

2.3.2 Adaptive morphological filters

The elementary operators of dilation and erosion use reflected SEs in order to satisfy the morphological adjunction. In order to get this adjunction without considering reflected SEs, the symmetric strong GANs $\{N^h_{m_O}(x)\}_{x \in D}$ are used as Adaptive Structuring Elements (ASEs).

The elementary adjunct operators of adaptive dilation and adaptive erosion are defined accordingly to the ASEs:

$\forall (m_O, h, f, x) \in E^{\oplus} \times \mathcal{C} \times \mathcal{I} \times D$

$$D^h_{m_O}(f)(x) = \sup_{w \in N^h_{m_O}(x)} f(w) \tag{9}$$

$$E^h_{m_O}(f)(x) = \inf_{w \in N^h_{m_O}(x)} f(w) \tag{10}$$

Therefore, the most elementary adaptive morphological filters can be defined: the GAN closing and the GAN opening.

$\forall (m_O, h, f) \in E^{\oplus} \times \mathcal{C} \times \mathcal{I}$

$$C^h_{m_O}(f) = E^h_{m_O} \circ D^h_{m_O}(f) \tag{11}$$

$$O^h_{m_O}(f) = D^h_{m_O} \circ E^h_{m_O}(f) \tag{12}$$

In the case where luminance is selected for the analyzing criterion ($h \equiv f$), these adaptive morphological filters are connected operators (for all (x, y) neighboring points - with the usual Euclidean topology on $D \subseteq \mathbb{R}^2$ - if $h(x) = h(y)$ then $N^h_{m_O}(x) = N^h_{m_O}(y)$ and therefore

$D^h_{m_\bigcirc}(x) = D^h_{m_\bigcirc}(y))$, which is an overwhelming advantage compared to the usual ones that fail to this strong property. Therefore, the building by composition or combination with the supremum and the infimum of these filters define connected operators, such as adaptive closing-opening and opening-closing filters:

$\forall (m_\bigcirc, h, f) \in E^\oplus \times \mathcal{C} \times \mathcal{I}$

$$CO^h_{m_\bigcirc}(f) = C^h_{m_\bigcirc} \circ O^h_{m_\bigcirc}(f) \tag{13}$$

$$OC^h_{m_\bigcirc}(f) = O^h_{m_\bigcirc} \circ C^h_{m_\bigcirc}(f) \tag{14}$$

The example of Fig. 4 illustrates the application of the usual and adaptive morphological operators of dilation and erosion on a human retinal vessels image. The adaptive operators do not damaged the spatial structures contrary to the usual ones.

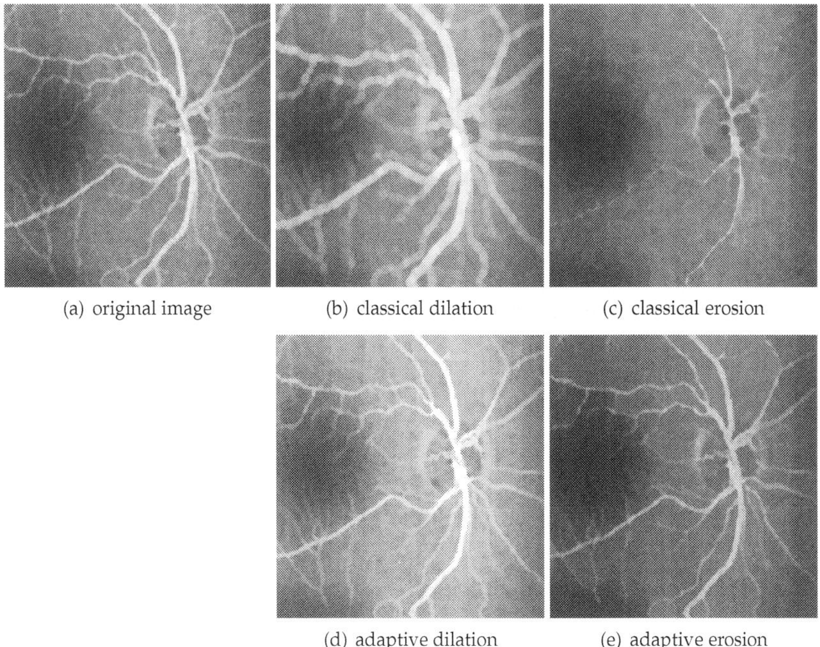

(a) original image   (b) classical dilation   (c) classical erosion

(d) adaptive dilation   (e) adaptive erosion

Fig. 4. Original image of human retinal vessels (a). Usual dilation (b) and erosion (c) of the original image using a disk of radius 2 as SE. Adaptive dilation (d) and erosion (e) of the original image using ASEs computed in the CLIP framework on the luminance criterion with the homogeneity tolerance value $m = 15$.

2.3.3 Adaptive sequential morphological filters

The families of adaptive morphological filters $\{O^h_m\}_{m \geq 0}$ and $\{C^h_m\}_{m \geq 0}$ are generally not a size distribution and antisize distribution (Serra, 1982) respectively, since the notion of semi-group is generally not satisfied. This kind of filters is largely used in image processing and analysis.

In the GANIP approach, such families can be built by naturally reiterate adaptive dilations or erosions. Explicitly, adaptive sequential dilation, and erosion are respectively defined as :
$\forall (m_O, h, f) \in E^\oplus \times \mathcal{C} \times \mathcal{I}$

$$D^h_{m,p}(f) = \underbrace{D^h_m \circ \cdots \circ D^h_m}_{p \text{ times}}(f) \tag{15}$$

$$E^h_{m,p}(f) = \underbrace{E^h_m \circ \cdots \circ E^h_m}_{p \text{ times}}(f) \tag{16}$$

The morphological adjunction of $D^h_{m,p}$ and $E^h_{m,p}$ provides, among other things, the two following adaptive sequential closing and opening filters:

$$C^h_{m,p}(f) = E^h_{m,p} \circ D^h_{m,p}(f) \tag{17}$$

$$O^h_{m,p}(f) = D^h_{m,p} \circ E^h_{m,p}(f) \tag{18}$$

Moreover, the families $\{O^h_{m,p}\}_{p \geq 0}$ and $\{C^h_{m,p}\}_{p \geq 0}$ generate size and antisize distributions, respectively. The extension to GANMM of the well-known alternating sequential filters (ASFs) can then be defined (Debayle & Pinoli, 2005a):
$\forall (m, n, h) \in E^\oplus \times \mathbb{N} \backslash \{0\} \times \mathcal{C}, \quad \forall (p_i) \in \mathbb{N}^{[\![1,n]\!]}$ increasing sequence

$$\text{ASFOC}^h_{m,n}(f) = OC^h_{m,p_n} \circ \cdots \circ OC^h_{m,p_1}(f) \tag{19}$$

$$\text{ASFCO}^h_{m,n}(f) = CO^h_{m,p_n} \circ \cdots \circ CO^h_{m,p_1}(f) \tag{20}$$

2.3.4 Adaptive toggle contrast filters

The usual toggle contrast filter (Soille, 2003) is an edge sharpness operator. This filter is defined from the classical dilation and erosion using a disk of radius r as structuring element. This (non-adaptive) filter is here defined in the GANIP framework using a local 'contrast' criterion, such as the local contrast defined in Jourlin et al. (1988). The LIP contrast at a pixel $x \in D$ of an image $f \in \mathcal{I}$, denoted $c(f)(x)$, is defined with the help of the gray values of its neighbors included in a disk $V(x)$ of radius 1, centered in x:

$$c(f)(x) = \frac{1}{\#V(x)} \, \overset{\triangle}{\triangle} \sum_{y \in V(x)}^{\triangle} (\max(f(x), f(y)) \, \overset{\triangle}{\triangle} \, \min(f(x), f(y))) \tag{21}$$

where $\overset{\triangle}{\sum}$ and $\#$ denote the sum in the LIP sense (Jourlin et al., 1988), and the cardinal symbol, respectively. The LIP contrast is here defined in the discrete case, but a continuous definition has been proposed by Pinoli (1991; 1997b). The so-called adaptive toggle contrast filter is the image transformation denoted $\kappa^{c(f)}_{m_O}$, where $c(f)$ and m_O represent the criterion mapping and the homogeneity tolerance within the GLIP framework (required for the GANs definition), respectively. It is defined as following:
$\forall (f, x, m_O) \in \mathcal{I} \times D \times E^\oplus$

$$\kappa^{c(f)}_{m_O}(f)(x) = \begin{cases} D^{c(f)}_{m_O}(f)(x) \text{ if } D^{c(f)}_{m_O}(f)(x) \ominus f(x) < f(x) \ominus E^{c(f)}_{m_O}(f)(x) \\ E^{c(f)}_{m_O}(f)(x) \text{ otherwise} \end{cases} \tag{22}$$

where $D_{m_\bigcirc}^{c(f)}$ and $E_{m_\bigcirc}^{c(f)}$ denote the adaptive dilation and adaptive erosion computed with the criterion mapping $c(f)$.

More details on the GAN-based morphological filters can be found in Debayle & Pinoli (2006b); Pinoli & Debayle (2009).

2.4 GAN Choquet filtering

Fuzzy integrals (Choquet, 2000; Sugeno, 1974) provide a general representation of image filters. A large class of operators can be represented by those integrals such as linear filters, morphological filters, rank filters, order statistic filters or stack filters (Grabisch, 1994). The main fuzzy integrals are Choquet integral (Choquet, 2000) and Sugeno integral (Sugeno, 1974). Fuzzy integrals integrate a real function with respect to a fuzzy measure.

2.4.1 Fuzzy integrals

Let X be a finite set. In discrete image processing applications, X represents the K pixels within a subset of the spatial support of the image (i.e. an image window). A fuzzy measure over $X = \{x_0, \ldots, x_{K-1}\}$ is a function $\mu : 2^X \to [0,1]$ such that:

- $\mu(\varnothing) = 0; \mu(X) = 1$

- $\mu(A) \leq \mu(B)$ if $A \subseteq B$

Fuzzy measures are generalizations of probability measures for which the probability of the union of two disjoint events is equal to the sum of the individual probabilities.

The discrete Choquet integral of a function $f : X = \{x_0, \ldots, x_{K-1}\} \mapsto \tilde{E}$ with respect to the fuzzy measure μ is (Murofushi & Sugeno, 1989):

$$C_\mu(f) = \sum_{i=0}^{K-1} (f(x_{(i)}) - f(x_{(i-1)}))\mu(A_{(i)}) = \sum_{i=0}^{K-1} (\mu(A_{(i)}) - \mu(A_{(i+1)}))f(x_{(i)}) \qquad (23)$$

where the subsymbol (.) indicates that the indices have been permuted so that: $0 = f(x_{(-1)}) \leq f(x_{(0)}) \leq f(x_{(1)}) \leq \ldots, \leq f(x_{(K-1)}), A_{(i)} = \{x_{(i)}, \ldots, x_{(K-1)}\}$ and $A_{(K)} = \varnothing$.

An interesting property of the Choquet fuzzy integral is that if μ is a probability measure, the fuzzy integral is equivalent to the classical Lebesgue integral and simply computes the expectation of f with respect to μ within the usual probability framework. The fuzzy integral is a form of averaging operator in the sense that the fuzzy integral is valued between the minimum and maximum values of the function f to be integrated.

2.4.2 Choquet filters

Let f be in $\mathcal{I}$, W a window of K pixels and μ a fuzzy measure defined on W. This measure could be extended to all translated window W_y associated to a pixel y: $\forall A \subseteq W_y \;\; \mu(A) = \mu(A_{-y}), A_{-y} \subseteq W$. In this way, the Choquet filter associated to f is defined by:

$$\forall y \in D, \quad CF_\mu^W(f)(y) = \sum_{x_i \in W_y} (\mu(A_{(i)}) - \mu(A_{(i+1)}))f(x_{(i)}) \qquad (24)$$

The Choquet filters generalize (Grabisch, 1994) several classical filters:

- linear filters (mean, Gaussian, ...):
  $LF_W^\alpha(f)(y) = \sum_{x_i \in W_y} \alpha_i f(x_i)$ where $\alpha \in [0,1]^K, \sum_{i=0}^{K-1} \alpha_i = 1$

- rank filters (median, min, max, ...):
  $RF_W^d(f)(y) = f(x_{(d)})$ where $d \in [0, K-1] \cap \mathbb{N}$

- order filters (n-power, α-trimmed mean, quasi midrange, ...):
$$OF_W^\alpha(f)(y) = \sum_{x_i \in W_y} \alpha_i f(x_{(i)}) \text{ where } \alpha \in [0,1]^K, \sum_{i=0}^{K-1} \alpha_i = 1$$

The mean, rank and order filters are Choquet filters with respect to the cardinal measures: $\forall A, B \subseteq W \quad \#A = \#B \Rightarrow \mu(A) = \mu(B)$ (#B denoting the cardinal of B). Those filters, using an operational window W, could be characterized with the application: $\#A \mapsto \mu(A), A \subseteq W$. Indeed, different cardinal fuzzy measures could be defined for each class of filters:

- mean filter: μ is the fuzzy measure on W defined by $\mu(A) = \#A/\#W$

- rank filters (of order d): μ is the fuzzy measure on W defined by:
$$\mu(A) = \begin{cases} 0 & \text{if} \quad \#A \leq \#W - d \\ 1 & \text{otherwise} \end{cases}$$

- order filters: μ is the fuzzy measure on W defined by: $\mu(A) = \sum_{j=0}^{\#A-1} \alpha_{\#W-j}$

For example, the median filter (using a 3x3 window) is characterized by the following cardinal measure:
$$\forall A \subseteq W \quad \mu(A) = \begin{cases} 0 \text{ if } \#A \leq \lfloor \#W/2 \rfloor \\ 1 \text{ otherwise} \end{cases}$$

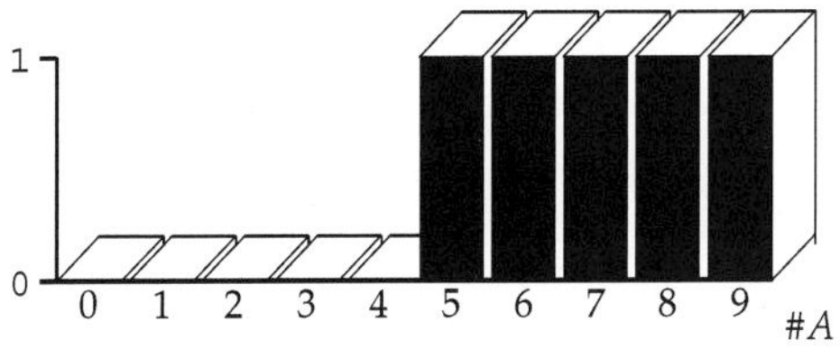

where $\lfloor s \rfloor$ denotes the round down of the real number s.

2.4.3 Adaptive Choquet filters

In order to extend Choquet filters with the use of GANs, the neighborhoods $V_m^h(y)$ are used as operational windows W. Since the GANs are spatially-variant, a set of fuzzy mesures has to be locally determined: $\{\mu_y : V_{m_O}^h(y) \to [0,1]\}_{y \in D}$. In this way, the GAN-based Choquet filter is defined as follows:
$$\forall (m_O, h, f, y) \in E^\oplus \times C \times I \times D$$

$$CF_{m_O}^h(f)(y) = \sum_{x_i \in V_{m_O}^h(y)} (\mu_y(A_{(i)}) - \mu_y(A_{(i+1)}))f(x_{(i)}) \tag{25}$$

Several filters (Grabisch, 1994), such as the mean filter, the median filter, the min filter, the max filter, the α-trimmed mean filter, the n-power filter, the α-quasi-midrange filter and so on, could consequently be extended to GAN-based Choquet filters (Amattouch, 2005). In the following, a few fuzzy measures μ_y attached to the GAN $V_{m_O}^h(y)$ are illustrated with respect to specific GAN-based filters.

- GAN-based mean filter:

$$\forall A \subseteq V_{m_O}^h(y), \quad \mu_y(A) = \frac{\#A}{K}, \quad \text{where } K = \#V_{m_O}^h(y) \tag{26}$$

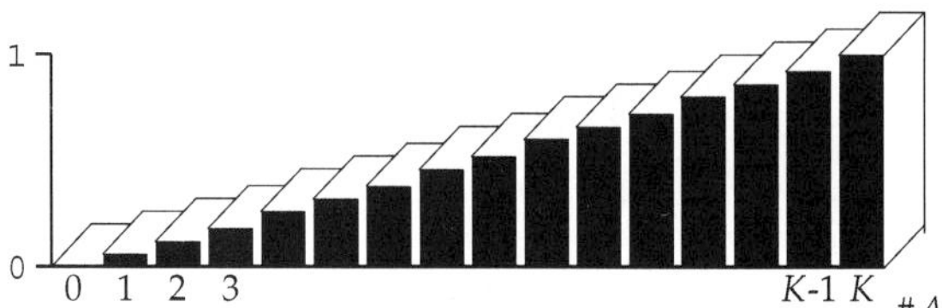

- GAN-based max filter:

$$\forall A \subseteq V_{m_\bigcirc}^{h}(y), \quad \mu_y(A) = \begin{cases} 0 \text{ if } \#A = 0 \\ 1 \text{ otherwise} \end{cases}, \quad \text{where } K = \#V_{m_\bigcirc}^{h}(y) \tag{27}$$

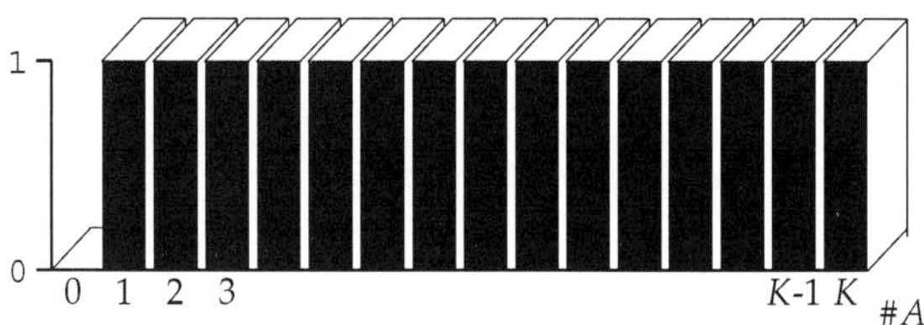

- GAN-based n-power filter:

$$\forall A \subseteq V_{m_\bigcirc}^{h}(y), \forall n \in [1, +\infty[\quad \mu_y(A) = \left(\frac{\#A}{K}\right)^n, \quad \text{where } K = \#V_{m_\bigcirc}^{h}(y) \tag{28}$$

Figure 5 shows an application example, on a magnetic resonance (MR) image of the human brain, of classical Choquet filtering with an operating window W (of size 5×5 pixels) using different fuzzy measures μ corresponding to the max and power filters, respectively.

Those GAN-based Choquet filters provide image processing operators, in a well-defined mathematical framework. More details on these GAN-based Choquet filters can be found in Debayle & Pinoli (2009a;b).

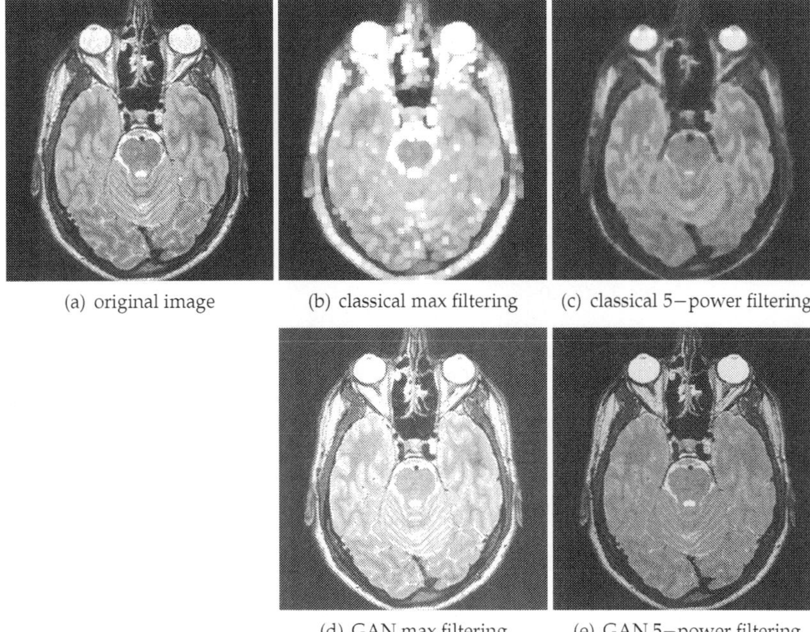

(a) original image   (b) classical max filtering   (c) classical 5−power filtering

(d) GAN max filtering   (e) GAN 5−power filtering

Fig. 5. Classical (b,c) and adaptive Choquet filtering (d,e) of the original brain magnetic resonance (MR) image (a) using different fuzzy measures corresponding to the max filter and the 5−power filter. The classical filters use a 5x5 operating window, while the adaptive filters use GANs computed with the luminance criterion using the homogeneity tolerance value $m = 50$ within the CLIP framework.

3. Biomedical application examples

GANIP-based processes are now exposed and applied in the field of image restoration, image enhancement and image segmentation on practical biomedical application examples.

3.1 Image restoration

The purpose of image restoration is to "compensate for" or "undo" defects which degrade an image. Degradations can come in many forms such as motion blur, noise, and camera misfocus. This restoration process is generally needed before segmenting and analyzing and measuring the regions of interest. In the following, two examples of image restoration are exposed using GAN mathematical morphology and GAN Choquet filtering.

3.1.1 Application to CerebroVascular Accident (CVA) diffusion MR images

This first application example addresses CerebroVascular Accidents (CVA). A stroke or a cerebrovascular accident occurs when the blood supply to the brain is disturbed in some way. As a result, brain cells are starved of oxygen causing some cells to die and leaving other cells damaged. A multiscale restoration of a human brain image f is proposed with a GANIP-based process using adaptive sequential openings $O_{m_{\bigcirc},p}$ (Fig. 6), using the GANs structuring elements with the luminance criterion mapping f and the homogeneity tolerance $m_\triangle = 7$ within the LIP framework. Several levels of decomposition are exposed: $p = 1, 2, 4, 6, 8$ and 10 (see Paragraph 2.3.3). The main aim of this restoration process is to smooth the image background for highlighting the stroke area, in order to help the neurologist for the diagnosis of the kind of stroke, and/or to allow a robust image segmentation to be performed.

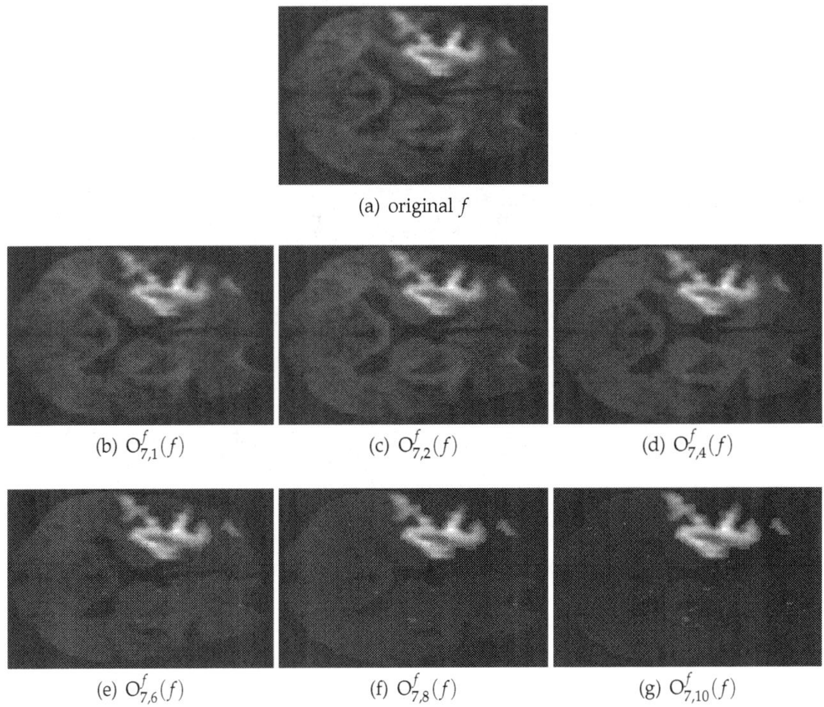

(a) original f

(b) $O^f_{7,1}(f)$ (c) $O^f_{7,2}(f)$ (d) $O^f_{7,4}(f)$

(e) $O^f_{7,6}(f)$ (f) $O^f_{7,8}(f)$ (g) $O^f_{7,10}(f)$

Fig. 6. Image restoration of CerebroVascular Accidents. A multiscale process (b-g) is achieved with the GAN-based morphological sequential openings (within the LIP framework) applied on the original image (a). The detection of the stroke area seems to be reachable at level $p = 10$.

These results show the advantages of spatial adaptivity and intrinsic multiscale analysis of the GANIP-based operators. Moreover, the detection of the stroke area seems to be reachable at level $p = 10$, while accurately preserving both its spatial and intensity characteristics which are needed for a further robust image segmentation.

3.1.2 Application to human brain MR images

This second application example is focused on the restoration of a human brain MR image (Fig. 7). This process is generally required before segmenting the different anatomical structures of the brain. The following GAN mean filter is both performed in the classical and adaptive framework in order to compare the two approaches: The adaptive filtering is applied with the luminance criterion using the homogeneity tolerance value $m = 30$, while the classical filtering uses a disk of radius 2 as operational window.

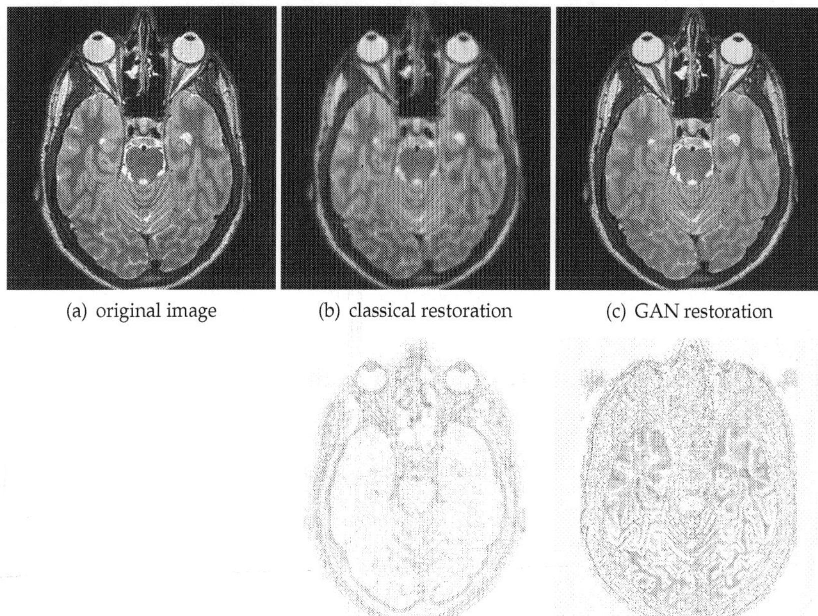

(a) original image	(b) classical restoration	(c) GAN restoration

(d) residue of the classical filtering	(e) residue of the GAN filtering

Fig. 7. Image restoration of a MR brain image (a) using a classical Choquet mean filtering (b) (with a disk of radius 2) and a GAN Choquet mean filtering (c) (within the CLIP model using the tolerance value $m = 30$). The residues of the resulting filtered images are shown in (d) and (e) with a gray tone inversion for a better visualization.

This example shows that the GAN filtering smooths the image while preserving spatial and intensity structures. On the contrary, the classical filtering acts on the different gray levels in the same way and consequently damages the region transitions. This difference is clearly shown in the filtering residues. Indeed, in the classical case, only the image transitions are highlighted. Consequently, the classical filtered image is blurred contrary to the adaptive filtered image.

3.2 Image enhancement

Image enhancement is the improvement of image quality (Gonzalez & Woods, 2008), wanted e.g. for visual inspection. Physiological experiments have shown that very small changes in luminance are recognized by the human visual system in regions of continuous gray tones, and not at all seen in regions of some discontinuities (Stockham, 1972). Therefore, a design goal for image enhancement is often to smooth images in more uniform regions, but to preserve edges. On the other hand, it has also been shown that somehow degraded images with enhancement of certain features, e.g. edges, can simplify image interpretation both for a human observer and for machine recognition (Stockham, 1972). A second design goal, therefore, is image sharpening (Gonzalez & Woods, 2008).

3.2.1 Application to human retina optical images

The following example (Fig. 8) is focused on human retinal vessels. The aim of this application is to highlight the vessels in order to help the ophtalmologists to make a diagnosis. For example, some retinal pathologies affect the tortuosity or the diameter of the blood vessels. The considered image enhancement technique is an edge sharpening process: the approach is similar with unsharp masking (Ramponi et al., 1996) type enhancement where a high pass portion is added to the original image. The contrast enhancement process is here realized through the GAN-based toggle contrast filter (Eq. 22). This adaptive process will be compared with the classical toggle contrast filter, whose operator κ_r is defined as follows (Soille, 2003):

$$\forall (f, x, r) \in I \times D \times \mathbb{R}^+, \quad \kappa_r(f)(x) = \begin{cases} D_r(f)(x) & \text{if } D_r(f)(x) - f(x) < f(x) - E_r(f)(x) \\ E_r(f)(x) & \text{otherwise} \end{cases} \tag{29}$$

where D_r and E_r denote the classical dilation and erosion, respectively, using a disk of radius r as structuring element.

This image enhancement example confirms that the GANIP operators are more effective than the corresponding classical ones. Indeed, the adaptive toggle contrast performs a locally accurate image enhancement, taking into account the notion of homogeneity within the spatial structures of the image. Consequently, only the transitions are sharpened while preserving the homogeneous regions. On the contrary, the usual toggle contrast enhances the image in an uniform way. Thus, the spatial zones around transitions are rapidly damaged as soon as the filtering becomes too strong.

3.2.2 Application to osteoblastic cell fluorescence optical images

A second application example addresses the study of interactions between osteoblastic cells and some biomaterials for biocompatibility purposes which are essential for bone tissue engineering (orthopedic implants). For this application, the biologists study the adhesion of osteoblastic cells of bones with hydroxyhapatite-based biomaterials. In this aim, some images of cells are acquired by fluorescence optical microscopy. Unfortunately, the images show a low contrast. In this way, an image enhancement process is proposed using the GAN max Choquet filtering (within the CLIP framework) followed by a stretching of the gray-tone range.

The cells are more and more highlighted according to the homogeneity tolerance value of the GANs. This GAN-based image enhancement is very useful for helping the biologists to identify the cells and characterize its interactions with the biomaterials on such images.

3.3 Image segmentation

The segmentation of an intensity image can be defined as its partition (in fact the partition of the spatial support D) into different connected regions, relating to an homogeneity condition (Gonzalez & Woods, 2008). A common segmentation process is based on a morphological transformation called watershed (Beucher & Lantuejoul, 1979). It will be illustrated on the two following examples.

3.3.1 Application to protein gel electrophoresis optical images

This first application example of image segmentation is focused on the proteomic expression analysis of colorectal cancer by two-dimensional differential gel electrophoresis (2D-DIGE)

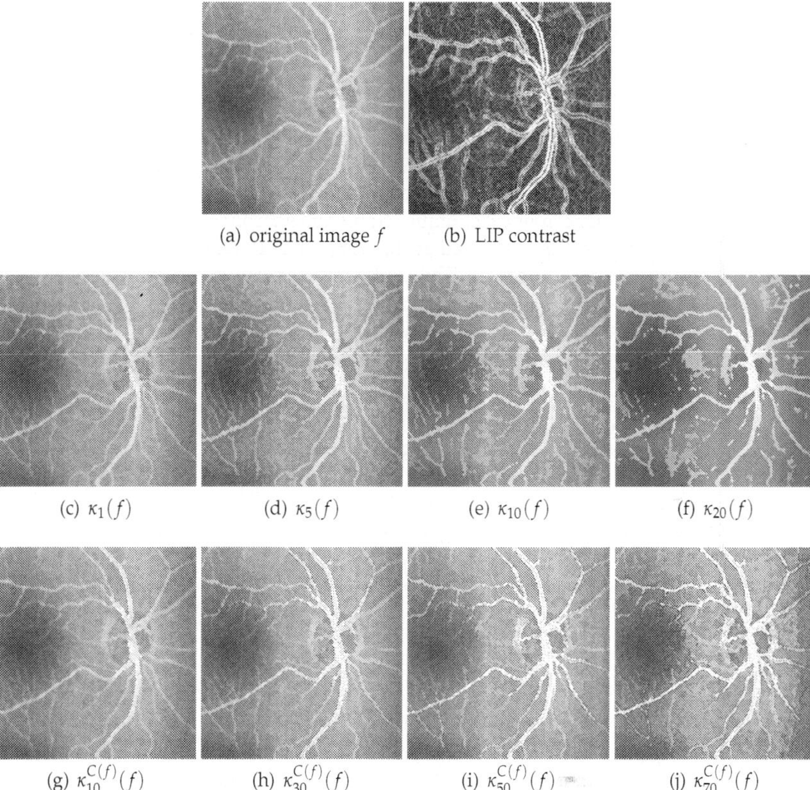

(a) original image f (b) LIP contrast

(c) $\kappa_1(f)$ (d) $\kappa_5(f)$ (e) $\kappa_{10}(f)$ (f) $\kappa_{20}(f)$

(g) $\kappa_{10}^{C(f)}(f)$ (h) $\kappa_{30}^{C(f)}(f)$ (i) $\kappa_{50}^{C(f)}(f)$ (j) $\kappa_{70}^{C(f)}(f)$

Fig. 8. Image enhancement of human retinal vessels through the toggle contrast process. The operator is applied on a real (a) image acquired on the retina of a human eye. The enhancement is achieved with the usual toggle contrast (c-f) and the GANIP-based toggle contrast (g-j), respectively. Using the usual toggle contrast, the edges are disconnected as soon as the filtering becomes too strong. On the contrary, such structures are preserved and sharpened with the GANIP filters.

(Bernard, 2008). The identification of specific protein markers for colorectal cancer would provide the basis for early diagnosis and detection, as well as clues for understanding the molecular mechanisms governing cancer progression. The objective is to identify the proteins differentially expressed in tumoral and neighboring normal mucosa. For this purpose, a segmentation process using GAN mathematical morphology is performed on 2D-DIGE images (Fig. 10). More precisely, a GAN-based opening-closing is used within the CLIP framework using the homogeneity tolerance value $m = 10$. Therafter, a constrained watershed process (Soille, 2003) is applied on the filtered image.

The result shows a satisfying segmented image obtained from a very poor contrasted original image. Despite a few errors, the following segmentation process could be used for a specific statistical analysis on a great number of 2D-DIGE images.

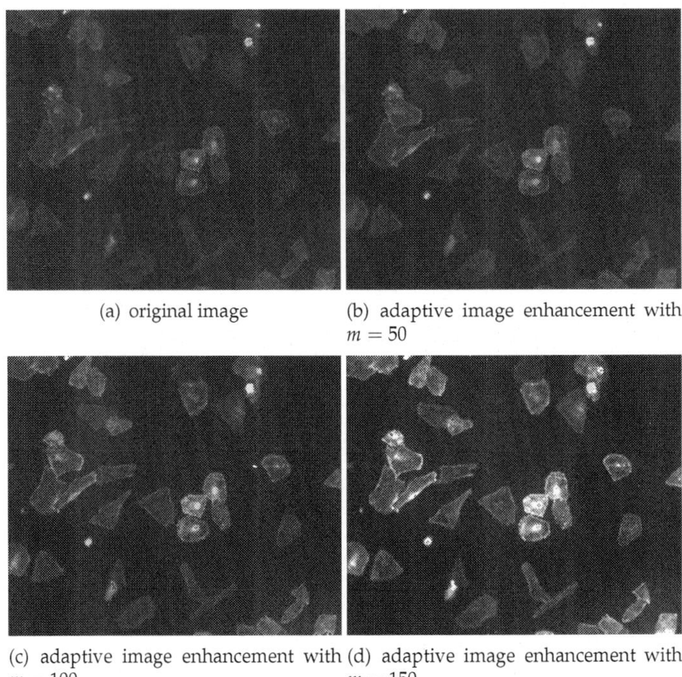

(a) original image

(b) adaptive image enhancement with $m = 50$

(c) adaptive image enhancement with $m = 100$

(d) adaptive image enhancement with $m = 150$

Fig. 9. Image enhancement of osteoblastic cells (a) by a GAN Choquet max filtering in the CLIP model using different homogeneity tolerance values (b-d).

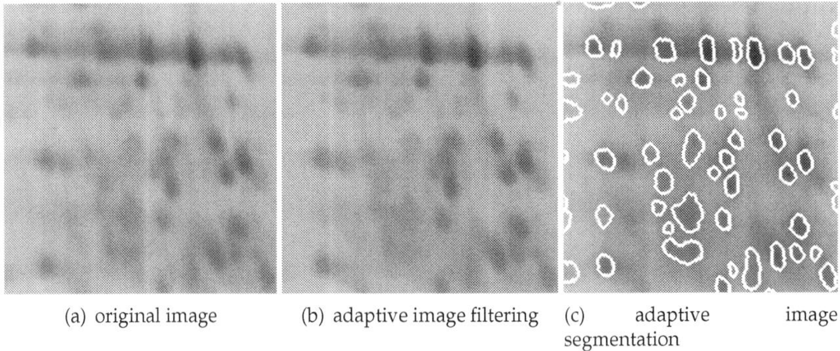

(a) original image

(b) adaptive image filtering

(c) adaptive image segmentation

Fig. 10. Image segmentation of a protein gel electrophoresis optical image (a) using a GAN opening-closing filtering (b) followed by a constraint watershed process (c).

3.3.2 Application to human endothelial cornea cell optical images

The second application example is focused on the cornea cell analysis. The cornea is the transparent surface in the front of the eye. It has a role of protection of the eye, and with the lens, of focusing light into the retina. It is constituted of several layers, such as the epithelium (at the front of the cornea), the stroma and the endothelium (at the back of the cornea). The endothelium contains non-regenerative cells tiled in a monolayer and hexagonal mosaic. This layer pumps water from the cornea, keeping it clear. A high cell density and a regular morphometry of this layer characterize the good quality of a cornea before transplantation, the most common transplantation in the world. Herein lays the importance of the endothelial control. Ex vivo controls are done by optical microscopy on corneal button before grafting. That image acquisition equipment give gray tones images which are segmented (Gavet & Pinoli, 2008), for example by the SAMBA™ software (Gain et al., 2002), into regions representing cells. These ones are used to compute statistics in order to quantify the corneal quality before transplantation.

The authors proposed a GANIP-based approach to segment the cornea cells. The process is achieved by a closing-opening morphological filtering using the GAN sets with the luminance criterion in the CLIP framework, followed by a watershed transformation. A comparison with the results provided by the SAMBA™ software, whose process is achieved by thresholding, filtering and skeletonization (Gain et al., 2002), is proposed (Fig. 11). The parameter m of the adaptive morphological filter has been tuned to visually provide the best possible segmentation.

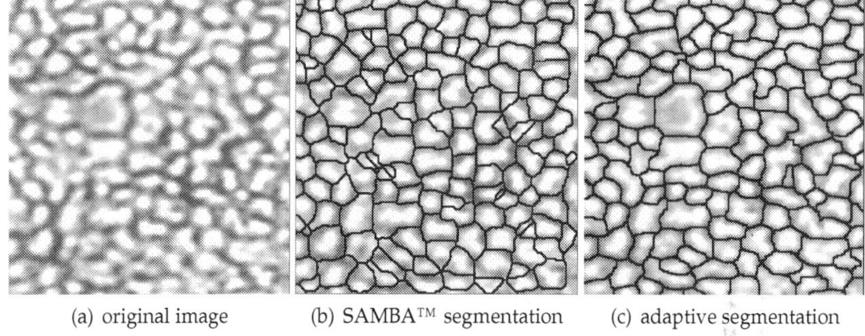

(a) original image(b) SAMBA™ segmentation(c) adaptive segmentation

Fig. 11. Image segmentation of human endothelial cornea cells (a). The process achieved by the GANIP-based morphological approach (c) provides better results (visually and from the point of view of ophthalmologists) than the SAMBA™ software (Gain et al., 2002) (b).

The detection process achieved by the GANIP-based morphological approach provides better results (from the point of view of the ophthalmologists) than the SAMBA™ software. Those results highlight the spatially-variant adaptivity of the GANIP-based operators.

4. Conclusion and prospects

The General Adaptive Neighborhood Image Processing (GANIP) approach allows efficient gray-tone image processing operators to be built. Those GAN-based operators are fully adaptive and enable to process an image in a consistent way with the image formation model, while preserving its regions without damaging its transitions. The theoretical aspects have been practically highlighted on real biomedical application examples (ophtalmology, microbiology, neurology, proteome biology) by using several image processing techniques in various biomedical fields, namely image restoration, enhancement and segmentation.

Different scales of biomedical structures have been investigated (proteins, cells, organs, tissues) with a resolution ranging from nanometres to centimetres.

In its current state of progress, the GANIP approach only deals with image transformations as well in image processing as in image analysis. Novel GANIP-based image processing techniques have been recently proposed by the authors (Debayle & Pinoli, 2011). Image quantitative analysis now appears clearly as a strong need. Therefore, the authors are currently working on combining geometric measurement concepts with GANIP (Rivollier et al., 2009; 2010d). Indeed, in the GANIP image representation an image is described in terms of particular subsets within the spatial support: the GANs. Thus, topological, geometrical and morphological measurements (Rivollier et al., 2010a;b;c) can be applied to the GANs associated to a given image. In this way, a local adaptive geometric quantitative analysis can be performed on gray-tone images without a segmentation step, classically required in image analysis.

5. Acknowledgments

The authors would like to thank the different partners from the University Hospital Center of Saint-Etienne and from the LPMG CNRS Unit in France who have kindly supplied different original images studied in this paper.

6. References

Amattouch, M. (2005). *Théorie de la Mesure et Analyse d'Image*, Master's thesis, Ecole Nationale Supérieure des Mines, Saint-Etienne, France.

Bernard, F. (2008). *IDADIGE : Procédé de traitement des images de gels electophorèse bidimensionnelle différentielle dans le contexte de la recherche de marqueurs protéiques*, PhD thesis, Ecole Nationale Supérieure des Mines, Saint-Etienne, France.

Beucher, S. & Lantuejoul, C. (1979). Use of watersheds in contour detection, *International Workshop on Image Processing, Real-Time Edge and Motion Detection/Estimation*, Rennes, France.

Bouannaya, N. & Schonfeld, D. (2008). Theoretical Foundations of Spatially-Variant Mathematical Morphology Part II: Gray-Level Images, *IEEE Transactions on Pattern Analysis and Machine Intelligence* 30(5): 837–850.

Choquet, G. (2000). *Cours de Topologie*, Dunod, Paris, France, chapter Espaces topologiques et espaces métriques, pp. 45–51.

Ciuc, M., Rangayyan, R. M., Zaharia, T. & Buzuloiu, V. (2000). Filtering Noise in Color Images using Adaptive-Neighborhood Statistics, *Electronic Imaging* 9(4): 484–494.

Debayle, J. & Pinoli, J. C. (2005a). Multiscale Image Filtering and Segmentation by means of Adaptive Neighborhood Mathematical Morphology, *IEEE International Conference on Image Processing*, Vol. 3, Genova, Italy, pp. 537–540.

Debayle, J. & Pinoli, J. C. (2005b). Spatially Adaptive Morphological Image Filtering using Intrinsic Structuring Elements, *Image Analysis and Stereology* 24(3): 145–158.

Debayle, J. & Pinoli, J. C. (2006a). General Adaptive Neighborhood Image Processing - Part I: Introduction and Theoretical Aspects, *Journal of Mathematical Imaging and Vision* 25(2): 245–266.

Debayle, J. & Pinoli, J. C. (2006b). General Adaptive Neighborhood Image Processing - Part II: Practical Application Examples, *Journal of Mathematical Imaging and Vision* 25(2): 267–284.

Debayle, J. & Pinoli, J. C. (2009a). General Adaptive Neighborhood Choquet Image Filtering, *Journal of Mathematical Imaging and Vision* 35(3): 173–185.

Debayle, J. & Pinoli, J. C. (2009b). General Adaptive Neighborhood Representation for Adaptive Choquet Image Filtering, *10th European Congress of Stereology and Image Analysis*, Milan, Italy, pp. 431–436.

Debayle, J. & Pinoli, J. C. (2011). General Adaptive Neighborhood-Based Pretopological Image Filtering, *Journal of Mathematical Imaging and Vision* . In Press.

Gain, P., Thuret, G., Kodjikian, L., Gavet, Y., Turc, P. H., Theillere, C., Acquart, S., LePetit, J. C., Maugery, J. & Campos, L. (2002). Automated Tri-Image Analysis of Stored Corneal Endothelium, *British Journal of Ophtalmology* 86: 801–808.

Gavet, Y. & Pinoli, J. C. (2008). Visual Perception based Automatic Recognition of Cell Mosaics in Human Corneal Endothelium Microscopy Images, *Image Analysis and Stereology* 27: 53–61.

Gonzalez, R. C. & Woods, R. E. (2008). *Digital Image Processing*, third edn, Prentice Hall.

Gordon, R. & Rangayyan, R. M. (1984). Feature Enhancement of Mammograms using Fixed and Adaptive Neighborhoods, *Applied Optics* 23(4): 560–564.

Grabisch, M. (1994). Fuzzy Integrals as a Generalized Class of Order Filters, *Proc. of the SPIE*, Vol. 2315, pp. 128–136.

Jourlin, M. & Pinoli, J. C. (1988). A Model for Logarithmic Image Processing, *Journal of Microscopy* 149: 21–35.

Jourlin, M. & Pinoli, J. C. (2001). Logarithmic Image Processing : The Mathematical and Physical Framework for the Representation and Processing of Transmitted Images, *Advances in Imaging and Electron Physics* 115: 129–196.

Jourlin, M., Pinoli, J. C. & Zeboudj, R. (1988). Contrast Definition and Contour Detection for Logarithmic Images, *Journal of Microscopy* 156: 33–40.

Maragos, P. & Vachier, C. (2009). Overview of Adaptive Morphology: Trends and Perspectives, *IEEE International Conference on Imge Processing*, Cairo, Egypt, pp. 2241–2244.

Matheron, G. (1967). *Eléments pour une Théorie des Milieux Poreux*, Masson, Paris, France.

Murofushi, T. & Sugeno, M. (1989). An Interpretation of Fuzzy Measure and the Choquet Integral as an Integral with respect to a Fuzzy Measure, *Fuzzy Sets and Systems* 29: 201–227.

Oppenheim, A. V. (1967). Generalized Superposition, *Information and Control* 11: 528–536.

Pinoli, J. C. (1987). *Contribution à la Modélisation, au Traitement et à l'Analyse d'Image*, PhD thesis, Department of Mathematics, University of Saint-Etienne, France.

Pinoli, J. C. (1991). A Contrast Definition for Logarithmic Images in the Continuous Setting, *Acta Stereologica* 10: 85–96.

Pinoli, J. C. (1997a). A General Comparative Study of the Multiplicative Homomorphic, Log-Ratio and Logarithmic Image Processing Approaches, *Signal Processing* 58: 11–45.

Pinoli, J. C. (1997b). The Logarithmic Image Processing Model : Connections with Human Brightness Perception and Contrast Estimators, *Journal of Mathematical Imaging and Vision* 7(4): 341–358.

Pinoli, J. C. & Debayle, J. (2007). Logarithmic Adaptive Neighborhood Image Processing (LANIP): Introduction, Connections to Human Brightness Perception and Application Issues, *Journal on Advances in Signal Processing - Special issue on Image Perception* 2007: Article ID 36105, 22 pages.

Pinoli, J. C. & Debayle, J. (2009). General Adaptive Neighborhood Mathematical Morphology, *IEEE International Conference on Image Processing*, Cairo, Egypt, pp. 2249–2252.

Ramponi, G., Strobel, N., Mitra, S. K. & Yu, T. H. (1996). Nonlinear Unsharp Masking Methods for Image-Contrast Enhancement, *Journal of Electronic Imaging* 5(3): 353–366.

Rivollier, S., Debayle, J. & Pinoli, J. C. (2010a). Shape diagrams for 2D compact sets - Part I: analytic convex sets, *Australian Journal of Mathematical Analysis and Applications* 7(2-3): 1–27.

Rivollier, S., Debayle, J. & Pinoli, J. C. (2010b). Shape diagrams for 2D compact sets - Part II: analytic simply connected sets, *Australian Journal of Mathematical Analysis and Applications* 7(2-4): 1–21.

Rivollier, S., Debayle, J. & Pinoli, J. C. (2010c). Shape diagrams for 2D compact sets - Part III: convexity discrimination for analytic and discretized simply connected sets, *Australian Journal of Mathematical Analysis and Applications* 7(2-5): 1–18.

Rivollier, S., Debayle, J. & Pinoli, J. C. (2009). General Adaptive Neighborhood-Based Minkowski Maps for Gray-Tone Image Analysis, *10th European Congress of Stereology and Image Analysis*, Milan, Italy, pp. 219–224.

Rivollier, S., Debayle, J. & Pinoli, J. C. (2010d). Integral geometry and general adaptive neighborhood for multiscale image analysis, *International Journal of Signal and Image Processing* 1(3): 141–150.

Roerdink, J. B. T. M. (2009). Adaptivity and group invariance in mathematical morphology, *IEEE International Conference on Imge Processing*, Cairo, Egypt, pp. 2253–2256.

Rosenfeld, A. (1969). *Picture Processing by Computers*, Academic Press, New-York, U.S.A.

Salembier, P. (1992). Structuring Element Adaptation for Morphological Filters, *Journal of Visual Communication and Image Representation* 3(2): 115–136.

Serra, J. (1982). *Image Analysis and Mathematical Morphology*, Academic Press, London, U.K.

Soille, P. (2003). *Morphological Image Analysis. Principles and Applications*, Springer Verlag, New York, U.S.A.

Stockham, T. G. (1972). Image Processing in the Context of a Visual Model, *Proc. of the IEEE*, Vol. 60, pp. 825–842.

Sugeno, M. (1974). *Theory of Fuzzy Integrals ans its Applications*, PhD thesis, Tokyo Institute of Technology, Japan.